CANCER AND ITS MANAGEMENT

To Jessica and Gabriela

Cancer
AND ITS MANAGEMENT

ROBERT SOUHAMI
BSc MD FRCP,
Kathleen Ferrier Professor of
Clinical Oncology,
University College and
Middlesex School of Medicine,
London

JEFFREY TOBIAS
MA(Cantab) MD MRCP FRCR,
Consultant in Radiotherapy
and Oncology,
Department of Radiotherapy
and Oncology,
University College Hospital,
London

BLACKWELL SCIENTIFIC PUBLICATIONS

OXFORD LONDON EDINBURGH

BOSTON PALO ALTO MELBOURNE

First published 1986
Reprinted 1987

Printed in Great Britain
by Butler & Tanner Ltd,
Frome and London

DISTRIBUTORS

USA
    Year Book Medical Publishers
    35 East Wacker Drive
    Chicago, Illinois 60601

Canada
    The C.V Mosby Company
    5240 Finch Avenue East,
    Scarborough, Ontario

Australia
    Blackwell Scientific Publications
        (Australia) Pty Ltd
    107 Barry Street
    Carlton, Victoria 3053

British Library
Cataloguing in Publication Data

Souhami, Robert L.
    Cancer and its management.
    1. Cancer—Diagnosis
    I. Title   II. Tobias, Jeffrey S.
    616.99'4075   RC270

    ISBN 0-632-01373-7
    ISBN 0-632-02158-6

Contents

Preface

Cancer medicine is one of the most rapidly changing of all medical specialties. Not long ago most cancers were treated either by surgery or local radiotherapy, with almost no hope of success if the cancer had spread to involve local lymph nodes, or if distant metastases were present. Recent advances in chemotherapy, hormone therapy, radiotherapy and diagnostic imaging have transformed our clinical practice; and progress in cell biology has led to a far greater understanding of the process of malignant transformation.

We have written this book because we are aware that many busy physicians, surgeons and gynaecologists, who are not themselves cancer specialists, may find it difficult to keep abreast of areas which are of considerable importance to them. General surgeons, for example, spend a substantial portion of their time dealing with gastro-intestinal and abdominal tumours, yet have little working knowledge of non-surgical treatment of these conditions. Similarly, gynaecological surgeons need to know more about what the radiotherapist and medical oncologist can offer for gynaecological tumours.

Many medical schools still do not provide any integrated teaching in cancer medicine, and student knowledge of the management of malignant disease is often acquired from specialists whose main interest may not be related to cancer. Medical students may wish to know more about the disease which is the second largest cause of mortality in the Western world. We hope that trainees in medicine, surgery and gynaecology will also find the book of value, and that it will be of help to postgrad-

uates beginning a career in radiotherapy or medical oncology. Finally, we hope that general practitioners, all of whom look after cancer patients and who have an important role in management and in terminal care, will find this book helpful. If specialists in cancer medicine feel it is a useful digest of current thought in cancer management, so much the better. However this book is not primarily intended for them. There are several very large texts which give specialist advice. Although some of these details necessarily appear in our book, we do not regard it as a handbook of chemotherapy or radiotherapy. To some extent it is a personal view of cancer and its management today and, as such, it will differ in some details from the attitudes and approaches of our colleagues.

We have attempted to give a thorough working knowledge of the principles of diagnosis, staging and treatment of tumours and to do so at a level which brings the reader up to date. We have tried to indicate where the subject is growing, where controversies lie, and from which direction future advances might come. In the first nine chapters we have provided a review of some of the mechanisms of tumour development, cancer treatment and supportive care. In the remaining chapters we have given an account of the principles of management of the major cancers. For each tumour we have given details of the pathology, mode of spread, clinical presentation, and staging and treatment with radiotherapy and chemotherapy. The role of surgery is outlined, but details of surgical procedure are beyond the scope of this book. The references which we have included have been chosen because they are clear reviews or representative of many similar articles, and sometimes because they are historical landmarks or represent important recent work.

We are well aware that no two people can be expert in all branches of cancer, but we wished to achieve a uniformity of style and approach which is not possible in multi-author books. It is a great pleasure to record our grateful thanks to the following colleagues who kindly read parts of the manuscript, invariably adding valuable comments which have greatly improved the final result: Dr Thurston Brewin; Professor John Cawley; Dr Alan Craft; Dr Michael Cullen; Dr Charles Edmonds; Mr Lawrence Freedman; Dr Anthony Goldstone; Mr Henry Grant; Dr Alan Horwich; Professor Peter Isaacson, Dr John Millar; Professor Niall O'Higgins; Professor Julian Peto; Dr John Richards; Dr Marjorie Ridley; Dr Gordon Rustin; Dr Martin Sarner;

Dr Peter Selby; Mr Anthony Silverstone; Dr Maurice Slevin; Dr Stephen Spiro; Mr David Thomas; Dr Colin Trask; Mr Peter Worth and Professor John Wyllie. Professor Peter Isaacson and Dr Meryl Griffiths helped us with the pathology illustrations and Dr David Edwards provided many of the X-rays. Most of the age-specific incidence figures are derived from data from the South West Thames Cancer Registry through the kindness of Dr Richard Skeet.

We were greatly helped by Penny Smart of Blackwell Scientific Publications; and Clare Little and her colleagues at Oxford Illustrators drew the excellent line drawings from what were often confusing and rudimentary sketches. Ms Susie Andrews and Ms Maureen Henry typed much of the text and coped cheerfully with constant requests for correction of the manuscript.

Chapter 1

The Modern Management of Cancer: An Introductory Note

Cancer is a vast medical problem. As a cause of mortality it is second only to cardiovascular disease. It is diagnosed each year in 1 in every 250 men and 1 in every 300 women. The incidence rises steeply so that over the age of 60, 3 in 100 men develop the disease each year (Fig. 1.1). It is often a costly disease to diagnose and investigate, and treatment is time-consuming, labour intensive and usually requires hospital care. In the Western world the commonest cancers are of the lung, breast, skin, gut and prostate gland (Fig. 1.2).

In the past the main methods of treating cancer have been by surgery and radiotherapy. The control of the primary tumour has been seen as the major problem, since it is this which is usually responsible for the patient's symptoms. There may be exceedingly unpleasant symptoms due to local spread, and a failure to control the disease locally means certain death. For many tumours, breast cancer being a good example, the energies of those treating the disease have been directed towards defining the optimum methods of eradication of the primary tumour. This is a worthwhile and important aim, but it is perhaps not surprising that these efforts while improving management have not greatly improved the prognosis because the most important cause of mortality is metastatic spread. Although prompt and effective treatment of the primary cancer diminishes the likelihood of recurrence, metastases have often developed before diagnosis and treatment have begun. The prognosis is not then altered by treatment of the primary cancer even though the presenting symptoms may be alleviated.

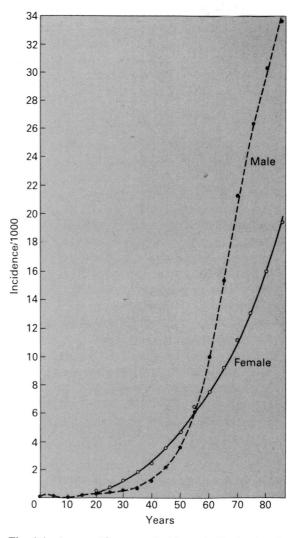

Fig. 1.1. *Age-specific cancer incidence in England and Wales.*

1

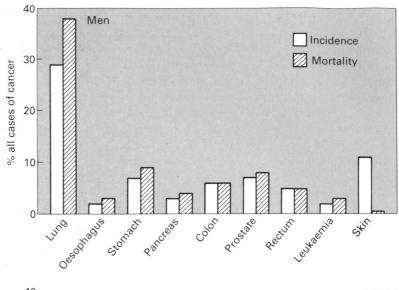

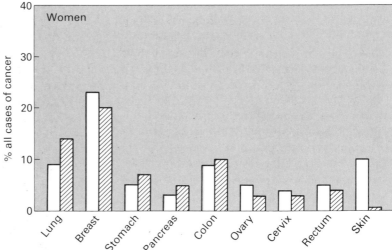

Fig. 1.2. *Incidence and mortality of cancer in men and women.* Lung cancers account for 29% of all cancers in men, but 38% of all male cancer deaths. Skin cancer accounts for 11% of all male cancers but less than 0.5% of all male cancer deaths.

Every medical specialty has its own types of cancer which are the concern of the specialist in that area. Cancer is a diagnosis to which every clinician is alerted whatever his field and, because malignant disease is common, specialists acquire great expertise in diagnosis, often with the aid of techniques such as bronchoscopy and other forms of endoscopy. On the other hand the management of cancer, especially the non-surgical management, once the diagnosis has been made, is not part of the training or interest of many specialists and the patient is often transferred to other hands at this point. While this is in some respects desirable, especially as cancer treatments become more complicated, it presents serious problems. For example, radiotherapists and medical oncologists are often asked to see patients who have had a laparotomy at which a tumour such as an ovarian cancer or a lymphoma has been found but the abdomen has been closed without the surgeon having made an attempt to stage the disease properly, or where appropriate, to remove the main mass of tumour. This poses considerable problems for the further management of the patient. At a more general level, lack of familiarity with the principles of cancer management and of what treatment can achieve, leads to a low level of recruitment into clinical trials. An understanding of the principles of investigation and treatment of cancer has become essential for every physician and surgeon if he is to achieve the best results for his patients.

Recent advances in the chemotherapy and radiotherapy of uncommon tumours such as Hodgkin's disease and teratoma of the testis have led to a more general awareness of the importance of a planned approach to the management of patients. This has been true not only for the problems of individual patients but also in the planning of clinical trials of treatment. It has become clear that for every cancer, an understanding of which patients can be helped, or even cured, can only come by attention to the details of disease stage and types. Patients in whom these details are unknown are at risk from inappropriate overtreatment or from inadequate treatment, resulting in the chance of cure being missed. Even though chemotherapy has not been of great benefit to patients with diseases such as squamous lung cancer or adenocarcinoma of the pancreas, it is now clearly essential that clinicians with a detailed and specialized knowledge of the risks and dangers of chemotherapy in these and other diseases are part of the staff of every oncology department. Knowing when not to treat is as important as knowing when to do so.

The improvement in chemotherapy of some cancers has greatly increased the complexity of management. Cancer specialists have a particular responsibility to validate the treatment which they give since the toxicity and dangers of some regimens means that the indications for treatment have to be established precisely. In a few cases an imaginative step forward has dramatically improved results and the need for controlled comparison with previous treatment is scarcely necessary. Examples are the use of combination chemotherapy in the management of advanced Hodgkin's disease and prevention of central nervous system relapse of leukaemia by prophylactic treatment. However, such clearcut advances are seldom made. In the main, improvement in treatment is made slowly in a piecemeal fashion and prospective trials of treatment must be undertaken in order to validate each step in management. There is always a tendency in dealing with cancer to want to believe good news and for early, uncontrolled but promising results to be seized upon and over-interpreted. Although understandable, uncritical enthusiasm for a particular form of treatment is greatly to be deplored, since it leads to a clamour for the treatment and the establishment of patterns of treatment which are improperly validated. An example is the widespread and uncritical acceptance of chemotherapy in the treatment of advanced lung cancer. The benefits of this approach are not proven, yet in some countries comparisons of such treatment with untreated control groups is regarded as unethical. The toxicity of cancer treatments is considerable and can only be justified if it is unequivocally clear that the end results are worthwhile either by increasing the cure rate or by improving the quality of life.

The increasing complexity of management has brought with it a recognition that in many areas it is necessary to establish an effective working collaboration between specialists. Joint planning of management in specialized clinics is now widely practised for diseases such as lymphomas, head and neck and gynaecological cancer. Some surgeons and gynaecologists are beginning to concentrate on the oncological aspects of their speciality. In this way patients can benefit from a coordinated and planned approach to their individual problems.

Before a patient can be treated not only must it be established that he has cancer, but the pathological nature of the tumour must be defined and the extent of the local and systemic disease determined. For each of these goals to be attained the oncologist must rely on colleagues in departments of histopathology, diagnostic imaging, haematology and chemical pathology. Every oncologist has patients referred where the diagnosis of cancer has not been definitely made pathologically but is based on a very strong clinical suspicion with suggestive pathological evidence, or where a pathological diagnosis of cancer has been made which, on review, proves to be incorrect. It is essential for the oncologist to be in close contact with histopathologists and cytologists so that diagnoses can be reviewed regularly. Many departments of oncology have regular pathology review meetings so that the clinician can learn of the difficulties which pathologists have with diagnosis and vice versa. Similarly, modern imaging techniques have led to a previously unattainable accuracy in pre-operative and postoperative staging, although many of these techniques are only as reliable as those using them (e.g. abdominal or pelvic ultrasound). The cancer specialist must be fully conversant with the uses and limitations of imaging methods. The techniques are expensive and the results must be interpreted in the light of other clinical information. The practice of holding regular meetings to review cases with specialists from the imaging departments has much to commend it.

Modern cancer treatment often carries a substantial risk of toxicity. Complex and difficult treatments are best managed in a specialized unit with skilled personnel. The centralization of high-dependency care means that staff can become particularly aware of the physical and emotional problems of patients undergoing treatments of this kind. Additionally, colleagues from other departments such as haematology, biochemistry and bacteriology can more easily help in the investigation and management of some of the very difficult problems which occur, for example in the immunosuppressed patient.

The increasingly intensive investigative and treatment policies which have been adopted in the last 20 years impose on the clinician the additional responsibility of having to stand back from the treatment of his patient and ask himself at each stage, what the aim of treatment is. Clearly radical and aggressive therapy is essential if the patient has a reasonable chance of being cured. However, palliative treatment will be used if the case is quite clearly beyond any prospect of cure. What is more difficult is to know when the intention of treatment must move from the radical to the palliative, with avoidance of toxicity as a major priority. For example, while many patients with advanced lymphomas will be cured by intensive combination chemotherapy, there is no prospect of cure in advanced breast cancer by these means and chemotherapy, must in this case be regarded as palliative therapy: a situation in which it makes little sense to press treatment to the point of toxicity. The judgement of what is tolerable and acceptable is a major task in cancer management. Such judgement can only come from considerable experience of the treatments in question and of the natural history of individual tumours.

Modern cancer management, therefore, often involves highly technological and intensive medical care. It is expensive, time-consuming and sometimes dangerous. Nowadays patients should seldom be in total ignorance of what is wrong with them or what the treatment involves. The increasingly technical nature of cancer management, and the change in public and professional attitudes towards malignant disease, has altered the way in which doctors who are experienced in cancer treatment approach their patients. There has been a decisive swing towards honest and careful discussion with patients about the disease and its treatment. This does not mean that a bald statement should be made to the patient about the diagnosis and its outcome, since doctors must sustain the patient with hope and encouragement through what is obviously a frightening and depressing period. One of the most difficult and rewarding aspects of the management of malignant disease lies in the judgement of how much information to give to each particular patient, at what speed, and how to incorporate the patient's own wishes into a rational treatment plan.

The emotional impact of the diagnosis and treatment can be considerable for both patients and relatives. Above everything else, treating patients with cancer involves an awareness of how patients think and feel. All doctors dealing with cancer patients must be prepared to devote time to talking to patients and their families, to answer questions and explain what is happening and what can be achieved. Because many patients will die from their disease the doctor must learn to cope with the emotional and physical needs of dying patients and the effects of grief and bereavement on their family.

The care and support of patients with advanced malignant disease and the control of symptoms such as pain and nausea have greatly improved in the last 10 years. This aspect of cancer management has been improved by the collaboration of many medical workers. Nurses who specialize in the control of symptoms of malignancy are now attached to many cancer units and social workers skilled in dealing with the problems of malignant disease and bereavement are an essential part of the team. The development of hospices has led to a much greater appreciation of the way in which symptoms might be controlled and to a considerable improvement in the standards of the care of the dying in general hospitals. Many cancer departments now have a symptom support team based in the hospital, but able to undertake the care of patients in their own homes, giving advice on control of symptoms such as pain and nausea and providing support to the patient's family.

There have been dramatic advances in cell and molecular biology in the last 10 years with the result that our understanding of the nature of malignant transformation has increased. This trend will continue and places an additional demand on the oncologist, namely to keep abreast both of advances in management and the scientific foundations on which they are based. The power of modern techniques to explore some of the fundamental processes in malignant transformation has meant that cancer is at the heart of many aspects of medical research and has led to an increased academic interest in malignancy. This in turn has led to a more critical approach to many aspects of cancer treatment. Cancer and its management is now one of the most complex and demanding aspects of medicine. More health care workers are seeing that cancer medicine is rewarding and interesting, and standards of patient care are improving as a result of these welcome changes.

Chapter 2

Epidemiology; Cure; Treatment Trials

The epidemiology of cancer, which concerns the study of the frequency of the disease in populations living under different conditions, has been illuminating in several ways. It has demonstrated variations in cancer incidence among different populations and by so doing has suggested possible aetiologies. It has allowed the testing of theories about the cause of a cancer by relating a particular characteristic, for example, cigarette smoking, to the occurrence of disease. It has suggested ways in which cancer might be prevented by changing the prevalence of a postulated aetiological agent, as shown by the decline of lung cancer in doctors who have given up smoking. Finally, epidemiological evidence has proved invaluable in planning cancer services.

TERMINOLOGY AND METHODS IN EPIDEMIOLOGY

When epidemiologists use the word *prevalence* they mean the proportion of a defined group having a condition at a single point in time. By *incidence* they mean the proportion of a defined population developing the disease within a stated time period. When they talk of *crude incidence* or *prevalence rates* they are talking of a whole population. *Specific rates* refer to selected groups, for example a defined age group. Crude rates cannot be used to compare populations of different or changing structure. For example, a higher crude fatality rate from breast cancer in one population might be due to more women being in the population in ques-

tion. *Standardized populations* should, therefore, be used when comparing incidence and prevalence.

In trying to find connections between a disease and a postulated causal factor, epidemiologists may construct either *case-control* or *cohort* studies. Take, for example, a study to determine if there is a connection between dietary fat and breast cancer. A case-control study would compare the dietary intake of people with the disease (cases) and those without (controls). Choosing appropriate controls is vital to the study design. Case-control studies are also suitable for studies of rare tumours in which cohort studies are impractical. A cohort study is a prospective study in which a group of people who are exposed to the putative aetiological agent are followed and the frequency of the disease is measured. The control group is unexposed, or exposed to a lesser extent. In the case of dietary fat and breast cancer a cohort study would compare the incidence of the disease in those with, say, a high fat and a low fat diet. If the cancer incidence is low, as it usually is, large numbers of women will be followed over many years before an answer is obtained. Other variables must be allowed for since eating habits, for example, are influenced by social class and profession and these may in turn be independently linked to the likelihood of developing breast cancer. Cohort studies take a long time, are very expensive, and are unsuitable for rare tumour studies.

There are considerable problems in the interpretation of data obtained from epidemiological studies. A possible relationship between a characteristic and a cancer may be discovered but there are several considerations which should influence us in deciding whether a causal connection really exists. First, is the relationship between the characteristic and the disease specific, or can a similar association be found with other diseases? An association with other diseases does not necessarily invalidate a causal connection but may suggest that both the characteristic and the cancer are themselves associated with another factor. For example, both lung cancer and coronary artery disease are commoner in social classes 4 and 5. The problem is then to decide if these diseases are due to social class itself or to the higher frequency of cigarette smoking in these social groups. Second, is the relationship a strong one? The likelihood of a causal connection is strengthened if, for example, the risk of cancer in the population showing the characteristic is increased ten-fold rather than doubled. Third, is there a gradation of risk with differing exposure? This is the situation with lung cancer and cigarette smoking. Such a gradation greatly increases the likelihood of a causal connection. Fourth, is the association biologically plausible? For example, it appears intuitively reasonable to accept an association between smoking and lung cancer but the relationship between smoking and bladder cancer is at first more surprising (see p. 326). It is, however, difficult to assess the biological basis for an association since often we do not know the explanation for these events until further investigation, perhaps prompted by the discovery of an association, reveals it. Finally, is there an alternative explanation for what has been found and do the findings fit in with other epidemiological data? The nature of epidemiological evidence is such that absolute proof that an association is causal is impossible to obtain except by randomized intervention studies in which, the suspected factor is altered or removed to see if the incidence of cancer then falls. Such studies are difficult, expensive and time-consuming.

GEOGRAPHICAL DISTRIBUTION OF CANCER

Clues to the aetiology of cancer have been obtained from studies of the difference in incidence of cancers in different countries, races and cultures although there are obvious difficulties in obtaining reliable data in many countries. Problems of different age distributions can to some extent be overcome by using age-standardized incidence and by restricting the comparison to the mature adult population aged 35–64 years. This age range excludes the ages where the figures are likely to be least reliable. A further difficulty lies in incomplete documentation of histological type. Usually the registration refers to the whole organ and may combine several different histologies.

Even allowing for some uncertainty in the reliability of the data, huge differences in incidence of various tumours between one country and another have been disclosed (Table 2.1). The very high incidence of liver cancer in Mozambique may be related to aflatoxin mould on stored peanuts, and the incidence is now falling since steps have been taken to store the peanuts under different conditions. In the Ghurjev region of Kazakhstan, carcinoma of the oesophagus is 200 times more common than in Holland and the same is true for the Transkei region

Table 2.1. Geographical variation in cancer incidence.

Cancer type	Ratio high:low rate	High incidence	Low incidence
Oesophagus	200:1	Kazakhstan	Netherlands
Skin	200:1	Queensland	India
Liver	100:1	Mozambique	Birmingham
Nasopharynx	100:1	China	Uganda
Lung	40:1	Birmingham	Ibadan (Nigeria)
Stomach	30:1	Japan	Birmingham
Cervix	20:1	Hawaii Columbia	Israel
Rectum	20:1	Denmark	Nigeria

where the incidence of the disease appears to have increased greatly in the last 30 years. The high incidence of carcinoma of the stomach in Japan is in contrast to Britain and the United States where the incidence of the disease is falling (1). The dietary factors which may be responsible are not understood.

Studies such as these provide strong evidence for environmental factors causing cancer but of course an interaction with possible genetic predisposition is also likely. An analysis of the genetic component can be made by studying cancer incidence in people who have settled in a new country and who have taken on a new way of life. Japanese immigrants in the United States, for example, have a similar incidence of colon cancer to native Americans but five times that of Japanese in Japan (2), see also Table 2.2, and it is therefore clear that this difference in rates is not primarily genetic.

Table 2.2. Cancer incidence* in Japanese immigrants compared with country of origin and residents of adopted country.

Cancer	Japanese in Japan	United States (mostly Hawaii) Japanese	White
Stomach	130	40	21
Breast	31	120	190
Colon	8.4	37	37
Ovary	5.2	17	27
Prostate	1.5	15	35

* Incidence = cases per year per 100 000

TEMPORAL DISTRIBUTION OF CANCER

The incidence of cancer in a given community may change with time providing further clues to aetiology. With rare tumours, this may be more dramatically apparent when a disease appears as a cluster in a given place at a given time. An example would be several cases of acute leukaemia occurring in close proximity in a town within a short space of time. Such clus-

tering has indeed been observed in acute leukaemia and has been suggested for Hodgkin's disease. The data are rather variable however, and not easy to verify, and chance effects make analysis difficult. However, in the case of Burkitt's lymphoma, outbreaks in Uganda have been shown to spread from one part of a district to another in a way which cannot be attributed to chance but which fits well with an infective aetiology widespread in the community while producing cancer in only a few.

CAUSES OF CANCER SUGGESTED BY EPIDEMIOLOGICAL STUDIES

The idea that cancer might largely be preventable has gained more widespread acceptance in recent years (3). While many substances present in the environment or in the diet have been shown to be carcinogenic in animals this does not mean that they will be so in man. One contribution of the epidemiological approach has been to try to verify the link between human cancers and substances which in animals are known to be carcinogens. Another has been to identify unsuspected carcinogens by observations on human populations without reference to previous animal experiments. Some of the factors which are known or strongly suspected to be carcinogenic in man are shown in Table 2.3.

Ionizing irradiation

Ionizing radiation has been well established as a human carcinogen. There has been an increased incidence of leukaemia (4) and breast cancer (5) in the survivors of the Nagasaki and Hiroshima atom bombs. Skin cancer frequently occurred on the hands of radiologists in the days before the significance of radiation exposure was understood. There is also an increased incidence of leukaemia in patients treated by irradiation for ankylosing spondylitis (6). Ultraviolet irradiation is probably responsible for the increased incidence of skin cancer on

Table 2.3. Some aetiological factors.

Ionising irradiation	
Atomic bomb (Nagasaki, Hiroshima)	Acute leukaemia, breast cancer
X-rays	
for ankylosing spondylitis	Acute leukaemia
in diagnostic and therapeutic radiologists	Squamous cell carcinoma of skin
Ultraviolet irradiation	Basal cell carcinoma
	Squamous cell carcinomas of skin
	Melanoma
Background irradiation	?Acute leukaemia
Inhaled or ingested carcinogens	
Cigarette smoking	Lung cancer
	Laryngeal cancer
	Bladder cancer
Atmospheric pollution with polycyclic hydrocarbons	Lung cancer
Asbestos	Mesothelioma
	Bronchial carcinoma
Nickel	Lung cancer and paranasal sinuses
Chromates	Lung cancer
Arsenic	Lung cancer
	Skin cancer
Aluminium	Bladder
Aromatic animes	Bladder
Benzene	Erythroleukaemia
Polyvinyl chloride	Angiosarcoma of the liver

exposed sites in those who work out of doors in strong sunshine, for example in Australia.

The level of background radiation in the environment is of course much smaller than that received in the examples given above. The doses are not only smaller in total, but are received at a much slower rate (< 100 millionth) than that of diagnostic X-rays. While there is no safe lower limit to radiation dose it is possible to calculate the approximate risk and it is generally accepted that for most cancers background radioactivity constitutes a small risk at present, although this may not be true of leukaemia where background radiation may be responsible for a slight increase in incidence.

Inhaled carcinogens

Cigarette smoking has been the subject of intense epidemiological investigation since the early work of Doll and Hill demonstrated the relationship between smoking and lung cancer (7). All studies have shown a higher mortality for lung cancer in smokers. This mortality has a dose-response relationship with the numbers of cigarettes smoked and diminishes with time after stopping smoking. This relationship is discussed further in Chapter 12. Cigarette smoking has also been implicated in the development of carcinoma of the bladder, larynx, pancreas and kidney and may be responsible for 35% of all cancer deaths.

Atmospheric pollutants such as chimney smoke and exhaust fumes have been widely suspected as a cause of lung cancer. Polycyclic hydrocarbons, such as 3:4-benzpyrene, are present in these fumes and are known to be carcinogenic in man (see p. 23). Several large scale studies have shown that the incidence of lung cancer in men in large cities is two or three times greater than those living in the country. This increase, which may or may not be attributable to air pollution, is probably present at all levels of cigarette smoking but is very small compared with the increase in incidence in smokers compared with non-smokers.

Occupational factors (Table 2.3)

Asbestos inhalation has been shown to be associated with two types of cancer: mesothelioma of the pleura and peritoneum, and bronchogenic carcinoma. Prolonged and heavy exposure is needed in the case of bronchogenic cancer and cigarette smoking further increases the risk (8). Mesothelioma is a rare tumour and there is often a clear history of asbestos exposure. Although the duration and intensity of the exposure is very variable, the relationship with this tumour is not in doubt. There is also an increased risk of lung cancer in workers in nickel refining and the manufacture of chromates and a possible association with haematite mining and gold mining. Lung cancer has also been described in workers in a sheep dip factory where there was a very high exposure to inhaled arsenic. These workers had signs of chronic arsenism and the risk of lung cancer with lower levels of exposure is probably very small.

Other human carcinogens have been identified as a result of industrial epidemiological evidence (see p. 24). Aniline dye workers were shown to have a greatly increased incidence of bladder cancer, and this observation led to the demonstration, in animals, of the carcinogenic effect of 2-naphthylamine. Benzidine and 2-naphthylamine have also been implicated in the pathogenesis of bladder cancer in these workers and those in the rubber industry who are also exposed.

Workers in the aluminium industry have been shown to have an increased incidence of bladder cancer. It has been estimated that about 4% of all cancers can be related to occupational factors.

Life-style and diet

What other factors in our environment or life-style might contribute to the development of cancer? Some American epidemiologists attribute a large proportion of cancers to as yet unspecified industrial poisons and claim that cancer incidence has increased in the last decade in the USA, an increase which is unrelated to tobacco consumption (9). The figures are disputed, however, since there is the confounding variable of improved diagnosis and registration among the poorer sections of American society during this period (see later). The issue is intensely political and the prevention and control of industrial pollution potentially involves large sums of money. The truth becomes obscured in a mass of conflicting epidemiological data.

The place of dietary factors in cancer causation is equally poorly understood. Recent studies have shown that in countries where there is a high average daily fat intake the age-adjusted death rate of breast cancer is also high and that the converse is true for populations consuming low fat diets. The problem here is of course that those countries where dietary fat intake is high also tend to be the most heavily industrialized. Furthermore, the total caloric intake is higher in these nations and a similar association exists for levels of dietary protein. Overnutrition has been shown to increase the incidence of spontaneous tumours in animals. Obesity appears to be an aetiological factor in cancers of the endometrium and gall bladder. Case-control studies relating dietary fat to cancer incidence have given conflicting results. Rather than being causally linked to the cancer, it may be that these dietary constituents are associated with other factors which are themselves causal. Other dietary factors which may be associated with the development of cancer are dietary fibre, which may protect against the development of cancer of the large bowel, and vitamin A analogues (retinoids). The incidence of many types of cancer appears to have an inverse relationship with serum vitamin A levels.

An appreciation of the difficulties involved in analysing the relative contributions of diet, life-style and occupational risk can be gained by reading the contradictory accounts of Epstein (9) and Peto (10).

Viral causes

Although many animal cancers are caused by viruses (feline leukaemia, murine sarcoma, polyoma) there is no epidemiological evidence to implicate viruses as a cause of the vast majority of human cancers. The clearest association is between Epstein-Barr (EB) virus and Burkitt's lymphoma (see Chapter 3) and the epidemiological evidence suggesting an infective aetiology preceded the demonstration of the association with EB virus infection. The disease mainly occurs in Africa and New Guinea in areas where the temperatures are above 16°C and with rainfall over 50 cm a year. Furthermore, in affected areas, cases occur in a non-random pattern moving from one district to another, presumably to susceptible populations.

Other possible viral causes are discussed in Chapter 3, but it may be noted here that chronic infection with hepatitis B virus is associated with an increased risk of hepatoma and that the viral genome has been demonstrated both in hepatoma cells and also in normal areas of the affected liver. It is of great interest that there is an increased risk of cancer in patients who are chronically immunosuppressed (11). These cancers are squamous carcinoma of the skin and cervix, lymphoma of B cell type (especially intracerebral), Kaposi's sarcoma and melanoma. Some of the tumours have an association with viral infection. It is possible that immunosuppression allows unchecked activity of oncogenic viruses.

CANCER STATISTICS

In recent years a number of registries have been established in Britain and in other industrialized countries, to record the number of patients developing cancer. The registry is usually notified of new cancer cases by the hospital where the diagnosis is made. In addition, it receives copies of all death certificates of patients within the region, where the diagnosis of cancer appears on a certificate. The quality of the data collected varies greatly from registry to registry and between countries. Incomplete information; changing patterns of registration and diagnosis; introduction of screening programmes and improved treatment, may all alter the number of patients being registered as dying of the disease in a given area in a given time. Minor fluctuations in incidence should, therefore, be viewed with caution. Consistent trends over several years require investigation before it can be accepted that a change in the incidence or mortality of a disease is occurring.

Even the most complete registries may have histological confirmation of the diagnosis in less than 60% of cases though the completeness of the records with respect to primary site of the tumour is much greater. The incidence figures for tumours of a defined histological type are,

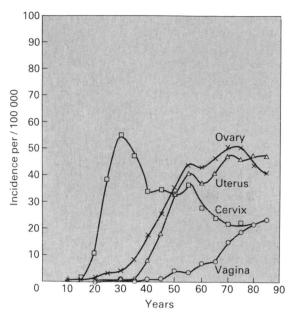

Fig. 2.1. *Age-specific incidence of female genital cancer.* The figures for cervical cancer include carcinoma *in situ*, diagnosed by screening examination, which accounts for the majority of cases in young patients.

therefore, usually much less reliable than those which describe its site of origin.

In spite of these reservations a glance at the age-specific incidence of various tumours is interesting and revealing. For example, the figures for female genital cancer (Fig. 2.1) show that cancer of the ovary and uterus follow a very similar pattern, the incidence rising sharply towards the end of the child-bearing years, reaching a peak postmenopause. An understanding of the causes of these cancers must clearly take into account these dramatic changes. This is not the pattern seen with all adenocarcinomas in women (Fig. 2.2). Indeed cancer of the ovary and uterus stand out as not showing the typical huge increase in incidence from the age of 60 onwards which characterizes other adenocarcinomas such as bowel, stomach and pancreas.

Cancer of the cervix and of the vagina, chiefly squamous cell cancers, are quite unlike each other in age of onset, that of the cervix being a

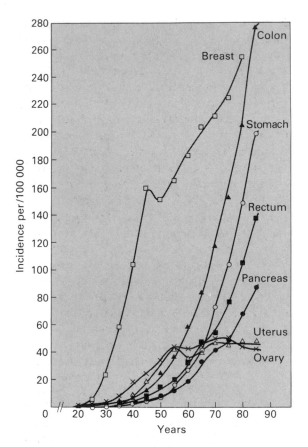

Fig. 2.2. *Age-specific incidence of female adenocarcinoma.* The incidence of cancer of the breast increases rapidly in premenopausal women and then slows. This change is more marked with ovarian and uterine adenocarcinoma. By contrast, the incidence of gastro-intestinal cancers shows no relation to menopause.

lem is discussed in more detail in Chapter 17 but it serves to illustrate how cancer statistics may be dramatically altered by early diagnosis.

The figures for other adenocarcinomas in women (Fig. 2.2) are revealing in another respect. The onset of cancer of the uterus and ovary is earlier than that of the gut and stomach, and does not increase in incidence with old age. Cancer of the breast, on the other hand, rises rapidly in incidence in early middle age, and then continues to rise in incidence postmenopause but at a somewhat slower rate compared to colonic cancer, so that the incidence over 80 years of age is less than that of the colon while at 40 years of age, breast cancer occurs 14 times more frequently. The factors responsible for the origin and growth of breast cancer clearly differ from those giving rise to gastro-intestinal malignancy.

SURVIVAL DATA AND DETERMINATION OF CURE IN CANCER

When results of cancer treatment are presented, a graph of survival is often shown or the proportion of patients alive at, say, 5 or 10 years is stated. It is often difficult to decide whether the results mean that some patients are cured, and unfortunately claims are often made on the basis of figures that are incomplete. An understanding of how survival figures are derived is therefore essential for judging the effectiveness of treatment.

A *survival curve* is a plot of the proportion of patients surviving as a function of time, Fig. 2.3; curve A gives the survival up to 10 years for all cases of cancer of the ovary. A *disease-free survival curve* is displayed in a similar manner but the x-axis represents the length of time before the disease reappears. Since some patients may be effectively treated on relapse the information is not the same as with a survival curve. This is especially true in a disease such as Hodgkin's disease where many patients can be cured on relapse.

disease of young and middle aged women, and that of the vagina a disease of elderly women (Fig. 2.1). There is an obvious problem in interpreting these data. The impact of screening programmes for cervical cancer has meant that many of these cases are diagnosed at a very early stage and study of the histology shows a large percentage of cases diagnosed *in situ*. Should we therefore conclude that the higher incidence of cervical cancer in young women is an artefact of early diagnosis and that these cancers would only have been clinically apparent, if at all, many years later? This prob-

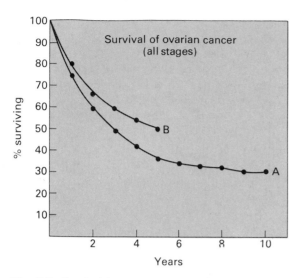

Fig. 2.3. *Survival in ovarian cancer.* Curve A represents survival of a group of patients where all patients had been diagnosed at least 10 years previously. Curve B is an actuarial survival curve: none of these patients had been diagnosed more than 5 years previously and some had been diagnosed only 2 years previously.

In constructing a survival curve a number of statistical methods may have been used. If, for example, the cases of ovarian cancer in Fig. 2.3 were all diagnosed between 1960 and 1970 and the results analysed in 1980, all the cases would have been followed for at least 10 years, that is, a 10 year follow-up would be complete. If the cases had been diagnosed between 1965 and 1975 then, in 1980, some cases would have been followed more than 10 years and other cases 5–10 years. The curve can nonetheless be constructed by dividing the follow-up period into fixed intervals, calculating the probability of surviving through each interval and combining these into an overall survival probability which is plotted as a function of time. This is an *actuarial survival curve* and may be thought of as a prediction of how the final survival curve will look if all the cases have similar survival characteristics to those which have been followed longest. These curves are less reliable in the 'tails' when the follow-up period for many patients is short and the number of late survivors is correspondingly small. Figure 2.3 curve

B is a hypothetical survival curve, for similar cases to curve A, of 40 patients where only 30 have been followed for 2 or more years and five for 4 or more years. The curve is similar in shape to curve A for the first 2 years (when there are most observations) but appears to show improved survival thereafter. Such a conclusion would be unwise, however, because of the small number of observations between 2 and 4 years on which the curve is based. It would not need many deaths to occur to alter the shape of curve B to that of curve A.

Can we judge whether patients are cured by looking at survival curves? The general answer is that cure can be assumed if the group of patients returns to a normal pattern of survival similar to those who have not had that cancer. In the case of ovarian cancer the comparison would be made with a large population of women with the same age distribution. The survival curve expected in such a population is the *age-adjusted expected survival curve*. An example is given in Fig. 2.4 for ovarian cancer

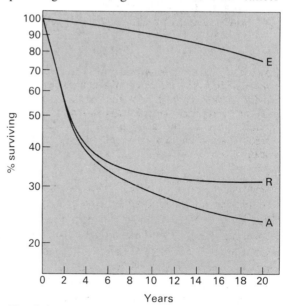

Fig. 2.4. *Survival in ovarian cancer.* Curve A shows observed survival, Curve E shows age-adjusted expected survival and Curve R shows relative survival. (Modified from Bush *et al.* (1982). In Stoll B. A. *Prolonged Arrest of Cancer*, John Wiley & Sons Ltd., England, with permission.)

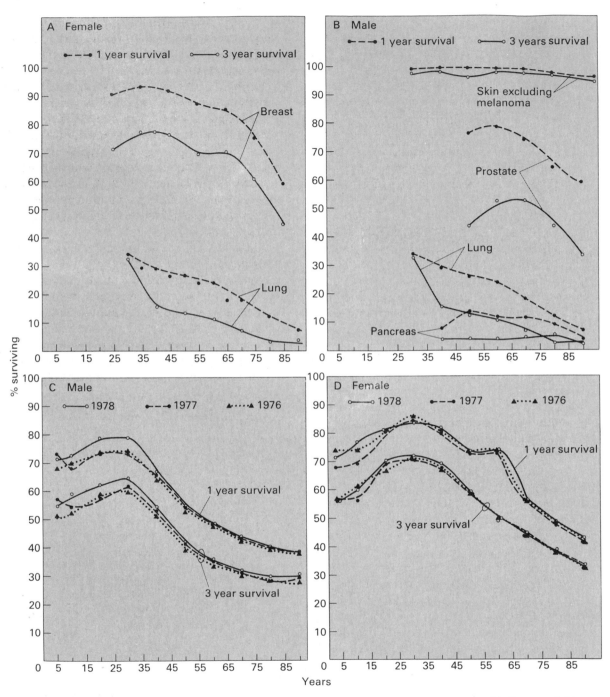

Fig. 2.5. *Age-related relative survival rates.* (A) Cancer of breast and lung in women (1978). (B) Cancer of skin, prostate, lung, and pancreas in men (1978). Figures are given for survival at 1 year and 3 years. (C) Cancer at all sites in men (resident in England and Wales) for 3 consecutive years. (D) Cancer at all sites in women for 3 consecutive years.

followed for 20 years. Curve A is the observed survival of the patients, curve E is the age-adjusted expected survival curve and it can be seen that A is approximately parallel to E at 15–20 years. The age-adjusted relative survival curve (R) is constructed by dividing the observed survival curve (A) by the expected curve (E). If there is no increased risk of dying due to the cancer this curve will run parallel to the abscissa. A difficulty might arise if the ability to cure the cancer were dependent on age, for example, if young women were more easily cured than elderly women. The age distribution of survivors would then change with time and the age distribution of the control population would, therefore, have to be adjusted accordingly.

Survival does depend on age for many tumours: Figure 2.5 shows *age-related survival rates* at 1 and 3 years for a variety of common tumours. For most cancers survival is worse in the elderly population at both 1 and 3 years. Curves C and D give the age-related survival

rates for all cancers for 3 successive years. There is no evidence of improvement in results; except in young men, due to better treatment of teratoma of the testis.

In Figures 2.3 and 2.4 the survival curves are given for all cases of cancer of the ovary but of course they could be plotted for individual ages at presentation, or stages of the disease. In this way one may investigate whether cure is being achieved only for certain age groups or stages of disease. In practice, however, data on very large groups of patients (thousands) is needed to demonstrate cure with any statistical certainty.

A linear scale plot of survival figures may suggest that a small proportion of patients are going to be long survivors. In Fig. 2.6, for example, the survival figures for a large trial in small cell bronchogenic cancer are shown on the linear scale. Curve A seems to flatten out at 2 years which might be interpreted as showing that a proportion of patients are cured. However, on a log/linear scale the curve (B) is shown

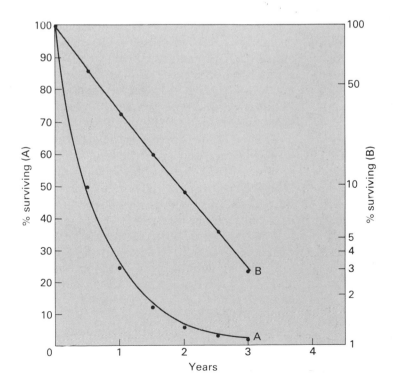

Fig. 2.6. *Survival in advanced small cell carcinoma of the bronchus.* There appears to be a flattening of the survival curve (curve A) but the rate of death is in fact exponential (curve B).

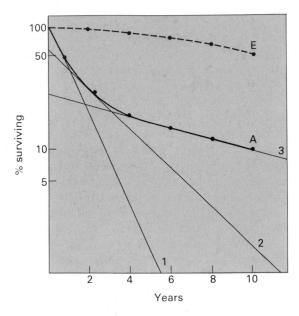

Fig. 2.7. *Survival following gastrectomy for carcinoma of the stomach.* Curve A can be considered to be a composite of 3 separate populations (1, 2 and 3) one of which is cured of the disease (3). Age-adjusted expected survival of a control population is shown by curve E.

to be a straight line, that is, exponential, indicating that the rate of death has remained constant with time; the slope of the line giving the rate. This shows that up to this point there is no evidence of cure in the group in question. Many survival curves do not however show an exponential shape on a log/linear scale. Figure 2.7 shows the survival after gastrectomy for carcinoma of the stomach, curve A, and the age-adjusted expected survival, curve E. The survival curve is not exponential. We might speculate that the curve consists of three separate components, a group (line 1) dying rapidly, another (line 2) whose rate of death is lower and third group (line 3) who appeared to be cured.

ASSESSMENT OF RESULTS: TRIALS OF TREATMENT

Many of the basic methods and techniques of treatment in cancer have been developed by ex-

perienced physicians and surgeons using their commonsense. When the treatment has resulted in a clear improvement, as was the case for example, when mastectomy was first introduced to treat patients with breast cancer, this approach has worked satisfactorily. When differences in treatment results have been less obvious, for example, in the case of simple versus radical mastectomy, the results are harder to evaluate.

The problem of assessment is made more complex by changing criteria for diagnosis and treatment during the period in question. For example, refined methods of detection of metastases at presentation (e.g. CT scanning) may result in patients being rejected for a treatment which in earlier days they would have received. This means survival may alter as a result of a *change in selection* which might then be falsely attributed to a recently introduced treatment.

Randomized trials

Many statisticians and oncologists take the view that the only way to avoid bias is to carry out a randomized prospective comparison of the new treatment with the best standard regimen, or in some cases, with no treatment. In this way hidden factors in case selection such as histological subtypes, presence of occult metastases and site of tumour, will be randomly distributed in the two groups. Similarly factors which are not known to be associated with prognosis at the start of the trial but which are later shown to be so, do not bias the results since these factors will apply equally to the randomly allocated groups.

When an analysis of the effect of different treatments is made, the data may be examined for effect on survival or disease-free survival. The results are typically presented as in Fig. 2.8 which illustrate the disease-free survival curves from a controlled trial of two treatments in breast cancer. Patient group A had received adjuvant chemotherapy and group B had not. There are several points to notice. Firstly, the

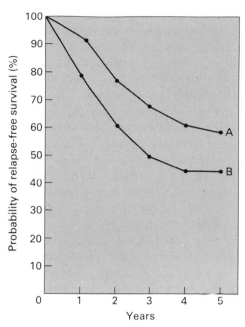

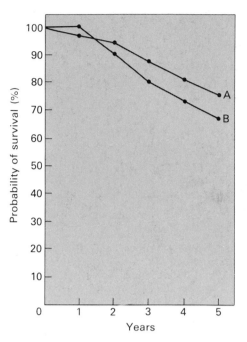

Fig. 2.8. *Actuarial relapse free survival in operable breast cancer.* Curve A: treated with adjuvant chemotherapy. Curve B: no adjuvant chemotherapy. (Reproduced from Rossi *et al* (1981) *BMJ*, **282**, 1427. With permission.)

Fig. 2.9. *Actuarial survival in operable breast cancer.* Curve A: treated with adjuvant chemotherapy. Curve B: no adjuvant chemotherapy. (Reproduced from Rossi *et al* (1981) *BMJ*, **282**, 1427. With permission.)

curves are actuarial curves, that is, not all the patients have been followed for 5 years. If the numbers of long term survivors are small the tails of the curves may be misleading. Secondly, a difference in favour of chemotherapy is apparent. The probability of this happening purely by chance can be assessed by statistical methods. The log-rank test is a convenient and commonly used method of comparing survival and disease-free survival curves. The test is sensitive to curves which separate to reveal a consistent survival difference. Other tests are more sensitive to early differences which are less apparent later. Thirdly, if the difference is genuine, it represents a delay in onset of recurrence. This may not be reflected in improved *survival*. The survival curves for the groups are shown in Fig. 2.9; it can be seen that the difference is much less striking. This apparent discrepancy may be due to a delay in onset of metastases in the chemotherapy treated group leading to an improved disease-free sur-

vival. Once metastases have appeared, the patients in the control group, who have not received chemotherapy, might benefit from its use so that the overall survival curves are less divergent. Early effects of this type on disease-free survival are often seen in cancer treatment. Delay of recurrence is certainly desirable, but one should bear in mind that for most treatments improved survival is the real objective.

A commonly used method of presentation of results is to quote *median* survival, that is, the time from randomization at which 50% of the patients will be alive. These figures are very unreliable unless the death rate in the 25–75% range is high and the numbers of patients in the study is large (Fig. 2.10). Average or *mean* survival times are often misleading because they can be greatly affected by one or two long term survivors. Analysis of the proportion surviving at a single point in time is myopic and a survival curve analysis is preferred because it makes use of the whole time span of the study.

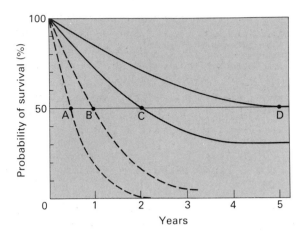

Fig. 2.10. *Median survival in cancer trials.* Trial 1 (dotted lines) median survival A = 6 months, B = 1 year. Trial 2 (continuous lines) median survival C = 2 years, D = 5 years. The differences are reliable in Trial 1 but less so in Trial 2.

It should be remembered that tests of significance merely provide estimates of the probability that an observed difference could have arisen by chance. There are many considerations besides the probability level which should affect one's judgement about whether the difference is interesting or important and whether or not it is solely the result of the treatment.

In designing a prospective randomized trial of treatment many factors must be taken into account, some of which may affect the value of the study:

1 *Can a single question be asked?* Wherever possible the hypothesis being tested should be as simple as possible. For example, can the study ask the question 'is treatment "A" better than no treatment at all?' A simple study design is always preferable but sometimes not possible. Is it ethically justified to give no treatment? If, for example, the effect of adjuvant chemotherapy on survival following mastectomy is being compared with no postoperative treatment, how will the no chemotherapy group be treated on relapse? A policy for treatment at each stage of the disease must be devised and agreed before the trial begins. Studies in which

there is a 'cross-over' from one treatment to another are usually hard to interpret. Studies which include several randomized groups will usually have to be very large if they are to detect realistic differences between the groups.

2 *Which patients will be included?* A precise statement must be made of the type of patient in which the treatments are to be tested.

3 *Are there known prognostic factors?* Patients with 'limited' stage small cell lung cancer (SCLC) have a better prognosis than those with 'extensive' disease. In trials of treatment in SCLC it is advisable to randomize limited and extensive category patients separately to ensure balanced numbers of each group in each arm of the study. This is *stratification* of patients prior to randomization. Major prognostic criteria should be stratified, but too many stratifications can cause confusion.

4 *What is the end-point?* Some trials will be concerned with differences in survival, others with disease-free interval, others with local recurrence. In some studies differences in median survival may be shown without any change in the final, long-term survival.

5 *Is the difference between the treatments in question likely to be large?* This is seldom the case in cancer where, if the effect of the therapy is dramatic, the trial would probably not be considered necessary or justified. To detect differences in survival of 10% with a significance level of 0.05, between 160 and 500 patients will be needed per patient group, the numbers varying with the proportion surviving. It requires fewer patients to show a 10% survival difference between 10% and 20% than a difference between 40% and 50%. Because of the large numbers of patients necessary to detect small differences with confidence, many cancer trials are collaborative efforts between different centres. Indeed for rare diseases such as leukaemia or osteosarcoma, treatment trials are almost impossible without such collaboration. Those responsible for the trial have to decide what sort of difference they will consider clinically interesting (see p. 19).

6 *The difficulties of collaboration are consider-*

able. Doctors participating in the study must agree on what is the most important question to be asked; how the treatment should be administered (including details of surgery, radiotherapy and chemotherapy); what the documentation should be and how it should be organized; who will pay for the study; who will analyse the data and so on. In a disease like breast cancer where the rate of death is low, the answers may not be available for 10 years or more. Doctors are usually, to put it kindly, 'individualistic' in their approach to treatment and large-scale trials sometimes acquire a design which proves an unsatisfactory compromise. Exceptionally intensive treatments cannot be carried out in every hospital and may not be of the same quality as when undertaken by a few specialized units. Such treatments may be 'watered down' in order to include more centres, possibly weakening the intention of the study.

7 *Even if the differences in survival are small they may be clinically worthwhile.* Dramatic advances in treatment are rare and come from an imaginative step forward by a few individuals, for example, CNS prophylaxis in acute leukaemia or combination chemotherapy in Hodgkin's disease. Large randomized studies are usually carried out where it is not clear if one treatment is better than another and differences are therefore likely to be small. A small difference may however lead to a change in clinical practice. For example, if it could be shown that following mastectomy, treatment with a drug such as tamoxifen led to a 5% improvement in long-term survival this would be a major contribution to management because in 20 000 women this could mean 1000 lives saved with negligible toxicity. On the other hand many would regard a 5% improvement achieved with cytotoxic chemotherapy as much less compelling, bearing in mind the greater toxicity of the treatment.

The confident detection of a 5% difference in mortality, requires very large numbers of patients. Statisticians are constantly urging doctors to unite into large collaborative groups for this purpose and international collaboration may sometimes be necessary. The design and execution of a large multinational study in cancer treatment is expensive, time-consuming and provides little gratification for the ego of participants. There is a marked tendency for doctors to lose interest after a few years. If a small survival difference will not be clinically important it is better not to ask the question.

ANALYSIS OF THE RESULTS OF RANDOMIZED TRIALS

Just as it is essential not to be over-impressed by dramatic results from uncontrolled studies, it is important not to be intimidated by the authority which randomized clinical trials appear to possess. A critical approach is needed. Some points to watch out for are:

1 *Is it likely that a false-positive result (type 1 or alpha error) has occurred?* Such errors are uncommon. False-negative errors (type 2 or beta errors) are commoner, but negative trials are not published as frequently as positive ones because journal editors seem to prefer 'positive' results. Does the trial accord with other studies addressing the same point?

2 *Were the treatments genuinely randomized?* Authors sometimes claim their study was randomized but a closer inspection of the method reveals it was not. These studies are nearly always misleading.

3 *Did one particular group of patients benefit?* This is an important matter because it allows treatment to be offered selectively and suggests future directions for study. However, it is almost impossible to draw firm conclusions about subgroups from a single study unless it contains thousands of patients.

4 *Have all the patients been included in the analysis, and if not, why not?* Sometimes patients who are not able to be evaluated are discarded from the report. One should beware of this, particularly if it occurs for large numbers of patients. One reason sometimes given is that the patient only completed one cycle of chemotherapy before deteriorating. The patient is discarded as not having had a fair trial of treatment. This practice will of course greatly improve the apparent results because early failures are not included.

5 *Has the trial run for sufficient time to allow enough events (deaths, relapses) to have occurred?* What are the confidence limits for the treatment difference? A statement of the 95% confidence limits for the treatment difference allows the reader to judge the result being presented and is more informative than a 'p' value from a significance test.

INFORMED CONSENT

Before starting any treatment most doctors will want to discuss the benefits and problems of treatment and the possible different approaches which might be used. In a clinical trial doctors also have to discuss the reason for the study, the meaning of randomization and the right of the patient not to be involved. This creates problems for both doctors and patient. Their relationship may be upset by these disclosures especially the admission that the results of the treatments are not known with certainty. There may have to be discussion of failure rates in the disease. The patient may become confused, and this and the time the explanation takes may deter many doctors from becoming involved in trials.

In most studies the patient is asked if he will take part. If he declines, he is not entered into the study. If he agrees to take part randomization proceeds. In order to avoid some of the difficulties posed by this procedure Zelen (12) has proposed a randomized consent design. In this system patients are randomized to A (conventional treatment) or B (new treatment). No consent is sought for A. For those randomized to B, consent is sought. If it is not given, the patient undergoes treatment A.

Several problems are posed with Zelen's system. Is this really informed consent? What if those patients randomized to B accept or refuse for reasons relating to their illness? For example more patients with large tumours might opt for radical surgery than those with small ones.

This would bias the distribution of cases. To meet these objections the method has been further modified. It is too soon to judge the usefulness of this approach. One problem is that if patients drop out of the study the trial efficiency is considerably weakened.

Non-randomized studies of treatment

The difficulties of controlled trials of treatment have led many investigators to embark on uncontrolled studies and to report survival with a given treatment in the hope that a clear advantage over the best current methods of treatment will be shown. The result has been a plethora of misleading small-scale studies where the numbers have been too small, the follow-up too short and with many omissions and exclusions from analysis. There is an important role for well conducted pilot studies but the results must be intepreted cautiously.

A compromise has been sought between the cumbersome controlled trial and the unreliable uncontrolled study. This has involved the use of *historical control* which compares present treatment to patients treated in the past. An attempt is normally, but not always, made to match the controls for age, sex, site and stage of tumour and other known prognostic factors such as histological grade and menopausal status. The problems are of course that staging methods are changing continually, that selection of control cases may not be impartial, and that not all prognostic factors will be known.

There is a place for studies in which the comparison is made with historical control groups, but such trials must be designed and interpreted with great care. These studies may point the way in management and indicate which questions should be asked in large scale prospective studies.

SCREENING FOR CANCER

The aim of screening a population for cancer is to make the diagnosis early and thereby increase the cure rate. So far, the practical benefits have been small or non-existent, with the outstanding exception of carcinoma of the cervix. The objective of screening is simple yet there are many problems and assumptions involved:

1 *What is the sensitivity of the test used?* Highly sensitive tests are essential if the disease is curable early and if the consequences of a false-positive test are not serious for the patients physically or psychologically. The Papanicolaou's smear is a sensitive test for cervical cancer and the diagnosis can be easily confirmed on biopsy. By contrast, abdominal ultrasound is an insensitive test for carcinoma of the pancreas and the diagnosis is difficult to confirm. This test is therefore of no value as a screening investigation. Self-examination for breast cancer is relatively insensitive but the finding of a lump can lead to early confirmation of the diagnosis.

2 *Is the disease curable if diagnosed early?* Carcinoma *in situ* or locally invasive carcinoma of the cervix are curable diseases. It remains to be proven, however, whether earlier diagnosis of colorectal cancer using screening by sigmoidoscopy or faecal occult blood testing will increase cure rate. Tumours such as colorectal cancer present late in their natural history and the limit of detection by screening may be only one or two doublings earlier than when the tumour would be clinically apparent. The question is whether the potential for metastasis is significantly less at the time when such a tumour is detectable by screening methods compared with the stage at which it is clinically apparent. It is true that, in breast cancer for example, small tumours have a better prognosis than large ones. This may, however, be more a reflection of the biological behaviour of small tumours rather than the tumour being detected earlier in its natural history. There is nothing to suggest that carcinoma of the head of the pancreas carries a better prognosis if diagnosed early since the results of treatment are poor at any stage.

3 *Is the disease common?* Cancer of the breast, cervix and lung are so common at certain ages and in certain individuals that screening is a practical proposition. Screening a general population for a disease such as gastric carcinoma is not practicable in Britain, but it is in Japan where the disease is 30 times more common. Clearly the incidence of the tumour has to be high enough to justify the screening programme.

4 *How frequently should the examination be undertaken, and in which population?* In some countries cervical smears are recommended every 3 years in women aged 20–65 years. In Britain on the other hand, the recommended lower age is 35 years (despite the falling age of incidence) and the recommended frequency 5-yearly. Breast self-examination can be carried out frequently, but investigations such as mammography are not currently recommended as a routine except in certain screening programmes. It is not clear what recommendations should be made for other investigations such as pelvic examination (for ovarian and uterine cancer) and sigmoidoscopy. The group at greatest risk from ovarian cancer includes nulliparous women over the age of 40 years; and for colorectal cancer, men and women over 50 years. Routine chest X-rays, even in smokers, have failed to show any benefit from early detection of lung cancer. Clearly patients with a genetic predisposition to certain cancers (e.g. polyposis coli, xeroderma pigmentosum) should have regular checks by the appropriate specialist.

5 *What are the disadvantages of screening?* Routine screening examinations can produce anxiety in the mind of the public at large and in certain individuals in particular. If applied to the whole population they would require a great expenditure of time and money. The benefits may be small and achieved at great expense. If the yearly incidence of breast cancer in women aged 50–70 years is taken at 2 per 1000, by screening 10 000 women each year, 20 new cases may be expected. If this is done by mammography and trained nurses in a clinic the cost might be in the region of £5 per visit. Even if the cure rate were improved from 30% to 60% by this procedure then six women would have been saved at a cost of £50 000. Screening of this type is, therefore, more expensive than most 'high technology' medicine.

At present the only well established screening procedure in Britain is the cervical smear for carcinoma of the cervix. Screening procedures which have been proposed, but not always convincingly validated, are listed below and are discussed in the appropriate chapters:

Breast cancer (see Chapter 13)	Self examination Nurse or doctor examination Mammography
Colorectal cancer (see Chapter 18)	Occult blood testing Rectal examination Sigmoidoscopy
Ovarian and Uterine cancer (see Chapter 17)	Pelvic examination Pelvic ultrasound
Skin cancers (see Chapter 22)	Self examination
Gastric cancer—Japan (see Chapter 14)	Radiological examination

REFERENCES

1 Devesa S. S. & Silverman D. T. (1978) Cancer incidence and mortality trends in the United States: 1935-1974. *Journal of the National Cancer Institute* **60**, 545-71.

2 Haenszel W. & Kurihera M. (1968) Studies of Japanese migrants: 1 Mortality from cancer and other diseases among Japanese in the United States. *Journal of the National Cancer Institute* **40**, 43-68.

3 Doll R. (1980) The epidemiology of cancer. *Cancer* **45**, 2475.

4 Bizzoreo O. J., Johnson K. G. & Ciocco A. (1966) Leukaemia in Hiroshima and Nagasaki. *New England Journal of Medicine* **274**, 1095.

5 Tokunaga M., Land C. E., Yamanisho T., Asano M., Tokuokas Ezaki H. & Nishimori I. (1982) Breast cancer in Japanese A-bomb survivors. *Lancet* **ii**, 924.

6 Court-Brown W. M. & Doll R. (1957) *Leukaemia and aplastic anaemia in patients treated for ankylosing spondylitis* (Medical Research Council Special Report Series, No. 295), HMSO, London.

7 Doll R. & Hill A. B. (1952) Study of aetiology of carcinoma of the lung. *British Medical Journal* **ii,** 1271.

8 Doll R. (1978) An epidemiological perspective of the biology of cancer. *Cancer Research* **38,** 3573.

9 Epstein S. S. & Swartz J. B. (1981) Fallacies of life-style cancer theories. *Nature* **289,** 127.

10 Peto R. (1980) Distorting the epidemiology of cancer: the need for a more balanced overview. *Nature* **284,** 297.

11 Shiel A. G. R. (1984) Cancer in organ transplant recipients: part of an induced immune deficiency syndrome. *British Medical Journal* **288,** 659.

12 Zelen M. (1979) A new design for randomized clinical trials. *New England Journal of Medicine* **300,** 1242.

FURTHER READING

Peto R. Pike M. C. Armitage P. Breslow N. E. Cox D. R. Howard S. V. Mantel N. McPherson K. Peto J. & Smith P. G. (1976, 1977) Design and analysis of randomized clinical trials requiring prolonged observation of each patient. *British Journal of Cancer* **34,** 585 (1976); **35,** 1-29 (1977).

Spodick D. H. (1982) The randomised controlled clinical trial: scientific and ethical bases. *American Journal of Medicine* **73,** 420-5.

Pocock S. J. (1983) *Clinical trials*. Wiley, Chichester.

Chapter 3
Biology of Cancer

INTRODUCTION

When thinking about cancer many scientists and physicians, and members of the public, perceive cancer as being 'foreign' to the body. Analogies with infections caused by parasites and germs are often drawn, and many infectious agents have been proposed as aetiological agents. As knowledge has progressed it has however become apparent that in many respects cancer cells are similar to normal cells and that there is considerable diversity of function and structure within a single neoplasm. Even greater diversity exists between tumours of the same type in different individuals and between tumours of different types. The fundamental property of cancer which distinguishes the disease from normal tissues, and which makes treatment so difficult, is metastasis. We are still ignorant of the mechanisms which underlie this remarkable process.

In this chapter some of the mechanisms of oncogenesis; tumour immunity; growth and spread of tumours are briefly reviewed.

PHYSICOCHEMICAL CAUSES OF CANCER

Chemical carcinogens

It has long been suspected that cancers might have a chemical cause. In 1775, Sir Percival Pott noticed an unusually large number of cases of cancer of the scrotum in chimney sweeps and in 1895, Rehn pointed out the high frequency of bladder cancer in dye factory workers. A

Table 3.1. Chemical carcinogens.

Polycyclic hydrocarbons:	3:4 benzpyrene 1:2, 5:6 dibenzpyrene
Nitrosamines:	Dimethylnitrosamine
Aromatic animes and azo dyes:	Beta-naphthylamine 2-acetylaminoglurorne Dimethylamino azobenzene Benzidine
Plant products:	Aflatoxin Senecis (producing pyrrolozidium)
Alkylating agents:	Nitrogen mustard Melphalan Nitrosourea
Inorganic chemicals:	Arsenic Nickel Asbestos Cadmium

wide variety of carcinogens have been described and some of these are shown in Table 3.1.

Some of the mechanisms of chemical carcinogenesis have now been elucidated. There are several types of carcinogen which are candidates for causing cancer in man (see below). For a more detailed account the reader is referred to references 1 and 2.

POLYCYCLIC HYDROCARBONS

These chemicals are among the products of combustion of carbon-containing materials. They are present in coal tar (from soot), cigarette smoke, car exhaust fumes and some cooked foods. One of the major developments in understanding the relationship between cancer and the environment was when Kennaway and his co-workers showed that benzanthracene was present in coal tar and subsequently that it was carcinogenic. Later 3:4 benzpyrene was isolated from coal tar and was also shown to be carcinogenic and capable of inducing skin cancers in animals. Not all polycyclic hydrocarbons are carcinogens. It appears that the carcinogenic property resides in one region of the molecule, the K-region, to which oxygen is added in a reaction catalysed by cellular enzymes (e.g. aryl hydrocarbon hydroxylase). This epoxide portion of the molecule reacts with cellular DNA: especially with guanine bases. It is this reaction with DNA which is thought to be responsible for its carcinogenic effect.

NITROSAMINES

Dimethylnitrosamine was shown to cause liver cancer in animals when added to their food. Nitrites, which are present in many foods, are converted to nitrous acid in the stomach and may then react with amines in food to produce nitrosamines. Thus a mechanism exists for the formation of a potential carcinogen from food. It must be stated however that there is no definite evidence that the formation of nitrosamines is important in carcinogenesis in man.

AROMATIC ANIMES AND AZO DYES

Following Rehn's original observation of the increased frequency of bladder cancer in aniline dye workers, the aniline derivatives β-naphthylamine and benzidine were shown to be carcinogens. Later azo dye derivatives were also found to be carcinogenic including dimethylamino azobenzene (butter yellow) which was used to add colour to margarine (Table 3.1). When ingested these substances produce cancers at sites remote from the gut. They are first metabolized to an active form which is the carcinogen. For example β-naphthylamine is hydroxylated to a carcinogen which is then glucuronated to an inactive water soluble form in the liver and excreted in the urine. Glucuron

idases in the bladder mucosa liberate active carcinogen (an aminophenol) again and the cancers develop only in those species which possess this bladder enzyme.

The aminophenol reacts directly with guanine bases on DNA and, as with polycyclic hydrocarbons, this is presumed to be the basis of their carcinogenic action. In man there is a 20 year latent period between exposure and the development of bladder cancer. Cigarette smoke also contains β-naphthylamine (see Chapter 12) and bladder cancer is associated with smoking.

AFLATOXIN

This toxin is produced by *Aspergillus flavus* which may contaminate staple foods. It causes hepatic necrosis in turkeys. It may be a carcinogen in hepatic cancer and there is an association between dietary aflatoxin and the high frequency of hepatic cancers in Mozambique; though direct proof is lacking. The hepatitis B virus is more likely to be involved in the development of a hepatoma, aflatoxin perhaps acting as a promoter (see below). The toxin is a complex molecule which is metabolized by the same pathway as polycyclic hydrocarbons and the hydroxy product reacts with DNA.

ALKYLATING AGENTS

Drugs used in the treatment of cancer are also carcinogens. Alkylating agents bind directly to DNA (see pp. 86–90) and their use has been associated with the development of second malignancies, for example, acute leukaemia in patients successfully treated for Hodgkin's disease or ovarian cancer.

Ionizing and ultraviolet irradiation

The effects of ionizing irradiation on the cell are discussed in Chapter 5. Irradiation produces breaks in DNA strands and chromosomal abnormalities such as fragmentations, deletions and translocations. These abnormalities lead to cell death in dividing cells; the mechanisms of carcinogenesis are however poorly understood. There is no doubt that cancers can be caused by ionizing radiation. Skin cancers developed on the hands of the early radiologists and there is a significant and dose-related increase in acute and chronic myeloid leukaemia and in breast and thyroid cancer in the survivors of the atom bomb explosions at Hiroshima and Nagasaki.

Ultraviolet light increases the likelihood of development of skin cancer (see Chapter 22). DNA absorbs photons and it seems likely that alterations in thymine bases occur with the formation of dimers. In xeroderma pigmentosum the DNA repair process is faulty leading to an excess of skin cancers (though not cancers at other sites).

Initiators and promoters in carcinogenesis

Some agents appear to act as 'initiators' (Fig. 3.1): they produce a *permanent* change in the cells they come in contact with, but do not themselves cause cancer. This contact may result in a gene mutation. Other agents act as 'promoters' producing *transient* changes and only causing cancer when they are repeatedly in contact with cells which have been 'initiated' by another compound (2). Promoters work over a long period of time and do not appear to be mutagenic themselves, while initiators may only require a brief exposure. The distinction is, however, not clear-cut since some initiators can themselves cause cancer. Mutagenic agents tend to act as initiators; and other factors, such as hormones or dietary constituents (e.g. cholesterol), as promoters. From a clinical point of view, cancers are more likely to arise as a result of long-continued exposure to an agent and removal of the agent may result in stabilization or even diminution of the increased risk. Cessation of cigarette smoking is an example of how the risk of developing cancer can be reduced by removal of the stimulus.

Repair of damage to DNA

Cells are able to repair damage to DNA. The process of repair is through two general mechanisms. In the first the abnormal piece of DNA is excised enzymatically firstly by endonucleases which cleave the DNA strand, then by exonucleases which remove the abnormal segment, followed by the action of a polymerase which resynthesizes the missing segment which is then joined to the strand by a ligase. This repair process, or 'unscheduled' DNA synthesis, is an essential mechanism for all living cells. The second process is called 'post-replication repair'. After the cell has undergone division, if any unrepaired lesions remain on the DNA, the DNA is replicated up to the point of damage and this damaged segment is then resynthesized using the other strand as a template.

These repair mechanisms are under enzymatic control and the ability of the cells of an individual to repair DNA damage varies and may itself be under genetic control. Thus susceptibility to cancer may depend on the genetic control of enzymes which convert carcinogens to their active form and on other enzymes which are responsible for the repair process.

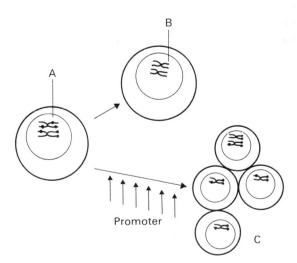

Fig. 3.1. *Initiators and promoters in carcinogenesis.* In A: chromosomal damage is caused by an initiator. This might be repaired, as in B, or, under the influence of a promoter, give rise to neoplastic growth, stage C.

VIRAL CAUSES OF CANCER

Since some animal cancers are known to be virally induced, the possibility that human cancers might also be caused by a virus has led to research to find candidate viruses and evidence of infection. Since attempts to induce cancer by viruses cannot be made in man the evidence is, of course, largely circumstantial.

Viruses causing tumours in animals were discovered at the turn of the century. In 1910, Peyton Rous showed that a cell-free filtrate made from avian sarcomas could induce new sarcomas in chickens, and at the same time the disease avian myeloblastosis was shown to be viral in origin. Much later it was realized that viruses might require a long latent period before the tumour appeared. However, it was not until the 1960s that it was appreciated that incorporation of viral DNA into the host genome was usually a prerequisite of malignant transformation, and that infectious virus might not be isolated from the cancer cell.

Two patterns of viral oncogenesis have been described. In both instances the viral genome is incorporated into the cellular DNA. In the first, the virus has a gene, *oncogene*, which quickly 'transforms' the cell in culture and causes tumours *in vivo*. The action of the oncogene dominates the cell. In the second, the virus acts slowly and tumours take longer to appear. These viruses do not transform cells in culture.

RNA viruses

RNA viruses are implicated in the production of a wide variety of tumours in animals notably lymphomas, leukaemias and sarcomas. In the virus there are two identical RNA molecules within a glycoprotein envelope together with the enzyme reverse transcriptase. Through the action of this enzyme the viruses are able to make the cell synthesize a sequence of DNA, complementary to their RNA, which is incorporated into host DNA. The action of the DNA leads to the manufacture of new viral proteins, envelope and reverse transcriptase.

They are therefore sometimes called *retroviruses*. They are of similar appearance on electron microscopy and are the smallest of the tumour viruses.

Some retroviruses, for example, avian leukosis, feline and murine leukaemia, have only three genes and have a long incubation period before producing the tumour in animals. Others rapidly transform cells and are usually isolated from tumours in culture. They produce tumours quickly after inoculation, an example being the Rous sarcoma virus (RSV). RSV has been shown to contain a gene (now called V-src) which appears to be the gene responsible for transformation of fibroblasts in culture. This gene appears to code for a protein-kinase which phosphorylates tyrosine, but it is not clear how this enzyme might be involved in malignant transformation.

Viral and cellular oncogenes

In the last few years it has become apparent that normal and malignant cells contain DNA sequences which are similar or identical to the oncogenic sequences of RNA tumour viruses (3). These are known as *cellular proto-oncogenes*, as distinct from viral oncogenes. It is postulated that it is these cellular oncogenes which, when activated by carcinogens, cause the events which lead to malignant transformation (Fig. 3.2). It has been suggested that retroviruses have incorporated these cellular genes into the viral genome during evolution. The genes involved in this form of oncogenesis are therefore of two types:—

1 *Viral oncogenes (derived from cellular oncogenes) which are inserted into cells and which lead to cancer.* Examples are Rous sarcoma virus (src), rat sarcoma virus (ras), avian erythroblastosis virus (erb A and erb B), simian sarcoma virus (sis). The products of gene activation are now receiving increasing attention. As mentioned above, a phosphokinase is produced by src and other viral oncogenes; epidermal growth factor receptor by the v-erb B gene; a platelet derived growth factor fragment by the

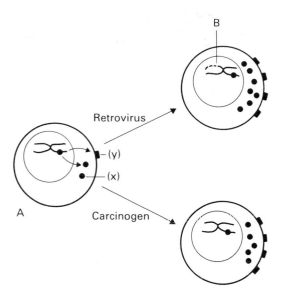

Fig. 3.2. *Oncogenes and malignant transformation.* In stage A, a normal cell has a low level of proto-oncogene activity producing a growth factor (x), or a differentiation protein or a receptor (y). Carcinogens increase the activity of the proto-oncogene and give rise to neoplastic transformation. Infection with a reterovirus leads to insertion of viral promoter sequences or oncogenes, stage B, and excess onco-gene activity, also resulting in neoplastic transformation.

v-sis gene and a variety of nuclear-binding proteins by avian leukaemia virus. The connection between these viral gene products and malignant transformation remains to be determined. Until recently it was felt that retroviruses did not have a definite role in human neoplasia but provided considerable information about the action of the cellular proto-oncogencs (see Fig. 3.3). A considerable impetus to research into retroviruses has been provided by the isolation of the Human T cell leukaemia-lymphoma virus (HTLV). The relationship of this virus to non-Hodgkin's lymphoma is discussed in Chapter 27. The first virus isolated (HTLV 1) appears to immortalize T cells and has been isolated from T cell leukaemias and lymphomas grown in culture. Several subtypes of HTLV 1 have now been isolated (4).

A new virus, HTLV 3, also with tropism for T cells, has been isolated from patients with acquired immune deficiency syndrome (AIDS). This virus appears to be cytopathic rather than immortalizing. It enters T cells bearing the T_4 molecule (helper T cells) and destroys them. Characteristically patients with AIDS have low levels of circulating helper T cells.

2 *Cellular oncogenes which are the cellular homologues of the viral oncogenes.* These genes have been identified by DNA transfer experiments, by their homology with known retro-viral genes and by gene rearrangements. The mechanism of activation of the cellular proto-oncogene has been the subject of much investigation. Possible mechanisms are shown in Fig. 3.3. This includes insertion of a promoter sequence causing an increased rate of transcription, insertion of an enhancer near the oncogene, and mutations or deletions in the oncogene itself.

Oncogene sequences from transformed cells (but not from normal cells), when inserted into susceptible cell lines, such as the 3T3 line, will cause transformation. Not all oncogene sequences will do this however, so the relationship between oncogene activity and transformation is not yet clear. The products of the cellular-oncogene (c-onc) appear to be the same as the equivalent viral-oncogene (v-onc). When

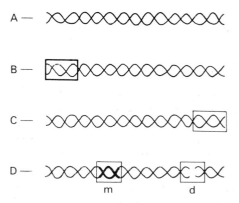

Fig. 3.3. *Possible mechanisms of cellular proto-oncogene activation.* A: proto-oncogene. B: insertion of a promoter sequence. C: insertion of an enhancer sequence. D: mutation (m) or deletion (d) of part of a gene.

these products are growth factors, or cell surface receptors for growth factors, they may be responsible for cell proliferation.

In Burkitt's lymphoma there is reciprocal translocation of part of chromosome 8 with chromosomes 2, 14 or 22. The 8:14 translocation is commonest. The c-myc oncogene is adjacent to the part of the chromosome 8 which is translocated, and the translocation is accompanied by reorganization of the c-myc gene. In chronic granulocytic leukaemia the c-abl oncogene is adjacent to the site of the chromosomal translocation (the Philadelphia chromosome: see p. 35).

Although it is by no means clear that activation of a single proto-oncogene can lead to malignancy, increased expression of cellular oncogenes has been found in many human cancer cell lines, for example, c-myc in small cell lung cancer and Burkitt's lymphoma, and N-myc in neuroblastoma.

DNA viruses

DNA viruses have also been implicated in the production of cancer. The largest in size is the Herpes group which can cause malignancies in animals. Epstein-Barr virus (EBV) was first demonstrated in cultured cells from a patient with Burkitt's lymphoma. Virally coded proteins are present on the surface of Burkitt's lymphoma cell lines in tissue culture, and EBV will cause proliferation of human B cells *in vitro*. Antibody titres to viral capsid antigen and membrane antigen are higher in patients than in controls. Nevertheless, many African children are infected with EBV at some time though Burkitt's lymphoma develops in very few so that its role in oncogenesis is not clear. In addition, some non-African cases of Burkitt's lymphoma are not associated with the virus. More recently EBV has been implicated in the pathogenesis of nasopharyngeal carcinoma.

Cytomegalovirus (CMV) is another DNA virus of the Herpes group which has been implicated in the pathogenesis of Kaposi's sarcoma. Chromosomes of cells from this rare hae-mangiosarcoma of the skin have been shown to contain viral DNA sequences. Recently, Kaposi's sarcoma has been described as a feature of a syndrome of chronic immunosuppression (AIDS) occurring in male homosexuals. In this disease the patients have a high incidence of infection with CMV.

The DNA virus herpes simplex (HSV) type 2 causes recurrent ulceration of the genital tract. Recent seroepidemiological data has linked HSV2 with cervical carcinoma, and viral antigens have been shown in the cytoplasm of carcinoma *in situ*. However, a direct causal connnection has not been established. Infection with HSV may be necessary, but not sufficient, to cause malignant transformation.

Other viruses

Of the other types of DNA virus which cause cancer in animals, adenoviruses have not been implicated in any human tumour. Human papilloma viruses are associated with *insitu* carcinoma of the cervix (see Chapter 17), and also cause benign papillomata.

Hepatitis B is associated with the development of hepatocellular carcinoma (see Chapter 15). It is not clear if the virus is a cause of malignant transformation; whether the viral infected cells are more susceptible to other carcinogens, for example, aflatoxin, or whether the association exists because the virus can cause cirrhosis which is associated with the development of hepatocellular cancer.

The case for RNA and DNA viruses having a causal role in oncogenesis in man has not yet been established but is tantalizing and immensely important. Populations can be immunized against viral infections. Furthermore, if viral coded proteins are on the surface of cancer cells this may render them susceptible to attack by the immune system. Similarly, tumour associated antigens might be the same in different individuals which would greatly facilitate an immunological approach to treatment.

Table 3.2. Constitutional (inherited) genetic factors in cancer.

Abnormality	Cancer	Abnormality	Cancer
Chromosomal abnormalities		*Immune deficiency disorders*	
Trisomy 21 (Down's syndrome)	Acute leukaemia	X-linked lymphoproliferative syndrome (XLR)	Lymphoma
47 XXY (Klinefelter's syndrome)	Breast cancer	Ataxia-telangiectasia (AR)	Lymphoma Gastric cancer
Mosaicism (45X0/46XY)	Gonadoblastoma	Sex-linked agammaglobulinaemia (Bruton) (XLR)	Lymphoma
11p– (aniridia-Wilms' syndrome)	Wilms' tumour	Wiscott-Aldrich syndrome (XLR)	Lymphoma
13q– (multiple malformations)	Retinoblastoma	IgA deficiency (S, AD, AR)	Adenocarcinomas
Inherited bowel disorders		*Miscellaneous syndromes*	
Polyposis coli (AD)	Carcinoma of colon	Hemihypertrophy (AR)	Wilms' tumour Hepatoblastoma
Gardner's syndrome (AD)	Carcinoma of colon	Beckwith's syndrome (gigantism, macroglossia, mental retardism, visceromegaly) (S)	Wilms' tumour Hepatoblastoma
Peutz-Jegher's syndrome (AD)	Duodenal cancer		
Tylosis palmaris (AD)	Oesophageal cancer	Multiple enchondromata (Ollier's syndrome) (S)	Chrondrosarcoma
Neurological-cutaneous disorders		Bloom's syndrome (telangiectases, short stature, chromosome fragility) (AR)	Leukaemias Numerous other cancers
Von Recklinghausen's neurofibromatosis (AD)	Sarcomata Glioma Acoustic neuroma Medullary thyroid cancer		
Retinal/cerebellar angiomatosis (AD) (Von-Hippel-Lindau syndrome)	Phaeochromocytoma Hypernephroma Ependymoma	Fanconi's anaemia (skeletal abnormalities, mental retardation, pigmented patches)	Acute leukaemia
Tuberous sclerosis (AD)	Gliomas		
Skin disorders (see Chapter 9, Table 9.2)			

AD = autosomal dominant	AR = autosomal recessive	XLR = X-linked recessive	S = sporadic

GENETIC FACTORS IN THE DEVELOPMENT OF CANCER

Inherited genetic factors

There are numerous inherited genetic abnormalities which predispose to the development of malignancy. The major syndromes are shown in Table 3.2. Refer to Table 24.1 for childhood cancers and Table 9.2 for skin cancers. It can be seen that a wide variety of genetic abnormalities predispose an individual to malignancy including chromosomal abnormalities, autosomal dominant and recessive disorders and X-linked syndromes. Most cancers probably arise from an oncogenic event in a single cell which forms a clone of cells (see p. 34) and it is by no means clear what is the relationship between the diverse inherited genetic abnormalities and the origin of malignancy. It has been suggested that in these inherited syndromes a 'two-hit' process is necessary. The first is an initial, germinal, mutation or abnormality, and the second an acquired, somatic, genetic event (5).

Acquired genetic abnormalities

Chemical carcinogens are often assumed to act by combining with DNA and cause mutations and viruses by altering the genetic structure of the cell. The simple view that genetic mutation leads to malignant transformation does not, however, explain the long latent period between exposure to an initiator (or virus) and the development of a cancer, or the need for promoters. In xeroderma pigmentosum, the mutation leads to a defective DNA repair mechanism in all the cells of the body, making them more susceptible to the mutagenic effects of UV light and chemicals. Although one might expect an excess of cancers of all types in these patients, the increase is in fact limited to UV induced skin cancers.

In many cancers large scale transposition of genetic material can be demonstrated in the mature tumours. In some tumours these are predictable, such as the translocation from chromosome 9 to 22 in chronic granulocytic leukaemia and the translocation affecting chromosome 14 in ataxia telangiectasia which is associated with lymphoblastic leukaemia. In cells from mature solid tumours, and acute leukaemia, karyotypic abnormalities are often observed. These observations have led some biologists (6, 7) to suggest that genetic transpositions might be important in carcinogenesis. The difficulty lies in knowing whether these genetic alterations are the result of malignant transformation, or its cause. At any rate, single point mutations in a chromosome do not appear to be the sole cause of cancer although they may make the cell susceptible to a subsequent oncogenic event.

Cancer in families

Certain families are clearly affected by specific cancers, such as familial phaeochromocytoma, hereditary retinoblastoma, aniridia-Wilms syndrome, etc. However, there appear to be some families in which there is an unusually high incidence of cancer but not of the same neoplasm. Although the cancers are the common cancers of adults they tend to occur at an earlier age than usual, and one person may have two or more different primary tumours in his life. More than 25% of the descendants are affected and the inheritance may approximate to an autosomal dominant characteristic. Two broad categories have been defined. In one there is a tendency for the cancers to be adenocarcinomas of various sites, and in the other a mixture of leukaemia, sarcoma, breast, and other cancers. The nature of any underlying abnormalities is ill-understood.

TUMOUR IMMUNOLOGY

The idea that human tumours might be recognized as foreign to the host has obvious attractions, since if an immune response to the tumour occurred as part of the disease, or could be provoked artificially, there would be opportunities for using such an immune response diagnostically or therapeutically (8). Early experiments in which tumours were transplanted from one animal to another often showed regression of the transplant. However, since these transplants were done in non-identical animals, all that was being recognized was transplantation immunity and graft rejection. Later it was shown that methylcholanthrene-induced tumours, when transplanted to identical mice, sometimes regressed and that 'regressor' mice had resistance to further tumour transplants. This was shown to be tumour specific, i.e. resistance was only to the original tumour and not to an unrelated one. The antigens responsible were called tumour specific transplantation antigens (TSTA). Similar regression has been seen in virus-induced sarcomas in mice and here the antigen being recognized is a virally coded product on the tumour surface.

In the early 1970s many laboratories reported that lymphocytes from human peripheral blood would kill, or inhibit the growth of, human tumour cells grown as cell lines and used as targets. At first it was felt that the killing was specific for the tumour type so that lymphocytes from patients with lung cancer would kill lung cancer targets but not, say, breast cancer. This killing and specificity was demonstrable even though the tumour target and lymphocytes were from different individuals, and was thought to be mediated by T lymphocytes. That tumour specific killing could be demonstrated on a foreign target, was, on the face of it, a surprising result. Furthermore, it led to the obvious question: if there is immunity why is the cancer still there? To answer this, the concept of 'blocking' of the immune response was invoked. 'Blocking factors' were present in serum and were said to be specific for the tumour type. Serum from lung cancer patients would only block killing of lung cancer targets. The nature of the blocking factors was never well understood. At first it was assumed to be antibody, borrowing the concept from enhancement of allo-transplants by antibody, but later antigen–antibody complexes were suggested to be responsible. However, in animal systems, such complexes were not consistently found and on the contrary, free antigen was sometimes present in the serum. However, with more rigorous analysis of the systems of target cell killing, and the recognition of natural killer cells and other types of effector cell, this approach was abandoned. When careful measurements are made there are no grounds for believing that tumour-specific killing of allogeneic (same species) targets is a property of blood lymphocytes from patients with cancer.

The demonstration of possible T cell reactivity to cancer had nevertheless led to attempts to try to treat cancer by intradermal inoculation of killed allogeneic tumour cells as an adjuvant to other treatments such as surgery or chemotherapy. The aim was to provoke an antitumour response by this means and to prevent recurrence. This approach was in general not shown to work except in poorly controlled trials. In addition, there were assumptions about the existence of tumour antigens on human cancers which are now known to be invalid. 'Active' immunization with allogeneic cells has now largely been discontinued as a mode of 'therapy'.

In the last few years there has been steadily increasing optimism that immunology might yet have a role to play in diagnosis and possibly treatment. This time the experiments underlying the optimism appear to be more soundly based. The recent advances which have led to the reawakening of interest have been mainly due to the development of new techniques in human immunology.

T cell cytotoxicity

T lymphocyte reactivity against human tumours is being reinvestigated now that it is possible to identify types of lymphocytes reliably, using antibodies, (usually monoclonal—see below), to lymphocyte surface antigens which relate to function. Thus sub-populations of T cells with cytotoxic, helper and suppressor function can be identified in blood, lymph nodes and the infiltrates in tumours. T cells can be separated from natural killer cells in cytotoxicity experiments. It has now become clear that, in many cytotoxic systems, T cell killing will only take place if there is genetic identity between the effector T cells and the targets. This leads to difficulty in demonstrating specific T cell anti-tumour cytotoxicity in man, because the effector and target cells need to be derived from either the same individual, or one identical with respect to histocompatibility antigens.

This problem may be surmounted by recently developed techniques whereby antigen-specific T cells can be grown and multiplied in culture using a growth factor (interleukin 2) which allows T cells with both specific and defined functions to be propagated for long periods of time *in vitro*. If T cells from blood, draining lymph nodes, or better still, from tumours, can be isolated, expanded in number and cloned, then a precise definition of their properties and target specificity should become possible. It is likely that much information will come from the many attempts to do this which are now being made in several laboratories.

Monoclonal antibodies

The older techniques whereby antisera to tumours were raised in animals and then extensively absorbed with normal tissues, led to results which were hard to repeat or interpret, because of confusing cross-reactivities since all the antibodies in the sera were polyclonal in origin. The recent development of somatic cell hybridization promises to allow a serological definition of the tumour cell's surface with an hitherto unattainable precision. Monoclonal antibodies can now be prepared by this technique (Fig. 3.4). The B-cell fusion partner is usually a murine myeloma, but human B-cell hybrids producing monoclonal human immunoglobin are being developed. Some of the potential uses of monoclonal antibodies are listed in Table 3.3.

So far monoclonal antibodies to human tumours have not been shown to define an anti-

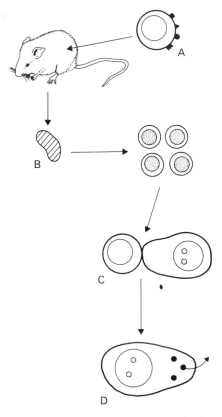

Fig. 3.4. *Making mouse monoclonal antibodies.* Stage A: a tumour cell, with many surface antigens is injected into a mouse. Stage B: later the mouse spleen is removed. Each of the disaggregated B-lymphocytes can make antibody against one antigen only. These B-cells are fused with an immortal mouse myeloma (stage C) and a clone of cells secreting antibody of defined specificity is produced (stage D).

Table 3.3. Potential uses of monoclonal antibodies in cancer.

Classification of tumours in tissue sections.
Identify 'undifferentiated' tumours in tissue sections.
Diagnosis and classification of leukaemias.
Diagnosis of metastatic tumour cells in low frequency e.g. in bone marrow.
Elimination of unwanted cells from bone marrow, e.g. metastatic tumour cells, residual leukaemic cells.
Tumour localization by isotopically labelled antibody.
Measurement of tumour products and 'markers', e.g. α-fetoprotein, CEA, peptide hormones.
Coupled with cytotoxic agents or isotopes to kill tumour cells.

---

gen exclusively associated with malignant proliferation. For example, a monoclonal reagent to common acute lymphoblastic leukaemia was later shown to react with a small number of normal marrow cells as well. Other antigens may be expressed as a result of rapid cell division and while they may be demonstrable in some cancers, using monoclonal reagents, they may also be present on some normal tissues such as bone marrow cells. The 'anti-cancer' monoclonals thus far produced appear to be identifying antigens which are expressed at a particular stage of differentiation of the cell type and it remains to be seen whether a truly cancer-associated antigen will be identified.

Even if this does not happen it is already clear that monoclonal reagents will be very useful in helping in the classification of cancer, in the diagnosis of undifferentiated tumours (Fig. 3.5), and possibly of therapeutic value in clearing sites such as the bone marrow of unwanted cells as part of the technique of antologous or allogeneic bone marrow (Table 3.4). Coupling radioisotopes to these antibodies may be of

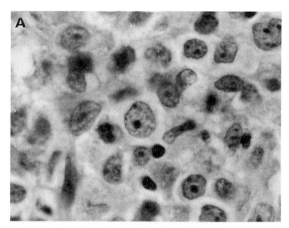

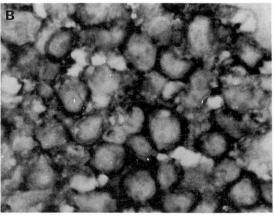

Fig. 3.5. *Use of monoclonal antibodies for immunocytochemical diagnosis.* (A) Undifferentiated nasopharyngeal tumour. Differential diagnosis would include anaplastic carcinoma, lymphoma and melanoma. (B) Same tumour as in A, stained for common leucocyte antigen using a monoclonal antibody. The tumour cells show dark membrane staining indicating that the tumour is a lymphoma.

Table 3.4. Possible approaches to immunotherapy of cancer.

Non-specific methods

Immune stimulants	Immune 'modulators'
BCG	Interferon
C Parvum	Transfer factor
Levamisole	

Anti-tumour antibody
To eliminate cells from unwanted sites *in vitro*, e.g. bone marrow.
To eliminate tumour cells *in vivo*, e.g. anti-idiotype antibody in B-cell malignancies such as CLL or non-Hodgkin's lymphoma.

Anti-tumour T lymphocytes
Actively generated *in vivo* by immunization with autologous tumour.
Generated *in vitro* from T cell lines, followed by passive reinfusion.

value in tumour localization, while coupling of a cytotoxic agent to the monoclonal may provide a means of specific immunotherapy if the antibody can be shown not to identify vital host cells such as gut or marrow stem cells.

Non-specific immunotherapy

Non-specific 'stimulation' of the immune response with bacteria has led to disappointing clinical results. The usual method has been the administration of BCG or *Corynebacterium parvum*, in patients in whom the primary tumour has been removed in an attempt to prevent recurrence, and in patients with acute leukaemia in remission. Using these methods delay of recurrence has been claimed in melanoma, breast cancer and colorectal cancer. Prolongation of duration of remission in acute lymphoblastic leukaemia has also been suggested. These findings have seldom been based on carefully controlled prospective comparisons but usually on the basis of historical control groups. Where randomized studies have been carried out the effect of BCG has not been confirmed. While there are differences relating to strain of BCG and method of administration the consensus of opinion is moving away from the belief that non-specific immunotherapy is worthwhile.

BCG scarifications are painful and unpleasant and fever, rigors and dissemination of the organisms may occur. *C. parvum* is associated with severe febrile reactions. BCG has also been introduced into the pleural space in an attempt to prevent local recurrence of operable lung cancer. Later studies have failed to confirm the early suggestions that this procedure had a beneficial effect.

Non-specific stimulation of the immune response with interferon or thymic hormones has been attempted in many forms of cancer. Interferon (IFN) is the term given to a group of proteins produced by cells in response to viral infection. Various interferons have now been produced commercially from cultured cell lines of fibroblasts and other cell types, from leucocytes, and by recombinant DNA techniques. Three main classes have been described: IFN derived from leucocytes; IFN from fibroblasts, and IFN or immune interferon derived from lymphoid cells stimulated with mutagens. The classical interferons are α and β which are induced by viral infection and are acid stable. Many functions have been ascribed to interferons apart from inducing resistance to viral infection, including alteration in cellular differentiation, modulation of expression of cell surface glycoproteins, inhibition of growth of tumour cell lines and increase in T cell cytotoxicity and natural killer cell activity. Some tumours such as Hodgkin's disease and chronic lymphatic leukaemia are associated with defective interferon production.

Attempts have been made to use interferons in cancer therapy. Regressions have been seen in non-Hodgkin's lymphoma and claims made for its use as an adjuvant to surgery in osteosarcoma. Alpha interferon may be the most effective agent in the treatment of metastatic hypernephroma. Most interferon preparations produce considerable toxicity, including fever, leucopenia and neurological effects.

THE DEVELOPMENT AND GROWTH OF CANCER

The three major characteristics of malignant neoplasms in man are first, that growth is not subject to the normal constraints of the parent tissue. Second, that cancers always show a degree of anaplasia, which is a loss of cellular differentiation. This is associated with a lack of some of the functions of the normal, differentiated parent tissue. Third, that cancers have the property of metastasis, that is the ability to spread from the site of origin to distant tissues.

While these features are present in most human malignant neoplasms, some of these properties are not absolutely distinct from normal tissues. Thus it is true that the normal regulatory mechanisms controlling growth are defective in cancer, but that is not to say that there is no check or constraint on the pattern of growth of human neoplasms (see below). Similarly, although we regard the most anaplastic of cancers as 'undifferentiated' in the sense that they seem to be more primitive precursors of the differentiated tissue from which they have arisen, many cancers nonetheless do perform some of the functions of parent tissues and our understanding of what we mean by differentiation is changing. Metastasis is however a property unique to cancer. Furthermore, it is metastasis which in most instances kills the patient and understanding the biology of metastasis is one of the central problems of cancer research.

In previous sections we have considered stimuli to the development of cancer either by viruses or chemical agents. This section is concerned with the events which follow the carcinogenic event and which lead to the development of an invasive, metastasising malignancy.

Monoclonality and heterogeneity in cancer

There is now a considerable body of evidence that most human neoplasms are monoclonal in origin. This means that the original oncogenic event affected a single cell, and that the tumour is the result of growth from that one cell. There are two major lines of evidence which have led to this conclusion. First, certain women are heterozygotes for two forms of the enzyme glucose 6-phosphate dehydrogenase (G6PD). These forms can be recognized by their different electrophoretic mobilities. The gene for the enzyme is carried on the X chromosome and, in female heterozygotes, either the maternal or paternal form is present on either one of the X chromosomes. In a female, each cell loses activity of one or other X chromosome and therefore, in a heterozygote for this enzyme, every cell in the body will either have one form of the enzyme or the other. In studies on haematological malignancies arising in heterozygotes for G6PD, the cancers are found either to contain the maternal form of the enzyme or the paternal form is present, implying that the original cancer arose from one cell which either had one form of the enzyme or the other (9).

In chronic granulocytic leukaemia the restriction of the enzyme expression is found in cells of the granulocyte series and, importantly, in red cells and platelets as well implying that a stem cell is affected by the malignant process. Interestingly if a remission is obtained with loss of the Ph[1] chromosome marker from the marrow cells, the marrow cells are still restricted to one form of the enzyme. This important result implies that the clonal expansion comes first and the Ph[1] chromosome is acquired at a later stage in the disease.

In Burkitt's lymphoma the lymphoid cells are also restricted in enzyme expression. If a remission is induced and the patient relapses quickly the same isoenzyme will be present indicating a failure to eradicate the disease. With later relapse the other form of the isoenzyme may be present alone, implying that the 'relapse' is really a new malignant clone.

The technique is much harder to apply to carcinomas and the results in solid tumours may prove to be different from those in haematological malignancies. It is still possible that some carcinomas arise from a 'field of change' in a tissue with many clones arising at the same time. More recent investigations have cast some doubt on the monoclonal origin of some carcinomas using data derived from studies with enzyme mosaicism and this issue is not finally settled.

The second line of evidence pointing towards the monoclonal origin of human neoplasms comes from lymphomas and other lymphoid malignancies in which it can be shown that the immunoglobulin produced by the lymphoid neoplasm (on its surface, or exported into the blood in the case of myeloma) is nearly always monoclonal, being of a single class and showing light chain restriction (see Chapter 27).

The problem with the notion of monoclonality is that it has led investigators to believe that there is a far greater uniformity of behaviour of cancer than is in fact the case. In spite of the monoclonal origin of neoplasms, significant heterogeneity appears to arise during the course of development of the tumours. This has important implications for treatment and for understanding the nature of metastases.

How does heterogeneity arise? If the tumour is *polyclonal* in origin then diversity can be explained on this basis. If *monoclonal*, other explanations are needed. It has been postulated that the occurrence of malignancy confers an inherent genetic instability on the clonogenic cells and that during the course of the growth of the tumour, phenotypic differences in clonogenic cells develop. Thus there is the development of mutants, some of which survive and undergo still further changes, whereas others, depending on their ability to survive hormonal, biochemical or immunological adversity, die. The mature tumour can therefore be envisaged as being composed of cells which are monoclonal in origin, but diverse in capacity to metastasise and to resist cytotoxic drugs and immune attack (10).

Diversities within the cells of a single tumour in both man and in animals have been described with regard to growth rate, cytoplasmic constituents, hormone receptor status, radiosensitivity and susceptibility to killing by cytotoxic agents. For example, in the case of small cell carcinoma of the bronchus, different levels of cytoplasmic calcitonin, histaminase and L-dopa decarboxylase have been found in the primary tumour compared with a metastasis. Primary and secondary tumours may also show karyotypic differences. Heterogeneity of neoplasms presents a formidable problem for the cancer therapist. If a single tumour shows diversity in cell phenotype and antigenic expression, it becomes hard to imagine how immunological attack can be successful. Likewise, a single tumour may contain cells with a wide variation in susceptibility to cytotoxic agents, thus providing the means for drug resistance to become clinically evident with repeated drug treatment. Evidence for the genetic instability of cancer cells has come from karyotype studies where chromosome deletions, breaks and translocations are frequently seen when cells from human tumours are examined.

The growth of cancer

Following mitosis, (see Chapter 6, Fig. 6.1) cells may rest in the early growth phase (G_1) for a long period of time, but then enter a phase of DNA synthesis (S phase) and subsequently a later, shorter, G_2 phase. This is a prelude to mitosis which then takes place over a period of 30–90 minutes. The two daughter cells then enter G_1. Some cells of both normal tissues and cancer are not in cycle, and the term G_0 has been used to describe these cells.

Normal tissues vary greatly in both the rate of cell division and the numbers of cells which are actively proliferating. Examples of rapidly proliferating cells are the intestinal mucosa, the bone marrow, the hair follicle cells, and normal tissue regenerating after injury, for example after surgical resection or infections.

An idealized representation of the way in which proliferation occurs in a normal tissue is shown in Fig. 3.6. This figure shows the stem or progenitor cell supplying a proliferating pool of cells which follow a particular differentiation pathway. These become mature cells which are held to be incapable of further division and subsequently die. While this model may apply to human cancers, it is possibly an oversimplification. Tumours probably do contain progenitor and mature cells but it is not clear whether cell renewal in a tumour comes from a small progenitor fraction. Nevertheless the model is useful in explaining many aspects of tumour

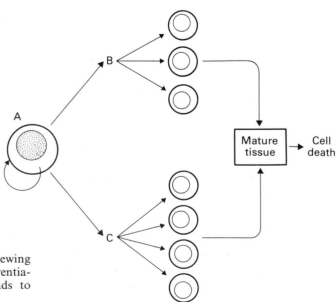

Fig. 3.6. *Normal tissue renewal.* The self renewing stem cell (A) produces cells committed to differentiation path B or C. Cellular proliferation leads to mature tissue and then to cell death.

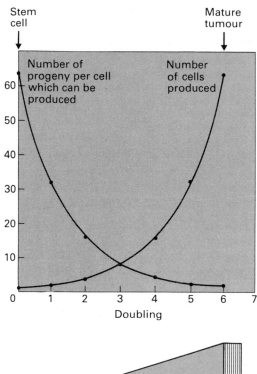

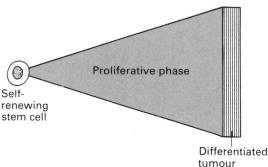

Fig. 3.7. *A model of tumour growth.* The progeny of the stem cells divide, increasing the tumour size but gradually losing their proliferative capacity.

growth (11). In Fig. 3.7 the stem cell is shown as self renewing. While the progeny of stem cell division go through successive divisions their number increases, but the number of further divisions they are 'programmed' to make declines concomitantly.

When cells are extracted from a tumour and placed in a nutrient agar the early cells (with many divisions still ahead) will form large colonies while the later cells will form small colonies or none at all.

When a tumour is treated with radiation or cytotoxic drugs it may shrink in size. This response may be entirely at the expense of later, non-self-renewing cells, in which case the tumour will regrow. To prevent regrowth it is probably essential to kill the progenitor or stem cells responsible for tumour growth. The growth fraction of a tumour—the proportion of cells in active proliferation—is often determined over a short time period. However, many cancer cells have prolonged cycle times and calculations of the growth fraction may seriously underestimate the proliferative capacity of the tumour as a whole. These slow growing cells are probably less susceptible to chemotherapy, particularly using cycle active agents. It is possible that the cell cycle time in these cells may shorten as a result of cytoreductive treatment, e.g. surgery.

A normal tissue grows and develops to a point when cell proliferation is balanced by cell loss and the tissue remains static in size, unless subjected to a changing environment, for example the normal breast ductular tissue during the menstrual cycle or during pregnancy. In a cancer, on the other hand, the regulatory mechanisms appear to be defective and the tumour gradually increases in size. Nevertheless, it must be emphasized that this does not necessarily mean a rapid growth. Figure 3.8 shows the volume doubling time of an almost spherical squamous carcinoma from one of our patients observed, untreated, over 4 years. Slow exponential growth can be seen with a volume doubling time of one year. During their growth, tumours undergo cell loss as well as cell renewal. This cell loss is partly due to the vascularization of tumours being somewhat defective. It appears that there is inadequate nutrition in the centre of tissues when they are more than 150 μ from a nutrient capillary. Sometimes the centres of human cancers are grossly necrotic where the tumour has clearly outstripped its blood supply. Other possible causes of cell loss are unsuccessful mitosis (possibly due to chromosomal aberrations), and death of tumours by immune or inflammatory

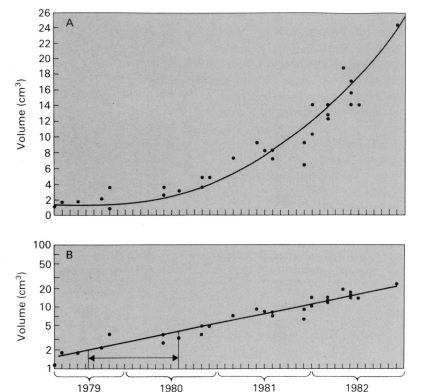

Fig. 3.8. *Growth of a squamous carcinoma.* Patient X had a peripheral squamous carcinoma untreated because of dementia and hypertension. Over 4 years this almost spherical tumour increased slowly in size exhibiting exponential growth with a doubling time of just over 1 year.

attack as a result of both specific immunity and non-specific processes excited by the tumour.

Doubling times of human tumours are enormously variable and Table 6.1 shows some of the measured volume doubling times in common human cancers. It is not clear whether tumours exhibit a consistent rate of growth from the origin of the cancer to the time when the patient has a massive tumour and is about to die. Certainly one can observe exponential growth (Fig. 3.8) in some human malignancies. In the case shown, if one were to extrapolate back to the origin of the tumour, it would prove to have arisen some 30 doublings (30 years) before the clinical presentation if the growth had been exponential at the same rate throughout this time. We have no way of knowing whether spontaneously arising tumours grow faster when they are small and then slow down. For *visible* tumours, there is some evidence that a progressive slowing of the rate of growth may

occur in some cases—a type of growth pattern known as Gompertzian (Fig. 3.9). At any rate, it is obvious that a clinical cancer is late in its natural history by the time it presents, and this of course has profound implications for the possible success or failure of screening programmes to detect cancer early. Similarly, in a tumour with a volume doubling time of 70 days a treatment which caused a reduction of 5 doublings would delay its reappearance for over a year if the growth rate was unchanged. This might lead to erroneous claims for the treatment if the follow-up time was short. This is shown diagrammatically in Fig. 3.10. These examples are obvious over-simplifications but serve to make the point that in the treatment of clinically apparent tumours, we are in fact dealing with the disease late in its natural history. The processes regulating tumour cell growth and death are complex and ill-understood. What we view as a clinical response to

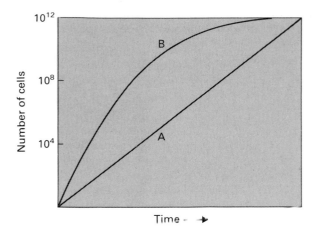

Fig. 3.9. *Two models of kinetics of tumour growth.* In curve A the growth is exponential. In curve B there is progressive slowing of growth rate with increasing size, termed Gompertzian growth.

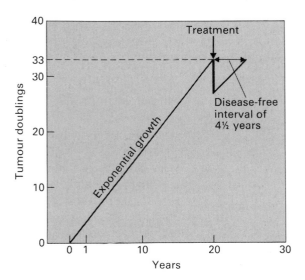

Fig. 3.10. *The lifespan of a tumour.* The tumour is clinically apparent after 33 doublings. Treatment reduces the tumour mass but the disease is again clinically detectable after $4\frac{1}{2}$ years.

treatment is clearly no more than a crude assessment of events within the tumour.

Differentiation in normal tissues and cancer

In a normal tissue the progeny of stem cells develop into the mature cells (Fig. 3.6). During this process the cells acquire specialized structures and functions and this process is known as differentiation. The phase of cellular proliferation may be some way along the maturation sequence from the stem cell which itself may be dividing only infrequently. During this process of differentiation, the cell acquires specialized biochemical properties, for example hormone responsiveness in the case of breast ductular epithelium, phagocytosis in the case of mononuclear phagocytes or synthesis of immunoglobulin in the case of plasma cells.

Although cancer cells differ from their normal tissue counterparts in many respects, these differences are often one of degree. When a pathologist talks of an *undifferentiated* tumour, he means one which does not look morphologically like the normal tissue. Some of the histological features will be present but the arrangement of cells appears chaotic and disorganized with variation in nuclear size and shape. An anaplastic carcinoma is one in which all the characteristic morphological appearances have disappeared to the extent that the primary tissue of origin cannot be determined.

The term 'undifferentiated' often carries the implication that the neoplasm has somehow reverted to a more primitive state. It is, however, possible that the oncogenic event has occurred early in the cell's differentiation pathway (e.g. in the stem cell) and that the neoplastic proliferation is occurring in a phase of cell development at which the cell has not yet acquired the mature functional characteristics of the final tissue. The neoplastic counterpart might therefore be morphologically and functionally similar to the stage of cellular differentiation at the point where the malignant proliferation occurred.

In recent years it has been recognized that, associated with the structural and functional alterations are changes in the surface properties of cells, with the acquisition of glycoproteins which serve as markers for various stages in the cell's differentiation pathway. An example is the antigen first identified on the surface of common acute lymphoblastic leukaemia, but subsequently recognized as also being present on early progenitor cells which are present in the bone marrow of normal individuals and therefore not a leukaemia-specific marker at all. A variety of other markers has been found, some of which are differentiation-linked, and others which are expressed on the cell surface in increased amounts when the cell is undergoing division but are not detectable in the resting phase.

Invasion and metastasis

The malignant cell is able to escape from normal control of growth. When normal tissues proliferate, they do so to the point where cell-to-cell contact appears to be able to exert an inhibiting role on further mitosis. In contrast, transformed cells continue to grow after they have become confluent, that is to say there is a loss of contact inhibition of cell division.

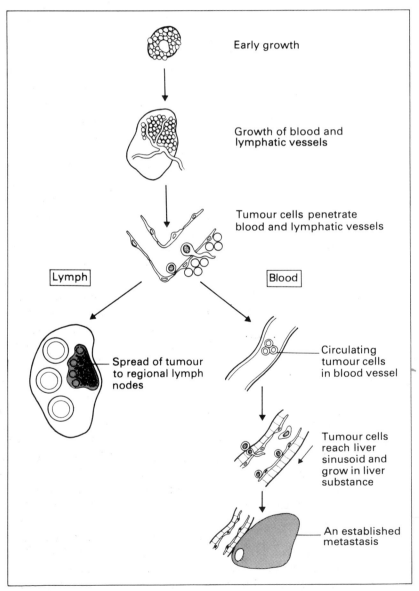

Fig. 3.11. *Tissue invasion and the development of metastasis.*

Tumours will grow and increase in size when planted subcutaneously in immune suppressed mice while normal tissues will not. The nature of the cell surface glycoproteins differs from normal cells with an increase in sialic acid content, and alterations in the surface charge. The locomotor apparatus of cells (microfilaments and microtubules) become disorganized and the cells alter their shape and show membrane movement at sites of contact with normal cells.

As the tumour grows, capillaries proliferate into it, possibly under the influence of tumour angiogenesis factors which stimulate blood capillary formation. At the same time the cells become locally invasive, though the biochemical basis of this property is ill understood. Alteration in surface charge may be one factor and there is also evidence from tissue culture that some tumour cells have decreased adhesiveness and attachment to normal cells. Secretion of enzymes by tumour cells may also play a part. There is evidence for production of trypsin-like enzymes as well as hyaluronidase and collagenases. It is however, unclear to what extent the production of enzymes is responsible for the property of invasiveness and destruction of normal tissues. Certain tissues are characteristically resistant to invasion, for example compact bone, large blood vessels and cartilage.

One of the results of local invasion is that tumour cells can enter vascular and other channels of the body and metastasise. The sequence of events is shown in Fig. 3.11. Lymphatic spread, which is particularly common with carcinomas, follows invasion of lymphatic channels and the tumour cells grow in cords and clumps in the lymphatic vessels and lymph nodes. From there spread to distal lymph nodes readily occurs. Haematogenous spread occurs after tumour cells have entered the vessels near the primary tumour or have been shed into the blood from the thoracic duct. Tumour cells are then trapped in the next capillary network, that is, in the lung or liver. Certain tumours characteristically spread to some structures while others do not; for example, sarcomas typically metastasise to lungs, and breast cancer to the axial skeleton. Local anatomy is often important, for example, gastro-intestinal cancers typically spread via the portal venous system to the liver. Tumours may also metastasise via a tissue space, for example those arising in the peritoneal cavity may seed widely over the peritoneal space, and lung cancer may spread over the pleura.

Regional lymph nodes may form a barrier to further metastases from the primary site. It is not clear if lymph nodes create a barrier to spread of tumour by virtue of specific immune mechanisms or not.

Having penetrated the vascular compartment, tumour cells must withstand the process of arrest in the capillary bed of an organ and then start to divide. At this site the tumour cell must leave the capillary bed of the new tissue. To do this the tumour cell must pass through the capillary endothelium and survive attack by host defence mechanisms such as phagocytic cells and so-called *natural killer* (NK) cells.

The capacity for invasion and colonization of distant tissues varies with different classes of tumour. Likewise, a given tumour type has a different tendency to metastasise in different individuals. More disconcertingly, there may be heterogeneity in the metastatic potential of its constituent cells, even within a single tumour in an individual. In experiments using the B16 melanoma, it has been shown that cloned sublines from a single tumour differ markedly in their ability to metastasise. This suggests that the parent tumour is heterogeneous in this respect. The basis of this variability is not known but it is possible that it may reflect differences in the surface properties of the neoplastic cells.

It is apparent that the problems of tissue invasion, metastatic spread and tumour heterogeneity are amongst the most fundamental in cancer research and clinical management of cancer patients. The lack of homogeneity of tumours, the similarities between tumours and their parent tissue and the lack of a single identifiable lesion in cancer cells which distinguishes them from normal, means that many of our simple assumptions about tumour immunity and the mode of action of cytotoxic drugs must be looked at critically, particularly if they are derived from experiments using homogeneous tumours.

REFERENCES

1 Miller E. C. & Miller J. A. (1981) Mechanisms of chemical carcinogenesis. *Cancer* **47,** 1055.
2 Farber E. (1981) Chemical carcinogenesis. *New England Journal Medicine* **305,** 1379.
3 Bishop J. M. (1982) Oncogenes. *Scientific American* **246,** 68.
4 Gallo R. C. & Wong-Staal F. (1984) Current thoughts on the viral aetiology of certain human cancers. *Cancer Research* **44,** 2743.
5 Knudson A. G., Strong L. C. & Anderson D. E. (1973) Heredity and cancer in man. *Progress in Medical Genetics* **9,** 113.
6 Klein G. (1981) The role of gene dosage and genetic transpositions in carcinogenesis. *Nature* **294,** 313.
7 Cairns J. (1981) The origin of human cancers. *Nature* **289,** 353.
8 Beverley P. C. L. (1983) Malignant disease. In Holborow E. J. & Reeves W. G. (eds) *Immunology in Medicine*. Academic Press, London.
9 Fialkow P. J. (1976) Clonal origin of human tumours. *Biochimica et Biophysica Acta* (Reviews on Cancer) **3,** 283.
10 Nowell P. C. (1976) The clonal evolution of tumour cell populations. *Science* **194,** 23.
11 Buick R. N. & Pollack M. N. (1984) Perspectives of Clonogenic Tumour cells, stem cells and oncogenes. *Cancer Research* **44,** 4909.

Chapter 4
Staging of Tumours

Although the overall prognosis of a tumour type can be summarized by stating the proportion of patients alive at 5 or 10 years, it is of course true that such figures usually conceal a wide variation in survival, ranging from cures to deaths within a few months of diagnosis. The search for indicators of prognosis has occupied the attention of oncologists for many years. The object is to identify those patients for whom a treatment strategy (e.g. surgery alone) is likely to be successful and those in whom it will fail and for whom another approach must be adopted.

Staging the extent of the disease at presentation is one aspect of the identification of factors which will influence prognosis in an individual patient. The purposes of careful staging of the extent of the tumours are:

1 To give appropriately planned treatment to the individual patient.

2 To be able to give the best estimate of prognosis.

3 To compare similar cases in assessing and designing trials of treatment (see Chapter 2).

STAGING NOTATION

For many tumours a useful staging notation is the TNM system developed by the 'American Joint Committee on Cancer Staging and End Result Reporting' (1). This system has the virtue of simplicity drawing attention as it does to the prognostic relevance of the size or local invasiveness of the primary tumour (T), lymph node spread (N) and the presence of distant metastases (M). Such a system has obvious drawbacks for some tumours such as diffuse lymphomas where the disease is often generalized, and it is clearly inappropriate for leukaemias. Even in some solid tumours, such as small cell carcinoma of the bronchus and ovarian cancer, the practicality and usefulness of the system is limited. In these diseases different approaches must be used for staging, which are described in the appropriate chapters. However, in the majority of solid tumours including cancers of the breast, head and neck, non-small cell lung cancer and genitourinary system, the TNM system has found wide acceptance.

The primary tumours (T)

In some cancers the *size* of the primary tumour relates to prognosis. This is well illustrated by some cancers of the head and neck, such as larynx and tongue (see Chapter 10). In other tumours the T stage relates not to size but to *depth of invasion*, for example in melanoma, colon and bladder cancer (Fig. 4.1). In squamous lung cancer the *size and site* of the primary tumour are both factors of prognostic importance (see p. 205). In some diseases the mode of spread is such as to make T status largely irrelevant. Examples are ovarian cancer, soft tissue sarcoma and small cell carcinoma of the lung. In such tumours 'stages' of spread are used which are often composites of tumour size and local invasion.

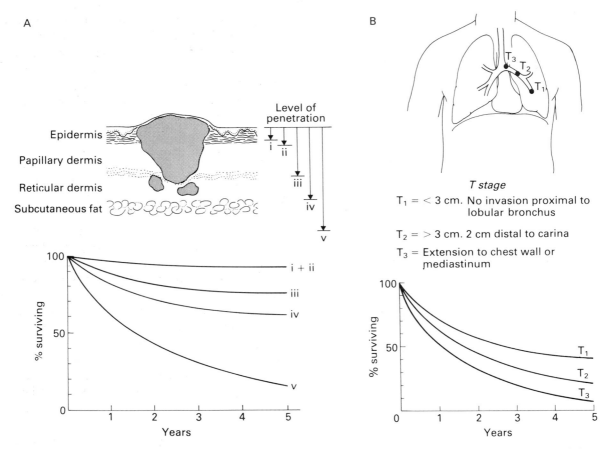

Fig. 4.1. *Prognosis related to local extent of primary tumour.* (A) Melanoma. (B) Squamous carcinoma of the lung.

Lymph node involvement (N)

Nodal involvement has important prognostic influence in many solid tumours (Fig. 4.2). In bladder cancer, for example, it is probably the most important determinant of survival (see p. 331). In most types of cancer fixed (N3) lymph nodes, which are surgically inaccessible, carry a far worse prognosis than mobile ipsilateral (N1) nodes.

Presence of Metastases (M)

This clearly defines a group of patients who are surgically incurable. Metastases may have been detected by clinical examination alone, or have been found by meticulous investigation using specialized techniques.

STAGING TECHNIQUES

Many techniques are available for determining the extent of spread of a tumour at the time when a patient first presents. Much information can be obtained by investigations such as chest X-ray, full blood count and liver enzyme tests. Many of these investigations are performed routinely in a patient who has been diagnosed as having cancer or where the diagnosis is suspected.

A chest X-ray may show metastases in the lungs or the bones or extension of a bronchogenic carcinoma into the pleura or overlying ribs. Hilar or paratracheal lymph enlargement may also be present. These findings indicate that the tumour has spread beyond its site of

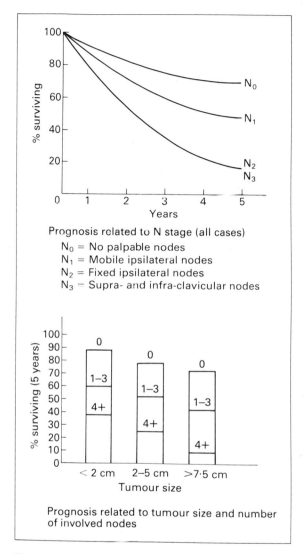

Prognosis related to N stage (all cases)

N₀ = No palpable nodes
N₁ = Mobile ipsilateral nodes
N₂ = Fixed ipsilateral nodes
N₃ = Supra- and infra-clavicular nodes

Prognosis related to tumour size and number of involved nodes

Fig. 4.2. *Breast cancer.* Prognosis related to N Stage and to number of involved nodes and tumour size.

cursors present in the blood. This finding is typical of widespread bone marrow infiltration with cancer and is most frequently caused by adenocarcinomas, particularly adenocarcinoma of the breast. Further haematological investigation may include bone marrow examination if infiltration is suspected. In some tumours, for example small cell carcinoma of the bronchus, a marrow examination is often part of the staging investigation if there is no other evidence of spread and if a localized treatment is contemplated, since the chance of occult marrow involvement being detected by aspiration and trephine biopsy is of the order of 5%. In other diseases such as cancer of the ovary or colorectal cancer, marrow examination is seldom rewarding and the investigation is not routinely performed.

Measurement of the liver enzymes may confirm a clinical suspicion of liver metastases, but more precise methods are now available and are discussed later. A raised plasma calcium may indicate bone metastases but isotope scanning (see p. 51) is the most sensitive investigative technique.

In recent years diagnostic imaging has been revolutionized by technical advances and has led to a previously unattainable degree of precision in staging of the extent of the primary tumour and in assessing whether there has been metastatic spread. Many of these investigations are time-consuming and expensive, and should therefore be used judiciously in order to answer specific questions which are designed to alter management. It must also be remembered that some investigations, for example ultrasound examination, are very much dependent on the skill and enthusiasm of the radiologist and it is important to have a healthy degree of scepticism about equivocal or uncertain findings, especially if these are not in accordance with the clinical circumstances.

Ultrasound investigation

Diagnostic ultrasound has been greatly refined

origin, and will considerably alter the approach to management.

A full blood count may show anaemia of an iron deficient type, or a normochromic anaemia typical of the anaemia of chronic diseases, and commonly found in patients with advanced cancer. More specifically the blood count may show leuco-erythroblastic anaemia in which there are immature white cells and red cell prein the last 15 years. It was first introduced into clinical practice in the 1950s and relies on the differing echo patterns which tissues create when bombarded by sound from an ultrasonic transducer. The echoes are generated at interfaces of tissues whose density differs, then recorded, interpreted and presented as a two-dimensional display. The orientation of the slice or 'cut' is determined by the operator who places the probe in the position most appropriate for demonstrating the organ and abnormality suspected (Fig. 4.3). This flexibility allows images to be obtained in many planes. Ultrasound echoes cannot be obtained if the organ is shielded by an area of bone or gas since these reflect all the sound from the beam and no echoes can be obtained from beyond these structures. For this reason ultrasound has its main diagnostic use in the abdomen and soft tissues. A great advantage of ultrasound is that it is cheap, quick and non-invasive. It can therefore be used to monitor the responses to treatment with measurements being made between chemotherapy cycles. Other techniques, such as CT scanning, which are more accurate, are far too expensive to be used in this way and the dose of radiation is too high.

Ultrasound is a useful investigation for diagnosis of liver metastases (Fig. 4.3). The type of echo obtained varies depending on the kind of

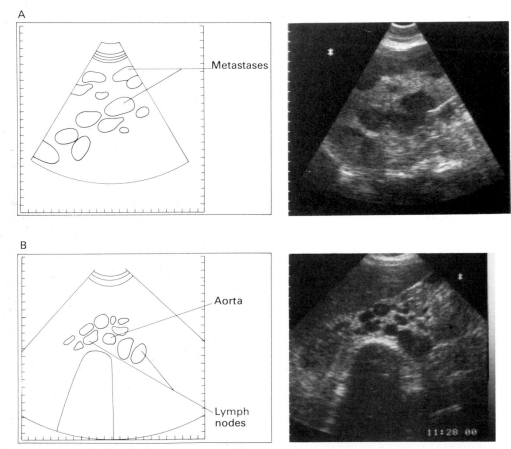

Fig. 4.3. *Diagnosis of hepatic metastases and lymph node enlargement by ultrasound.* (A) Hepatic metastases. Several large metastases are shown in this transverse scan of the liver. (B) Para-aortic lymph nodes. These are demonstrated lying in front of and behind the aorta. (We are grateful to Dr K. Walmsley, UCH, London, for providing these scans.)

metastases which are present. Thus echo-poor areas are often associated with lymphomas and sarcomas, while gastrointestinal metastases produce a more echo-dense appearance. In colorectal cancer the accuracy of ultrasound approaches that of CT scanning. Ultrasound is particularly useful in visualizing lesions in the pancreas, but it is usually only able to define a relatively large tumour. It is therefore of value in the investigation of patients with obstructive jaundice. The ability of ultrasound to define intra-abdominal metastases, for example in retroperitoneal nodes, is fairly limited. If it is important to know whether there is node involvement in the abdomen, CT scanning and lymphography are better techniques. In the kidney, ultrasound examination is frequently able to detect a renal carcinoma and distinguish this from cysts. The accuracy in this differential diagnosis is said to be of the order of 90% and the resolving power is approximately 2–3 cm. Ultrasound has been helpful in assessing the response to chemotherapy in ovarian cancer. Ultrasound of the thyroid is useful in making the distinction between solid and cystic lesions, and in the testis it can sometimes demonstrate an occult or doubtfully palpable tumour.

Computed tomography

Modern CT scanners are able to demonstrate normal anatomy, in detail which would have been thought impossible in the early 1970s. The accuracy of the technique has been greatly improved and its use in staging is gradually being defined. There are, however, limitations to the use and interpretation of CT scans, and it is important to be aware that they can give both false-positive and false-negative results. For example, in the abdomen, false-positive results are usually due to confusion with non-specified bowel loops and false-negatives due to the inability of CT to detect malignant infiltration of normal-sized nodes. Clarity of the CT scan image depends partly on the presence of the normal fat planes which surround anatomical structures. If these are lost, alteration of the

anatomy is less easily detected and the investigation loses reliability. The tomographic technique can demonstrate a tumour by showing distortion or enlargement of an organ, or a change in its density. In cancer the CT scan is of use in demonstrating both the extent of infiltration of the primary tumour ('T' staging) and to delineate metastatic spread to adjacent lymph nodes and to other structures such as liver or lung ('N' and 'M' staging).

CT scanning is of great importance in the definition of the spread of tumours within the chest. Several studies have shown that chest X-ray and conventional tomography greatly underestimate the extent of infiltration of lung cancer within the chest, particularly in the mediastinum (Fig. 4.4). Oesophageal cancer is also well demonstrated by CT scanning and the technique is of particular value in planning oesophageal resection. The CT scan has been of great help in demonstrating the full extent of infiltration of tumours arising in the head and neck particularly in the paranasal sinuses (Fig. 4.5). For retroperitoneal structures, CT scanning remains the most reliable pre-operative investigation and is particularly useful in

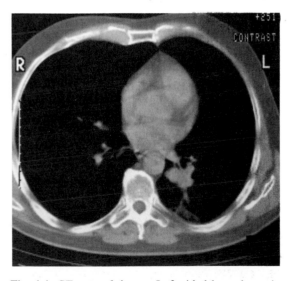

Fig. 4.4. *CT scan of thorax.* Left-sided bronchogenic carcinoma behind the heart. The tumour extends to the pleura. The chest X-ray was normal.

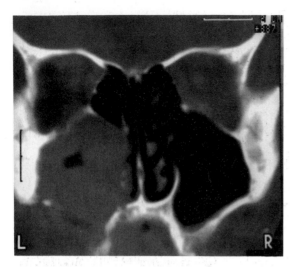

Fig. 4.5. *CT scan (coronal plane) through the nose and maxillary antrum.* A large tumour fills the left maxillary antrum, destroying its walls and extending medially into the nasal fossa.

demonstrating both lymph node enlargement and abnormalities of the adrenal and pancreas. Using fine flexible needles CT-guided aspiration may help in the distinction between a benign and malignant neoplasm (Fig. 4.6), or between an inflammatory mass and a carcinoma, for example in the pancreas. The extent of retroperi-

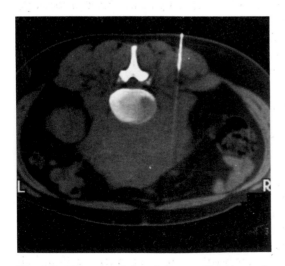

Fig. 4.6. *CT scan of the abdomen.* Showing a large para-aortic mass. The track of a CT scan-guided biopsy needle is shown.

toneal tumours such as sarcomas and lymphomas can be assessed with CT scanning, as can the size of malignant tumours of the kidney. In the pelvis, CT scanning frequently demonstrates the extent of advanced carcinomas of the cervix, bladder, prostate and rectum (Fig. 4.7). However, interpretation requires considerable expertise. CT scanning is also used to determine the degree of lymph node involvement. In the chest, the CT scan is more reliable than

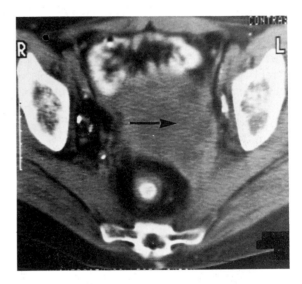

Fig. 4.7. *CT scan of the pelvis.* Shows a large central mass (arrowed) anterior to the rectum. This was an advanced carcinoma of the cervix.

chest X-ray or lung tomography in demonstrating mediastinal and hilar node involvement. In the abdomen, CT scanning delineates pelvic and abdominal lymph nodes. The nodes are less clearly outlined than in the chest and must usually be enlarged to more than twice their normal size before they can be confidently assessed as pathological. In the pelvis lymphography is a more sensitive technique, since it demonstrates the fine anatomical detail of the lymph node, while CT scanning merely shows enlargement. However, lymphography does not outline upper para-aortic nodes and CT scanning is therefore of more value at this site.

Although CT scanning has largely replaced lymphography as the primary imaging procedure in the lymphomas, the two techniques can give complementary information and lymphography is valuable when CT is equivocal, occasionally demonstrating involvement of normal sized nodes.

CT scanning is the most sensitive method available to assess pulmonary metastases (2). It has been widely employed for this purpose in osteogenic sarcoma, where occult pulmonary metastases may be demonstrated in patients whose chest X-ray is normal (Fig. 4.8). Because

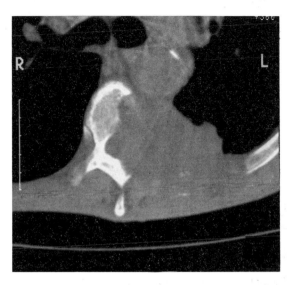

Fig. 4.9. *CT scan of thoracic vertebra at level of carina.* The vertebra and rib are largely destroyed by local extension of a bronchogenic carcinoma.

A CT scan is of little practical value in the search for an occult primary tumour presenting with distant metastases. Similarly, it has very limited value in detecting bone metastases— isotope scanning is much better for this purpose. Occasionally, CT scanning may be helpful in showing the extent of destruction in a bone lesion which is causing pain. This is particularly likely to be the case in vertebral deposits where infiltration of the soft tissues and surrounding structure is difficult to demonstrate on conventional X-rays (Fig. 4.9).

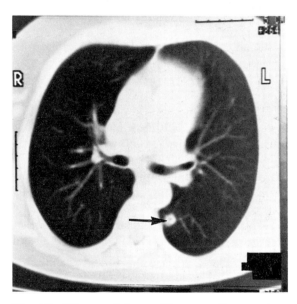

Fig. 4.8. *CT scan of thorax.* Shows a solitary metastasis (arrowed) behind the heart. In this patient with osteosarcoma, the chest X-ray was normal.

a transverse section of the chest is shown, the technique is particularly valuable in demonstrating metastases which lie in front and behind the heart or sub-pleurally, and which are not visible on plain X-ray. In the liver CT scanning is now more sensitive than ultrasound examination, but is very much more expensive. The technique is made more accurate by using intravenous contrast material. CT scanning remains the most sensitive method of demonstrating brain metastases.

Nuclear magnetic resonance (NMR)*

Nuclear magnetic resonance is likely to provide a further step forward in imaging particular areas of the body, especially the brain and spinal cord. In this technique the patient lies within an intense magnetic field which produces magnetization of atomic nuclei in the patient, in the direction of the field. Electromagnetic pulses are then applied to the patient to change the direction of this nuclear magnetization. Fol-

* Now often referred to as magnetic resonance imaging (MRI).

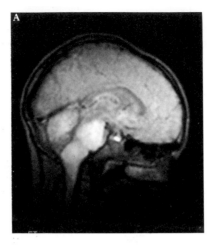
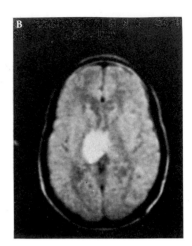

Fig. 4.10. (A) MRI scan (sagittal view) showing large brain-stem tumour. The CT scan was normal. (B) MRI scan of brain showing deep-seated thalamic tumour which was not clearly shown on the CT scan.

lowing the cessation of the pulse the nuclei return to their original orientation within the static field. This recovery time, which is measured by the scanner, depends on exchange of energy between protons and surrounding atoms and molecules. The original observation was that this recovery time might be different in tumours compared with normal tissues. In the last few years it has become apparent that this is indeed the case in human tumours, and the technique has proved particularly valuable in the brain where deep seated primary tumours can be readily visualized. The technique has been able to detect tumours in the brain stem, cerebellum and deep midline structure when CT

scanning has been inconclusive. Examples are shown in Fig. 4.10.

Lymphography

This technique is described in Chapter 25. Contrast material is injected into lymphatics in the dorsum of the feet, and nodes are opacified in the pelvic, iliac and para-aortic regions. Occasionally, lymphography of the arm and neck has been carried out, but such techniques are now rarely used, having been replaced by other less invasive investigations. One advantage of lymphography over CT scanning is that it may allow abnormal internal anatomy of the lymph

Fig. 4.11. (A) Lymphogram showing bilateral para-aortic lymphadenopathy, with the typical lace-like structure often seen in lymphoma. (B) Lymphogram (oblique view) and IVU showing obvious ureteric displacement by a large lymph node mass which is not itself opacified.

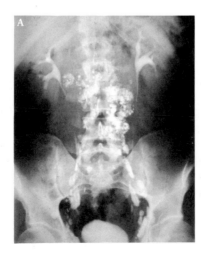
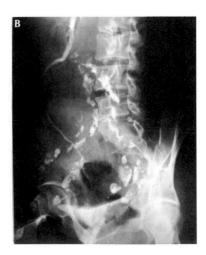

nodes to be shown at a time when overall enlargement has not taken place. There are two 'classical' patterns of abnormality. In lymphomas the nodes are often very large with a lace-like texture (Fig. 4.11A), whereas in carcinoma the appearances are usually those of a filling defect in a moderately enlarged node.

The disadvantages of lymphography are that it is invasive; that many nodes are not outlined in the abdomen (particularly mesenteric, high para-aortic, splenic and porta hepatic nodes); that false-positive filling defects or equivocal abnormalities occur, and that lymph nodes which are totally replaced by tumour sometimes do not opacify at all (Fig. 4.11 B). The technique has been particularly valuable in the pre-treatment assessment of Hodgkin's disease and other malignant lymphomas, in testicular tumours and in tumours of the cervix and bladder. In lymphomas the overall accuracy of the technique is of the region of 80% with a false-positive rate of approximately 15%. With other tumours the accuracy is less. It is sometimes stated that follow-up films of the abdomen will be useful in assessing the response to treatment and will allow a better assessment of whether minor abnormalities were due to tumour or not. The problem with this approach is that contrast material may disappear relatively quickly following lymphography and that the purpose of the technique is to stage the patient before treatment begins. Knowledge of the lymphographic changes during treatment seldom influences management.

Isotope scanning

Scanning with radioactive isotopes is a simple and widely available technique for assessing metastatic spread. In certain sites it has a rather poor accuracy, that is, a low percentage of correct results. This is due to both a poor *sensitivity* of detection (the percentage of positive tests in abnormal tissues) and poor *specificity* (percentage of negative tests in normal tissues). However, the dose of radiation is small, the technique is safe and reproducible and it is relatively inexpensive.

In the liver, scanning is performed with ^{99m}technetium-labelled sulphur colloid. This substance is taken up by the Kupffer and endothelial cells in the liver and spleen, and metastases appear as areas of diminished uptake. With modern techniques metastases of 1.5 cm can be detected, but this depends on whether the filling defect is near the surface of the liver, or deep in its interior. Most studies have shown that the isotope liver scan is less accurate than ultrasound or CT scanning, but comparisons of this type are somewhat difficult since details of techniques and experience of the operator are major determinants of accuracy.

In the brain there is no doubt that isotope scanning has been replaced by CT scanning as the most accurate method of showing metastases; however an isotope scan may be adequate and is much cheaper. In the absence of neurological symptoms or signs, isotope scanning of the brain is unlikely to be rewarding.

Skeletal metastases are best demonstrated by isotope scanning. Technetium-labelled phosphate compounds are usually used. The isotope is rapidly taken up into bone, rate of uptake being related to both blood flow through the bone and the amount of new bone formation. Metastases cause increase in blood flow and an increase in osteoblastic activity, usually sufficient to be demonstrable as areas of increased uptake of isotope (Fig. 4.12). An exception to this is in multiple myeloma where osteoblastic activity is minimal.

Because of the non-specific nature of the uptake, a variety of other conditions will cause increased uptake. Rib fractures, arthritis and vertebral collapse from osteoporosis may all give rise to increased uptake and be misinterpreted as due to metastases, in a patient with a malignancy. Single areas of increased uptake in an otherwise fit patient should therefore be interpreted with extreme caution. X-rays of the affected region should be taken and if necessary a CT scan should be obtained if the presence of a metastasis would materially alter the therapeutic decision. This is especially important if the single site is in the vertebral column, since

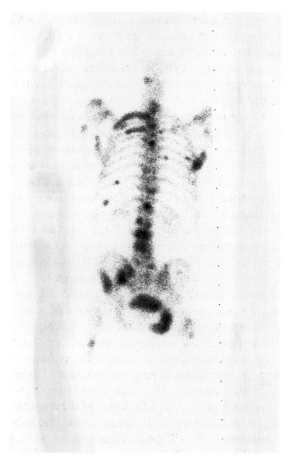

Fig. 4.12. *Isotope bone scan.* Shows multiple bone metastases. This patient had a carcinoma of the prostate.

degenerative disease is common at this site. In spite of these problems an area of increased uptake in a patient with cancer is likely to be due to a secondary deposit and should be carefully evaluated. Multiple areas of increased uptake are almost certainly due to disseminated tumour.

DIAGNOSIS OF METASTASES BY SITE

Pulmonary metastases

A chest X-ray is the most widely used method for screening. Lung tomography will increase the sensitivity of the test from about 35% to 50%. CT scanning will add to this figure, bringing the overall sensitivity up to 60–65%. Doubtful lesions such as sub-pleural deposits and isolated opacities can be examined by percutaneous needle aspiration.

Bone metastases

Bone scanning is the most accurate and rapid means of screening for bone metastases (3). Skeletal X-rays are used to demonstrate the degree of bone erosion at a site of metastasis if an alternative explanation for increased isotope uptake such as trauma or infection is possible. Percutaneous needle aspiration of bone can be undertaken safely at many sites and is helpful when the diagnosis is uncertain.

Hepatic metastases

Biochemical tests of liver function are the most widely used screening procedure. The most widely used imaging technique is scanning either with ultrasound or ^{99m}technetium-labelled sulphur colloid. The sensitivity is approximately 65%, the specificity rather higher at 75%, with an overall accuracy of 70%. Ultrasound scanning has a sensitivity of approximately 55%, a specificity of 85%, with an overall accuracy of 70%.

Brain metastases

CT scan is the investigation of choice. An isotope brain scan is of much lower sensitivity but is cheaper, and if positive may avoid the need for a CT scan. Isotope scans are rarely positive in patients without neurological symptoms or signs.

THE ROLE OF SURGERY IN DIAGNOSIS AND STAGING

Traditionally, surgery has been the most effective local treatment for patients with cancer.

The importance of surgery was based not only on the uniqueness of the cancer operation for controlling the primary tumour, but also on the general view that most cancers tended to recur at the original site making wide local excision essential. This concept is perhaps best illustrated by the evolution of operative techniques for breast cancer surgery. In the past 30 years there has been an increasing trend towards more conservative surgery (see Chapter 13), though some surgeons have, in recent years, preferred radical mastectomy. This has come about because radical mastectomy, with full axillary dissection, gives superior information on the state of the axilla and is being recommended in order to determine which patients might benefit from adjuvant chemotherapy—a situation which could not have been predicted 20 years ago when radical operations seemed to hold no future. Whether it is right to pursue such a radical approach, for the sake of obtaining staging information whose therapeutic value is perhaps questionable, is a point hotly debated by surgeons, radiotherapists and medical oncologists.

In the past, the surgical roles of diagnosis, staging and cure have been understandably confused. For example, a patient with a carcinoma of the large bowel might present with constipation, rectal bleeding and an abdominal mass; at laparotomy, the diagnosis would be confirmed and the appropriate operation carried out. This has led to the common practice of surgical removal of the primary tumour before consultation with a non-surgical specialist, which can certainly lead to difficulties where there are competing approaches for control of the primary tumour; breast cancer is again a good example. With the increasing precision of simpler diagnostic techniques, such as aspiration cytology, percutaneous needle biopsy and CT-guided fine needle biopsy; major surgical procedures are sometimes unnecessary simply to establish the diagnosis. In carcinoma of the pancreas for example, it has been difficult in the past to obtain histological confirmation without laparotomy. The increasing use of non-surgical techniques often leads to a pre-operative tissue diagnosis. This may allow new therapeutic approaches to be considered in the future, in which planned surgery might be undertaken following pre-operative radiotherapy or chemotherapy.

With the emphasis on tailoring of treatment to the extent of the disease, the cancer surgeon is now frequently called upon to perform staging operations which are not in themselves therapeutic but are intended to assist radiotherapists and medical oncologists in deciding their therapeutic strategy. Perhaps the best example is the use of laparotomy, splenectomy and lymph node sampling in patients with Hodgkin's disease (see Chapter 25). The contribution of the cancer surgeon is to define the extent of disease, enabling a rational decision to be made regarding the use of radiotherapy or chemotherapy as definitive treatment. Furthermore, a great deal of useful information has been obtained as a result of these operations, concerning patterns of spread of Hodgkin's disease and the likelihood of intra-abdominal disease as a function of the different histological subtypes. It seems likely that subsets of patients will be identified in whom the risk of abdominal disease is so low that laparotomy is not justified. In ovarian cancer, an important part of the initial procedure is the careful examination of the peritoneal cavity with particular attention to subdiaphragmatic spaces, which have been shown to harbour secondary deposits in patients otherwise thought to have only pelvic disease. In carcinoma of the colon, excision of the tumour should be accompanied by surgical staging since the presence of lymph nodes and hepatic metastases have considerable prognostic significance.

Surgical procedures are often performed for reassessment of patients who have undergone treatment, particularly with intensive drug and irradiation schedules. The aim is to determine if treatment can be discontinued if there is no evidence of disease, or changed if disease persists. In advanced ovarian cancer, laparoscopy has been widely employed as a means of confirming a complete response following treatment with chemotherapy or irradiation (see Chapter 17). Based on these findings, it may sometimes be appropriate to proceed to laparotomy and resection of residual tumour deposits.

THE EFFECTS OF STAGING ON TREATMENT AND PROGNOSIS

It is self-evident that the results of staging investigations will alter management. Radical operations are clearly inappropriate in patients with disseminated disease and attempts to cure these patients with local radiotherapy will also fail. What may be less apparent is that the introduction of staging investigations as a routine will appear to alter the results of treatment and invalidate historical comparisons.

If we consider a tumour diagnosed and treated in the 1950s when many staging investigations were not available we might find the results shown in Table 4.1. Many patients with stage I disease had occult stage 2 or 3 disease (i.e. they were 'understaged'). The 5-year survival is only 50%. Similarly patients with stage 2 disease have occult stage 3 disease and 5-year survival is poor (20%). Only patients with clinically obvious metastases are included in stage 3 with a dismal prognosis (2%). By introducing staging investigations but keeping the treatment the same, stage I patients have a

better prognosis (because investigation has placed many into stage 2 or stage 3) and the same is true for stage 2. Even stage 3 now has a better prognosis because patients with small, clinically inapparent metastases are now in this category and more of them (10%) survive 5-years (Table 4.1). However, the overall prognosis of the tumour has not changed. The 5-year survival was 28.5% in 1950 and 29% in 1980. All that has happened is that patients have been reassigned to different categories.

TUMOUR MARKERS

Some malignant tumours produce substances which can be detected in the blood and which may serve as a marker both of the presence of the tumour and sometimes of its size. Measurement of these tumour markers has become an important part of the management of testicular and ovarian germ cell tumours, choriocarcinoma and hepatoma. The ideal requirements for a tumour marker are as follows:

1 *The markers should always be produced by the tumour type.* This is not the case for the great majority of markers (Table 4.2). In teratoma, α-fetoprotein (AFP) and human chorionic gonadotrophin (HCG) are present in serum in 75% of cases and HCG is present in almost all choriocarcinomas. Apart from CEA (carcinoembryonic antigen) and acid phosphatase, most other markers are of little value in diagnosis or staging.

Table 4.1. Effects of staging on survival.

	(a) Tumour diagnosed in 1950s, but with only clinical staging; treated with surgery for stages 1 and 2.		(b) Same tumour diagnosed and carefully staged in 1980s; treated with surgery for stages 1 and 2 as in 1950s.	
	% of all cases	5-year survival %	% of all cases	5-year survival %
Stage 1: Local disease	40	50	10	80
Stage 2: Modes involved	40	20	40	40
Stage 3: Distant metastasis	20	2	50	10
Overall 5-year survival (%)		28.5		29

Table 4.2. Circulating tumour markers.

Marker	Tumour
Placental products	
Human chorionic gonadotrophin	Choriocarcinoma Teratoma
Placental alkaline phosphatase	Ovarian cancer, seminoma
Placental lactogen	Choriocarcinoma
Oncofoetal antigens	
Carcinoembryonic antigen	Gut cancer, breast, pancreas
α-fetoprotein	Germ cell tumours, Hepatoma
Pancreatic oncofetal antigen	Pancreatic carcinoma
*Tissue or organ antigens**	
Antigens of ovarian cancer	Cancer of ovary
Antigens of cervical cancer	Cancer of cervix
Lung tumour antigens	Lung cancer
Thyroglobulin	Thyroid cancer
Ectopic hormones	
Calcitonin	Medullary carcinoma of thyroid
ACTH	Small cell carcinoma of bronchus
ADH	Small cell carcinoma of bronchus
Isoenzymes	
Alkaline phosphatase	Osteosarcoma and variety of other cancers
Lactic dehydrogenase	Neuroblastoma
Prostatic acid phosphatase	Cancer of prostate

*The antigenic specificity of some of these markers is questionable.

2 *The marker should give an accurate and sensitive indication of tumour mass.* This is the case with the β subunit of human chorionic gonadotrophin and α-fetoprotein in germ cell tumours. In other tumours the marker is inconsistently produced or is too insensitive to be a useful guide to treatment although acid phosphatase is of value in monitoring progress in prostatic cancers and CEA in colorectal cancer.

3 *The marker should be produced by recurrent and metastatic disease.* One of the major uses of markers is to diagnose recurrence early. Occasionally in teratomas recurrent disease is associated with a rise in either HCG or AFP, even though the original tumour produced both. Marker negative recurrences (from a previously positive tumour) are rare. Similarly a rise in CEA or acid phosphatase may precede clinical evidence of recurrence in bowel or prostatic cancer respectively.

4 *The tumour should be amenable to therapy.* There is little value in detecting recurrence early if no treatment is available. For example, recurrence of colorectal or pancreatic cancer is seldom curable and early diagnosis of metastasis may serve only to alarm the patient. In teratoma on the other hand, a rise in AFP or HCG is a firm indication for full investigation since curative treatment is available.

5 *The marker should be specific for the disease and easy to measure.* Some markers, for example AFP and HCG (β subunit), are seldom present unless there is a tumour. However, AFP may be raised in pregnancy and with liver disease. CEA can be produced in inflammatory bowel disease as well as in colorectal and pancreatic cancer, and raised levels are found in smokers. The advent of sensitive radioimmunoassay techniques has led to the measurement of AFP and HCG as a routine in germ cell tumours and hepatoma. Other markers, for example ovarian cancer antigens, are being evaluated. Some peptide hormones, for example ADH, are extremely difficult to measure accurately.

Examples of tumour markers are given in Table 4.2. Some of these are in daily clinical use and justify more detailed consideration. *Human chorionic gonadotrophin (HCG).* The β subunit is measured to avoid cross reactivity with lutenizing hormone. HCG is measured by radioimmunoassay. It is used to detect and monitor therapy in choriocarcinoma and testicular and other germ cell tumours. The half-life is 24–36 hours, and it is measurable in both blood and urine (where it gives a positive pregnancy test).

Alpha fetoprotein (AFP). This protein is similar in size to albumin and is a major serum component before birth. It may cross the placenta and be detected in maternal blood. It is produced during liver regeneration and is elevated in viral hepatitis and cirrhosis. AFP is produced by malignant yolk-sac elements in germ cell tumours (see Chapter 19) and by the malignant hepatocytes in hepatomas. It is present in small amounts in some patients with pancreatic carcinoma and occasionally in gastric carcinoma. The plasma half-life is 5–7 days.

Carcinoembryonic antigen (CEA). CEA refers to a family of glycoproteins produced by many epithelial tumours, the molecule usually being demonstrable at the cell surface rather than at the cytoplasm. It is produced by normal colonic epithelium but is not usually present in the blood unless there is inflammation or neoplasia involving the epithelium. It is also found in plasma in pancreatitis, heavy smokers, ulcerative colitis and gastritis, thus limiting its usefulness in diagnosis. It is of little value in early diagnosis of bowel cancer and its value in early diagnosis of recurrent disease is limited by the lack of successful therapy in the majority of patients.

REFERENCES

1 American Joint Committee for Cancer Staging and End Result Reporting (1978) *Manual for Staging of Cancer*. American Cancer Society, Chicago.
2 Chang A. E., Schaner E. G., Conkle D. M. *et al* (1979) Evaluation of computed tomography in the detection of pulmonary metastases. *Cancer* **43**, 913.
3 Fisher B., Slack N., Katrych D. *et al.* (1975) Ten year follow-up results of patients with carcinoma of the breast in a cooperative trial evaluating surgical adjuvant chemotherapy. *Surgery, Gynecology and Obstetrics* **140**, 528.

FURTHER READING

Husband J.E. & Golding S.J. (1982) Computed tomography of the body: when should it be used? *British Medical Journal* **4**, 284.
Fraley E.E., Lange P.H. & Kennedy B.J. (1979) Germ cell testicular cancer in adults. *New England Journal of Medicine* **301**, 1370, 1420.
Peterman S.B., Steiner R.E., Bydder G.M., Thomas D.J., Tobias J.S. & Young I.R. (1985) Nuclear magnetic resonance imaging (NMR), (MRV), of brain stem tumours. *Neuroradiology* **27**, 202.

Chapter 5
Radiotherapy

Ever since the discovery of X-rays by Roentgen in 1895, attempts have been made not only to understand their physical nature but also to use them both in the biological sciences and in a variety of human illnesses. Within 20 years, the development of the X-ray tube led to a variety of clinical applications, first as a diagnostic tool and later as a means of therapy for patients with malignant disease. The discovery of radium by Marie and Pierre Curie in 1898 also led to a rapid growth of interest in the use of radioactive materials for the treatment of cancer, since surgery was the only treatment available at that time. Over the past 80 years our understanding of the physical characteristics, biological effects and clinical roles of ionizing radiation has greatly increased.

To understand the nature of radioactivity, it is important to grasp the concept of a natural spectrum of electromagnetic waves whose energy varies widely, in inverse proportion to the length of the wave itself. This spectrum (Fig. 5.1) includes X-rays (very high energy and very short wavelength), visible light rays (of intermediate wavelength and energy) and also the radio waves (of generally longer wavelength and lower energy) which are responsible for modern telecommunications and include the transmission signals for radio and television. Of these various types of electromagnetic waves, only X-rays and gamma rays (the terms are almost interchangeable) are of sufficiently high energy to produce the ionization of atoms, which will occur when a beam of radiation passes through tissue.

In the process of ionization, the essential event is the displacement of an electron from its orbital path around the nucleus of the atom. This creates an unstable or ionized atom, and a free electron which is normally 'captured' by a neighbouring atom, which then becomes equally unstable because of its possession of an extra negative electric charge. When radiation beams pass through living tissue, the intensity, duration and site of these ionization events can be controlled by varying the characteristics of the radiation source. This permits a deliberate and controlled cellular destruction in the case

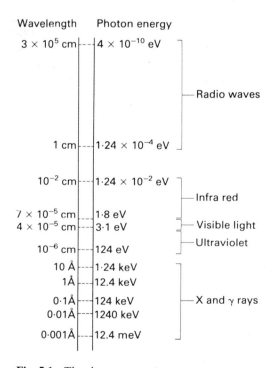

Fig. 5.1. *The electromagnetic spectrum.*

of therapeutic radiation (radiotherapy), or in the case of diagnostic radiation, trivial and short-lived alterations which usually have no permanent biological effect. The creation of the radiographic image is due to the differential alteration of the X-ray beam by biological tissues containing atoms of differing atomic weights.

SOURCES AND PRODUCTION OF IONIZING RADIATION

Radioactive isotopes

Radioactivity is an unalterable property of many naturally occurring atoms which exist in a relatively unstable state. Although the identity of any given atom is defined by the number of protons and electrons it possesses; the atoms of any one element may contain differing numbers of nuclear neutrons, so that their atomic weights (as determined by the proton and neutron component) differ. Such atoms or *isotopes* occur naturally in fixed proportions, and most pure substances (particularly metals such as iron, manganese or cobalt) consist of mixtures of these isotopes. Emission of radioactivity is one of the consequences of physical decay of unstable atoms resulting in a final and more stable state. The rate and intensity of these emissions varies with each element.

There is a wide variety of naturally occurring radioactive materials, whose chief characteristic is the emission of electromagnetic waves of a frequency which can produce ionization within

biological materials. Historically, these emissions have been divided into alpha, beta or gamma waves, depending on the wavelength or energy of the emission. At this point it is worth remembering that although many of the properties of radioactive emission are better understood in terms of their characteristic wave forms, the 'wave' also has features of a particle. Alpha and beta emission is best understood in terms of these features since alpha particles are positively charged helium nuclei, with a substantial mass, and beta particles are no more than electrons, with a negative charge but almost no mass. Gamma rays, on the other hand, are uncharged.

Although alpha, beta and gamma rays can all produce ionization in tissues it is the gamma rays which have the greatest application in radiation therapy. For example, in a reaction of great clinical importance, the unstable isotope of cobalt, with an atomic number of 60, disintegrates to a more stable isotope (atomic number 59) by discharging one of its nuclear neutrons, together with gamma rays. The characteristics of the emitted gamma radiation are constant for this particular reaction, and the rate of the nuclear disintegration is unalterable, such that after 5.33 years, exactly half of the original radioactive material still remains, thus defining the radioactive 'half-life' of cobalt-60. The half-life is an important concept in theoretical and clinical work, and varies between a fraction of a second, and hundreds or thousands of years (Table 5.1). Radium, widely

Table 5.1. Therapeutically useful isotopes.

Isotope	Type of Radiation	Energy (MeV)	Half-life
Cobalt-60	β,γ	1.17 (β) and 1.33 (γ)	5.3 years
Caesium-137	β,γ	0.51 (β) and 0.66 (γ)	30 years
Iodine-131	β,γ		8 days
Gold-198	β,γ	0.96 (β) and 0.41 (γ)	2.7 days
Phosphorus-32	β		14 days
Iridium-192	γ	0.36–0.6 (γ)	
Radium-226 (decays to radon, then Ra A,B,C)	α then β, γ	1.0 (γ)	1620 years for radium but 3–27 mins for Ra A,B,C

used before the introduction of more suitable radioactive materials, has a half-life of 1620 years, which meant that radioactive sources for therapeutic use never needed replacing. Beta particles, or electrons, however, are increasingly being used as their characteristics are more suitable in certain clinical situations. In addition, other atomic fragments are being studied since they have theoretical advantages as a result of their different biological effects. These include neutrons, protons and pi-mesons (see below).

Although the early radioactive substances discovered by the Curies and others were all naturally occurring, modern high energy physics has provided ready access to many new materials, or artificially manufactured isotopes. These substances, *radionuclides*, are generally manufactured in nuclear reactors by heavy particle bombardment of natural materials. The chief advantage is that their properties more closely resemble the theoretical ideal for radioactive half-life, gamma ray characteristics and intensity, than any natural substance. The changing demands of both diagnosis, for example, in radioisotope imaging, and therapy have led to ever increasing attempts at producing new radioactive isotopes with differing radiation characteristics. For therapeutic work, this will include the production of both sealed and unsealed sources. For sealed sources, the radioactive material will be physically enclosed by an impenetrable barrier or casing such as the platinum casing of a typical radium or caesium needle (Fig. 5.2), so that the radioactive material can be inserted into the tissue to be irradiated, and then removed at some predetermined time. With unsealed sources, such as iodine-131, the isotope is physically ingested either by mouth or by injection, passes via the bloodstream to the end organ and is taken up (in this case, by the thyroid) where the effects of the radioactivity are directly deposited and the isotope cannot be recovered.

Unsealed sources are widely used in diagnostic work such as the radioactive bone or brain scan. In therapeutic work, the most specific and ideal application is for carcinoma of the thyroid, where radioactive isotopes of iodine (usually ^{131}I) are given by mouth, and selectively taken up by the thyroid gland and thyroid cancer cells providing 'internal' irradiation to a high intensity without compromising other organs by the delivery of an unacceptable dose of radiation at an unwanted site. Use of injectable radioactive phosphorus (^{32}P) for bone marrow irradiation in polycythaemia rubra vera is another well-known example. Other less specific instances of the therapeutic use of unsealed sources, include the intraperitoneal or intrapleural use of radioactive gold colloids for malignant ascites or pleural effusions.

For use in clinical work, the choice of either naturally occurring or artificially produced radioactive isotopes will depend on the clinical requirement. For example, in interstitial implantation work where radioactive needles are directly placed adjacent to or even within the malignant tissue, caesium needles have increasingly been employed in preference to radium, because of the more suitable characteristics of the emitted radiation from this material. This is because the specific activity (number of radioactive disintegrations per second) is so high with radium that protection for doctors, radiographers and nurses has always been a major problem. With caesium, however, the specific

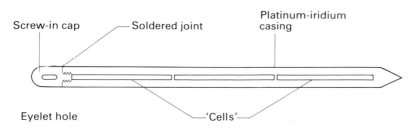

Fig. 5.2. *A radium neeedle.* (From Meredith W. J. & Massey J. B. (1972) *Fundamental Physics of Radiology.* Williams & Wilkins, Baltimore. With permission.)

activity is substantially lower, making protection easier.

Radioactive isotopes are also used as a source of external radiation (teletherapy). All clinical departments place a heavy clinical reliance on their external therapy techniques since the majority of tumours are deeply situated and inaccessible to irradiation by direct implantation (brachytherapy). Nowadays when gamma irradiation from a major radioactive source is employed, the most common choice of material is cobalt-60, a material which emits a high energy gamma ray (mean energy 1.2 MeV) of sufficient penetration to allow for treatment of deeply situated tumours. Cobalt-60 has a reasonably satisfactory half-life of 5.3 years so that major source replacement will not be required more than every 3–4 years.

A modern cobalt unit is in essence no more than a cylindrical source of ^{60}Co produced artificially within a nuclear fission pile, placed in a protective shell made of lead, and supplied with a simple mechanism for moving the source into the treatment position when required (Fig. 5.3). In this position, the radioactive cobalt source is still protected by a lead sphere, though a cone of the protective material has been removed and moveable jaws fitted allowing the beam of gamma rays to be altered in size to suit the clinical requirements. This extremely simple

piece of equipment is still the most widely used high energy apparatus in the world today, and has the advantage of reliability, simplicity, and longevity, as well as being relatively inexpensive both to purchase and to maintain. Its disadvantages are that there is a substantial 'penumbra' of scattered radiation, which forms a significant part of the edge of the beam and that treatment times can be lengthy. This is particularly the case when the source has started to age, since radioactive decay results in a loss of residual radioactive material and treatment time increases proportionately.

Artificial production of X-rays and particles

Shortly after the discovery of radium by the Curies, Roentgen constructed the first X-ray apparatus, consisting of a sealed glass vacuum tube containing an electrode at one end and a target at the other. Heating the electrode resulted in a discharge of electrons which travelled relatively easily through the vacuum, to bombard the target at the other end of the tube. This produced characteristic rays which, like those of radium, could create an image on a photographic plate. The nature of these rays was uncertain; *X-rays* therefore seemed the most suitable title. It gradually became clear that X-rays and gamma rays were fundament-

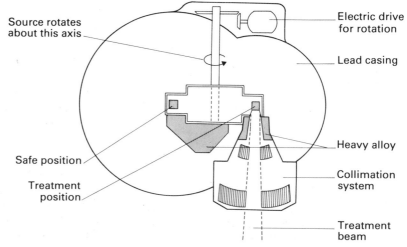

Fig. 5.3. *Schematic representation of a typical* ^{60}*Cobalt treatment unit.* The treatment unit is usually mounted on a counterbalanced gantry capable of rotation through 360° permitting treatment from underneath the patient where necessary. (From Meredith W. J. & Massey J. B. (1972) *Fundamental Physics of Radiology.* Williams and Wilkins, Baltimore. With permission.)

Source rotates about this axis

Electric drive for rotation

Lead casing

Safe position

Treatment position

Heavy alloy

Collimation system

Treatment beam

ally similar though their method of production is quite different. Unlike the gamma irradiation from radioactive materials whose characteristics cannot be changed other than by altering either the choice or the purity of the material, X-rays of quite different properties can be produced simply by varying the voltage input to the cathode of the X-ray tube.

For instance the X-rays used in diagnostic radiology are generated in a low voltage machine (e.g. 50 kV) have a longer wavelength and less penetrating power. In contrast, therapeutic X-rays are produced by equipment of higher voltage varying from 50 kV up to 30 MV, a 600 fold increase. As voltage is increased, X-rays of shorter wavelength are produced, which have greater penetrating power.

For therapeutic use, one of the chief criteria for successful treatment is the availability of X-rays of sufficient penetrating power, or depth dose, to deal effectively with deep-seated tumours. For this reason, most X-ray departments have a range of equipment with a wide-spectrum of clinically useful X-ray beams available to deal with both superficial tumours such as skin cancers and those more deeply situated, such as tumours of the media-stinum or pelvis. With conventional or *ortho-voltage* X-ray equipment, the maximum deposition of radiation energy is in the superficial tissues, with a steep fall-off (Fig. 5.4), such that the dosage received by a deep tumour which may be 10 cm or more below the skin surface is low, and limited by the skin reaction that this treatment will inevitably cause. The physical and electromagnetic problems of safely in applying a very high tension (voltage) input had to be overcome before further progress could be made.

Fortunately, most of these problems were solved in the 1960s with the advent of an entirely fresh approach to the generation of high energy megavoltage beams. Instead of the traditional X-ray tube, with its cumbersome, fragile construction and somewhat unpredictable emission, a new means of X-ray production was developed, which depended on the acceleration of electrons down a cylindrical 'wave guide', terminating in the deliberate bombardment of a fixed target by electrons travelling almost at the speed of light and resulting in a harder beam, of higher intensity (Fig. 5.5). As well as possessing much greater depth-dose, these beams typically have far less in the way of scattered radiation, leading to a much cleaner beam with narrower penumbra than with traditional cobalt apparatus. In addition, the beam output (or dose rate) is usually greater, leading to shorter treatment times. Unfortunately, the drawbacks of very high initial expenditure and maintenance costs, combined with slightly lower reliability than cobalt equipment, have yet to be fully overcome. Nevertheless, the linear accelerator has become the standard work-horse of most sophisticated radiotherapy departments. A further important advantage of this equipment is that the target can be moved out of position, yielding a beam of high velocity electrons (instead of X-rays) of up to 30 MV

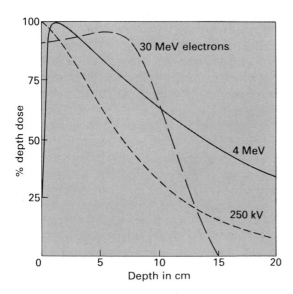

Fig. 5.4. *Typical depth-dose curves for radiotherapy equipment (kilovoltage, megavoltage and 30 MeV electron beam).* There is skin 'build-up' over the first centimetre for megavoltage therapy but not for kilovoltage or electron treatment. Depth dose for both megavoltage and electron beam therapy is much superior to kilovoltage treatment.

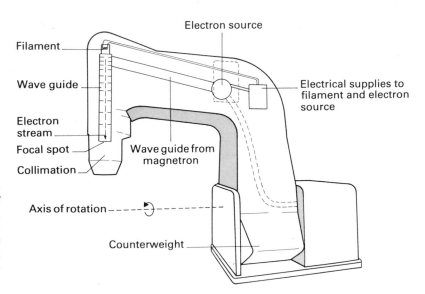

Fig. 5.5. *Schematic representation of an isocentrically mounted 4–8 MeV linear accelerator.* (From Meredith W. J. & Massey J. B. (1972) *Fundamental Physics of Radiology.* Williams and Wilkins, Baltimore. With permission.)

energy or more which can be useful therapeutically in certain clinical situations (see later).

To the clinician, the fundamental difference between X-ray and electron therapy lies in their entirely different depth-dose characteristics (Fig. 5.4). With X-ray or gamma ray therapy, the amount of radiation energy deposited at any given depth of tissue (the depth-dose) falls off exponentially which means that however powerful the source and whatever the distance, unwanted areas of tissue will be irradiated, both superficial to the tumour area, and also beyond it. The entrance and exit dose will irradiate a substantial volume of normal host tissue, and this unavoidable characteristic is usually the limiting factor in a course of treatment. With electron therapy this disadvantage is at least partly overcome, since the beam decays completely at a depth entirely dependent on the energy of the electron beam.

With low and medium voltage X-rays, the energy deposited in the tissues is critically dependent on the mean atomic number of the tissue in which this deposition is occurring. With high voltage X-rays, γ rays and electrons, the energy absorbed by the tissue is much less dependent on the atomic number, so that the drawbacks of very high bone absorption

(with its twin problems of dosage inhomogeneity and radionecrosis) is largely avoided. Radiotherapists are therefore very careful when irradiating superficial lesions situated over bone or cartilage, which require treatment with low voltage (superficial) beams. For this reason, electron therapy is often preferred in these cases, particularly for skin tumours which overlie an area of cartilage. A common example is a basal cell carcinoma on the nose, or pinna of the ear.

A further intriguing possibility under active clinical trial at present, is the use of heavy charged and uncharged particles, including neutrons, protons and pi-mesons. All of these beams have theoretical advantages, though the capital expenditure required for the development and building of neutron and charged particle generators is substantially greater than the cost of more conventional equipment. Only a few centres throughout the world have these resources available at present. With neutron beam therapy the major theoretical advantage is that tumour cells appear equally sensitive whatever their state of oxygenation, a critically important characteristic since local tumour recurrence after conventional radiotherapy is thought to be largely due to the relative ineffectiveness of X-ray treatment on hypoxic malignant cells (see later). If this is so, then treatment by neutron therapy could perhaps prove curative with localized but relatively radioinsensitive tumours such as glioma, sarcoma, salivary tumours and malignant melanomas. Preliminary work has been encouraging, but further large scale clinical trials will undoubtedly be necessary, with careful prospective comparisons between neutron therapy and conventional X-ray treatment, before firm conclusions can be drawn. Irradiation with protons or pi-mesons requires even more expensive equipment and is not available in Britain at present, though there are centres both in the United States and Europe which are currently carrying out clinical trials. The particular theoretical advantage with these beams is that the energy is deposited at a defined narrow level in tissue, which is determined by the energy of the beam. Very little of the beam energy is deposited in superficial tissues, and virtually none in tissue deep to the chosen volume. This phenomenon, known as the Bragg effect after its discoverer, naturally makes the concept of heavy charged particle irradiation particularly attractive to the radiotherapist, since it might perhaps be possible to irradiate a given tumour to a very high dosage without compromising host tissues. With increasingly sophisticated methods of tumour imaging and localization, the precision use of this kind of beam would seem to approach an ideal form of radiation therapy.

BIOLOGICAL PROPERTIES OF IONIZING RADIATION

Tumour sensitivity

Ever since the turn of the century, clinical scientists have been interested in understanding the extraordinary cellular events which occur when living tissue is exposed to a beam of ionizing radiation. It is now clear that radiation-induced damage to the cell may be lethal, resulting in death, or sublethal, in which case the cellular damage can be repaired. In general, the degree of radiosensitivity of any given tumour type will depend not only on the immediate damage sustained by the cell (a measure of its true 'intrinsic' sensitivity) but also on its ability to repair the sublethal damage that has been caused. Although a high degree of radiosensitivity is generally required if there is to be any hope of a radiation cure, other factors may prevent the realization of this aim; radiosensitivity is not in itself sufficient. Acute lymphoblastic leukaemia, for instance, is highly radiosensitive, since small malignant lymphoblasts are permanently damaged by a relatively low dose of radiation. However, the widespread nature of this disease, which by definition affects the whole of the bone marrow and therefore every organ supplied by the peripheral bloodstream, made it impossible until recently to deliver curative radiotherapy without fatal over-irradiation. The modern technique of allogeneic bone marrow transplantation has resulted in safe delivery of total body irradiation to a sufficiently high dosage for total irreversible ablation of the malignant marrow elements. It is not the bone marrow transplant itself which is the therapeutic event, but the lethal radiation damage inflicted on the leukaemic cell population.

The physicochemical events which take place within the radiation-damaged cells are far from understood. Although there is little doubt that the important target site is the nuclear DNA, it is certainly uncommon for the damage to be inflicted as a result of a 'direct hit', though this mechanism will certainly produce irreversible cleavage of the DNA strands. More commonly the effects are indirect, resulting in the production of unstable, highly reactive and short lived free-radicals which in turn produce destruction of the normal DNA molecule with which they rapidly react. The probability of a lethal cell injury varies not only with the quantity of radiation energy deposited in the tissues (a function of the output of the radiation beam) but also with the intensity of the beam and with its 'type', that is whether the radiation is produced by gamma rays, electrons, neutrons or other particles. These differences give rise to the concept of linear energy transfer, LET, which refers to the amount of radiation energy transferred to the tissue by the particular beam. In general, kilovoltage beams of X-rays have a higher LET than megavoltage beams, and neutron beams have a very much higher LET than X-rays or gamma rays. Thus appropriate adjustments in total doses will have to be made if neutron therapy, for example, is being offered as an alternative to conventional treatment. Another important principle is that the relatively protective effect of hypoxia is particularly apparent with beams of relatively low LET; this is one of the reasons why neutron therapy should be effective regardless of the state of oxygenation of the malignant tissues and might be superior to X-ray therapy if, indeed, anoxia is genuinely as critical as it appears to be from the mass of radiobiological literature that has accumulated during the last 50 years.

In other clinical circumstances, failure of radiation therapy may occur because of the recurrence of disease after apparently successful radiation treatment. This is a frequent event, for example in squamous cell carcinoma of the bronchus, where careful assessment by chest X-ray and even bronchoscopy may well demonstrate an apparently satisfactory response to treatment. When relapse occurs, often 1–2 years after primary treatment, what can we suggest by way of explanation? One widely held view, for which there is a good deal of experimental evidence, is that at the time of the initial treatment, there is a spectrum of cellular sensitivity to the radiation, and that the degree of oxygenation of each cell is the key determining factor. A great deal of radiobiological work has gone into defining and characterizing this phenomenon, and almost all studies (both with experimental animals and *in vitro* tissue culture systems) have shown that well oxygenated cells are substantially more radiosensitive than those which are anoxic.

This difference in sensitivity may be reflected in a two- or three-fold increase in the dosage required for tumour eradication in an anoxic environment (Fig. 5.6), and the clinical impor

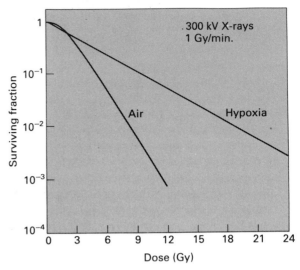

Fig. 5.6. *Effect of oxygen concentration on cytotoxicity of X-rays.* The survival of Hela cells are shown under conditions of hypoxia and in air. (From Duncan W. & Nias A.H.W. (1977) *Clinical Radiology.* Churchill Livingstone, Edinburgh. With permission.)

tance of this observation is thought by many to be critical, since cells far removed from a good arterial supply will inevitably be relatively anoxic. In large tumours with a relatively rapid growth rate and in areas of necrosis where vascularization is poor, anoxia may be a major cause of radioresistance, and experiments using microelectrodes for measurement of oxygen tension have confirmed these theoretical predictions.

Quite apart from the oxygen effect, the progenitor cells will not be equally radiosensitive so that recurrence after apparently successful treatment may be due to repopulation through regeneration of the radioresistant stem cells within the tumour. This can take place either after a complete course of radiotherapy, or rapidly, even between fractions given, say, on daily basis. There is at least some evidence that regrowth through repopulation may be more delayed with malignant tissues than with normal host cells, and that this may be an important basis for the difference between the relatively adequate regenerative capability of many normal tissues, in contrast to the more permanent destructive effects on malignant tumours.

This is analogous to the effects of chemotherapy on normal and malignant tissue (see Chapter 6).

Fractionation and cell death

Fractionation, the use of repeated dosage of radiation within a course of treatment, has been the subject of considerable interest. Early radiation workers rapidly realized that repeated use of modest radiation doses seemed to be the best method of safely delivering a higher total dose of radiation than would be possible with a single large treatment, and that this, in general, led to a greater likelihood of cure. The interest in fractionation has developed not only because of a natural desire to understand the mechanisms of radiation-induced cell damage, but also to understand how best to exploit this phenomenon and to advise the clinician as to the optimal choice of fraction size, overall treatment time and other important details which might make the difference between success and failure. In most single dose experiments, the degree of damage to the malignant cell (usually measured by inhibition of cell division) is directly proportional to the radiation dose, in a log-linear fashion (Fig. 5.6). The important

additional feature is that at low dosage, the steep curve is flattened to form a characteristic 'shoulder'. With relatively more radioresistant cells (such as malignant melanoma) the shoulder will be broader, and the rest of the curve less steep.

Most theorists agree that the shoulder region represents an area of sublethal damage, from which repair is possible. With repeated or fractionated treatment, further radiation damage can be inflicted before completion of this repair, though naturally the degree of cell recovery between fractions will depend on the interval and intensity of each fraction of treatment. If recovery outweighs the degree of newly inflicted damage by each succeeding fraction of radiation, then the total effect might well be less satisfactory than treatment employing a single large fraction. Although most experimental work suggests that with each daily fraction of treatment, the shoulder region is reproduced (Fig. 5.7), the clinical superiority of fractionated treatment may, in large part, be due to the relatively slow rate of recovery in malignant cells. Other possible advantages of fractionated treatment relate to the rapid improvement in oxygenation of the tissues following early treatments, which, by reduction of the tumour mass,

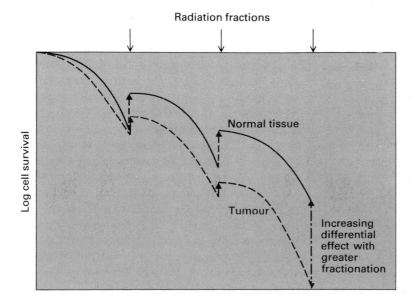

Fig. 5.7. *Fractionation: the effect of repeated doses of radiation.* Fractionation increases the differential cytotoxic effect on normal and malignant tissue. (From Duncan W. & Nias A. H. W. (1977) *Clinical radiobiology.* Churchill Livingstone, Edinburgh. With permission.)

leads to relief of vascular obstruction, a more effective blood supply and greater sensitivity to subsequent doses of irradiation, again due to the oxygen effect. In addition to these theoretical advantages, fractionated treatment has other benefits since the earlier fractions may produce a significant improvement in clinical well-being, allowing better tolerance of the total course. Other advantages include the diminution of radiation sickness by comparison with a single large dose of treatment, and the much greater flexibility which results from a course rather than a single treatment, allowing, for example, for a change in radiation volume and/or dose rate, which may well be called for as the tumour begins to resolve.

Despite these general comments, there have been very few satisfactory studies comparing different fractionation regimes, and most radiotherapists rely on approaches which have been empirically tested and found acceptable in terms of both effectiveness and toxicity. For example, lengthy fractionation regimens of 6 weeks of daily treatment are sometimes used for squamous carcinomas, while other radiotherapists will offer treatment which take no more than 3 or 4 weeks. Very careful estimates of dose equivalents have to be employed when comparing treatment regimens since all radiotherapists know that, for example, the radiobiological effect of a single dose of 10 Gy (1000 rad) is greatly in excess of the effect produced by 10 daily doses of 1 Gy (100 rad). A yardstick for measurement of dose equivalence is therefore essential, not only for prospective trials of fractionation regimens but also for the radiotherapist who quite often has to deviate from his standard regimen for a whole host of reasons including the personal needs of the patient, unexpected machine breakdown, pressures on equipment, staff shortages and so on.

Although no system can accurately predict dose equivalence, the most satisfactory approach so far has been that of Ellis, who introduced the concept of a *nominal standard dose* (NSD), or single dose which produces a clinical reaction as close as possible to that pro-duced by any given fractionation regimen. The important parameters of his NSD equation were the total dose of radiation, the number of fractions and the total length of the treatment from first to last fraction. Use of the NSD concept has at least permitted an attempt at comparing the clinical effectiveness of differing treatment approaches, and has been helpful in confirming the importance of the dose response concept for optimal tumour control at a variety of sites.

RESPONSE OF TISSUES TO RADIATION
Normal tissues

Since the adverse effects of radiation limit the clinician in his choice of dosage, an understanding of the radiation tolerance of normal host tissues is an important facet of the radiotherapist's training and practice. The study of radiation response in normal tissues has become a major area of specialized research, and very wide discrepancies of the radiation tolerance of different organs have been demonstrated (Table 5.2). In general, the most radiosensitive tissues are those with a rapid cell division which include the bone marrow, the stem cells of the gonads and the epithelial lining cells of the alimentary tract, all of which are damaged by relatively low doses of radiation.

Clinically, there is an important distinction to be drawn between early, *acute*, effects and later, *chronic*, damage. It is not necessarily the intensity of the acute reaction which determines the probability and duration of the more chronic effects. Even where recovery from acute irradiation appears complete, the 'reserve' of stem cells in these organs is often permanently depleted, so that further treatment either with radiation therapy or cytotoxic drugs may well produce a surprising degree of tissue damage including, for example, marrow suppression. Understanding of this long term but latent (invisible) damage is of increasing importance since many patients with cancer are likely to be offered both these forms of therapy.

Table 5.2. Radiosensitivity of normal and malignant tissue.

Radiosensitivity	Normal	Malignant
Highly sensitive	Marrow Gonads Gut (mucosa) Lymphatic tissue Eye (lens)	Lymphoma Leukamia Seminoma Ewing's sarcoma Some embryonal tumours
Moderately sensitive	Liver Kidney Lung Skin Breast Gut wall Nervous tissue	Small cell lung cancer Breast cancer Squamous carcinomas (including gynaecological, head and neck, and skin tumours) Adenocarcinomas of the gut
Relatively insensitive	Bone Connective tissue Muscle	Sarcoma of bone and connective tissue Melanoma

Highly radiosensitive tissues

HAEMOPOIETIC TISSUES

The bone marrow is exceedingly sensitive to irradiation. In man, a single total body dose of 4 Gy (400 rad) would prove lethal to about half of all patients and the majority of these deaths would be due to early myelosuppression producing anaemia, neutropenia and thrombocytopenia. With localized treatment at high dose (a much more common clinical situation) long lasting inhibition of myelopoiesis occurs, but usually without appreciable affect on the blood count. Lymphopenia is a well recognized complication of localized radiotherapy at any site, resulting from irradiation of the blood as it passes through the beam—a consequence of the extreme radiosensitivity of the small lymphocyte. Allogenic bone marrow transplantation has permitted total body irradiation to a higher dose (often up to 10 Gy, 1000 rad) as part of the therapy for acute leukaemia. In addition, large areas of the body can now be treated with therapeutic irradiation for widespread and painful bony metastases (e.g. from myeloma or carcinoma of the prostate) without recourse to marrow transplantation techniques since the unirradiated marrow is able to compensate by increased production. This is the basis of so-called 'hemi-body irradiation', an increasingly used method of simple palliation for patients with widespread metastatic disease, which can be repeated on the opposite half of the body providing a suitable gap of 6–8 weeks is allowed between each fraction of treatment.

THE GONADS

In the testes and ovary, small single doses of radiotherapy can permanently damage reproductive function, though the testis is undoubtedly more sensitive. It is likely that some of the primitive spermatogonia (the precursors of the spermatocytes) may be sensitive to a dose of as little as 1 Gy (100 rad) though a dose as low as this would be unlikely to reduce the human sperm count to zero. The radiation sensitivity of the hormone-producing testicular Leydig cell is very much less, so that large doses of radiotherapy to the human testis do not result in loss of secondary sexual characteristics. In the female, single doses of 4–5 Gy (4–500 rad) have been used to induce artificial menopause, though some 30% of women appear to continue regular menstruation following this single fraction of radiation. Fractionated treatment to 10–12 Gy (1000–1200 rad) results in complete cessation of menses in virtually every patient.

Moderately radiosensitive tissues

This group is characterized by relatively low cell turnover rates which are paralleled by a relative, but by no means complete insensitivity to radiation; these include nerve cells, including the brain itself, as well as the spinal cord and peripheral nervous system, skin, kidney, gut and other sites, (Table 5.2).

NERVOUS TISSUE

The nervous system is of great concern partly because the sequelae of damage to the central nervous system can be both profound and irreversible, and also because for the large majority of malignant brain tumours, radiation therapy is the most valuable modality available (see Chapter 11). During the early acute phase of radiation response, the blood vessels, nerve cells and supporting glial structures are all injured directly; sufficiently large doses may result in acute cerebral oedema and a sudden rise in intracranial pressure. These changes will gradually subside, but chronic effects include demyelination, vascular damage, with proliferation of subendothelial fibrous tissue, and, eventually, brain necrosis if the dose is sufficiently high. It is generally accepted that the hypothalamus, brainstem and upper cervical spine are rather more sensitive to radiation than other parts of the brain and it is also thought that concurrent administration of chemotherapy (chiefly methotrexate and vincristine) may also reduce radiation tolerance.

Irradiation of the spinal cord may pose even more problems, particularly since this may be unavoidable in, for example, the palliation of painful bony metastases of the spine. The radiation tolerance of the spinal cord is governed by a variety of important details such as the length of cord irradiated, the fractionation employed, and the total dose given. It is widely held that for a 10 cm length of cord, a total dose of 40 Gy (4000 rad) in 4 weeks is safe though many clinicians err on the side of great caution since radiation myelitis, leading to irreversible paraparesis, is such an appalling complication. Recent work with total body irradiation has shown that a single dose of about 10 Gy (1000 rad) delivered to the whole length of the spinal cord very rarely produces significant neurological sequelae, though the mildest (reversible) late complication, that of Lhermitte's syndrome of paraesthesiae in the extremities on flexion of the neck, is often encountered. Moreover, with prophylactic spinal cord irradiation in children with medulloblastoma, the risk of clinically significant neurological sequelae, after doses as high as 30 Gy (3000 rad) applied over 5–6 weeks to the whole of the spinal cord, seems acceptably low. In general, careful fractionation should be employed wherever a significant length of cord is likely to be irradiated in a patient whose survival may be prolonged. For palliative radiation treatment it seems prudent to recommend the lowest effective dose which is compatible with durable pain relief, particularly since further treatment may well be required, inevitably adding to the possibility of cord damage.

THE SKIN

A portion of skin will be irradiated in all patients treated by external methods of X-ray therapy. Historically, the skin reaction was the chief guide in determining the total radiation dose. With modern high-energy (megavoltage) equipment, far fewer severe skin reactions are seen, since the scattered radiation component of these beams is almost exclusively in the forward direction so that maximum energy deposition takes place well beneath the skin surface (Fig. 5.4). Nonetheless, clinically important skin reactions can still pose major problems

Table 5.3. Skin reactions to radiotherapy.

Early changes	Later changes
Erythema	Fibrosis
Dry and moist desquamation	Loss of pigment
Pigmentation	Telangiectasia
Epilation	Loss of skin appendages
Loss of sweat gland function	Loss of connective tissue
Tissue oedema	

both with orthovoltage and even with megavoltage beams (Table 5.3). Typically, the changes consist of an erythema of increasing severity, leading to dry and then moist desquamation, followed (if the radiation therapy is discontinued) by a repair process associated with progressive fibrosis, hyperplasia of vascular elements (sometimes resulting in telangiectasia much later on) and also by excessive pigmentation which may be permanent, though depigmentation can also occur. If the skin is further irradiated at a time when moist desquamation is evident, then extensive skin and subcutaneous necrosis may occur; this may take place when the further treatment is separated by months or even years. It is therefore unwise to attempt re-irradiation of recurrent skin carcinomas, since the risk of necrosis is ever-present and such cases are usually much better treated by surgery. It is also worth remembering that the skin 'appendages' such as sweat glands, sebaceous glands and hair follicles are also damaged directly by radiation. Radiation-induced epilation of the scalp is an inevitable drawback of whole brain irradiation for cerebral metastases, which is in other respects an effective technique with few side-effects. Both single doses (as in total body irradiation) and fractionated treatment will cause complete epilation of the scalp if the dose is high enough, though hair regrowth will usually occur, given time, even when a radical dose has been used as, for example, in children with medulloblastoma.

THE EYE

The eye is frequently irradiated, particularly during the treatment of carcinomas of the maxillary antrum and paranasal sinuses, and of course in the definitive radiation therapy of orbital lymphomas, rhabdomyosarcomas, retinoblastomas and other orbital tumours. It is often not appreciated that for the most part, the eye is relatively radioresistant, and careful attention to detail can result in a healthy eye with very adequate vision even after whole orbital irradiation. However, there are two important points to remember. First, that the greatest danger to the eye is posed by dryness of the cornea, leading to keratoconjunctivitis sicca. This generally results from lack of tear formation, following irradiation of the lacrymal gland which can be avoided in most instances by the use of a small lead shield. Second, the most radiosensitive structure of the eye is the lens, which is particularly sensitive to large single fractions of irradiation. Cataract formation can often be prevented by the use of a pencil-shaped corneal shield, though there is always the danger of under-irradiation of important structures deep to the protected cornea and lens. Fortunately, radiation-induced cataracts can be removed without difficulty; only a small proportion give rise to significant visual symptoms.

THE KIDNEY

The kidney is frequently irradiated during treatment of abdominal or retroperitoneal tumours, and is a relatively radiosensitive structure. Both glomerular filtration rate and renal plasma flow are reduced after modest radiation doses, and it is often a year or more before recovery begins. Acute radiation nephritis can occur when the dose to both kidneys is no greater than about 25 Gy (2500 rad) in 5 weeks. The acute clinical syndrome includes proteinuria, uraemia and hypertension which can be irreversible and even fatal. More chronic changes include persistent albuminuria and poor glomerular and tubular function, which may be lifelong even in patients who recover from the acute syndrome. These complications are particularly likely to occur after whole abdominal irradiation.

THE GUT

Although both small and large bowel tissues are sensitive to radiation, the rectum deserves special mention since this is frequently the organ of limiting tolerance when treating carcinomas of the cervix and other pelvic tumours. Acute radiation reactions, accompanied by diarrhoea, tenesmus and occasional rectal haemorrhage, are encountered both with external irradiation of the pelvis and also with intracavitary treatment. When intracavitary sources are used, careful attempts must be made to reduce the rectal dose by packing the vagina in order to keep the rectum well away from the high doses of radiation. The later radiation effects are of greater importance, and include oedema and fibrosis of the bowel, which once again may be responsible for diarrhoea, painful proctitis and rectal bleeding, sometimes progressing to stricture, abscess or fistula formation. Occasionally these complications will be severe enough to warrant temporary or even permanent colostomy or may cause difficult diagnostic problems by mimicking symptoms of recurrence of the cancer. Fortunately these severe radiation sequelae have become less frequent with better understanding of radiation dosimetry within the pelvis, coupled with increased attention to technical details. Radiation damage to the small bowel is pathologically similar to that of the rectum and may limit treatment of intra-abdominal tumours. Late sequelae include stricture formation which may cause intestinal obstruction.

Less radiosensitive tissue

BONE

Therapeutic radiation of bone is a particular problem in children since normal growth may be interrupted, especially when the epiphyseal plate is included in volumes taken to radical dosage, since this area is responsible for the increase in length of any growing long bone. Direct irradiation of the epiphysis interferes with the high mitotic rate of the cartilaginous cells adjacent to the shaft. Radiation damage to the metaphysis may also be severe, though apparently fully reversible provided that the dose of radiation is moderate. The severity of radiation-induced deformity and/or growth disturbance is much greater with high rather than low dosage, particularly where large volumes have been irradiated. The advent of megavoltage irradiation has been particularly helpful in this respect. Nonetheless in children treated for medulloblastoma, where the whole spine is irradiated to a minimum dose of 30 Gy (3000 rad) in 5-6 weeks, the majority of survivors have some deficit in the sitting height. As many as one-third remain persistently below the 3rd centile for height. Younger children are at particular risk but this has to be accepted when radiotherapy is essential for cure, as in medulloblastoma.

OTHER CONNECTIVE TISSUES

Muscle, tendon and connective tissue are all relatively insensitive to radiation and do not usually limit dosage. Fibrosis may occur when high or repeated doses are used and this may lead to loss of joint mobility and contractures.

LATE SEQUELAE OF RADIATION

In addition to the specific effects on the various organs as described above, there are a number of important long-term hazards following the use of radiotherapy. These include carcinogenicity, mutagenicity and teratogenicity, and are all attributable to a fundamental property of ionizing radiation, namely its biological effect on nuclear DNA with consequent damage to genetic material.

Carcinogenesis

This is a well documented phenomenon. Survivors from Hiroshima have an increased incidence of neoplasia, particularly leukaemia. Recently an increased incidence of breast cancer has been reported, 35 years after the acute radiation damage was inflicted. Analysis of a large series of patients with ankylosing spondylitis treated by low doses of radiotherapy, has demonstrated a ten-fold increase in the incidence of leukaemia. Occasionally malignant change develops at the site of previous localized irradiation, for example osteosarcoma of the scapula following radiation for carcinoma of the breast. In children treated for retinoblastoma, late orbital neoplasms may occur and there is evidence of a steep dose-response relationship.

These studies illustrate the general points that neoplasia tends to occur within an organ directly affected by the radiation beam, that there is usually a latent period of at least 10 years before neoplasia develops, and that even moderate doses of irradiation such as those which used to be employed for benign disease during childhood or young adult life may lead to a radiation-induced malignancy later on. Much higher doses of radiation are usually given to patients with cancer but the patients are usually older and with a far smaller likelihood of long survival, so that the true risk of late radiation carcinogenesis is much less amenable to study. In addition it is now widely accepted that patients with cancer have a higher probability of developing a second neoplasm. This is sometimes due to common risk factors, for example, patients cured of early laryngeal carcinomas who continue to smoke and then succumb to carcinoma of the bronchus. Patients with cancer also have an inherent increased probability of developing a second ma-

lignancy for reasons which are currently unclear. Increasingly, patients are being treated with radiation and cytotoxic chemotherapy, the latter adding to the risk of carcinogenesis. This is well demonstrated by the higher risk of acute leukaemia following treatment of Hodgkin's disease (see Chapters 6 and 25). As more patients are treated with, and cured by, combinations of radiation and chemotherapy, we must expect the incidence of second neoplasms to rise. Although the risk of radiation carcinogenesis is low, it should cerainly deter radiotherapists from treating benign skin and other disorders, particularly in children, which could be better and more safely dealt with by other means.

Teratogenicity

The teratogenic effects of ionizing radiation are well known. Minimal exposure even to 'soft' X-rays in pregnant women, is hazardous because of the risk of growth retardation and serious malformation in the developing embryo. Irradiation during the last trimester, well after organogenesis is complete, is safer though growth retardation may still occur. Radiation treatment of pregnant women should be avoided wherever possible. This may well lead to difficult points of judgement especially when the diagnosis of malignancy is made early in the pregnancy. For example, in patients with pelvic tumours (usually carcinoma of the cervix which is becoming increasingly common in the childbearing age group) there is general agreement that during the first trimester of pregnancy, treatment should be given as if the patient were not pregnant. Spontaneous abortion will always occur but few would feel justified in delaying therapy for perhaps 6 months until the pregnancy is over (see Chapter 25).

Mutagenicity

This refers to genetic alteration in somatic or germ cells resulting from their direct irradiation. In somatic cells these mutations may be the basis of radiation induced carcinogenesis. In germ cells mutation may lead to foetal death or abnormality although in man, most germ cell mutations are thought to be non-viable. For these reasons abnormal births following scattered irradiation to the testis are very uncommon.

THE RADIOTHERAPY DEPARTMENT

In order to deal adequately with both surface and deep-seated tumours, departments of radiotherapy must possess a suitable range of equipment, comprising superficial (low energy), orthovoltage (medium energy) and supervoltage (high energy) machines. In general, a depart-

ment will need to draw on a population of at least half a million in order to have a sufficient throughput of new cases. At least 40% of cancer patients require treatment with radiotherapy at some point. Important additional features of the modern department include facilities for planning the radiation treatment, closely liaising with departments of medical physics. For many patients, multifield techniques are used and the physics staff, in conjunction with the radiotherapist, will decide (usually with the aid of a planning computer) on the most appropriate field arrangement. Modern computing techniques have enormously improved the tasks of defining and comparing the alternative plans; drawing out the isodose curves (similar to contour lines on an ordnance survey map) defining points of equal radiation depth-dose and mak-

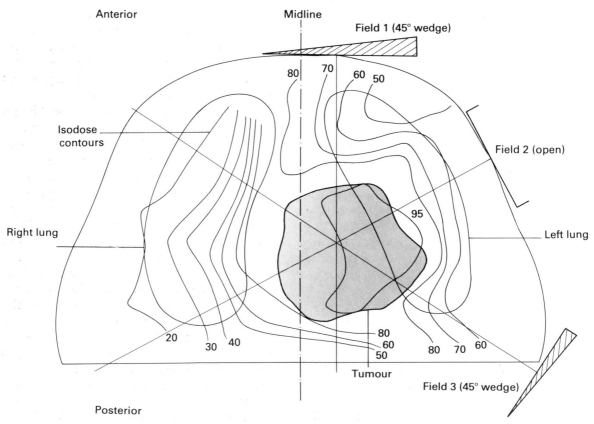

Fig. 5.8. *Typical plan for multifield irradiation of carcinoma of left main bronchus showing site of tumour, position of lungs and isodose contours.*

ing suitable corrections for tissues of unusual density such as lung or bone (Fig. 5.8). In many departments, a treatment simulator is available. This is able to mimic the radiation therapy apparatus in its geometry, capability and limitations, and is useful in 'setting-up' patients without actually delivering any treatment, allowing the careful appraisal of both the tumour volume to be irradiated and the best alternative techniques. In addition, a mould room, often separately staffed, will be necessary if there is a sizeable demand for treatment immobilization devices such as individually manufactured perspex head shells for use in head and neck or brain tumour work. Mould room staff are often responsible for manufacturing templates which might be necessary either for superficial irradiation of irregularly shaped skin cancers, or when individualized shaped fields are used such as the 'mantle' or 'inverted-Y' fields for irradiation of patients with Hodgkin's disease.

It is the radiotherapist's responsibility not only to judge whether radiotherapeutic treatment is indicated but also to decide upon the best technique, field arrangement, choice of therapy unit, total dose and fractionation. Although these technical aspects of radiotherapy are often thought to be synonomous with the total workload of the radiotherapist, they in fact form a limited part of the task. Perhaps even more important is his continuing and ever-present role as the clinician responsible for diagnosis, management and follow-up of patients with cancer. In Britain, where the division of radiotherapy from diagnostic radiology occurred early, departments of radiotherapy have been entirely clinical (i.e. nondiagnostic) for well over 30 years, and have assumed the complete care of cancer patients.

RADIOTHERAPY PLANNING AND TREATMENT TECHNIQUES

Non-radiotherapists are often puzzled by the technical vocabulary which radiotherapists use, making it difficult for them to understand the intentions, achievements and limitations of the techniques employed. A short glossary follows:

Treatment prescription. The total dose and treatment time is normally prescribed at the outset of treatment, though in certain circumstances the radiotherapist may prefer to prescribe, say, the first week's treatment and then make a further decision as to whether to continue or not. Total absorbed dose is given in rad (r), Gray (Gy), or centiGray (cGy). 1 rad = 100 ergs per gram and 1 Gy = 1 J/kg of absorber. The Gray is increasingly preferred as it is the S.I. unit of dose; 1 Gy = 100 rad and some radiotherapists prefer centiGrays to Grays since 1 centiGray = 1 rad, so that total dose in centiGray is identical to total dose in rad. For most treatments, the total dose is split into a number of equal fractions given either on a daily basis or intermittently. The number of fractions of treatment is also prescribed by the radiotherapist. The *treatment volume*, that is the volume of tissue to be covered by the prescribed radiation dose, is determined by the radiotherapist using whatever radiological and imaging aids he feels to be necessary.

Maximum, minimum and modal dose. Since it is impossible to achieve homogeneous irradiation of the desired volume without irradiation of surrounding normal tissue, the radiotherapist must decide on the appropriate compromise. One traditional approach was to prescribe to a *maximum* dose, that is, a dose which would not be exceeded, even if this particular dose level was reached only in a small part of the tumour. The opposite approach, to prescribe to a *minimum* dose which represented the lowest possible dose level was also commonly used. The problem with prescriptions of this kind is that neither maximum nor minimum dosage is necessarily representative. A more suitable prescription is made with reference to the *modal* dose, that is, the particular dose level occurring with the greatest frequency in the prescribed volume, which by definition, is a more representative dose level. The *applied dose* is used where the radiotherapist wishes to prescribe the dose at the surface of the skin. If he wishes to state more precisely what the dose at a certain depth should be (e.g. when treating spinal metastases where the dosage at certain depth is of greater interest than the surface dose) a *depth dose* prescription may be preferable. The radiotherapist may specify a certain dose at 4 cm depth for metastases in the upper spine, but at 7 cm depth for those in the lower spine.

Open (direct) and wedged fields. An open or direct field is usually applied perpendicular to the patient's skin surface and the beam emerging from the treatment machine is not modified in any way. In treatments using several fields (multifield techniques), a number of fields, usually two to four, are used and, by inserting wedges of various dimensions into the beam and using radiation fields applied obliquely, the tumour volume can be irradiated to a more homogeneous level (Fig. 5.8). The use of mul-

tifield arrangements, often employing wedged fields, has permitted safer megavoltage irradiation of deeply seated tumours to a high dose level.

Parallel opposed fields. The simplest type of multifield technique is provided by a two field arrangement where the fields are opposed in opposite directions, usually applied to the anterior and posterior skin surface (Fig. 5.9) and irradiating the block of tissue in between. This technique is widely used and if necessary, the fields can be shaped so that important structures are avoided, for example, the use of the 'mantle' irradiation technique for patients with supradiaphragmatic Hodgkin's disease where the lungs are protected from over-irradiation (see p. 444). For parallel opposed pairs of fields, the dose prescribed is normally the *midplane dose* since this will define the dose achieved at a point midway between the two fields and in-

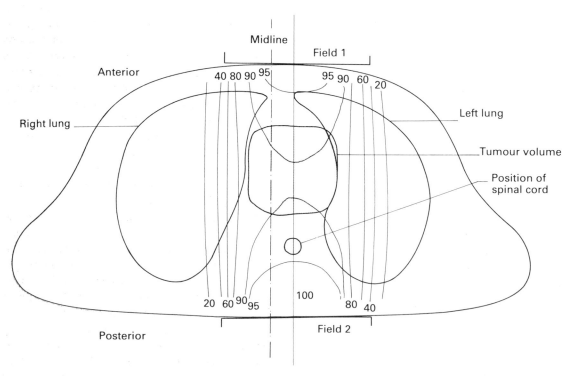

Fig. 5.9. *Typical antero-posterior parallel pair field arrangement.* This is often used for treating thoracic or pelvic tumours. In this instance the patient had an inoperable carcinoma of the bronchus and the tumour position and size were determined by CT scanning. The spinal cord is also shown since irradiation of this structure is often dose-limiting with this set-up.

deed midway between the anterior and posterior skin surface of the patient.

Shrinking field technique. During a course of treatment it is sometimes desirable to reduce the treatment volume so that part of the initial treatment volume is treated to a certain dose level and a smaller area taken to a higher dose. This is often done, for example, in pelvic tumours such as carcinomas of the bladder or prostate where the original treatment volume might include pelvic lymph nodes with the intention to treat these to a 'prophylactic' dose of irradiation to deal with microscopic disease, whilst the primary site requires a higher dosage. A further good example is the irradiation technique often employed in a primary bone sarcoma such as Ewing's tumour where the whole of the long bone might be irradiated to a moderate dose, the field being reduced during treatment so that the primary tumour site receives the full total dose.

Immobilization devices. For precision work, particularly treatment of head and neck cancers, it is essential that the patient be absolutely still, and in a reproducible position throughout the whole of the lengthy treatment period. The best means of achieving this is to use an im-

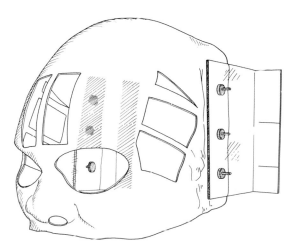

Fig. 5.10. *Perspex head shell.* Shells are individually made to ensure accurate positioning. These are widely used in treatment of tumours of the head and neck.

mobilization device such as a perspex headcast (Fig. 5.10) which is individually made by obtaining a plaster impression, which is then used to produce a perspex shell which fits the patient snugly and can be screwed to the treatment couch. Use of these devices also carries the advantage that field markings can be made on the cast rather than the patient, thereby avoiding unsightly ink marks or tattoos, and ensuring accurate reproduction for each day's treatment.

INTEGRATION OF RADIOTHERAPY AND CHEMOTHERAPY

Remarkable changes in the therapy of cancer have occurred over the past 25 years. Whereas it was once unusual for patients to be treated both with radiotherapy and also with cytotoxic chemotherapy, it has now become commonplace. This trend is almost certain to continue for at least two reasons. First, radiation therapy is being increasingly used as an alternative to surgery for treatment of the primary tumour, particularly with carcinoma of the larynx and other head-and-neck sites, carcinoma of the cervix, and, over the past few years, with some carcinomas of the breast, bladder and prostate. Second, there is increasing use of chemotherapy both for palliation and, in some tumours, as adjuvant therapy immediately preceding or succeeding the initial local treatment.

There are important disadvantages to the simultaneous use of both treatments. Some cytotoxic agents act as radiation sensitizers, increasing the local reactions from radiotherapy and occasionally even producing 'recall' of previous skin reactions. The most important agent is actinomycin D, though there is evidence that other drugs such as doxorubicin may also interact with radiotherapy in this way. For example, oesophageal stricture has been documented in patients undergoing mediastinal irradiation and concurrent treatment with this drug. Doxorubicin-induced cardiomyopathy may occur at a lower dosage in patients who have undergone mediastinal or chest wall radiation, if a significant volume of cardiac muscle has been included. For patients undergoing wide-field irradiation, particularly if a substantial volume of bone marrow is involved (such as in children with medulloblastoma), the use of adjuvant chemotherapy may lead to more troublesome myelosuppression than the radiation alone. Certainly, with 'synchronous' use of combination chemotherapy during radical irradiation for squamous carcinomas of the head and neck region, the mucosal toxicity is much greater than with radiotherapy alone. Our feeling is that radiotherapy and concomitant cytotoxic chemotherapy should be avoided wherever possible since there are real risks in patients already undergoing intensive treatment with radiotherapy, which in many instances must be given at near tolerance doses for maximum effect.

Despite these drawbacks, there are many theoretical advantages to combined use of radiotherapy and chemotherapy as initial treatment, even if not administered synchronously. Radiotherapy as a powerful local tool is often able to produce tumour control with minimal physiological disturbance, though without effect on occult metastases. It may not be possible to ensure satisfactory irradiation of the primary tumour and its lymph node drainage area if nodal metastases are known to be present, for example, in gynaecological, testicular or bladder tumours with known para-aortic involvement. Chemotherapy, on the other hand, can seldom be relied upon to deal adequately with the primary tumour, though it does at least offer hope in dealing with occult metastatic disease. Combined therapy should then represent a logical approach in a disease which by its very nature has often spread widely.

Use of chemotherapy with curative intent after radiation failure represents a different form of combined therapy, since the treatments are separated in time. This approach is only likely to be successful in highly chemosensitive tumours such as Hodgkin's disease, in which chemotherapy for radiation failure is as successful as it is for primary therapy. A newer concept, as yet relatively unexplored, is the use of 'adjuvant' radiotherapy in patients treated primarily by chemotherapy. In small cell carcinoma of the bronchus, chemotherapy is now widely employed as the mainstay of treatment. We now have to ask whether mediastinal irradiation, formerly the most widely used method of treatment, still has a role to play. Radiotherapy may also be valuable in a slightly different adjuvant fashion as, for example, in the use of cranial irradiation as prophylaxis for children with acute lymphoblastic leukaemia in whom meningeal relapse is substantially reduced by routine irradiation, since the CSF is poorly penetrated by the drugs used for systemic control.

Because many radiotherapists in Britain have no access to specialist medical oncologists, most regard themselves as specialists in chemotherapy as well, though there is substantial local variation. It is probably fair to say that with the advent of more specialist medical oncologists, and increasingly complex and taxing regimens often including new and hazardous drugs, many radiotherapists are increasingly prepared to pass this aspect of their work to those more thoroughly trained in cancer chemotherapy, though most would be unhappy to forego this role entirely.

In our view, boundary disputes between these specialties are for the most part pointless and are best solved by the radiotherapist and medical oncologist working closely together, preferably from within a single department. It seems increasingly counter-productive to maintain distinct departments of radiotherapy and medical oncology often with an uneasy relationship, rather than to create a single unified department of Clinical Oncology which is responsible for all non-surgical aspects of cancer treatment.

FURTHER READING

Gilbert H. A. & Kagan A. R. (1978, 1983) *Modern Radiation Oncology: Classic Literature and Current Management*, Vol. 1 (1978), Vol. 2 (1983). Harper & Row, New York.

Duncan W. & Nias A. H. W. (1977) *Clinical Radiobiology*. Churchill Livingstone, Edinburgh.

Fowler J. (1983) La Ronde—Radiation Sciences and Medical Radiology. *Radiotherapy and Oncology* **1**, 1–22.

Dutreix A. (1984) When and how can we improve precision in radiotherapy? *Radiotherapy and Oncology* **2**, 275–92.

Fletcher G. H. (1980) *Textbook of Radiotherapy*, 3rd edn. Lea & Febiger, Philadelphia.

Easson E.C. & Pointon R.C.S. (1985) *The Radiotherapy of Malignant Disease*. Springer-Verlag, Berlin.

Chapter 6
Systemic Treatments for Cancer

Over the past 30 years there has been little change in the 5-year survival rate for most common cancers. There has been a modest improvement in some tumours, for example in bladder cancer and cancer of the rectum, which is related in part to earlier diagnosis, but other tumours such as breast and pancreatic carcinoma have nearly as bad a prognosis now as in 1950. While there have been advances in the surgical and radiotherapeutic control of the primary tumour during this period, failure to improve survival is due to the fact that the major cause of death is lymphatic and blood borne metastasis. Better control of the primary site has in general a small effect on metastatic spread, which has often occurred by the time of surgery.

For this reason any hope of improvement in survival lies in the development of better methods of treatment of metastases. The systemic treatment of cancer has, in the last 15 years, become an important part of cancer management. In some uncommon tumours such as lymphomas and teratomas great progress has been made with the use of cytotoxic drugs. Sadly, in other more common cancers, the results have been less impressive. Since the treatments are often toxic and usually expensive, a clear understanding of the uses and limitations of chemotherapy and other forms of medical treatment is essential. If there is a reasonable chance of cure, toxicity and expense can usually be accepted. If there is not, then the potential benefits of palliative treatment with cytotoxic agents must be carefully weighed against unwanted effects.

CHEMOTHERAPY

In 1946 Gilman and Philips published a review of their data on the use of nitrogen mustard (1). The effectiveness of this class of compound in producing regression in lymphomas was rapidly established, as was the gastro-intestinal and haematological toxicity they produced, and they became the first cytotoxic agents to be introduced into clinical practice. In 1947 Farber introduced the antifolates and showed that aminopterin could produce remissions in acute leukaemia. This was followed by the production of the closely related drug methotrexate in 1949. Development of other drugs followed swiftly: 6-mercaptopurine by Elion in 1952, and the antitumour antibiotic actinomycin D in 1954. Since 1965, numerous new antimetabolites, alkylating agents and antibiotics with significant activity have been developed, many of which are related to the parent molecules discovered over 20 years ago.

The development of an anti-cancer drug

Before a new agent is introduced into clinical practice it undergoes routine evaluation in both experimental systems and early clinical trials. Potentially useful agents may be synthetic analogues of existing drugs, or new classes of chemicals thought worthy of testing because of clinical or laboratory data. The preclinical screening is usually carried out on a murine leukaemia (L1210 or P388) and agents active against these tumours are carried over for further testing against other mouse tumours and human tumour xenografts (usually established in immune suppressed or 'nude' mice). It is, however, by no means clear if this method of initial screening is appropriate. The murine leukaemias are rapidly growing, uniform, multiple passaged tumours, quite different from slowly growing heterogeneous human neoplasms. The active drugs are then tested in rodents and larger vertebrates to determine toxicity and to establish the basic pharmacological data with respect to dose, absorption, tissue distribution, plasma half-life, pathways of metabolism and excretion.

If a drug shows activity it then may be tested in Phase I clinical studies. The patients selected have cancers resistant to conventional therapy and a wide variety of tumours is studied. The aims at this stage are to elucidate details of dosage, toxicity, the route of administration and the pharmacology of the drug in man, and to document any responses which may occur. Active drugs are then taken to Phase II testing where toxicity is further studied, and larger groups of patients with a single tumour type are treated. Usually these patients have been unresponsive to previous treatment. Effective agents are then taken to Phase III studies where the patients have tumours which have not been treated previously. An attempt is made to compare the response with other effective agents and at this stage the response rate is quantified and related to dose and method of administration. When reading reports of the effectiveness of drugs as single agents it is important to bear in mind that the response rate will largely depend on whether the patients are previously untreated, and on details of the dose and schedule. Since the next phase (Phase IV) is the incorporation of the drug into primary treatment, often in combination with other agents, it is important that these data are reliable. The validity of these response rates depends on the number of patients studied. For example if no responses are seen in 15 patients, there is only a 1 in 20 chance that a 20% response rate will have been missed. If occasional responses occur, larger groups (over 30) are needed; confidence increas-

ing with group size. Phase IV studies usually require many hundreds of patients to assess the new approach to treatment (unless the effects are exceptional). The design and conduct of these studies is further discussed in Chapter 2.

Principles of cancer chemotherapy

Many of the recent advances in cancer chemotherapy have come from a greater understanding of the best way to use cytotoxic agents rather than the appearance of new agents with superior efficacy. A knowledge of the way in which normal cells and tumours grow is important in order to understand the way in which cancer chemotherapy is used.

THE CELL CYCLE

After cell division each cell enters a growth phase, G_1, (Fig. 6.1) which lasts for a variable period of time in different tissues. Cells which are not dividing at all are said to be in G_0 phase but it is not clear if this differs fundamentally from the G_1 phase of dividing cells. After G_1 the cells move into the phase of DNA synthesis, S phase, in which the amount of chromosomal material is doubled. The cell then passes

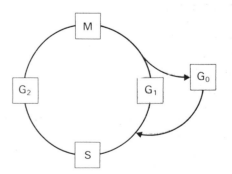

M = Mitosis (prophase → metaphase → anaphase → telophase)
G_0 = Resting phase
G_1 = Early growth phase
S = DNA synthesis
G_2 = Later growth phase

Fig. 6.1. *The cell cycle.*

through a pre-mitotic phase, G_2, and then into mitosis, M, in which the pairs of chromosomes separate and the cell divides.

As with other tissues, tumours are heterogeneous with respect to cell division; some cells proliferating, others dying or dormant. The tumours probably contain progenitor or 'stem' cells which are capable of cell division, continuously renewing and increasing the tumour mass. The rate of cell division in human tumours, and the speed with which their size increases, varies considerably from one disease to another as is shown in Table 6.1. The majority of common cancers increase in size very slowly in comparison with sensitive normal tissues such as bone marrow and gastro-intestinal epithelium. Even rapidly dividing tumours, such as acute myeloblastic leukaemia, do not divide as rapidly as normal myelopoietic precursors. The visible growth of solid tumours appears to vary with tumour size, slowing as the tumour becomes larger. The reasons for this are not completely understood. Vascularisation of large tumour masses is often defective and the rate of cell death is high in those areas of tumour more than 150μ from a capillary. The tumour growth rate also depends on the proportion of cells dividing at any given time, called the *growth fraction*. In experimental tumours the growth fraction falls as the tumour becomes larger, but in man, direct proof that small tumours have a higher growth fraction is lacking.

The potential importance of these considerations lies in the fact that some cytotoxic drugs are thought to be effective only against cells which divide. If the growth fraction is indeed higher for small tumours, these would be more susceptible to chemotherapy and this concept is often used as a rationale for adjuvant chemotherapy. Similarly if surgical removal of massive disease led to increased cell division in the remaining cells, this might also be exploited therapeutically.

Cytotoxic drugs produce their effect by damaging the reproductive integrity of cells. In general the more rapidly growing tumours with a high growth fraction are more likely to respond to drug treatment. This, however, is a generalization. The explanation of why some types of cancer (lymphoma, testicular cancer, leukaemia) are sensitive to cytotoxic drugs and other types are not (pancreatic, colonic cancer) is almost certainly not solely a matter of cell kinetics. Most cytotoxic regimens have been derived empirically, not on the basis of cell kinetics. Some drugs (for example methotrexate) are only effective at a particular phase of the cell cycle such as DNA synthesis, while others, such as alkylating agents, exhibit some action even against resting cells. Table 6.2 shows the phase specificity of some anti-cancer drugs.

The relationship between cell cycle and cell death is modified by repair mechanisms. For example in a resting cell, DNA damage by an

Table 6.1. *Approximate volume doubling times of human tumours.*

Tumour	Doubling time (days)	
	mean	range
Burkitt's lymphoma	—	2–5
Acute lymphoblastic leukaemia	—	3–5
Small cell lung cancer	50	20–100
Squamous carcinoma of lung	90	30–300
Adenocarcinoma of lung	130	25–350
Colon cancer	100	50–250
Late breast cancer	150	25–500
Lymphoma	25	10–200
Seminoma	20	10–100

Table 6.2. Phase specificity of anti-cancer drugs.

Phase of cell cycle	Effective agents
S phase	Cytosine arabinoside Methotrexate, 6MP, Hydroxyurea
Mitosis	Vinca alkaloids
Phase non-specific	Alkylating agents, nitrosoureas antibiotics, procarbazine, cisplatin

alkylating agent may be repaired before the cell moves into cycle, if the repair mechanisms are efficient and if the interval between drug exposure and onset of DNA synthesis is long. In a previously treated slowly growing tumour, damage to resting cells from alkylating agents will be repaired before cell division occurs, so the drug will prove ineffective.

Attempts have been made with human cancers to time drug administration in such a way that the cells are synchronized into a phase of the cell cycle which tenders them especially sensitive to the cytotoxic agent. For example, in experimental systems, vinblastine can be used to arrest cells in mitosis. These 'synchronized' cells enter cycle together and can be killed by a cycle active S phase specific agent, such as cytosine arabinoside (2). While these ideas are attractive in theory and can be shown to work in rapidly dividing, susceptible, experimental tumours, there is no evidence that any successful regimen in human cancer is effective by virtue of cellular kinetic considerations such as these.

KINETICS OF CELL KILLING BY CYTOTOXIC DRUGS

Some of the principles on which modern methods of chemotherapy are based, stem from an understanding of the kinetics of killing of tumour cells by cytotoxic agents. In the 1960s several workers showed that a given dose of a cytotoxic drug killed a given *proportion* of cells and not a given number (3). This fractional cell

kill hypothesis is shown diagrammatically in Fig. 6.2. A single dose of a drug might for example kill 99% of cells and will do so whether 10^{12} cells are treated (leaving 10^{10} cells) or 10^4 cells (leaving 10^2 cells). If true for solid human cancers the implications are that a small tumour will be killed by fewer chemotherapy cycles than a large one. Because fewer exposures to drugs will be needed there will be less chance of resistance emerging. Drugs should then be scheduled in such a way as to produce maximum killing. This will depend on the rate of regrowth of the tumour and on the rate of recovery of the normal tissues which have been most damaged by the drug. In man these tissues are usually the gut and marrow

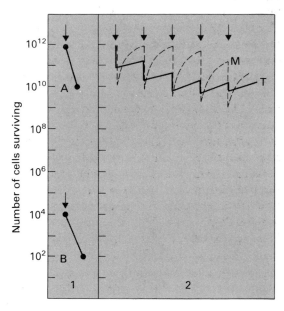

Fig. 6.2. *The fractional cell kill hypothesis.* In part 1 of the figure a given dose of drug is shown killing 99% of cells in both case A and case B. In case A the tumour is reduced from 10^{12} to 10^{10} cells and in case B from 10^4 to 10^2 cells. In part 2 of the figure, T shows the effect of repeated drug administration (arrowed) on tumour growth. With repeated doses there is less killing of tumour, indicating the emergence of drug resistance. M shows the effect of drug administration on marrow progenitor cells. The marrow recovers quickly but with repeated doses this is less complete and myelosuppression becomes clinically evident.

which regenerate quickly in comparison with most cancer tissue (Fig. 6.2). For this reason pulsed intermittent therapy, with time for normal tissues to recover, is the usual method of drug administration.

This approach has both theoretical and practical limitations: (a) the fractional cell kill hypothesis was validated in homogeneous rapidly growing (doubling time less than one day) experimental tumours. Extrapolation to slowly growing human cancers (doubling times up to one year) has obvious dangers; (b) experimental tumours grown as ascites or in body fluids (such as leukaemias) can be assumed to have uniform exposure to a drug. This is obviously not the case for poorly vascularized solid neoplasms, so that the kinetics of killing will be a much more complex function than the first order kinetics of experimental systems; (c) the proportion of inherently resistant tumour cells may be a function of size of the tumour (see drug resistance, below), being greater with large tumours; (d) the rate of regrowth of the tumour may change with repeated chemotherapy. Although this does not appear to occur with tumours such as L1210 the situation may be different for solid tumours; (e) the recovery of normal tissues, as judged for example by blood count, may appear complete after the first few cycles, but becomes less so as treatment proceeds (Fig. 6.2); (f) there is very little clinical data on the dose/response relationship for a given cytotoxic drug in a particular tumour. The clinical pharmacology of cytotoxic drugs is extremely complex and varies from drug to drug. There is clinical evidence that an antitumour effect of a drug will only be seen if a maximum dose is given and in practice the range from ineffective to maximum tolerated dose may be quite small.

These considerations notwithstanding, pulsed intermittent therapy is the schedule of drug administration most widely employed in cancer chemotherapy.

THE USE OF DRUGS IN COMBINATION

Even in sensitive tumours, such as Hodgkin's disease, single agent chemotherapy is rarely curative. It is, therefore, logical to try and improve response rate and duration by the use of drugs in combination. This approach soon proved effective in childhood leukaemia and adult lymphomas (4) and has been adopted for a wide variety of other tumours.

The development of a combination chemotherapy schedule should follow a number of general principles:

1 Only drugs which are known to be effective as single agents should be used.
2 Wherever possible it is preferable to use drugs of non-overlapping toxicity.
3 Pulsed intermittent treatment should be used, to allow gut and marrow recovery.
4 Ideally, each drug should be used in its optimal dose and schedule.
5 Where possible drugs with synergistic killing effects should be used (normally not known in practice).
6 Drugs which work at different phases of the cell cycle are used if practicable.
7 Most schedules are derived from an informed empiricism.

The improved efficacy of these combination regimens has several possible explanations, for example:

i Since the tumour is exposed to a wider variety of agents, chances of resistance are smaller.
ii A maximal killing effect is achieved without undue toxicity.
iii There may be less opportunity for the early emergence of a resistant cell population.

DRUG RESISTANCE

The cells in a solid tumour are not uniformly sensitive to a cytotoxic drug before treatment starts. Nowell (5) has suggested that genetic instability increases as cancers grow and that greater heterogeneity develops accordingly, both with respect to cell surface properties and resistance to drugs. This concept provides a partial explanation for greater drug resistance in large tumours (as judged by diminished extent and duration of response). In addition the penetration of cytotoxic agents into large tumours is less uniform than into small ones. There is also evidence to suggest that, as with radiotherapy (see Chapter 5) cellular hypoxia may be a determinant of resistance to cytotoxic agents. The biochemical bases for drug resistance are varied and differ with each class of drug. They are discussed in more detail with each drug. The general mechanisms are shown in Table 6.3.

The position can be summarized as follows: As the tumour grows in size the frequency of development of resistant cells increases so that large tumours have a greater number of intrinsically resistant cells. This resistance is produced by one or more of the mechanisms shown in Table 6.3 and its fundamental cause is an alteration in genetic control of enzyme concentration or transport proteins. An example is the increase in gene copy number resulting in increased concentrations of dihydrofolate reductase and which causes resistance to methotrexate (p. 91). The use of cytotoxic drugs exerts a selection pressure encouraging the survival of the resistant cells which grow and multiply. In addition to this type of cellular resistance at least two other mechanisms are important. The first is diminished vascularity of parts of the tumour as it gets larger resulting in hypoxia and decreased drug penetration. The second is that only a small proportion of cells may be in cycle, allowing time for repair from cytotoxic damage before cell division. This mechanism may be very important in slowly growing tumours.

MAINTENANCE THERAPY

Following the induction of a remission in acute leukaemia, chemotherapy of a less intensive type is used to 'maintain' the remission. In acute lymphoblastic leukaemia this has been shown to contribute to survival. The term is somewhat confusing since the improvement comes from continued cytotoxic effect on the tumour when the induction therapy has not completely eradicated the disease. In this sense the treatment is not really 'maintenance' but continued treatment.

In most tumours maintenance therapy has not been shown to improve the results of cyclical combination chemotherapy given over a period of several months. In Hodgkin's disease for example, survival is not improved by treating the patient with further cycles of MOPP chemotherapy after six cycles have been given. A similar lack of effect has been found in small cell lung cancer and testicular tumours. In these diseases the patient is cured (or not) during the early phase of treatment and maintenance treatment of long duration has no value.

Table 6.3. Cellular mechanisms of resistance to anti-cancer drugs.

Mechanism	Drug
Efficient repair to damaged DNA	Alkylating agents
Decreased uptake by cell	Methotrexate
	Doxorubicin
Decreased intracellular activation	6 Mercaptopurine, 5FU
Increased intracellular breakdown	Cytosine arabinoside
Bypass biochemical pathways	Methotrexate
	6 Mercaptopurine
	Asparaginase
Gene amplification of blocked enzyme	Methotrexate

ADJUVANT CHEMOTHERAPY

Following resection of an operable cancer (for example of the breast or stomach) many patients will develop local or distant recurrence even if no evidence of spread was found at operation or during pre-operative investigations. It is therefore logical to consider the use of cytotoxic chemotherapy as an adjuvant to surgery. The aim is to eradicate micrometastases at this early stage. There are theoretical reasons to believe that chemotherapy may be more effective on these small tumours than it will be when they have become clinically detectable (pp. 80–81).

There is little doubt that this approach has been very effective in sensitive paediatric tumours such as Wilms' tumour, Ewing's sarcoma and rhabdomyosarcoma. With the less chemosensitive solid tumours of adults the situation is less clear. The benefits of chemotherapy when given to all patients may be to increase survival by, say, 5%, but the toxicity is significant. This issue is discussed in more detail with respect to breast cancer (Chapter 13). With each tumour the degree of improvement in survival must be weighed against the toxicity of the regimen for those patients who will not benefit.

Predicting sensitivity to anti-cancer drugs

The wide variety of anti-cancer agents and the variable response of tumours to them has led to an interest in developing methods by which the individual sensitivity of a tumour might be tested. Such a system would have great advantages in the rational selection of therapy in an individual patient. In the last 20 years there has been a great deal of work designed to develop *in vitro* systems allowing prediction of the clinical response of malignant neoplasms. Such systems have, however, run into serious technical and logistic problems, some of which are outlined below.

1 *The pharmacology of the anti-cancer agent in vitro may be entirely different from the in vivo situation.* There are many reasons for *in vivo* drug resistance including inadequate concentration and duration of drug exposure, poor penetration of drug into the tumour, a low growth fraction at the time of administration and heterogeneity of drug action within the primary neoplasm. By contrast, in the *in vitro* system, the dose and time of the drug used in the test is necessarily somewhat arbitrary and artificial, and essential differences between sensitive and resistant tumours may be obscured. Alternatively, a tumour may be deemed sensitive *in vitro* under circumstances which do not pertain in the patient.

2. *Most systems depend on the production of single cell suspensions or explants of tissue.* Single cell suspensions are often technically very difficult to prepare, particularly from fibrous neoplasms, and the viability of the culture may be poor. Explants of small fragments of tumour may grow but certain tumours, for example breast cancer, are notoriously difficult to culture in this way. In any case, even if the tumour grows in culture, there must always be doubt as to the degree to which the cultured cells are truly representative of the entire tumour.

3 *It is by no means clear what parameter of cell death or injury should be used in predictive tests.* The test systems have used morphological assessment of cytotoxic effect in culture, incorporation of radioactive precursors of DNA, measurements of protein synthesis, and inhibition of colony growth.

All of these methods have advantages and disadvantages and the relevance of these end points of drug effect to the clinical regression of a tumour, is often rather tenuous.

TECHNIQUES

Despite the above objections the following techniques have been used in recent years:
1 *Incorporation of radioactive precursors into tumour cells or explants.* In this technique pieces

of tumour or cell suspensions are incubated in culture with a radioactive precursor of DNA or RNA. This technique is relatively straight-forward and fairly quick. The disadvantage is that it assumes that the block of the incorporation of the labelled precursor into DNA caused by the drug, is a true reflection of the response of the *in vivo* neoplasm to the agent.

2 *Clonogenic cell survival.* In this technique cell suspensions are prepared from solid tumours or malignant effusions and, after incubation with the cytostatic agent, are then cultured in soft agar. Many tumours will grow in soft agar forming colonies of about 50 cells. The degree to which this is inhibited by the agent in question, is the basis of the assay. Some disadvantages of this technique are: Firstly, not all tumours form colonies easily and many tumours will only do so if they are taken from pleural effusions or bone marrow aspirates. This severely restricts the applicability of the system. Secondly, the efficiency of the procedure is very low. Often only one in 10 000 cells which are cultured will form colonies and the degree to which these are representative of the main tumour mass must be open to question. Thirdly, it is likely that many of the proliferating cells are in the S phase of cell cycle and that it is these cells which are being damaged by exposure to the drug.

3 *Human tumour xenografts.* In this technique a small piece of tumour is implanted subcutaneously in an immune deprived or 'nude' mouse where it will grow. Drug sensitivity can then be tested by injecting the mouse with the anti-cancer agent. There are several drawbacks with this method: the proportion of tumours which 'take' successfully is relatively low at about 20% and some tumour types grow much better than others; the kinetics of growth of a tumour in animals are different from those which would normally occur in the host; the metabolism of the cytotoxic agent is that of the mouse and not of the human; it is very expensive, and the process is very slow so that clinicians must treat the patient long before the results are known. On the other hand, this technique has allowed

the testing of drug combinations and also the assessment of drugs such as cyclophosphamide which must be activated *in vivo* to form their active principles.

4 *Cellular damage in tissue culture.* Here, the tumour is grown in tissue culture over a period of several days and the drugs are then added, their effects being measured by morphological and cytological changes. The problems here are that the tumours do not always grow well in culture and the number of 'takes' is relatively small. Furthermore, there is the usual problem as to the degree to which the cultured line is representative of the primary tumour.

In summary, when carried out systematically, using defined criteria, in large numbers of patients with a given tumour, it has generally been found that these tests indicate resistance with a high degree of certainty. That is to say, if there is no effect of the cytotoxic drug in tissue culture, it is unlikely that there will be any effect on the patient. The converse, however, is not true. Demonstration of an effect of the agent *in vitro* is not necessarily a pointer to its effect *in vivo*. Nevertheless, it would still be useful to have techniques which allowed us to exclude certain drugs with confidence, but regrettably with all these techniques only small numbers of patients can be tested, and most of the procedures are time-consuming and expensive. Much more work needs to be done but it does not seem likely that such tests will become available for routine assessment of tumour sensitivity in the way that bacteriological testing is used in selecting the choice of an antibiotic (6).

What cancer chemotherapy has achieved

The curable cancers are uncommon tumours such as childhood cancers, leukaemias, lymphomas and testicular tumours. Other cancers are partially responsive but the impact of chemotherapy on survival is small or unproven. These include cancer of the breast, small cell lung cancer, ovarian cancer and cancer of the stomach. Figure 6.3 shows that the cure rate with chemo-

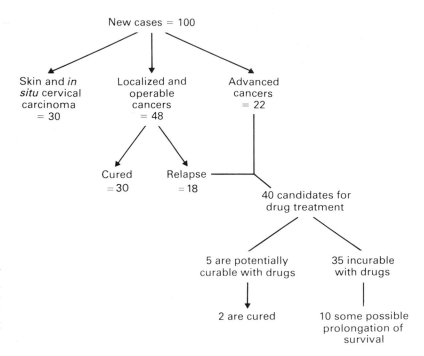

Fig. 6.3. *The impact of cancer chemotherapy.* The flow diagram gives the proportion of new cancer cases which might be expected to benefit from drug treatment.

therapy is very low and that the proportion of all cancer patients who need, or will benefit from, current drug treatments is relatively small.

Classes of cytotoxic drugs, mode of action and toxicity

ALKYLATING AGENTS AND NITROSOUREAS

These very reactive compounds probably produce their effect by covalently linking an alkyl group $(R—CH_2—)$ to chemical moieties in proteins and nucleic acids. Nitrogen mustard for example has two chlororethyl side chains (Fig. 6.4A) and one of these forms a cyclical, highly reactive immonium ion which binds to nucleic acid constituents such as the 7-nitrogen group of guanine. After forming this bond, if there is another side chain, as there is with nitrogen mustard, another link can be formed which may result in DNA strands being cross-linked, either within a strand or between strands.

Many other molecules may be attacked including cytoplasmic proteins and RNA. At therapeutic doses however, it seems that impairment of DNA replication is the major mechanism of the cytotoxicity. Alkylating agents which are bifunctional (with two alkylation products) are more cytotoxic than monofunctional compounds by virtue of the cross-linking they produce. The cell can repair itself against this kind of damage of excision of the damaged segment of DNA with formation of a new segment of DNA which is then linked to the strand. Although DNA alkylation occurs at any stage in the cell cycle, it seems to have more serious consequences if it occurs during S phase, possibly because there is less time for DNA repair before cell division begins. For this reason, alkylating agents usually have greater effect on proliferating cells but are not cycle phase specific.

Nitrosoureas seems to act in part as alkylating agents linking an alkyl (Fig. 6.4B) or carbamoyl group to cell proteins. The compounds are unstable and decompose in water to liberate alkylating and carbamoylating groups. It seems probable that damage to cell proteins occurs with both types of reaction but alkylation is

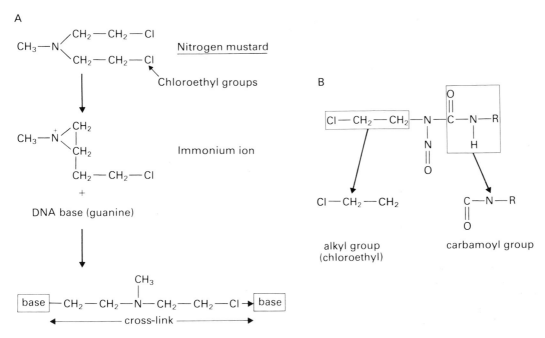

Fig. 6.4. *The alkylating action of nitrogen mustard* (A) *and chloroethylnitrosourea* (B).

probably the main mechanism of damage to DNA.

Other alkylating agents have different structures. Busulphan is a methane-sulphonate ester which also binds to guanine in DNA and cross-links DNA strands. Dacarbazine (DTIC) is an analogue of an intermediary in purine metabolism but acts by alkylation, after enzymatic cleavage, to form a carbonium ion which again binds to guanine and other bases. Thiotepa, and other related compounds, are ethyleneimines which act similarly to nitrogen mustard, forming an immonium ion which is the initial step in alkylation. Both nitrosoureas and other alkylating agents are associated with leukaemia in long term administration, and nitrosoureas cause brain and other tumours in animals.

Mechlorethamine (mustine, HN$_2$) (Fig. 6.4) This drug is given by intravenous injection and undergoes such rapid transformation that within minutes it is no longer present in active form. It must be given within a few minutes after it has been made up into a fast flowing intravenous drip and is an intense irritant outside a vein. The usual dose is 6 mg/m^2 and the drug is mainly used in the treatment of Hodgkin's disease. The toxic effects are nausea and vomiting, leucopenia, thrombocytopenia, thrombophlebitis and tissue necrosis if extravasated. This can be modified by subcutaneous isotonic sodium thiosulphate.

Cyclophosphamide (Endoxana, Cytoxan) *(Fig. 6.5)* This is a stable compound which is well absorbed when given orally. It is activated in the liver by the cytochrome P450 system to 4-hydroxycyclophosphamide and thence to phosphoramide mustard and acrolein (Fig. 6.5). The latter is responsible for the haemorrhagic cystitis which is a complication of prolonged or high dose administration. Recently it has been shown that 2-mercaptoethane sulphonate, which binds acrolein in the urine, will prevent this complication. After oral administration maximal plasma concentrations are reached in one hour, and the plasma half-life of the drug

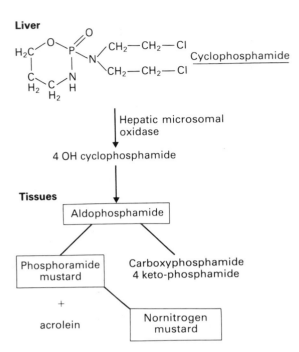

Fig. 6.5. *The metabolism of cyclophosphamide.* The boxed compounds are alkylating agents. Acrolein is the major cause of haemorrhagic cystitis.

is 5–6 hours. Very little unchanged drug is excreted. The dosage, route and schedules of administration are very variable. In solid tumours such as small cell lung cancer, single intravenous dosage of the order of 1 g/m² are often used, but in breast or ovarian cancer and some lymphomas it is often given orally in lower dose (e.g. 100 mg/m² daily). There are numerous tumours in which the drug has been found to be useful, and it is the most versatile alkylating agent in terms of activity and method of administration. There is increasing interest in the use of very high dose cyclophosphamide (10 g/m²) in solid tumour chemotherapy and in allogeneic marrow transplantation for leukaemia and aplastic anaemia. Because the drug must be converted to an active form in the liver, it is not suitable for local use, for example intrapleural administration.

Haematological toxicity is common, but thrombocytopenia is less marked than with other alkylating agents. Nausea and vomiting accompany intravenous administration, and nausea may also occur when it is given orally. The drug is not vesicant if extravasation occurs. Haemorrhagic cystitis and bladder fibrosis commonly occur and alopecia is frequent with higher doses. Pulmonary fibrosis occurs, as it does with other alkylating agents. High doses may be complicated by inappropriate secretion of ADH leading to hyponatraemia. As with all alkylating agents male infertility is usual. Haemorrhagic carditis has been reported with very high doses.

Melphalan (Alkeran) (Fig. 6.6) This is a stable alkylating agent in which the two chloroethyl groups are linked to phenylalanine. It was

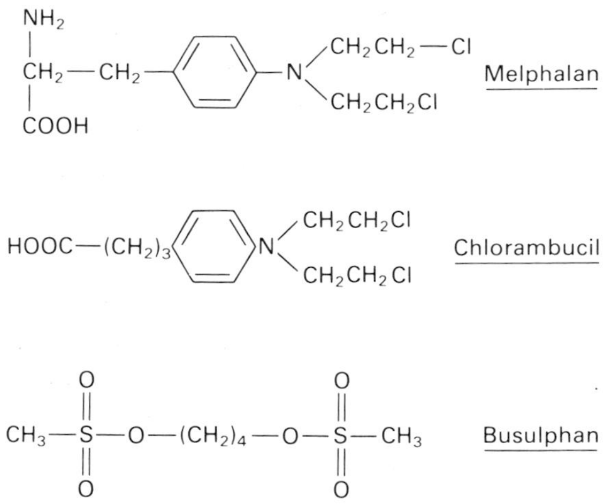

Fig. 6.6. *The structure of other commonly used alkylating agents.*

originally hoped that this would result in selective activity against melanoma, but in conventional doses, this has not proved to be the case. It is usually given orally, (for example 10 mg daily to an adult for 7 days every 4–6 weeks). It is well absorbed, not vesicant and has a half-life of 90 minutes. Delayed leucopenia and thrombocytopenia occur but nausea, vomiting and alopecia are infrequent. The drug is often used in myeloma, ovarian and breast cancer and has a similar activity to cyclophosphamide in these tumours. With prolonged continuous use there is an appreciable risk of the development of myeloid dysplastic states leading to acute leukaemia. As with cyclophosphamide there is interest in its use at very high dose as treatment for neuroblastoma, melanoma and myeloma (7).

Chlorambucil (Leukeran) (Fig. 6.6) In this compound the two chloroethyl groups are linked to a phenyl group. It is a stable compound, well absorbed orally with a plasma half-life of 90 minutes. The drug is usually given in low continuous dose (e.g. 4 mg daily) or as a higher intermittent dose (e.g. 10 mg for 2 weeks). It produces its antitumour effects slowly and its myelosuppressive effect is gradual in onset but persistent. Thrombocytopenia is frequent but haemorrhagic cystitis rarely occurs. It is generally well tolerated and is widely used in the treatment of ovarian cancer and low grade lymphomas particularly in the elderly.

Busulphan (Myleran) (Fig. 6.6) This compound differs in structure from other alkylating agents being an alkyl sulfonate. It is exceptional in that it has very little action apart from bone marrow depression. Thrombocytopenia is frequent and pancytopenia develops which may be irreversible. Pulmonary fibrosis is a complication of long-term administration, which occurs with other alkylating agents but is especially frequent with this drug. Other side-effects include skin pigmentation, glossitis, gynaecomastia and anhidrosis. It is particularly used in the treatment of chronic granulocyte leukaemia.

BCNU (Carmustine) (Fig. 6.7) BCNU (bis-chloroethylnitrosourea) was the first nitrosourea to be used clinically. It has a wide spectrum of activity similar to the alkylating agents. It is lipid soluble and penetrates the blood/brain barrier which is assumed to exist for primary brain tumours. However, the response rates are low in primary tumours and the effect usually transient. It has also been used in the treatment of small cell lung cancer and lymphoma, but does not have major activity in these disorders.

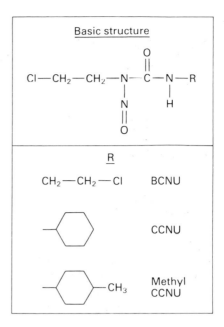

Fig. 6.7. *The structure of nitrosoureas.*

It is usually given intravenously and the half-life is very short, i.e. less than 5 minutes. The major toxic effect is bone marrow depression which is characteristically delayed for 5–6 weeks. Nausea and vomiting are frequent, renal and hepatic damage may occur as does pulmonary fibrosis, oesophagitis and flushing. It is not vesicant.

CCNU (Lomustine) (Fig. 6.7) CCNU (cis-chloroethylnitrosourea) is rapidly absorbed and metabolized, and is usually given by mouth. The products of metabolism have a plasma half-life of 1–2 days, and the metabolites can be detected in the CSF. As with BCNU the major toxic effects are nausea, vomiting and delayed bone marrow depression. For this reason the drug is given at 6 week intervals. Nausea and vomiting can be reduced by spreading the dose over 2 or 3 days. Its spectrum of activity is similar to alkylating agents. It has been widely used in the treatment of primary and secondary brain tumours as well as in lymphomas and small cell bronchogenic cancer.

Dimethyltriazenoimidazole carboxamide (DTIC)
This drug probably produces its cytotoxic effect by functioning as an alkylating agent. It is administered intravenously and is vesicant if extravasated. There is an initial rapid clearance followed by slower clearance (t/2 five hours). Much of the drug is excreted unaltered in the urine. It was initially introduced as a treatment for melanoma but the results have proved disappointing. It is sometimes used in combination chemotherapy for soft tissue sarcoma but evidence for its value is meagre. It is also included in some regimens for Hodgkin's disease. It causes severe nausea and vomiting, and myelosuppression is frequent. Damage to liver and peripheral nerves occurs as does flushing and myalgia.

ANTIMETABOLITES: FOLIC ACID ANTAGONISTS

Several folic acid antagonists have been developed since the introduction of aminopterin in 1947, but only one, methotrexate, is now widely used. The antifolate action is complex and includes inhibition of the enzyme dihydrofolate reductase. This enzyme is essential for reducing dihydrofolate (FH_2) to tetrahydrofolate (FH_4), which in turn is converted to a variety of coenzymes that are essential in reactions where one carbon atom is transferred in the synthesis of thymidylate, purines, methionine and glycine. The critical effect in preventing cell replication appears to be the blocking of synthesis of thymidine monophosphate as shown in Fig. 6.8. The block of thymidine monophosphate synthesis results in inhibition of DNA and RNA synthesis and the drug is therefore S phase specific. The block in activity of dihydrofolate reductase can be bypassed by supplying an alternative intermediary metabolite. This is N^5-formyl-FH_4, variously termed leucovorin, citrovorum factor or, more commonly, folinic acid. It is converted to the FH_4 coenzymes, needed for thymidylate synthetase to function.

The most important mechanism of methotrexate resistance appears to be by production of large amounts of dihydrofolate reductase (8). In methotrexate resistant cells there is a considerable increase in the number of copies of the gene coding for dihydrofolate reductase. Molecular probes for the dihydrofolate reductase gene have been used to demonstrate this gene amplification. An increase in gene copy number is shown by dense homogeneous staining regions on chromosomes or in small

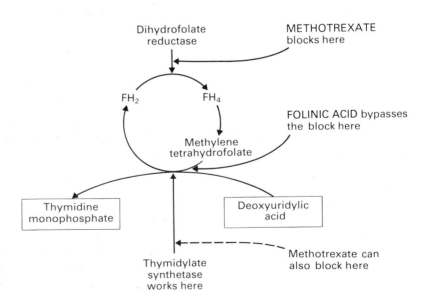

Fig. 6.8. *The action of methotrexate and folinic acid.*

chromosome fragments called double minute chromosomes. Double minute chromosomes do not appear to be passed to daughter cells but the homogenous staining regions appear more stable and may be responsible for the continuation of methotrexate resistance in subsequent cell divisions.

Other described mechanisms are the production of variants of the enzyme with decreased affinity for methotrexate, and impaired transport into cells.

Methotrexate (amethopterin) (Fig. 6.9) This drug is readily absorbed from the gut at low

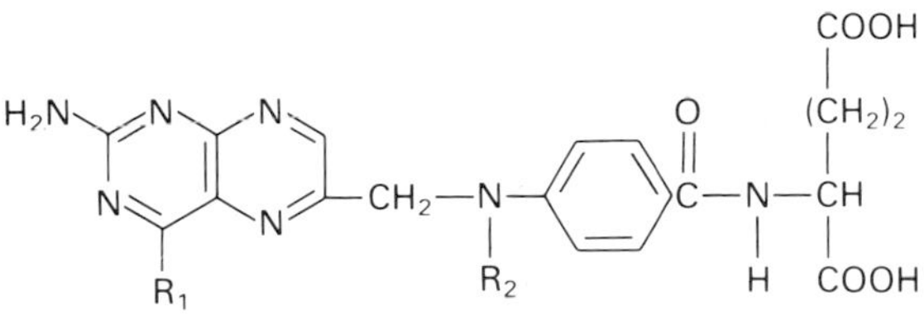

Folic acid R_1 = OH R_2 = H
Methotrexate R_1 = NH_2 R_2 = CH_3
Aminopterin R_1 = NH_2 R_2 = H

Fig. 6.9. *Folic acid analogues.*

dosages, but higher doses are incompletely absorbed. After i.v. injection there is an initial rapid distribution phase (t/2 45 minutes), then a slower phase of renal excretion (t/2 2–3 hours) followed by a very slow phase when the drug concentration is low. It is this latter prolonged phase of clearance that is responsible for toxicity to marrow, gut and mucous membranes. If there is ascites or a pleural effusion the drug may accumulate in these sites and then be slowly released from the 'reservoir' (or third space) causing unexpected toxicity even from a low dose. The drug is 50% bound to albumin from which it can be displaced by drugs such as salicylates, sulphonamides, tetracycline and phenytoin. It is not metabolized significantly but is mainly excreted unchanged in the urine especially in the first 8 hours both by glomerular filtration and tubular secretion. Drugs which

compete for tubular secretion, or the presence of renal failure, may greatly delay the excretion of the drug and thereby increase toxicity. The drug may remain bound to dihydrofolate reductase in kidney and liver cells for several weeks, only being released when these cells die. When given in very high dose renal excretion must be promoted by i.v. fluids and possibly by alkalinization of the urine.

In conventional doses the drug does not penetrate significantly into the CSF, but when given at high doses the CSF concentrations can achieve cytotoxic levels of up to 10% of the plasma concentration. The drug can also be administered intrathecally, usually at a dose of 10 mg/m^2, and high CSF levels are thereby achieved, especially in the spinal CSF.

The toxicity is mainly haematological and to epithelial surfaces. Pancytopenia develops rapidly after a large dose. After 4–6 days there is oral ulceration, diarrhoea which may be bloody, and erythematous skin rashes. Other toxic effects include alopecia; renal failure with high doses; hepatic toxicity (occasionally leading to cirrhosis); pneumonitis, and osteoporosis after long-term therapy. The drug has a wide spectrum of activity and is part of the established treatment of acute lymphoblastic leukaemia. It is also widely used in non-Hodgkin's lymphomas; breast and ovarian cancer; soft tissue sarcomas and osteogenic sarcoma. It is the most effective single agent for choriocarcinoma. Attempts have been made to overcome methotrexate resistance by using very high doses followed by folinic acid rescue. Encouraging results have been claimed in osteogenic sarcoma but the value of this approach is still disputed (see Chapter 23).

ANTIMETABOLITES: PYRIMIDINE ANTAGONISTS

Drugs in this category either antagonize or mimic natural pyrimidine metabolites and thereby interfere with nucleic acid synthesis. The most important members of this group are 5-fluorouracil and cytosine arabinoside.

5-fluorouracil (*5FU*) (Fig. 6.10) The fluorine atom which is substituted for hydrogen on the uracil molecule is similar in size to the hydrogen atom so that the 5FU molecule can enter into

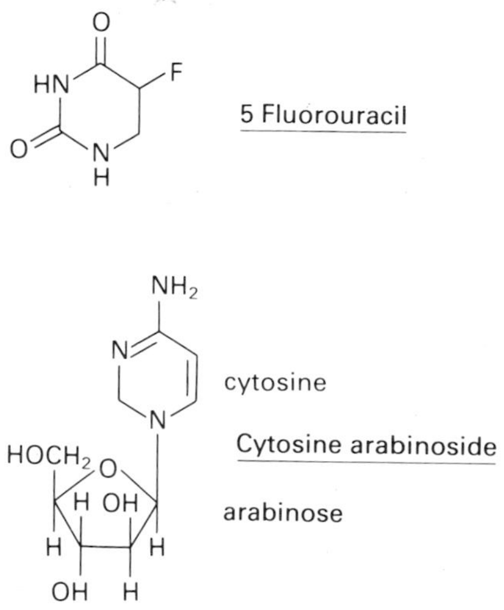

Fig. 6.10. *The structure of the pyrimidine analogues.*

many reactions where uracil would be the normal participant. 5FU has first to be activated to 5-fluoro-2 deoxyuridine monophosphate (FdUMP). This is the active form of the drug. The conversion of 5FU to FdUMP can proceed through a variety of pathways, and resistance to the drug is associated with decreased activity of the enzymes necessary for this conversion. FdUMP interferes with DNA synthesis by binding to the enzyme thymidylate synthetase and inactivating it (Fig. 6.8). The effect of the block can to some extent be overcome if thymidine is given (similar to the effect of folinic acid rescue for methotrexate). 5FU is also incorporated into RNA but the importance of this for its antineoplastic effect is not certain. 5FU is more toxic to proliferating cells, that is, it is cycle specific, but it does not seem to have an effect at a particular phase of the cycle. Recovery from 5FU involves the synthesis of both thymidylate synthetase and the normal substrate deoxyuridine monophosphate.

The intestinal absorption of 5FU is erratic so the drug is normally given intravenously. Plasma clearance is rapid (t/2 15 minutes). Much higher plasma concentrations are achieved by rapid i.v. injection than by continuous infusion, and the toxicity of the drug is greater when given by bolus injection. The drug penetrates the CSF well. The usual schedule of administration is 12 mg/kg daily for four days, then every 2–3 days at a dose of 6 mg/kg unless the patient develops diarrhoea or stomatitis. Myelosuppression is commonest between 10 and 15 days. Full doses are usually necessary to get a tumour response. Care is necessary in the presence of hepatic dysfunction. Intra-arterial infusion of 5FU sometimes produces good results in hepatic metastases from gut cancer. The drug has activity against adenocarcinoma of the gut, breast and ovary, but responses are infrequent and tend to be transient.

The drug is generally well tolerated but toxic effects include nausea, diarrhoea, stomatitis, alopecia, myelosuppression, cardiac disturbances and a cerebellar syndrome.

Cytosine arabinoside (*cytarabine, ara-C*) (Fig. 6.10) In this analogue of cytidine the pyrimidine base is unchanged but the sugar moiety differs by an alteration in the position of a hydroxyl group. This leads to impaired mobility of the pyrimidine base so that it cannot be effectively incorporated into DNA. The drug is converted by a series of enzymic steps to its active form known as ara-CTP. This is an inhibitor of DNA polymerase but it is not clear if this is the mechanism of its cytotoxic action. It would explain why the drug is markedly cell cycle, S phase, specific. Resistance to the effect of the drug could either be due to low levels of one of the converting enzymes (deoxycytidine kinase) or to increased rates of deamination. The former seems to be the major mechanism.

The drug is very poorly absorbed from the intestine. After i.v. injection there is a fast phase of clearance (t/2 20 minutes) followed by a slower phase (t/2 2 hours) and the clearance is largely determined by the speed of deamination in the liver and other tissues. The drug penetrates well into the CSF and deamination occurs slowly at this site. Because it is S phase specific it is usually given as multiple i.v. injections or as a continuous intravenous or subcutaneous infusion.

The agent is mainly of use against acute myeloblastic leukaemia (AML) but has been used in acute lymphoblastic leukaemia (ALL) and poor prognosis lymphomas as well. It is of little use in solid tumours which usually have a low growth fraction.

The toxic effects include marrow suppression, oral ulceration, diarrhoea, nausea and vomiting and, uncommonly, CNS toxicity It is particularly toxic in the presence of hepatic dysfunction since the liver is the chief site of deamination.

ANTIMETABOLITES: PURINE ANTAGONISTS

There are several cytotoxic agents which are analogues of the natural purine bases and nucleotides. They are in wide use as cytotoxic and immunosuppressive agents. Mercaptopurine and thioguanine are derivatives of hypoxanthine and guanine respectively but with the keto group on carbon-6 replaced by a sulphur atom. In many cases, the drugs of this class must undergo enzymatic conversion to the active form.

6-Mercaptopurine (6MP, Puri-nethol, Fig. 6.11) 6MP must be converted to the nucleotide to become active. This is done by the enzyme hypoxanthine-guanine phosphoribosyltransferase (HGPRT). The resultant nucleotide is 6-mercaptopurine ribose phosphate (6MPRP). 6MPRP accumulates in the cell and inhibits several important metabolic reactions in the formation of normal nucleotides. The cytotoxicity of the drug cannot be ascribed to disruption of a single metabolic pathway and cell death probably results from multiple biochemical abnormalities. However, inhibition of purine nucleotide biosynthesis is a major action of the drug. 6MP is also incorporated into DNA as 6-thioguanine but the contribution of this reaction to cytotoxicity is not clear.

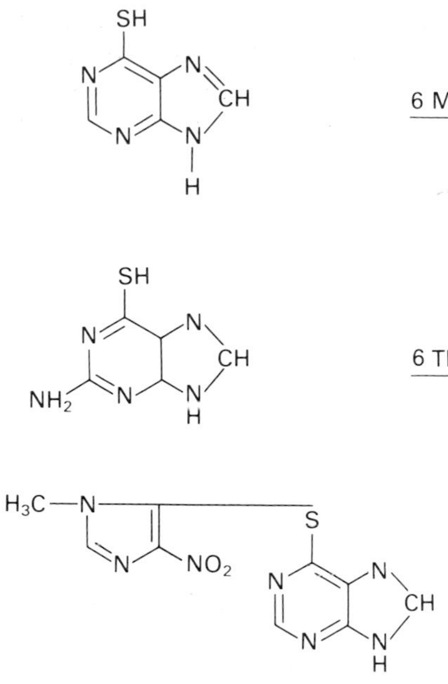

Fig. 6.11. *The structure of commonly used purine analogues.*

Resistance to the action of 6MP is often due to low levels of the converting enzyme HGPRT, and such cells also show resistance to 6-thioguanine and azaguanine. There is evidence however, that in leukaemia cells, deficiency of HGPRT is not the main mechanism of resistance, and that increased rates of drug breakdown are more important. Intracellular alkaline phosphatase levels rise in treated patients, and dephosphorylation may be a mechanism of resistance to 6-thiopurines generally (9).

6MP is readily absorbed from the gut, and about half of an oral dose is excreted as antimetabolites in 24 hours. After i.v. injection the drug is rapidly cleared from the plasma (t/2 90 minutes) due to distribution and metabolism. A major site of metabolism is the liver where xanthine-oxidase rapidly converts the drug to an inactive form. The xanthine-oxidase inhibitor allopurinol blocks this conversion but this increases toxicity as well as effectiveness and the therapeutic ratio is unchanged. Allopurinol is sometimes used in the early stages of treatment of ALL and non-Hodgkin's lymphoma, to prevent hyperuricaemia occurring during the rapid destruction of the tumour. If 6MP is used as part of the initial treatment, allopurinol will increase its toxicity. 6MP is widely used in remission mainenance in ALL and has been used in the treatment of chronic granulocyte leukaemia. Its use as an immunosuppressive agent has largely been superceded by azathioprine although there is evidence that 6MP is a more powerful immunosuppressive agent. The frequent occurrence of cholestatic jaundice with 6 MP has, however, made it less satisfactory for long-term administration. Its other toxicities are nausea and vomiting with gradual and reversible bone marrow suppression. The usual maintenance dose in ALL is 50–100 mg/day.

Azathioprine (Imuran) (Fig. 6.11) This drug was developed in an attempt to decrease the rate of inactivation of 6MP. The drug acts as a 'prodrug' whereby 6MP is slowly formed in the tissues. It is degraded in the liver by xanthine-oxidase, and allopurinol increases its toxicity. The drug is well absorbed orally and is partly excreted by the kidneys so that its toxicity is greater if renal failure is present. Reversible bone marrow depression is the major toxicity. It is most widely used as an 'immunosuppressive' agent in connective tissue diseases and renal allograft recipients. The usual dose is 1–2 mg/kg/day.

6-Thioguanine (6TG) (Fig. 6.11) This purine analogue has a mode of action similar to that of 6MP. It is well absorbed orally and peak concentrations are achieved in 6–8 hours. About half the dose is excreted in the urine as metabolites within 24 hours. Degradation by xanthine-oxidase does not appear to be an important aspect of detoxification and the drug can be used safely with allopurinol. The drug is widely used as part of remission induction and maintenance in AML. It has also been used as an immunosuppressive. The average oral daily dose is 2 mg/kg. Reversible bone marrow de-

pression is the major toxicity, but nausea and diarrhoea may also occur.

2-Deoxycoformycin (Pentostatin) This new drug is closely related to adenosine and is a potent inhibitor of adenosine deaminase. Deficiency of adenosine deaminase is a rare, inherited cause of immune deficiency in which lymphocyte function is defective but other cells are relatively normal. The drug may prove to be valuable both as an immunosuppressive and in treatment of lymphomas.

VINCA ALKALOIDS AND PODOPHYLLOTOXINS

Vinca alkaloids are extracted from the periwinkle, *Catharanthus roseus*, and were observed to cause granulocytopenia in animals. Subsequently they have been shown to be mitotic spindle poisons, and their mode of action is related to other agents such as colchicine and epipodophyllotoxin. To understand the action of these agents some knowledge of the events which occur during mitosis is essential.

In the *prophase* of mitosis the centrioles divide and move to opposite ends of the cell, the chromosomes appear as double strands and the nuclear membrane disappears. In the *metaphase* the chromosomes line up at the equator and the spindle of microtubules appears. In *anaphase* the chromosomes divide, are pulled to opposite ends of the cell and the cleavage furrow appears. In *telophase* the cells separate and the nuclear membrane forms. The vinca alkaloids and other mitotic inhibitors act by binding to tubulin which is the constituent protein of the microtubules. The assembly and function of the microtubules during metaphase is shown in Fig. 6.12. Colchicine and epipodophyllotoxin both bind to the same site on tubulin but vinca alkaloids bind differently. Exposure of the cell to vinca alkaloids leads to to rapid disappearance of the microtubules because no further assembly can take place (Fig. 6.12).

Microtubules are involved in other cell functions such as secretion of hormones, axonal

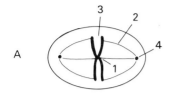

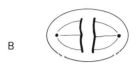

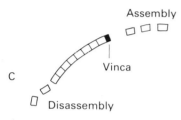

Fig. 6.12. *The assembly and function of microtubules during metaphase.* (A) The chromosome pair (1) is attached to a microtubule (2) which is assembled at the equatorial region (3) and disassembled at the centriole (4). (B) In metaphase the chromosome pair is divided and pulled to opposite ends of the cell. (C) A microtubule is a polymer of the protein tubulin which is made up of α and β subunits. Vinca alkaloids bind to tubulin, blocking further assembly, but disassembly continues.

transport and cell mobility. It is generally assumed however, that the cytotoxic activity of these agents is related to the effect on mitosis.

Very little is known about the mechanisms of resistance to these drugs. In some cell lines vinca resistance is associated both with the appearance of a 180 Kdalton membrane glycoprotein and resistance to many other agents (pleiotropic drug resistance). The relationship of this protein to resistance is not clear. There is often cross-resistance from one vinca alkaloid to another and between vinca alkaloids and podophyllotoxin.

Vincristine (Oncovin) The drug is administered intravenously usually in a dose of 1.5 mg/m² and can be repeated weekly when used as a single agent. The drug is poorly and unpredictably absorbed from the gut. It is vesicant if it escapes from the vein into the tissues. The pharmacokinetics are similar to those of vinblastine (see below).

The drug is useful in treatment of lymphatic malignancies such as Hodgkin's disease, non-Hodgkin's lymphoma and ALL. In these diseases it is usually used in combination with other drugs such as steroids and alkylating agents. It also has a place in treatment of other cancers such as breast cancers, small cell carcinoma of the bronchus and brain tumours.

The toxicity of the drug is mainly neurological and peripheral neuropathy is an almost invariable sequel to long term administration. It is especially likely to occur in the elderly and those with liver disease, and may be severe and incapacitating. Loss of reflexes and paraesthesia occur early and are not usually regarded as indications for cessation of treatment, but severe myalgic and neuritic pain and motor weakness and/or peripheral sensory loss are signs that treatment should be stopped. Nerve conduction is usually preserved even with severe neuropathy, but electromyography shows a pattern of denervation. Cranial nerve palsies are occasionally encountered. Neurons are rich in tubulin, which appears to be important for axonal transport. It is postulated that vincristine blocks the passage of tubulin from proximal to distal axonal sites. Autonomic neuropathy often occurs, with constipation and ileus; symptoms can be partially alleviated with bulk laxatives. Myelosuppression is mild, increasing the usefulness of the drug when used in combination. Alopecia occurs in 20% of patients and a syndrome of inappropriate release of ADH occurs. The drug sometimes causes thrombocytosis.

Vinblastine (Velbe) After intravenous injection the drug disappears from the plasma in three phases with half-lives of 4 minutes, 1 hour and 16 hours. Much of the drug remains tissue-bound for many days. In the blood it binds to platelets, red cells and plasma proteins. All vinca alkaloids behave in a similar manner and clinical differences cannot be explained on pharmacokinetic grounds.

Indications for the use of vinblastine are similar to those for vincristine. In addition, vinblastine is often used in high dose for the treatment of testicular teratoma in combination with cisplatin and bleomycin (see Chapter 19). In these high doses neutropenia and ileus are common. Vinblastine causes more myelosuppression but less neurotoxicity than vincristine. The usual intravenous dose is 6 mg/m² weekly. Extravasation leads to cellulitis. Alopecia and mucositis are infrequent side effects.

Vindesine (*Eldisine*) This new semisynthetic addition to the vinca alkaloids has a similar spectrum of activity but appears to have additional activity in non-small cell lung cancer making it a useful agent in diseases where response to chemotherapy is generally disappointing. The toxicity of the drug appears similar to that of vinblastine and vincristine. Myelosuppression and neurotoxicity both occur.

Epipodophyllotoxin derivatives—VP16-213 (etoposide) and VM26 (vepesid) These substances are semisynthetic derivatives of extracts of *Podophyllum peltatum*—the American mandrake. Epipodophyllotoxin itself binds to tubulin probably at the same site as colchicine. In contast the two derivatives, VM26 and VP16-213, seem to prevent the cells from entering mitosis from G_2. The drugs have an early rapid phase of clearance followed by a slower phase (t/2 11–39 hours for VM26 and 2–13 hours for VP16-213). They enter the CSF in low concentration. VP16-213 (etoposide) is the drug most widely used at present. It is absorbed erratically from the gut with a plasma availability of about 50% of the i.v. dose which must be adjusted accordingly. The drug can be infused at high dose and its efficacy may be increased by this. However, mucositis then becomes dose limiting. At conventional doses bone marrow suppression is the major toxicity. VP16-213 is highly protein bound and about half of the drug is excreted in the urine in 72 hours. Unopened ampoules are stable for 2 years. After dilution it is stable for about 24 hours depending on the concentration. A commonly used intravenous schedule is 120 mg/m² on days 1, 3 and 5 repeated every 4 weeks.

The drugs have a similar spectrum of activity to the vinca alkaloids and are useful in treatment of lymphomas, acute leukaemias, small cell lung cancer, testicular and brain tumours. Etoposide is one of the more active drugs in squamous cell lung cancer. The toxic effects are alopecia, leucopenia, nausea and vomiting, febrile reactions and peripheral neuropathy.

ANTITUMOUR ANTIBIOTICS

A wide variety of antitumour antibiotics has now been produced from bacterial and fungal cultures. They produce their effect by binding to DNA.

Actinomycin D (*dactinomycin*) This antibiotic was first isolated from *Streptomyces* in 1940. At low concentrations it blocks DNA-directed RNA synthesis and at higher concentration also blocks DNA synthesis. The drug does not react directly with RNA. The molecule intercalates between guanine-cytosine base pairs and the transcription of DNA is blocked. The drug inhibits the division of all rapidly dividing cells. Resistance appears to be associated both with impaired drug entry and a failure of retention of the drug within the cell.

It is given intravenously and is cleared within a few minutes. The usual daily dose is 15 µg/kg and this can be repeated daily for 4–5 days. A further course of injections can be given 3–4 weeks later. It is however, more usual to give the drug as a single injection of 15 µg/kg in combination with other agents (such as vincristine and cyclophosphamide).

Its main use has been in the treatment of childhood cancers, such as rhabdomyosarcoma, Wilms' tumour and Ewing's sarcoma. It is of less value in adult tumours. The toxicities are nausea and vomiting, myelosuppression, mucositis and diarrhoea. It sensitizes tissue to radiation and should not be given concomitantly with radiotherapy.

Doxorubicin (Adriamycin) and daunorubicin (Cerubidin) (10) These are anthracycline antibiotics produced from a species of *Streptomyces* fungus. Doxorubicin is a useful agent with a wide spectrum of activity against many tumours and differs from daunorubicin only in the substitution of an —OH group for a hydrogen atom.

Both drugs bind tightly to DNA, deforming the helical structure. The drugs intercalate between base pairs but there appears to be no base specificity in the binding. Breaks in DNA strands have also been shown to occur. The drugs also produce highly active intracellular free radicals and these may be important in producing some of the toxic effects, for example, cardiac toxicity. Resistance to the action of anthracyclines is poorly understood. Despite markedly different spectra of clinical activity there appears to be complete cross-resistance between these two drugs as well as some degree of cross-resistance with vinca alkaloids and actinomycin, possibly related to decreased entry into the cell. The drugs are effective mainly against cells in S phase.

Both drugs are injected intravenously into a fast-running drip, and are highly vesicant. They are cleared rapidly from the plasma, but there is a slow terminal clearance of doxorubicin. There is rapid uptake into spleen, kidney, lungs, liver and heart, but not into the brain. The drugs are metabolized in the liver and severe toxicity may result if they are given to patients with impaired liver function. With doxorubicin, 40% is excreted in the bile as free drug, adriamycinol and other metabolites. With both drugs the major and acute side effects are bone marrow depression, nausea and vomiting, mucositis, alopecia and gastro-intestinal disturbance. Alopecia can be lessened by cooling the scalp with ice packs for 25 minutes before and after drug administration. The most important chronic and dose limiting side-effect is cardiotoxicity causing arrhythmias and heart failure. It is related to the total dose administered and is not a major risk below a total dose of 500 mg/ m^2. There is some evidence that irradiation over the heart adds to this risk.

Daunorubicin is of value in the treatment of acute lymphoblastic and myeloblastic leukaemia. Dosage schedules vary but 50 mg/m^2 once weekly is often given. Doxorubicin has a wide spectrum of activity in childhood and adult tumours including lymphomas, small cell bronchogenic carcinoma, adenocarcinomas of ovary breast and stomach, bone and soft tissue sarcomas, liver and bladder cancer.

Mitoxantrone This is an anthraquinone related to doxorubicin which binds to DNA. When injected intravenously it has a terminal half-life of 36 hours. It is vesicant and has a spectrum of activity similar to doxorubicin with useful effects in metastatic breast cancer, lymphoma and leukaemia. The main toxicity is myelosuppression. It causes less alopecia than doxorubin and possibly less cardiotoxicity. The usual single dose schedule is 12–15 mg/m^2 repeated every 3 weeks.

Mithramycin This antibiotic is derived from *Streptomyces plicatus*. Its clinical use is mainly in the treatment of hypercalcaemia, but it also has activity against embyonal carcinoma of the testis. It inhibits RNA synthesis, possibly in a manner similar to that to actinomycin D. The drug is cleared rapidly from the circulation, chiefly by Kupffer cells and renal tubular cells. It crosses the blood-brain barrier and penetrates into brain tumours. It is locally irritant, is inactive orally, and is therefore given intravenously.

The hypocalcaemic effect of mithramycin appears to result from interference with bone resorption by osteoclasts. In full doses (25 μg/kg) it causes nausea, stomatitis, thrombocytopenia, a haemorrhagic tendency and impaired renal and liver function. The dose used to treat hypercalcaemia is lower and the drug has been successfully used to treat Paget's disease in doses of 15 μg/kg daily for 3 days. Weekly doses of 15 μg/kg can be given safely without serious toxicity and will often control hypercalcaemia refractory to steroids.

Bleomycin This antibiotic is a mixture of glycopeptides isolated from *Streptomyces verticillus* but has now been chemically synthesized. The commercial bleomycin consists mainly of bleomycin A_2. The drug inhibits DNA synthesis and causes breaks in the DNA chain. It arrests cells in G_2, and this has led to attempts to use it to synchronize cells for subsequent chemotherapeutic attack, though little therapeutic advance has come from this approach.

The drug can be given parenterally by any route. It disappears from the plasma with an initial t/2 of 1 hour and then more slowly (t/2 9 hours). It is excreted in the urine and caution is needed with impaired renal function. The drug concentration is very low in the brain and CSF and it appears to be concentrated mainly in skin and lung. Many tissues contain an inactivating enzyme which hydrolyses the drug, and the levels of this enzyme appear to correlated with resistance. It is active in squamous carcinomas of the head and neck, skin and cervix and against lymphomas and testicular tumours. Responses are short-lived when it is used as a single agent.

The drug is valuable in combination with other agents because it causes little bone marrow toxicity. Skin toxicity is characterized by pigmentation, erythema and vesiculation. It also causes mucosal ulceration, pulmonary infiltrates and fibrosis. These toxic effects are serious, sometimes disabling and are related to total dose, with a high risk when the dose exceeds 300 mg/m². Acute pyrexial reactions commonly occur, and can be relieved or prevented by hydrocortisone. Rarely, cardiorespiratory collapse occurs. A small subcutaneous test dose at the start of treatment is a wise precaution.

The dosage schedule varies considerably but is usually of the order of 15 mg/m² as a single dose which can be repeated weekly.

MISCELLANEOUS AGENTS

Cis-Diammine Dichloroplatinum (*cisplatin, DDP*) Following the observation by Rosenbergthat certain platinum complexes inhibited bacterial replication, cisplatin was synthesized and shown to be active in experimental tumours (11). The drug is only active in the *cis* form. It diffuses into cells and the chloride ions are then lost from the molecule. The compound then binds to DNA with cross-linking of the strands similar to an alkylating agent. The binding appears mainly to be guanine groups. The drug is administered i.v. and the early t/2 is about 40 minutes and the later phase of clearance is slow (t/2 60 hours). It is 90% bound to plasma protein, and it taken up in the kidney, gut, liver, ovary and testis but not in the CNS.

The drug is highly nephrotoxic, and when administered in high dose a high urine flow is essential with i.v. fluids being administered before the drug and for 24 hours after. Renal function may worsen during repeated cycles and the plasma creatinine level and clearance should be checked regularly. Nausea and vomiting are severe with higher doses, and ototoxicity may be irreversible so that pretreatment audiometry should be carried out if treatment is to continue. Myelosuppression is not severe.

The drug is highly effective in the treatment of testicular tumours, and, in combination with vinblastine and bleomycin has revolutionized the outlook in advanced disease (see Chapter 19). It is also effective in cancer of the ovary and bladder as well as in lymphomas and small cell carcinoma of the bronchus. It is active in osteosarcoma and squamous cancer of the head and neck. It is not clear, however, if the drug is more effective than large doses of conventional alkylating agents in these diseases. Recently new platinum analogues have been developed which appear to have similar activity but much less renal toxicity.

L-Asparaginase (Crasnitine, Elspar) When L-asparaginase was first shown to have antitumour effects, it was hoped that this might prove to be an agent acting exclusively on malignant cells. The enzyme is produced by *Escherichia coli* and *Erwinia carotovora* and its action is based on the observation that while most normal tissues synthesize asparagine, some tumour cells need an exogenous source which the enzyme removes. Resistance may be related to the appearance of asparagine synthetase in the tumour cells.

The drug is initially eliminated rapidly from the circulation but the later t/2 is 6–30 hours. It does not penetrate into the CSF. There is no marrow, gut, or hair follicle toxicity but anaphylaxis, pancreatitis, hyperglycaemia, raised liver enzymes with fatty change in the liver, confusion, somnolence, coma, and hypofibrinogenaemia all occur and the drug is extremely nauseating.

The main use of the drug is in remission induction in acute lymphoblastic leukaemia. The dosage schedules vary considerably with different combinations of drugs.

Procarbazine (Natulan) This drug is the most useful of the hydrazine derivatives which were originally synthesized as mono-amine oxidase inhibitors and found to have antitumour activity. It causes inhibition of action in DNA and RNA, and protein synthesis is depressed. The mode of action is, however, unclear. Metabolic activation is needed and the active product may be a methyldiazonium ion which acts as a alkylating agent. The drug oxidises at 37°C and hydrogen peroxide is formed but does not appear to be responsible for the cytotoxic effect. Interphase is prolonged and mitosis is suppressed with breakage of chromatin strands occurring.

The drug is very well absorbed from the gut, and rapidly equilibrates with blood and CSF. After i.v. injection the t/2 is 7 minutes and the drug is rapidly metabolized. The toxic effects are nausea and vomiting, leucopenia, CNS disturbances especially psychological upsets, flushing with alcohol, and hypertensive reactions to foods rich in tyramine.

The drug is usually given in a dose of 100 mg/m² daily for 1–2 weeks. It is especially useful in Hodgkin's disease and brain tumours.

Hydroxyurea (Hydrea) This drug was synthesized over 100 years ago, but was only found to have antineoplastic activity much later. It blocks the action of ribonucleoside diphosphate reductase and thereby interfers with DNA synthesis. It causes leucopenia and megaloblastic changes in the bone marrow. It is S phase specific, and has been used in attempts to produce cell synchrony.

The drug is well-absorbed orally and enters the CSF. It is excreted in the urine. The usual dose is 20–30 mg/kg/day, or 80 mg/kg every 3 days. Toxic effects are mainly marrow suppression and gut disturbances. Its main use is in chronic granulocytic leukaemia resistant to other forms of therapy.

Hexamethylmelamine Although this drug has a similar structure to the alkylating agent triethylene melamine, it does not act as an alkylating agent itself. Indeed its mechanism of action remains largely unknown. It is well-absorbed orally and is rapidly metabolized.

The drug is administered in 2–3 week cycles of 12 mg/kg/day and is active in ovarian and cervical cancer. Nausea, vomiting and neurotoxicity are major problems with its use. Abdominal cramps and diarrhoea occur and leucopenia may develop. CNS toxicity includes altered mental state, extra-pyramidal effects and convulsions.

Razoxane (ICRF 159) This drug is a chelating agent but little is known of its method of action. It appears to block the early phases of mitosis. Experimentally it has been observed that it may prevent metastases in certain animal tumours, for example, Lewis' lung carcinoma, possibly by interfering with the tumour vascular supply.

The drug is not well-absorbed, is extensively metabolized and is largely excreted by the kidney. It has some activity in lymphomas and leukaemia but its clinical role is not established. Its toxicity includes bone marrow depression, alopecia and gut disturbance and it has been found to be leukaemogenic in man.

The administration of cytotoxic agents

There is much to be said against the occasional chemotherapist. Most surgeons, gynaecologists and physicians are quite unfamiliar with cytotoxic agents and when they attempt to use them, often run into difficulty because of lack of experience and also because of the lack of an appropriate organization to give drugs, check on blood counts and inquire into side-effects. Just as hospitals concentrate expertise in other activities—diabetic clinics, endoscopy clinics, coronary care units—so, for best results, they should bring chemotherapy into the hands of those expert in its administration.

It is our practice to separate patients needing chemotherapy into three groups:

Patients on outpatient regimens. The majority of patients can receive their drugs in this way especially if the person giving them is the same each time and gets to know the best anti-emetic or sedative regimen *for that patient.* Some patients are not sick at all, others vomit several hours later and prefer to get home quickly and take a phenothiazine and sleep it off, others vomit at the sight of the needle and require a premedication with diazepam and prochlorperazine. There is little doubt that trained nurses are the best people to give the drugs. They become very expert in putting up intravenous infusions and noting side-effects from previous drug treatment, and there are seldom difficulties with extravasation. Newly qualified house staff are not nearly so capable or as accessible to the patient during the day.

Patients undergoing cytotoxic chemotherapy should be aware of the nature of the treatment and its possible hazards. It is easier to make sure that patients receive adequate information if the treatment is the responsibility of a single department. The patient should be told of the nature of the drugs, what the possible side-effects might be and which of these effects should lead him to contact the hospital. This can be done in a way which is not frightening. For example, he should be told to report fever or sore throat so that a blood count can be taken. It is often worthwhile supplying explanatory leaflets about chemotherapy, and drug cards giving the names, dosage and purposes of the drugs are very useful.

Patients staying overnight. Some regimens such as those containing platinum, or a methotrexate infusion, require an overnight stay. It is convenient and efficient to have designated overnight-stay beds for this kind of chemotherapy where the admission is planned in advance and is relatively informal. It is our practice to have the ward chemotherapy nurse give the drugs after the patient has been seen by a doctor, and to book the next admission.

Patients on lengthy regimens. These patients, many of whom are on treatments where there is a serious possibility of prolonged myelosuppression, are admitted in the usual way. They are under the care of a single team, experienced in the use of intensive cytotoxic regimens, familiar with the supportive techniques required (see Chapter 8) and in mitigating the side-effects of the drugs.

Thus organization should be the responsibility of a senior member of staff whose particular interest is the medical treatment of cancer. In some hospitals this will be a radiotherapist or a haematologist, in others a medical oncologist. A lot of hardship can be caused by inexpert treatment and inefficient organization.

Chemotherapy-induced vomiting

Vomiting appears to be initiated from a centre in the lateral reticular formation in the medulla. There are several stimulatory pathways including a chemotherapy trigger area adjacent to the fourth ventricle which contains histamine receptors (H1 and H2). H1 antagonists have anti-emetic properties. Drugs with dopamine-blocking activity are also anti-emetic.

Intravenous alkylating agents, doxorubicin and cisplatin typically produce nausea and vomiting 2–8 hours after injection and the symptoms persist for 8–36 hours. Other drugs do not cause vomiting so frequently. After one or two cycles of chemotherapy some patients suffer from anticipatory nausea and vomiting at the sight of the nurse, doctor, intravenous infusion or hospital or even on setting out on the journey to hospital. In these patients prophylactic anti-emetic therapy must be given a considerable time before chemotherapy.

There are several different types of drugs which can be used to prevent or treat vomiting (Table 6.4). None is satisfactory in all patients and most are only partially effective. Anti-emetic therapy should be started prophylactically and often a satisfactory regimen can be established in each individual patient by trial and error.

Piperazine phenothiazines. These include prochlorperazine and perphenazine. They are effective anti-emetics in some patients but need to be used near the maximum dose, at which point extrapyramidal reactions are common particularly with i.v. administration.

Aliphatic phenothiazines. The most commonly used agents are chlorpromazine and promazine. They have more sedative and less anti-emetic properties and are more liable to produce hypotension.

Metoclopramide. This drug appears to act on the trigger area, possibly through blocking dopamine receptors. It increases gastric emptying. The drug can be given i.m. or i.v. and may cause extrapyramidal side-effects, restlessness and diarrhoea. In low dose (10 mg orally or i.v.) it has little activity.

There has been recent interest in the use of metoclopramide in very high dose in the prevention of vomiting. It is probable that it is more effective at high dose and some studies have shown it to be more effective than phenothiazines.

Table 6.4. Anti-emetic agents

Drug	Dose	Action	Toxicity
Metoclopramide	10 mg p.o. or i.v. or 1–2 mg/kg i.v. repeated 3 hourly	Dopamine antagonist (central and peripheral)	Extrapyramidal symptoms, diarrhoea
Butyrophenones e.g. Haloperidol	0.5–1 mg p.o. or i.v. repeated 4–8 hours	?Dopamine antagonist	Extrapyramidal symptoms, akasthesia
Dexamethasone	10–20 mg i.v. before treatment	Unclear	Restlessness, mood changes
Phenothiazines e.g. Prochlorperazine	12.5 mg i.m. or 25 mg suppository	Dopamine antagonist	Extrapyramidal syndromes, drowsiness
Benzodiazepines e.g. Lorazepam	1–2 mg p.o. or i.v. every 4–6 hours	Cerebral cortex	Sedation, hypotension
Cannabinoids e.g. THC	5–10 mg/m² every 4–6 hours	? histamine receptor blocking agent	Hallucinations, dysphoria, dizziness, ataxia

Benzodiazepines. Although these drugs have no anti-emetic properties they may make the vomiting more tolerable by inducing a somnolent state in which the patient cannot remember the period of nausea clearly. Intravenous lorazepam is useful for this purpose.

Cannabinoids. Delta-9-tetrahydrocannabinol (THC) is an effective anti-emetic whose site of action is unknown. Synthetic analogues have been developed of which the first, nabilone, is under investigation. It seems probable that the anti-emetic effect becomes less powerful with repeated usage and that the dose of THC needs to be at least that which will also cause a mild euphoric state. Side-effects of hallucination and dizziness are troublesome.

Butyrophenone derivatives. These drugs are dopamine receptor blocking agents which work centrally. Haloperidol is the most widely used and is partially effective against cisplatin induced vomiting.

Long-term complications of cancer chemotherapy

More children and young adults are now surviving diseases such as acute leukaemia, lymphoma and testicular cancer which were formerly incurable. Survival has been achieved by intensive combination chemotherapy. It has become apparent that chemotherapy of this type is associated with long-term complications in some patients. The recognition of these sequelae has emphasized that treatment of great intensity may not always achieve the best long-term results and that such drug and radiation therapies must be restricted to those categories of patients in which they are essential for survival. Long-term follow-up of patients is essential since some of the complications may develop many years after treatment is discontinued.

IMPAIRED GONODAL FUNCTION

Suppression of spermatogenesis occurs in the majority of men being treated with combination chemotherapy (12). Procarbazine and alkylating agents seem to have the greatest adverse effect, methotrexate and doxorubicin less so. The degree of infertility and its permanence vary with different regimens. With MOPP therapy for Hodgkin's disease (Chapter 25) 95% of men will have long lasting infertility. With the ABVD regimen this is less so, and with the PVB regimen for teratoma there is frequent recovery of fertility. It is not yet clear how the suppression of spermatogenesis will be. Damage to the germinal epithelium is associated with a rise in serum FSH (which normally stimulates spermatogenesis). While pre-pubertal boys do not appear to experience long-lasting endocrine changes from chemotherapy, intensive chemotherapy during puberty damages Leydig cells and is accompanied by a rise in both FSH and LH, low testosterone levels and gynaecomastia.

Ovarian failure is often produced by combination chemotherapy and is more frequent the nearer the patient is to her natural menopause. Even if menstruation does not cease, subfertility is common. As with testicular failure, alkylating agents and procarbazine appear to be more likely to cause ovarian failure than antimetabolites.

PULMONARY FIBROSIS

Pulmonary damage is produced by many cytotoxic drugs (see Table 6.5). Most alkylating agents will produce pulmonary fibrosis with long-term impairment of diffusing capacity (13). Busulphan is however far more likely to do so than other drugs. Bleomycin causes pulmonary infiltrates, a total-dose related phenomenon which is very common over $300\,mg/m^2$. Usually these infiltrates will disappear when the drug is stopped but permanent fibrosis may follow.

LIVER DISEASE

Many drugs cause a transient rise in plasma enzymes (nitrosoureas, cytosine arabinoside) but permanent hepatic dysfunction is rare. Per-

Table 6.5. Pulmonary and hepatic toxicity of cytotoxic drugs.

Drug	Effect
Pulmonary	
Busulphan	Fibrosis
(*and other alkylating agents*)	
Bleomycin	Pulmonary infiltrates and fibrosis
Mitomycin C	Pulmonary infiltrates and fibrosis
Hepatic	
Methotrexate	Fibrosis
6MP and azathioprine	Cholestatic jaundice and necrosis
Asparaginase	Fatty infiltration

manent liver damage can occasionally occur with antimetabolites (Table 6.5).

SECOND CANCERS

Second malignancies have been noted after long-term administration of alkylating agents particularly melphalan and chlorambucil. Particularly in patients with ovarian cancer and myeloma (14). In both cases there is an increased risk of acute myeloid leukaemia.

In patients treated intensively for Hodgkin's disease there is also an increased risk of acute myeloid leukaemia. The risk appears to be greater for men over the age of 40 and for patients treated with both combination chemotherapy and radiotherapy where the risk is 18 times that of the normal population (15).

Bladder cancer is a reported complication of cyclophosphamide therapy but the risk appears to be very small.

Long-term immnosuppressive therapy in renal allograft recipients also predisposes to the development of cancer (16). Lymphomas are the commonest malignancy, particularly large cell lymphoma of the brain. The average time of onset is 2 years but the risk persists indefinitely.

The mechanisms whereby chemotherapy induces cancer are not known. Hodgkin's disease is associated with a slight increase in acute leukaemia even in patients not treated with chemotherapy. Postulated mechanisms are a direct carcinogenic effect of the drugs, diminished 'immune surveillance' and activation of oncogenic viruses in immune suppressed individuals.

CARDIAC DAMAGE

Anthracycline drugs produce cardiomyopathy. Doxorubicin binds to the membrane of myocardial cells and induces changes in function. Spectrin and cardiolipid appear to be the target molecules. The functional changes are not clear. Sodium transport may be affected and damage from free-radicals may occur.

There is no simple and accurate way of predicting cardiac damage in patients on treatment although a drop in voltage on the ECG does have some correlation with cardiomyopathy. Mediastinal irradiation and hypertension predispose to cardiac damage from doxorubicin.

Clinically arrythmias and conduction disturbances occur in acute toxicity as may acute myocarditis and pericarditis. With each dose of doxorubicin cardiac damage progresses and half of all patients will have functional damage by the time a dose of $500\,mg/m^2$ is reached. Only 5% of these patients will develop cardiac symptoms. Clinically evident cardiomyopathy is irreversible and progressive cardiac failure is frequent (17).

PRINCIPLES OF HORMONE THERAPY

The demonstration by Beatson in 1896 that inoperable breast cancer sometimes regressed after oöphorectomy was one of the most remarkable discoveries in the history of cancer treatment (18). Many years later Huggins demonstrated that metastatic prostatic cancer would regress with orchidectomy or the administration of oestrogens (19). A rational basis for the use of hormone manipulation in cancer treatment has, however, been hampered by lack of knowledge of how hormones act on cancer cells and of which cancer cells are likely to be affected. In the last 10 years, there has been a transformation in our understanding and in at least one tumour—breast cancer—knowledge of the hormone receptor status of the tumour has become clinically important.

Steroid hormone receptors

It is now clear that there are receptor proteins for steroid hormones both in the cytoplasm and the nucleus and that interaction between the hormone and its receptor modifies DNA activity and hence cell growth and replication. These events are depicted diagrammatically in Fig. 6.13.

The steroid hormone, unbound to plasma protein, crosses the cell membrane by a mechanism which is not well understood. The hormone then links to the cytoplasmic receptor protein and the complex undergoes a conformational change either in the cytoplasm or in the nucleus. This hormone/receptor complex binds to a nuclear protein which in turn exerts a controlling activity on DNA. There then follows an increase in RNA polymerase activity which results in the synthesis, first of messenger RNA (m RNA), and then cytoplasmic protein. After 24 hours DNA synthesis occurs, followed by cell division.

This model appears to be generally applicable to a variety of steroid hormones. There is also evidence that the synthesis of the receptor proteins is promoted by the hormone to which they bind and that other hormones can reduce the synthesis of receptor proteins; for example,

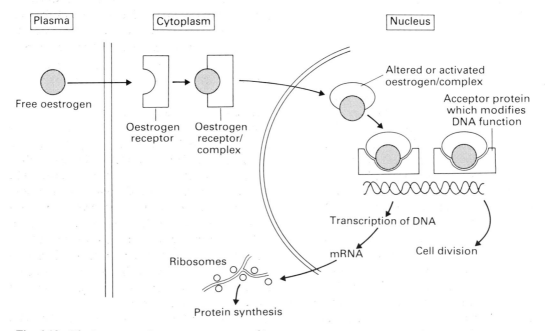

Fig. 6.13. *The interaction between oestrogen and its receptor.*

progesterone inhibits the synthesis of oestrogen receptor.

Using these concepts of hormone action, several strategies for modifying tumour growth can be developed: The plasma concentration of the stimulating hormone might be lowered by ablative therapy, either surgical, radiotherapeutic or chemical. Once the hormone has entered the cell it may be prevented from binding to the receptor either by competitive inhibitors or by reduction of receptor synthesis. It might also be possible to block the binding of the complex to the nuclear 'acceptor' protein.

In practise it is often difficult to determine the site of action of agents used in hormone therapy. Tamoxifen, for example, appears to bind to the oestrogen receptor but may also affect its synthesis and the tamoxifen/receptor complex may also block the acceptor site in the nucleus.

The situation may become clearer when it is possible to measure the concentration of receptor molecules independently of their hormone binding properties, for example, by monoclonal antibodies. It may then be possible to say whether lack of oestrogen binding, for example, is due to lack of receptor protein or to lack of free binding sites.

Hormone receptor assays

Attempts to use the presence of a hormone receptor to predict the responsiveness of an individual tumour to hormone manipulation have been only partially successful. To some extent this is due to the difficulties and lack of standardization of the assay techniques. The usual assay is a measure of uptake of isotopically labelled hormone by homogenized tumour cells. The degree of binding varies and an arbitrary cut-off point has to be made in what is in fact a gradation from negative to positive. In studies on tissue sections it can be shown that in breast cancer some cells are oestrogen receptor (ER) positive and others negative. The overall expression of ER status is thus an oversimplication of the position. Furthermore, the presence of hormone receptors does not prove that they are functionally active. Oestrogen promotes the synthesis of progesterone receptor (PR) in breast cancer cells, and measurement of PR may thus provide a better measure of functionally active oestrogen receptor than measurement of ER itself. At present it is clear that in, for example, breast cancer, the absence (or very low values) of an oestrogen receptor strongly predicts a lack of response to hormone manipulation, and that high levels of receptor are indicative of probable response. Intermediate values are associated with a variable response rate.

The role of hormone therapy in individual tumours is discussed in detail in the appropriate chapters.

Approaches to hormone therapy

1 *Lowering the plasma hormone concentration.* This may be done by surgical or medical means: *Surgical* Oöphorectomy (surgical or radiotherapeutic) will abolish oestrogen secretion by the ovary in premenopausal women and was widely used as a first step in hormone treatment of advanced breast cancer. Knowledge of the oestrogen receptor status is useful because the likelihood of response in ER +ve tumours is 50% compared with only 5% of ER −ve tumours in whom the procedure is not worthwhile.

Adrenalectomy sometimes produces further responses in premenopausal patients with advanced breast cancer responding to oöphorectomy. This is probably due to residual sex hormone synthesis by the adrenal. The tumour response occurs despite adequate glucocorticoid replacement. Hypophysectomy produces a similar effect. Both of these operations are less commonly performed since the advent of aromatase inhibitors (see below). Orchidectomy is effective in reducing plasma testosterone levels and is widely used as treatment for metastatic prostatic carcinoma.

Medical In premenopausal women the main source of oestrogens is the ovary, but some oestrogens are formed as a result of the peripheral conversion of androgens, formed in the adrenal. This conversion takes place in muscle, liver, and fat and is mediated by aromatase enzymes. After the menopause the adrenal becomes the main source of oestrogens by production of androgen (delta-4-androstenedione) which is converted in the peripheral tissues. However, the adrenal is not the only source of oestrogen precursors, and breast tissue itself can synthesize oestrogens. Aminoglutethimide blocks the action of aromatase enzymes and also depresses synthesis of androgens and cortisol in the adrenal itself. Premenopausal women (whose major source of oestrogen synthesis is the ovary which is not dependent on aromatase enzymes) do not respond to aminoglutethimide.

Approximately 30% of postmenopausal women will respond and the response rate of bone metastases is particularly striking (55%) while liver metastases are less responsive (20%). Toxicity includes somnolence, transient skin rash, and muscle cramps. Aminoglutethimide has been shown to be as effective as adrenalectomy in advanced breast cancer.

2 *Blocking the action of circulating hormones.* Anti-oestrogens, of which the most notable example is tamoxifen, have been a major advance in the treatment of metastatic breast cancer. The mode of action of tamoxifen is ill understood. The drug appears to exert its effect by binding with the cytoplasmic oestrogen receptor but its affinity for the ER is much less than that of oestrogen itself. Possibly the drug-receptor complex undergoes a conformational change which blocks its entry to nuclear sites of activity. Other receptor sites which bind tamoxifen but not oestrogen have also been described, however the balance of evidence at present suggests that tamoxifen exerts its effect by competitively binding with ER thus displacing oestradiol. Tamoxifen does not increase plasma oestradiol levels in postmenopausal women but does do so in premenopausal women. Tamoxifen has a prolonged terminal half-life in plasma and after 1 month of treatment the plasma concentration exceeds

that of oestradiol by up to a thousand fold. It is for this reason that a dose-response effect is not usually observed clinically. Toxic effects are uncommon the most frequent being mild nausea and hot flushes. Occasionally a flare-up of the breast cancer may be seen which is then sometimes followed by a response. Megestrol acetate is a synthetic anti-androgen. It blocks the synthesis of testosterone, reducing plasma testosterone levels. Adrenal androgens (androstenedione) are also reduced. The drug also blocks the action of testosterone on prostatic carcinoma cells and this is a further mechanism for its action in the disease.

3 *Additive hormone therapies.* In breast cancer these include oestrogens, androgens, glucocorticoids and progestogens. The fact that ER + ve breast cancers will regress with exogenous oestrogen indicates that we still have considerable gaps in our knowledge of the mechanism of action in hormone therapies. Medroxyprogesterone acetate and megestrol acetate produce responses in about 20% of patients. They possibly do this by lowering the cytoplasmic ER content and responses are usually only seen in ER + ve tumours, but appear independent of progesterone receptor status. Progesterone derivatives produce responses in about 30% of uterine carcinomas usually in cases which are ER + ve or PR + ve.

REFERENCES

1 Gilman A. (1963) The initial clinical trial of nitogen mustard. *American Journal of Surgery*, **105**, 574–8.
2 Frei E. (1972) Combination cancer therapy. *Cancer Research* **32**, 2593.
3 Skipper H. E., Schabel F. M. & Wilcox W. S. (1964) Experimental evaluation of potential anticancer agents XIII on the criteria and kinetics associated with 'curability of experimental leukaemia, *Cancer Chemotherapy Report* **35**, 1.
4 De Vita V. T., Serpick A. A. & Carbone P. P. (1970) Combination chemotherapy in the treatment of advanced Hodgkin's disease. *Annals of Internal Medicine* **73**, 891–5.

5 Nowell P. C. (1976) The clonal evolution of tumour cell populations. *Science* **194**, 23.

6 Selby P., Buick R. N. & Tannock I. (1983) A critical appraisal of the 'human tumour stem-cell assay'. *New England Journal of Medicine* **308**, 129–34.

7 Pritchard J., McElwain T. J. & Graham-Pole J. (1982) High-dose mephalan with autologous marrow for treatment of advanced neuroblastoma. *British Journal of Cancer* **45**, 86.

8 Alt F. W., Kellems R. E., Bertino J. R. & Schimke R. T. (1978) Selective multipheation of dihydrofolate reductase genes in methotrexate-resistant variant of cultured murine cells. *Journal of Biological Chemistry* **253**, 1357.

9 Rosman M., Lee M. H., Creasy W. A. & Sartorelli A. C. (1974) Mechanisms of resistance to 6-thiopurines in human leukaemia. *Cancer Research* **134**, 1952.

10 Young R. C., Ozols R. F. & Myers C. E. (1981) The anthracycline antineoplastic drugs. Medical progress review. *New England Journal of Medicine* **305**, 139.

11 Symposium on platinum analogues (1979) *Cancer Treatment Reports* **63**, (9) 1431.

12 Chapman R. M., Sutcliffe S. B. & Malpas J. S. (1981) Male gonadal dysfunction in Hodgkin's disease. *Journal of the American Medical Association.* **245**, 1323.

13 Weiss R. B. & Muggia F. M. (1980) Cytotoxic drug-induced pulmonary disease. *American Journal of Medicine* **68**, 259.

14 Bergsagel D. E., Bailey A. J., Langley G. R., McDonald R. N., White D. F. & Miller A. B. (1979) The chemotherapy of plasma-cell myeloma and the incidence of acute leukaemia. *New England Journal of Medicine* **301**, *743.*

15 Canellos G. P., De Vita V. T., Arseneau J. C. Whang Peng J. & Johnson R. E. C. (1975) Second malignancies complicating Hodgkin's disease in remission. *Lancet* **i**, 947–50.

16 Sheil A. G. R. (1985) Cancer in organ transplant recipients: part of an induced immune deficiency syndrome. *British Medical Journal* **288**, 659–60.

17 Van Hoff D. O., Rozencweig M., Layard D. W. et al (1977) Daunomycin induced cardiotoxicity in children and adults. A review of 110 cases. *American Journal of Medicine* **62**, 200–10.

18 Beatson G. T. (1896) On the treatment of inoperable cases of carcinoma of the mamma. *Lancet* **ii**, 104.

19 Huggins C. & Hodges G. V. (1941) Studies on prostatic cancer 1. The effect of castration on serum phosphatases in metastate carcinoma of the prostate. *Cancer Research* **1**, 293.

FURTHER READING

Gilman A. G., Goodman L. S. & Gilman A. (1980) *The pharmacological basis of therapeutics*, 5th edn., Chap. 55, 61, 62, 63. Macmillan, London.

Pratt W. B. & Ruddon R. W. (1979) *The anticancer drugs.* Oxford University Press, Oxford.

Furr B. J. A. (1982) Hormone Therapy. *Clinics in Oncology* **1**, (1).

Nesbit M. E. (1985) Late effects in successfully treated children with cancer, *Clinics in Oncology* **4**, 2.

Chapter 7

Supportive Care and Symptom Relief

PSYCHOLOGICAL ASPECTS OF CANCER MANAGEMENT

Talking about the diagnosis and treatment

Major disease brings anxiety and worry, but few diseases are associated with such dread as cancer, with its imagined inevitable sequel of certain death, of pain, lingering and suffering. One of the most difficult, and most rewarding tasks for the physician is to set the disease in its right context, to explain the treatment, to give enough information at the correct rate and time, to sustain hope, and to be accessible, competent, open minded and, above all, kind.

It is easy to forget that the patient has a life outside the consulting room and that he will interpret what is said in the light of his own experience and apprehensions. Cancer is commonest in the elderly. In the course of a long life many patients will have had friends or relatives who have died of the disease or may perhaps have cared for a member of the family with cancer. These experiences will have an important influence on a patient's outlook and expectations. In recent years cancer and its treatment has been widely discussed in the media of mass communication. Although patients are better informed now than 20 years ago, their knowledge is often fragmentary and disorganized. Some patients may have recognized the seriousness of a sympyom—haemoptysis, unexplained weight loss, a lump, or back-ache, but be too anxious (or too afraid of surgery, etc) to voice their suspicions. Other patients may have no idea of the possible diagnosis.

As with patients, the attitude of physicians is influenced by their experience and training. Frequently the diagnosis of cancer is made by a specialist in another area such as general surgery, gynaecology or chest medicine. Some of these doctors may themselves have a very pessimistic view of cancer and what can be achieved by treatment. Furthermore, in hospital medicine the specialist has often had little opportunity to get to know the patient before the diagnosis has been made. A lack of familiarity both with what can be achieved by treatment and also with the patient, combined sometimes, with the fear of the disease, may lead the physician or surgeon into euphemisms and half-truths. Words may be used such as 'growth' or 'ulcer' to soften or obscure the diagnosis, while the doctor often betrays his real meaning by appearing evasive or unclear.

This attitude means that, unless the patient is bold and asks for a more frank statement of the diagnosis, the doctor may be unable to assess what impact his words have had, though the patient's face is usually very revealing. Because the meaning of the diagnosis is being avoided it becomes difficult to allow the patient to express his or her fears or ask the appropriate questions. The patient may in fact be under the impression that the diagnosis is worse than it actually is, that he has only a short time to live, or that treatment will be to no avail. The doctor's evasions may then strengthen this opinion. Another failing is that there will be many clues to the patient as to where the truth lies. He may learn the diagnosis from a pathology request form, from a hospital porter, a well meaning friend or an overheard remark. If the diagnosis is discovered accidentally the patient may realize that the intention behind concealment was to spare him anxiety, but will usually feel let down by the doctor and be cautious in accepting any further reassurance.

In recent years the attitude of cancer specialists has moved decisively towards a fuller discussion of the diagnosis and treatment. What is said to the patient must, however, be well-judged and carefully delivered. Every physician makes errors of judgement which shake his confidence with the next patient he sees, but it is important not to retreat from these discussions when difficulties have occurred. It is important to learn from one's mistakes.

If possible it is useful to assess the attitude of the patient before the diagnosis is made. Questions such as 'what do you feel is wrong with you' or 'have you any particular anxieties about what might be wrong' are often very revealing since the patient will sometimes admit to a fear of malignancy and, if so, it allows the physician to ask the patient whether, if this proves to be the diagnosis, he would want to know the details of what is found.

It is sometimes possible to make the diagnosis before major surgery is undertaken; by bronchoscopy for lung cancer, needle biopsy in breast cancer, endoscopy for gastro-intestinal disease. When the diagnosis has been established pre-operatively and treatment by surgery is necessary, it is hardly possible, still less desirable, that the diagnosis is not discussed and the probable operative procedure described. Often the diagnosis only becomes apparent after an operation and the patient will be waiting to hear the result. In either case when talking to the patient about the diagnosis, the doctor needs to have a clear idea of what he is going to say and the words he will use, though he must be prepared to modify the approach if the situation demands it.

In explaining the diagnosis the word 'cancer' is the only word which unequivocally conveys the nature of the complaint. Many physicians use the words 'malignancy', 'tumour' or 'growth' with the best of intentions, but this carries the risk that the patient will fail to realize the true nature of the disease (indeed this is often what is intended). Many patients have only a vague idea of what cancer means and are surprised that the disease is nearly always treatable and sometimes curable. The explanation of the diagnosis must be combined with a realistic but hopeful account of what can be done. Few patients can exist without hope of any kind. It is nearly always necessary to hold out the hope of cure or at least of a long period of healthy normal life even when the prognosis is poor. This does not mean that a cure is promised but that the patient can feel confident that every attempt will be made to cure him and that there is a possibility of success. Naturally, if it is likely that the patient will be cured this must be stressed and a much more optimistic account of the disease can be given.

The manner in which the explanation is given is critical. The doctor should be unhurried, speak clearly and not technically, look at the patient's face while speaking, and show that he is not frightened or discomfited by the diagnosis and indicate by look and gesture that he is competent and prepared to disscuss the problem calmly. There is a limit to the number of facts which a patient can assimilate during one conversation, particularly under stressful circumstances. Too much information may progressively extinguish the understanding which a short account would achieve. Not infrequently the patient may seem to understand, but in fact be too anxious to take in anything of what is being said. This failure of understanding is not 'denial' but is due to confusion and anxiety. It is a good policy to stop frequently and enquire if what is being said is clear or if there are questions which the patient wants to ask. When the patient is able to ask questions it implies that he or she has understood at least part of the explanation. The doctor should make it quite clear that he or a member of the team will always be pleased to answer questions and that he will talk again in a day or two. One discussion is seldom enough. It may take a few days for the patient to start to understand and to take a realistic view of his situation and at that stage want to know more. It is usually advisable therefore to impart the details of the diagnosis and treatment, over a period of time. The facts of the diagnosis are given first with a brief outline of treatment, gradually giving more information as the patient begins to come to terms with his position.

Some physicians ask relatives for advice on how much to tell the patient, particularly when they are in doubt about the correct approach. This can be helpful but there is a risk that the relatives may misjudge the patient and, out of love and sympathy, suggest that the truth be withheld when the patient would have wished otherwise. It is of course essential that relatives have a clear understanding of what has been said and why, and that the medical team do not give contradictory accounts. For this reason, after talking to the patient, the doctor should explain to the medical and nursing team exactly what has been said, with an idea of the words that have been used together with what the reaction has been. The same information should be conveyed to the relatives but the discussion about prognosis may have to be more pessimistic with relatives. We think it almost always wrong to give patients a prognosis measured in a finite time because they tend to remember the stated number of months or years however many qualifications are made, and such predictions are often incorrect.

The patient's reaction may be a mixture of acceptance, anxiety, anger and grief. Some of this emotion may be directed at the doctor and this is one of the challenges of the job. It is essential to be understanding and not to be irritated by unjustified hostility if it occurs. This demands a lot from the doctor who must have enough self-confidence and maturity to realize that, in the end, the patient will come to trust his honesty and rely on his support.

At a later stage the physician, while discussing the details of investigation and treatment, may wish to explain that an illness such as cancer will alter the patient's perception of himself.

That is, he will tend for a while to view himself as 'ill' and minor aches and pains which would previously have been ignored, may be magnified in his mind and be interpreted as symptoms of relapse. In explaining that this is an understandable but usually temporary phase, the physician should make it clear that he will be seeing the patient regularly and, if symptoms occur which cause anxiety, the patient should get in touch. The best cancer departments operate an 'open-door' policy of this type, eliminating a lot of bureaucratic difficulty for the patient who may otherwise be given an appointment weeks ahead for a problem which is immediate. The ideal arrangement is where the hospital specialist works in close collaboration with the family doctor in providing support and reassurance. The family practitioner may have long and invaluable experience of the patient and his family.

Whenever a patient visits, either for a regular review or because of a symptom, the physician should give equal priority to discussion as to the technical aspects of examination and investigation. It is greatly to be regretted that some doctors, and most health administrators, regard heavily booked clinics as a sign of efficiency. A 5 minute consultation with a cancer patient is nearly always bad medicine. These are conditions which may be forced upon doctors but should never be accepted by them.

Many cancer treatments have a bad reputation. Before the era of megavoltage equipment, high dose radiotherapy required multiple fields if severe skin reactions were to be avoided (see Chapter 5). Fear of being burnt or scarred by radiotherapy is very common and a careful explanation of modern advances is sometimes needed. Alopecia, nausea and vomiting are unpleasant side-effects of chemotherapy and increasing numbers of patients have heard of these and, understandably, fear them. If chemotherapy is judged necessary, then the reasons should be explained. Patients will easily grasp the idea that cancer may not be localized and that a systemic treatment is being given to prevent or treat any recurrence from cancer cells which may have spread to other sites. Indeed they often find the idea of a systemic as well as a local treatment, reassuring. The ways in which the side-effects can be mitigated should be clearly explained.

Although patients will usually accept the need for radiotherapy or chemotherapy they may find the reality worse than they had imagined. This is particularly true for chemotherapy which often goes on for many months. There can be few things more miserable than repeated, predictable episodes of severe nausea and vomiting. Many patients begin to feel that they cannot go through with treatment and then find themselves in a frightening dilemma. On the one hand they are fearful of jeopardizing their chance of cure and of disappointing the doctor, but on the other the side-effects may produce progressive demoralization. In the case of a potentially curative treatment, for example for Hodgkin's disease, testicular tumours or acute lymphoblastic leukaemia, the doctor must try to sustain the patient through the treatment and do all he can to see it completed. For many cancers of adult life the benefits of chemotherapy are, however, much less clear. In these cases the worst outcome is that a patient is made to feel wretched by the treatment and guilty at stopping, and is then frightened of the prospect that he or she has jeopardized the chance of survival. If relapse occurs there may be self-blame and depression. The responsibility for this situation is as much the doctor's as the patient's. When chemotherapy is being given without a reasonable prospect of cure and the patient cannot continue, the physician should be sympathetic and reassuring and explain that he does not feel let down by the patient or that the prognosis has been materially worsened.

There are few other branches of medicine which demand simultaneously such technical expertise and kindly understanding as does cancer medicine. The strains on the doctor are considerable, especially if he takes the human aspect of his work seriously. It is a great failing in a doctor if he talks to his patients only about the physical and technical aspects of the illness, relies heavily on investigation in making treatment decisions and finds it difficult to give up intensive measures and accept that the patient cannot be cured. Technical prowess has then replaced a thoughtful analysis of the patient's feelings and what is in his best interests.

Treating patients with cancer demands great resources of emotional energy on the part of the doctor. In some units, part of the work of talking to patients is taken over by psychiatrists, psychologists, social workers or other counsellors. Invaluable though help from these persons may be, we do not think it desirable that doctors should see themselves as technical experts and that when human feelings intrude into the medical situation, the patient should be sent to talk to someone else about their problems. Sustaining and counselling a patient and his relatives is a matter of teamwork, but the doctor in charge of the case must make it clear that he or she regards the psychological aspects of the disease as being as important as the physical. The special problems of dealing with children with cancer are discussed in Chapter 24.

SUPPORT, COUNSELLING AND REHABILITATION

With any disease it is important to put oneself in the patient's position and try to anticipate the problems which are likely to arise. For example, it may seem obvious that mastectomy is a mutilating operation and that some psychological support pre- and postoperatively will be necessary. Nevertheless, many women do not receive adequate advice from their doctors. What may be less obvious (until one thinks of it) is that husbands of women with mastectomy may be in need of explanation too. Indeed the reaction of a partner to the operation may be of fundamental importance in helping the patient to recover from her illness. Such advice is seldom offered.

In addition many patients with cancer face specific problems of rehabilitation as a result of surgical and other treatments. Rehabilitation and counselling are an essential part of the general care of cancer patients. In recent years specialized support services have developed to help patients overcome the effects of the illness and its treatment, and to return as far as possible to a normal life.

Stoma care

Successful treatment of cancer of the bowel or bladder will sometimes require permanent colostomy or ileostomy. Similarly in the treatment of gynaecological cancers, there will be a few patients in whom a permanent colostomy, resulting from radiation damage to the large bowel, is the price of a radiotherapy cure (see Chapter 17). Although some patients manage their stoma without difficulty, others require a great deal of education and help, and the role of the stoma therapist has now become established. Patients must learn not only how to keep the stoma clean and healthy, but also how to recognize the complications that might demand further surgical review, such as prolapse or stricture. Although a left-sided colostomy is relatively easy to manage, there are considerable difficulties with an ileostomy because of the fluid loss of 4–500 ml/day which can lead to electrolyte disturbance, dehydration (especially if gastro-intestinal infection occurs) and greater aesthetic difficulties. Surgery advances may yet lead to continent ileostomies, but at present most patients need to wear an appliance. The Colostomy Welfare Group and Ileostomy Association offer support and practical help.

Breast prostheses

Most large hospitals should now have some form of mastectomy counselling service, to provide not only psychological support for patients who have undergone mastectomy, but also to offer expert advice regarding external prostheses. Almost all patients, including those with very radical operations, can now, when clothed, disguise their defects since a wide variety of prostheses, brassières and swimsuits are available. A nurse/counsellor specializing in the problems of mastectomy is of great help and many patients will benefit from the advice available from the Mastectomy Association. Nonetheless, an increasing number of women are unhappy with any form of external prosthesis and request prosthetic implantation surgery which they hope will give them a more normal contour and the opportunity for more adventurous dress. Part of the mastectomy counsellor's job is to advise such patients that, contrary to their expection, following surgery they cannot expect to look completely normal.

Laryngectomy rehabilitation

Following total laryngectomy, the patient has to be taught how to create an oesophageal voice, using techniques of air swallowing and careful phonation which can only be acquired with the help of an experienced speech therapist. Although some patients find this straightforward, the majority require careful tuition, and some never achieve a satisfactory voice. For these patients, a vibrating device or 'artifical larynx' should be available. The vibrating device is held against the neck, and permits a vibrating column of air to be produced which, with careful phonation by the patient gives montonous, barely acceptable but comprehensible speech. In a few centres, permanent valves are now being implanted which increase the power and durability of speech. Although these experimental techniques may well have a place in the future rehabilitation of laryngectomy patients, it should be stressed that well taught oesophageal speech can be very acceptable indeed. The National Association of Laryngectomy Clubs may provide further helpful advice.

Limb prostheses

The regional limb fitting centres are responsible for providing both temporary and permanent external prostheses for those who have lost limbs whether through trauma or surgery. Traditionally, amputation has been the mainstay of treatment for bone and soft tissue sarcoma. Most patients, including children, adapt remarkably well to the loss of a limb, and many are able to drive a car, participate in sport, and lead a full and active life. In children, the limb must be replaced as the child grows and care must be taken with the details of weight, length, construction and fitting in order to avoid unequal pressure on the spine which might lead to scoliosis.

Other prostheses

Other sophisticated prostheses may also be necessary, particularly for patients with facial defects following radical surgery of the head and neck region. In particular, radical surgery for tumours of the maxillary antrum, orbit and nasal fossa, though curative, may result in substantial disfigurement which can only be covered by external prostheses. Remarkable results can be obtained but the work is highly specialized.

Home support

Learning how to use a colostomy bag or walk with an artificial limb is the start of a much more complex process of rehabilitation, in which the development of self reliance and self esteem needs encouragement. Whilst many patients achieve this with the help of their family, some are more isolated and require more professional help. The importance of, for example, a modified bathroom with supporting rails and wheelchair access may well be underestimated compared with the surgical and oncological challenge that the patient represented, but may help to make independent existence at home possible. District nursing help may allow patients to leave hospital relatively early after major operations, improving morale and reducing both the cost of the operation and also its morbidity from postoperative complications.

National counselling organisations

In a general hospital the work of counselling patients and their families is made easier if much of the inpatient treatment is in a specialized unit. In such a unit the nursing staff become very skilled in anticipating the problems of the disease and its treatment. When frequent admissions are necessary, for example for chemotherapy, it is of great help to the patient to see familiar faces. There is also a considerable benefit to be gained by having medical social workers who are especially skilled and interested in the problems of cancer. Not only do they provide another source of advice and reassurance but they will be knowledgeable about the local availability of counselling groups, nursing support, bereavement organizations and facilities for the care of the dying.

Self-help groups have arisen in many counties, organizing themselves nationally. Such groups have an enormous amount to offer, provided that they take care to give well-balanced and sensible advice,. Many patients find it very helpful to talk about their problems with fellow sufferers and much detailed practical advice may be given which few doctors are in a position to match.

The following are examples of such organizations in Britain.

The Mastectomy Association. Women who have had a mastectomy and give advice.

Malcolm Sargent Cancer Fund for Children. Advice and financial support to children with cancer and their families.

The Leukaemia Society. Started by parents of children with leukaemia and now helping adults.

The Ileostomy Association.

The Colostomy Welfare Group.

The Stoma Advisory Service.

The Marie Curie Fund. Provides nursing care to cancer patients in nursing homes and at home.

The National Association of Laryngectomy Clubs.

CRUSE. This is a counselling service which helps with the problems of bereavement.

CANCER TREATMENT AND THE QUALITY OF LIFE

Most cancer treatments are unpleasant, producing short and long term side-effects which interfere with the patient's quality of life. Assessment of the quality of life in cancer patients is not straightforward. Obvious criteria include length of time spent in hospital, the ability to get back to work, or at least to an independent life after treatment, and the degree of relief from troublesome symptoms, particularly pain. These parameters give an incomplete description of morbidity, and fail to draw attention to important symptoms such as nausea, fatigue depression and anorexia.

Wherever possible, the distinction between *radical* and *palliative* treatment intent should be clear in the doctor's mind. For example, patients with widely metastatic breast cancer are often treated with combination chemotherapy, and remissions, often lasting several months, are frequently seen. However, since cure is never achieved, such treatment must be viewed as palliative and offered to patients with symptomatic deposits which are likely to respond. It is surprising how frequently this approach is not followed and patients with widely disseminated cancers (including far less sensitive tumours than carcinoma of the breast) are treated routinely with combination chemotherapy.

Where two types of treatment appear to give similar results, one should undoubtedly choose the less toxic. For example, chemotherapy for Hodgkin's disease has been made much more acceptable by the substitution of chlorambucil and vinblastine for mustine and vincristine (see Chapter 25). In certain situations, where there is a slight possible advantage to a more toxic treatment, the greater toxicity might outweigh the slight improvement in results. For example, in infiltrating carcinoma of the urinary bladder,

there may be a slight survival advantage in a combination of irradiation and radical cystectomy, compared with treatment by radiotherapy alone (see p. 329) However, the extra few months of median survival is obtained at the cost of both a permanent ileostomy and a high risk of impotence. Given a choice, many of us might opt for radiotherapy alone, despite the slightly greater risk, particularly since surgery is still possible if there is local recurrence.

The use of surgery when there is radiation failure at the primary site (salvage surgery), is now widely accepted as it has become apparent that the treatment of solid tumours by radiotherapy can give local control rates which are the equal of surgery. This is clearly shown by the increasing use of radiotherapy for carcinoma of the cervix, of the head and neck, bladder, prostate and breast. In each of these sites, there are important physiological and psychological advantages to treatment with radiotherapy. Radical surgery can usually be performed if relapse occurs. Finally one should remember that there are some patients with malignant disease in whom treatment may not be immediately necessary. Many patients with follicular lymphoma harbour a disease whose course is so indolent that treatment is unnecessary, often for several years. In patients with asymptomatic but inoperable squamous carcinoma of the bronchus, there is generally no advantage to early treatment with radiotherapy or chemotherapy since such treatment does not prolong life and may cause side-effects (see Chapter 12). Treatment is better withheld until a troublesome symptom such as haemoptysis, dyspnoea or pain from a secondary deposit becomes apparent.

For all these reasons, when trials of cancer treatments are undertaken, it is important to include some assessment of quality of life, especially if there is unlikely to be a substantial difference in cure rate. In this way, any advantage in terms of survival or local control can be set against the morbidity which the treatment has induced.

THE CARE OF THE DYING

It has become increasingly apparent that patients dying from cancer have particular needs which are often poorly served by traditional means of support. Even the most well-meaning of doctors frequently finds himself out of his depth either through inadequate training in the use of the appropriate drugs (particularly analgesics) or because of the difficulties of exploring the patient's needs. It is against this background that interest and expertise in the management of terminally ill patients has developed, and as so often happens, it has been the determined work of a few individuals which has identified the problem and developed principles which are now widely adopted.

First and foremost, it is always wrong for a doctor to say, or feel, 'there is nothing more that I can do'. The enthusiastic oncologist may feel that his work is over when the specific anti-cancer treatment is at an end. His patient will in general make a much less clear distinction between *active* and *supportive* treatment so that from the patient's point of view, careful treatment with analgesics, concern about appetite, constipation, mobility and so on, may be equally important. Second, it is largely through the work of hospice staff that we are beginning to learn the critical importance of adequate symptom control. The symptoms most commonly causing distress are pain, anorexia, nausea and vomiting, constipation, weakness and lassitude.

PAIN RELIEF WITH ANALGESICS

Relief of pain is a particularly important aspect of the care of the dying. There is no single ideal analgesic and most patients will require drugs of different strength and dosage during the course of their illness. It is convenient to group analgesics into the three classes according to their strength as shown in Table 7.1.

1 *Mild analgesics.* This group includes aspirin, paracetamol, dextropropoxyphene and non-steroidal anti-inflammatory agents. These can be valuable for considerable periods of time. Aspirin and the non-steroidal anti-inflammatory agents (indomethacin, ibuprofen etc.) are particularly helpful in bone pain. Side-effects include dyspepsia and gastro-intestinal bleeding. They can be combined with agents from a more powerful class (e.g. aspirin and papaveretum tablets). Dextropropoxyphene is sometimes combined with paracetamol and many patients prefer this to paracetamol alone. The combination has been criticized because of the possibility of habituation but this is not important in the present context.

2 *Moderate analgesics.* This group includes codeine derivatives, oxycodone, pentazocine and dipipanone. These agents are more effective than those in the mild analgesic group but at the cost of greater side-effects, particularly constipation. Oxycodone is particularly valuable as it is available in the form of suppositories. Pentazocine should be avoided because it commonly produces hallucinations. It has a partial antagonist action to morphine and should not be used in combination with opiates.

3 *Powerful analgesics.* These drugs, which include morphine and related compounds (synthetic and semi-synthetic derivatives), are powerful in their pain-relieving effects and are the mainstay of analgesic therapy for patients with unremitting pain. Almost all patients with terminal cancer pain require regular medication with analgesics of this type. Useful agents include morphine, diamorphine, methadone, pethidine, dextromoramide, papaveretum (often combined with aspirin as effervescent compound tablets) and buprenorphine. Ordinary morphine and diamorphine have activity only for 4 hours and should be given 4-hourly, but long-acting oral tablets of morphine sulphate are now available, as described below.

The choice of opiate analgesic and dosages should be determined by the patient's need. For example, many patients are comfortable and pain-free with small regular dosage (10–20 mg every 4 hours) of morphine or diamorphine where others require twenty times this dose. There are few other drugs with a dose-range

Table 7.1.   Analgesics

Drug	Duration of action	Toxicity
Mild Analgesics		
Aspirin	4–6 hours	Gastro-intestinal bleeding and abdominal pain.
Paracetamol	2–4 hours	Skin rash. Hepatic damage with overdose.
Propionic acid derivatives (e.g. ibuprofen)	2–6 hours	As asprin.
Indole derivatives (e.g. indomethacin)	8 hours	As asprin.
Moderate Analgesics		
Codeine and dihydrocodeine	4–6 hours	Constipation, excitement.
Oxycodone	8–10 hours	Constipation, hypotension, nausea, dysphasia.
Pentazocine	3–4 hours	Nausea, dizziness, palpitations, hypertension, dysphasia.
Dipipanone	6 hours	Constipation, mental confusion, respiratory depression.
Powerful Analgesics		
Morphine Sulphate	4–6 hours (longer with sustained-release preparations)	Constipation, hypotension, nausea, dysphasia.
Diamorphine	4–6 hours	As morphine sulphate.
Methadone	15–30 hours	As morphine sulphate, more nausea, cumulative.
Dextromoramide	6 hours	Dizziness, sweating, constipation, respiratory depression.
Pethidine	3 hours	Nausea, dry mouth, respiratory depression.

as wide. In most patients, oral medication is appropriate and effective though in those with, for example, complete obstruction from pharyngeal or oesophageal cancer, an alternative route will have to be found. Sublingual buprenorphine can be a useful alternative but it antagonizes the effect of morphine and should therefore not be abruptly substituted for morphine nor given with it concurrently. Treatment by rectal suppositories of oxycodone or morphine can be extremely effective. In very occasional cases, where both the oral and rectal routes are unavailable, suppositories can be given vaginally.

Regular intramuscular or intravenous treatment with opiates is almost never required though subcutaneous or intravenous infusions of diamorphine can be valuable if treatment by other routes proves unsatisfactory. Diamorphine is preferable because of its very high

solubility, allowing volumes for injection to be small. Very rarely, regular administration of subdural or intrathecal morphine may be necessary for pain relief, but this should never be considered as a long-term solution unless other methods of regular opiate administration have been tried.

A recent and important addition to the family of useful opiates is the long-acting morphine now available in oral tablets of 10, 30, 60, and 100 mg strength. The tablets are formulated in a long acting base and give sustained pain relief for 12 hours. Since both morphine and diamorphine must be given frequently thoughout the day, the availability of long acting morphine is of real value, particularly to the active patient who is disinclined to carry bottles of diamorphine elixir with him. It is important to remember, when changing the treatment from diamorphine elixir to long-acting morphine that the dose ratio of diamorphine to morphine is 2:3 so that a patient on say diamorphine 20 mg 4 hourly (i.e. total daily dosage 120 mg), will require 180 mg of morphine daily, or long-acting morphine 90 mg twice daily, given orally at a 12-hour interval.

All patients taking regular opiate medication will require advice regarding constipation. Regular laxatives are usually (but not always) necessary, and may need to be given in above normal doses. We usually recommend regular danthron-poloxamer mixture (Dorbanex) but the standard daily dose of 10–20 ml is often inadequate and up to 100 ml in divided daily doses may be required for patients on large doses of morphine or diamorphine elixir or tablets. Nausea, vomiting and sedation are the other important side-effects of opiate analgesics but are less consistent and often disappear rapidly. We do not find it necessary to offer routine anti-emetics with diamorphine elixir.

GUIDELINES FOR PAIN CONTROL IN TERMINAL CANCER PATIENTS

1 Use enough analgesia to be effective. Regular aspirin, or compound paracetamol/dextropropoxyphene tablets can be effective for many weeks. A change to dihydrocodeine will then usually give further pain relief. Use of morphine or related agents should be considered when drugs of lesser effect are inadequate for the patient's pain. At this stage less powerful agents such as dipipanone or aspirin can still be valuable, to supplement the regular morphine dose. A common useful starting dose of diamorphine elixir is 10 or 20 mg every 4 hours, but some patients need more than 1 g of diamorphine daily for adequate pain relief. Addiction is not a problem and opiates should not be withheld for fear of producing it. Dysphoria and loss of lucidity may occur and can be distressing. In such cases a lower dose may have to be accepted, even if pain relief is incomplete, and additional analgesia attempted by other means (see below).

2 Give analgesics regularly rather than on a 'when required' basis. This is one of the commonest of prescribing errors. Patients should not have to 'earn' their analgesia. Morphine and diamorphine need to be given every 4 hours to be effective.

3 Warn patients about side-effects. This particularly applies to constipation. High-fibre diet and regular laxatives are sufficient to deal with this important and painful problem in most cases. Metoclopramide, prochlorperazine or cyclizine can be useful if nausea is a persistent problem.

4 Keep drug prescriptions as simple as possible. Some opiates antagonize each other and should never be given together (e.g. sublingual buprenorphine and oral diamorphine).

5 Consider alternative methods of pain control.

(a) Alternative routes of analgesic administration. Oral, sublingual, rectal, vaginal or even (rarely) via colostomy; subcutaneous, intramuscular, intravenous, intrathecal.

(b) Alternative approaches. Consider radiotherapy for painful bone metastases, surgical internal fixation for pathological fractures and other procedures such as nerve block and neurosurgical approaches.

NERVE BLOCKS, SURGICAL PROCEDURES AND OTHER APPROACHES

Some patients with cancer have intractable pain at a particular site, which responds poorly even to high doses of opiates. In such cases, a nerve block which destroys pain and other sensations in the affected part of the body, can be extremely valuable. The technique requires great skill and is usually performed by an anaesthetist with special training. Local dorsal root block using fine needle insertions of phenol or absolute alcohol is the commonest method. Careful positioning of the patient is important and advantage can be made of the fact that phenol is heavier, and absolute alcohol lighter than CSF, so choice of agent and patient position can result in effective blockage of pain at different sites (Fig. 7.1). A similar technique can be used to produce coelic or brachial plexus block.

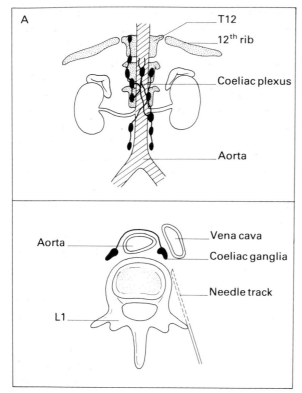

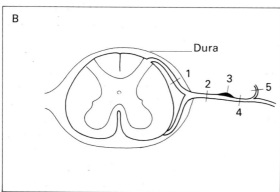

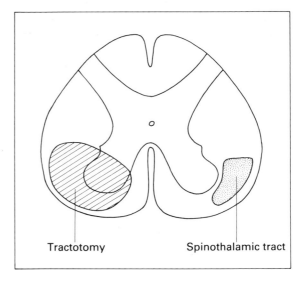

Surgical destructive procedures may have to be considered if all else fails. Spinothalamic tractotomy is an operation performed on the spinal cord in which the fibres carrying pain are divided. Anatomical specificity is often possible since the pain fibres are arranged in the lateral spinothalamic tract in an orderly fashion (Fig. 7.2). Pain relief may however not be complete

Fig. 7.2. *Spinal tractotomy*. Often carried out at T_1 or T_2. Included in the operation are vestibulospinal, rubrospinal, ventral corticospinal and ascending ventral spinocerebellar tracts. It is increasingly performed percutaneously.

since other spinal pathways may also subserve pain sensation. Operations can also be considered at higher levels (e.g. thalamotomy) if tractotomy is ineffective.

Alternative procedures include transcutaneous nerve stimulation and acupuncture analgesia, both of which can be valuable even in patients taking large doses of opiates. The mechanisms of these methods may involve a stimulation of endogenous endorphins at a central level.

ANOREXIA AND NAUSEA

Anorexia is a very common accompaniment of terminal cancer and there is of course no long

Fig. 7.1. *Coeliac plexus and dorsal root blocks to relieve pain.* (A) Anatomical relations of coeliac plexus. The plexus is comprised of a number of ganglia situated in front of T_{12} and L_1. The injection is made in front of the anterior border of the body of L_1. The needle is inserted below the 12th rib. (B) Dorsal root block and section. 1. Block of root inside dura. 2. Block of dorsal root outside dura. 3. Excision of dorsal root ganglion. 4. Coagulation of nerve trunk. 5. Coagulation of medial branch of primary ramus.

lasting remedy. There is however much that can
be done to relieve the anxiety which the patient
feels about the continued wasting. Small meals
should be offered, particularly the patient's favourite dishes, and a glass of wine or sherry
may stimulate appetite. One of the great cruel-
ties of faddish 'alternative' diets is the denial of
the simple pleasure of eating and drinking in
the final weeks of a patient's life. Steroids may
be extremely valuable and are underused in this
situation. Steroid side-effects will not be a problem if the prognosis is a matter of weeks. Dexamethasone is probably the drug of choice
(2 mg given three or four times a day) though
lower doses may be adequate.

Treatment of nausea (and vomiting) may be
difficult. If there is a mechanical cause, such as
intestinal obstruction from intra-abdominal
cancer, a fine bore nasogastric tube may have
to be passed for aspiration of stomach contents.
In most cases symptomatic treatment with
prochlorperazine, chlorpromazine or metoclopramide given regularly before meals may help.
Rectal administration may be necessary.

DEPRESSION AND ANXIETY

Most patients will have episodes of depression
and anxiety, and sympathetic conversation with
family, friends, doctors and nurses will usually
help the patient over bad days. Persistent, dis-
turbing or suicidal depression (fortunately very
uncommon) may require additional treatment
with tri- or tetra-cyclic antidepressants and occasionally skilled psychiatric help is needed.
Some authorities find amphetamines are helpful
in special circumstances. Benzodiazepines are
useful for acute or persistent anxiety.

Terminal care: home, hospice and support teams

Many patients like to remain at home for as
long as they can and to die there if possible.
Familiar surroundings and family life offer
great comfort. The care of a dying patient is
however extremely demanding and a great deal
of support is always required if home care is

to be achieved successfully. Women generally
look after dying men much better than men
care for their wives. There are many factors
which determine the feasibility of home care.
These include whether the patient lives alone;
the continued presence of family or friends to
provide support (the spouse or partner may
have to go to work); whether there are young
children at home to be cared for; the availability of adequate local support services such as
nursing, laundry, home helps and meals-on-
wheels; and the degree and nature of the
patient's disability and symptoms. It may be
necessary to provide specialized aids to nursing
and mobility, such as hand rails in the lavatory,
commodes, a ripple or water bed, a hoist or a
wheel chair.

A flexible approach is essential. Even if the
intention is to care for the patient at home, the
circumstances may change and the situation become more difficult, making hospital or hospice
care necessary. This may lead to feelings of guilt
or of defeat in the family and the doctor should
realize this and explain that continuous care of
the dying patient is a highly skilled task and
that professional help is often needed and the
change in plan is not a sign of failure.

Hospices for terminally ill cancer patients
have taught us the importance of careful pain
control, attention to the patient's physical and
spiritual needs, and the important ways in
which medical, nursing and other staff can
make enormous contributions by spending a
little more time with patients, often just by
listening or simply by being there. Nonetheless,
the hospice movement is itself aware of the disadvantages of hospice care. Hospices are
expensive to set up and maintain, and demand
a high staff:patient ratio. Some patients find the
concept of moving to a 'terminal home' difficult
to accept, even though the majority are content
once they arrive. Psychologically, many
patients find it difficult to accept that the doctor
who had been treating them, in whom they had
trust and confidence, no longer has any treatment to offer. Doctors with a genuine interest
in the management of terminally ill cancer

patients often find it upsetting if they are made to feel that they have no further role, as sometimes happens where hospice support teams take the view that they should be entirely responsible for the patient. For the general practitioner who will have to look after the family after the death of the patient with cancer, this sudden role change can create real difficulty.

The traditional alternative, and the place where many cancer patients die, has been the general hospital ward. Undoubtedly there are advantages, in particular the continuity of care afforded by familiar staff and surroundings. Some patients might gain comfort from the fact that many of the patients on the ward will be suffering from non-malignant conditions, and that the general atmosphere is likely to be brisk and active. However, most of us would agree that for patients in the final stages of their illness, the ideal environment would be more tranquil and the staff rather less busy so that there is more time for reflective discussion. It is well known that on many general medical or surgical wards, the cancer patient is all too often hurriedly passed by, particularly by the medical staff, who perhaps feel pressured and unable to help, and embarrassed or discomfited by this inadequacy.

A solution which is rapidly becoming more popular, is the setting up of community or hospital-based supportive care teams, which consist of medical and nursing staff, usually with a social worker. This team exists to help both hospital specialists and also the local general practitioners, by providing expertise, assistance and time for terminally ill cancer patients, maintaining continuity of support whether the patient has been admitted to a hospital bed or is at home under the care of the local practitioner. From our own experience of working with such a team it is apparent that there are benefits both for the patient and also for his family. Supportive care teams can assist by providing an expert service regarding, for example, choice of analgesic or anti-emetic, as well as arranging for essential facilities such as commodes, home oxygen, rapid installation of

telephone services and so on. Although all of these roles could be undertaken by general practitioners, district nurses or social workers, there is no doubt that the presence of a team entirely committed to the improvement of standards in terminal care enormously improves the efficiency of the service. Many teams also take on a bereavement counselling role, and remain closely in touch with bereaved relatives particularly if problems have been perceived before the death of the patient. Although there is no ideal time to refer patients to such a team, we feel that early referral is to be encouraged so that possible problems can be rapidly identified, and a close relationship quickly established.

CANCER QUACKERY

Quackery: the pretensions or practice of a quack.
Quack: shortened form of quacksalver—a charlatan.
Quacksalver: one who quacks about his salves (derived from Dutch).

Patients with cancer may decide to abandon medical treatment and opt for false or unproven remedies such as dietary manipulation, 'natural' or herbal medicines, homeopathy, faith healing, visualization therapy, immunizations, multivitamin supplements and enemas. They may be urged to do so by relatives or other cancer patients and they sometimes try these treatments in addition to conventional methods.

Patients who do this are usually frightened and anxious; some may see doctors as members of a conspiratorial establishment who have closed minds to any alternative approach. They may have strong ideas about the way their body works or what causes cancer, believing for example that the disease is the result of life-style, diet, psychological stress or pollution. However, even if dietary factors are important in aetiology it is illogical to expect that the cancer can therefore be cured by alterations in diet, emotional attitude, or by taking natural products such as herbal remedies. Sadly, giving up smoking does not cure lung cancer. Many august personages are prepared to lend their support to these notions, their names often being more impressive than their intellectual credentials.

There is also no shortage of doctors, naturopaths or homeopaths to support the public in these beliefs, as well as some more tough-minded charlatans out to make money. There are many damaging aspects to their activities.

First, there is no evidence that any of these remedies work. No evidence for antitumour activity is presented, no evaluation of results and no independent or critical assessment of data. Instead cases are quoted, anecdotes offered and spurious facts and figures are produced. In one of the few controlled studies of alternative cancer treatments, Laetrile (amygdalin), a 'harmless yet effective' remedy approved by most alternative cancer 'authorities' was found to be entirely without benefit and yet with significant side-effects when assessed in over 500 cancer patients treated at the Mayo Clinic.

Second, the proponents may say that they do not pretend to offer a cure-all, but it is clear that patients believe that they *will* be cured or the disease arrested. The process of mental adjustment to the diagnosis may be badly shaken by false optimism followed by despair at failure. The term *alternative medicine* is in itself a lie when it is used to imply that a proven method of treatment is being offered. Third, the patient may delay conventional treatment occasionally with tragic consequences in the case of a potentially curable tumour. Fourth, the treatment is often expensive and the patient may waste a lot of money. Finally, these 're-medies' may create a great deal of conflict within the family. Patients with advanced cancer can be cajoled or even bullied by their well-meaning relatives into taking an entirely 'natural' diet; then find it intolerable and lose what remaining interest they may have in nutrition. They may even feel that they have to continue in order not to let their children down.

It must be admitted however, that one reason that patients seek these remedies is a dissatisfaction with conventional medicine or with their doctor which may in part be well-founded. Patients will often say that they tried these treatments because they were given no hope or emotional support, because they found the prospect of radiotherapy or chemotherapy unnatural, because there was inadequate explanation and reassurance or because treatment was being unreasonably and thoughtlessly prolonged or aggressive without any hint of benefit. The first question a doctor should ask himself when faced with a patient who has decided to undergo a quack treatment is 'Have I given enough explanation and reassurance?'

If a patient or relative decides to discontinue treatment it is of course essential to say what the consequences might be but cruel to overstate the case in order to browbeat the patient into continuing. Much cancer treatment is palliative and no great harm may be done by stopping it. It is kind to make it clear that, although the proposed alternative is bogus, the patient will be welcome to come back at a later date.

FURTHER READING

Twycross R. G. (1984) Pain Relief in Cancer. *Clinics in Oncology* **3**, (1).
Saunders C. M. (1985) *The Management of Terminal Malignant Disease.* Edward Arnold, London.

Chapter 8
Medical Problems and Radiotherapy Emergencies

Acute and often life-threatening medical problems may arise as a result of the cancer and its treatment. Iatrogenic deaths are not infrequent because many treatments, particularly intensive chemotherapy, are inherently very dangerous. Nevertheless the majority of deaths are avoidable and many oncologists prefer to look after their patients in specialized cancer units with staff skilled in anticipating, avoiding and managing these problems.

BONE MARROW FAILURE AND ITS CONSEQUENCES

Cytotoxic drugs damage the reproductive integrity of cells. Bone marrow haemopoietic cells are among the most rapidly dividing cells in the body and are extremely sensitive to the action of most antineoplastic agents. Some drugs, for example, vincristine and bleomycin, produce only slight bone marow depression while the majority impair haemopoiesis. With drugs such as doxorubicin, myelosuppression is one of the major toxicities. There is some evidence that cytotoxic agents affect different proliferative compartments within the marrow. This leads to non-uniform patterns of toxicity even within the same class of cytotoxic agent. For example cyclophosphamide, administered as a single intravenous injection, causes predictable granulocytopenia 4–7 days later with a less marked effect on platelet count. In contrast, melphalan and busulphan produce a slower marrow suppression with onset at 7–8 days and maximum depression of white count at about 2–3 weeks. Nitrosoureas such as CCNU characteristically exert a delayed effect on the blood count occurring at about 4–5 weeks.

The speed of onset and the severity with which the marrow is affected also depend on dose and timing of drug administration. Although the platelet count does not fall significantly with cyclophosphamide given in conventional doses, it will do so at much higher doses. Similarly although neutropenia and thrombocytopenia usually occur at 4–5 weeks after CCNU administration in conventional doses, at very high doses such as those which have been used experimentally in the treatment of brain tumours, an earlier onset of neutropenia and thrombocytopenia may be seen, occasionally as early as 4–5 days after the drug has been given.

Although some agents (melphalan, busulphan, CCNU) may cause prolonged marrow suppression even when given on the first occasion, in a patient receiving intermittent cytotoxic chemotherapy for the first time, the marrow depression is usually transient and the blood count normal in 2–3 weeks when the next cycle can be given. With increasing duration of chemotherapy however, the proliferative compartments in the marrow may become progressively more depleted and the nadir of the white count then becomes lower and recovery less rapid, so that chemotherapy cycles may have to be delayed or the dose reduced. In order to avoid life-threatening marrow suppression a familiarity with the cytotoxic regimen is essential and the physician must be aware of the likelihood of increasing marrow depression with time.

However experienced the clinican, marrow depression does occur unexpectedly. With some treatment regimens, for example during the induction of remission in acute myeloblastic leukaemia, or with the use of very high dose chemotherapy in some solid tumours, pancytopenia is an inevitable consequence of treatment.

The symptoms of granulocytopenia are those of infection (i.e. fever, malaise, shaking, chills), sometimes accompanied by oral ulceration and perineal inflammation. If the platelet count is depressed the patient may develop epistaxis or purpura. It is unusual for symptoms of anaemia to occur acutely even if erythropoiesis ceases altogether as a result of cytotoxic agents, since the half-life of red cells (25 days) is such that the haemoglobin does not usually fall appreciably.

The management of marrow depression by blood component therapy

BLOOD TRANSFUSION (1,2)

Many patients undergoing combination intermittent chemotherapy for solid tumours develop moderate anaemia with a haemoglobin of 10–12 g/dl. The blood count will recover when treatment is discontinued and transfusion is not usually required unless the haemoglobin falls below 9 g/dl. In deciding whether to transfuse a patient, the symptoms of anaemia (i.e. fatigue, malaise and breathlessness) must be balanced against the risks of transfusion, in particular volume overload in elderly patients. If a patient is at risk of cardiac failure because of ischaemic heart disease, volume overload can be minimized by the use of packed cells and diuretics. There is some evidence that, in the presence of thrombocytopenia, a transfusion can precipitate episodes of bleeding, in particular intracerebral haemorrhage. For this reason, many physicians prefer to use a platelet transfusion before giving blood or packed cells in severely thromobocytopenic patients.

Many patients with advanced malignant disease become anaemic due to an effect of the tumour itself or to marrow infiltration (e.g. in myeloma, leukaemia or widespread bone secondaries). This occurs even when patients are not having treatment with chemotherapy or radiotherapy. Even if no active treatment for the tumour is planned, a patient may gain symptomatic relief from blood transfusion. Since the symptoms of anaemia will be similar to those of the tumour, it is often difficult to anticipate whether blood transfusion will help a patient. Precise guidelines cannot be drawn, but in general transfusion should be considered only if the haemoglobin falls below 9 g/dl.

PLATELET TRANSFUSION

The risk of bleeding is related to the platelet count and rises sharply below $20 \times 10^9/l$. Ecchymosis and purpura are characteristically found in pressure areas and on the shins. Major bleeding is life-threatening and intracerebral haemorrhage is often fatal.

The life span of platelets is approximately 10 days, but transfused platelets have a half-life of only a few days. Platelets have a variety of antigens on their surface including HLA antigens. Repeated transfusion may be accompanied by immunization against these antigens with the result that further platelet transfusions lead to rapid platelet destruction and a failure to elevate the platelet count. Nevertheless, platelet transfusion has been a major factor in decreasing the morbidity of intensive chemotherapy regimens and most patients can be protected during periods of hypoplasia without serious haemorrhage (3). A unit of platelets is derived from one fresh unit of whole blood and yields about 0.5×10^{11} platelets. Although theoretically a unit of platelets should raise the platelet count by $10 \times 10^9/l$ this seldom happens, particularly if patients have had many previous transfusions or if there is fever or infection.

There is no single level of platelet count at which transfusion should be given. Platelet transfusion is rarely required at counts above

$30 \times 10^9/1$. Indications for platelet transfusion are:

1 A rapidly falling platelet count following the start of intensive chemotherapy in which it can be predicted that the circulating platelets will fall below $20 \times 10^9/1$ within a 24 hour period. This is particularly important when making arrangements for the care of patients at weekends. The trend of the platelet count will help in deciding if a further transfusion will soon be necessary.

2 If there is evidence of bleeding (such as widespread ecchymosis, nose bleeds or gastro-intestinal bleeding), platelet transfusion is essential, even at levels higher than $30 \times 10^9/1$.

3 Platelet transfusions are sometimes necessary at higher levels of platelet count (above $30 \times 10^9/1$). If there are other complicating factors such as anaemia, peptic ulceration or infection which predispose to bleeding.

Occasionally, patients will become refractory to platelet transfusions, with little or no rise in platelet count. Fever, infection and splenomegaly may all contribute to this, but the usual cause is immunization to platelet antigens. This can be avoided by using HLA matched donors, generally obtained from the patient's family. In immunized patients a rise in platelet count can sometimes be produced by the use of corticosteroids.

GRANULOCYTE TRANSFUSION

A great deal of controversy has surrounded the use of granulocyte transfusion in the aplastic patient (4, 5). Granulocytes can now be collected using blood cell separators, and can be shown to function after injection into the recipient. However with the advent of modern broad spectrum bactericidal antibiotics, particularly of the aminoglycoside group, the frequency of granulocyte transfusion has diminished, particularly in patients where the aplasia is expected to be transient. From 5–25×10^9 cells are transfused which is less than one-tenth of the normal daily granulocyte produc-

tion. Early studies showed that granulocyte transfusion was of value in patients whose granulocyte count was less than $0.5 \times 10^9/1$. There is, however, little evidence that they are useful prophylactically in patients who do not have evidence of infection or fever. It is the practice in most oncology units to use granulocytes, when available, in patients with proven gram-negative septicaemia who are not responding to antibiotics and whose granulocyte count is $< 0.5 \times 10^9/1$, or where there is strong clinical suspicion of bacterial infection even if it has not been documented by blood culture. If recovery of the blood count is confidently expected within 1–2 days, then it is reasonable to withhold granulocyte transfusion.

Granulocyte collections must be taken from donors who are ABO and Rh compatible with the recipient. In most instances it is not possible to match for HLA antigens. Repeated granulocyte transfusions may therefore be associated with alloimmunization against HLA and other antigens on the surface of the granulocyte. For this reason if the marrow aplasia is occurring as a result of intensive therapy in which allogeneic marrow transplantation is being used, HLA matched granulocytes must be obtained.

INFECTIONS IN THE IMMUNE-COMPROMISED PATIENT

Infections are a major cause of death in cancer. Not only do they occur frequently, they are often more severe than in other patients, less responsive to therapy and are sometimes produced by organisms which are not pathogens in healthy people. This susceptibility results from depression of host defence mechanisms produced by the tumour and its treatment.

Host defence mechanisms in cancer

PHAGOCYTE FUNCTION

Advanced cancer is sometimes associated with reduced function of both neutrophils and monocytes. Depression of chemotactic, phagocytic and bactericidal activity have all been described. There is some evidence that chemotherapy can cause a deterioration in function as well as granulocytopenia.

CELL MEDIATED IMMUNITY (CMI) AND HUMORAL IMMUNITY

Anergy to delayed hypersensitivity antigens is common in advanced untreated Hodgkin's disease but less common in other malignancies. Lymphopenia is an invariable accompaniment of treatment with alkylating agents and radiotherapy—the effect of the latter lasting for many months. CMI is particularly important in host defence against fungi, viruses, tuberculosis and protozoa. Cytotoxic T cells and natural killer cells are especially important in the control of herpes virus infections. Several studies have shown that intensive cytotoxic chemotherapy leads to impaired production of antibody to bacterial and viral antigens (7).

RETICULOENDOTHELIAL (RE) FUNCTION

Circulating bacteria are cleared by the phagocytic cells lining the sinuses of the RE system especially in the liver and spleen. Antibody and complement are important for this clearance. Splenectomy increases the risk of severe bacterial infection, especially pneumococcal septicaemia in young children and to a lesser extent in adults (8).

THE MUCOSAL BARRIER

The skin and mucosal surfaces are a barrier to infection. Tumour infiltration and local radiotherapy may lead to damage to lymphatic or venous drainage, with resulting susceptibility to local infection. The turnover of gastro-intestinal epithelial cells is normally very rapid and this is depressed by chemotherapy leading to mucosal damage and ulceration which allows gut organisms to escape into the portal system. The skin is breached by intravenous needles and cannulae, and nasogastric tubes act as a focus for infection with *Candida albicans*.

Bacteraemia and Septicaemia (9)

Bloodstream infections are particularly frequent in granulocytopenic patients. Gram-negative bacteria (*E. Coli*, *P. aeruginosa*) staphylococci and streptococci are frequent pathogens. Fever in a neutropenic cancer patient is an indication for blood cultures, but an organism is often not isolated. Treatment should not be delayed in the neutropenic patient. An aminoglycoside (gentamicin) is usually given with penicillin and metronidazole or with a semi-synthetic penicillin such as ticarcillin. Cephalosporins and beta-lactamase resistant penicillins are valuable for gram-positive septicaemia. The prognosis depends mainly on the time it takes for the bone marrow to recover. In patients who are undergoing intensive chemotherapy or a bone marrow allograft, prophylactic gut sterilization is attempted with oral antibiotics. The use of granulocytes is discussed on p. 124. If there is an obvious source of the infection such as infected infusion sites, cultures should be taken and the cannula removed.

Respiratory infection

Fever with pulmonary infiltration is a common occurrence in the severely immunocompromised patient. The major causes are given in Table 8.1. The difficulties in making a diagnosis can be considerable because sputum and blood cultures may be negative, and more invasive procedures such as transbronchial biopsy may be impossible because of thrombocytopenia or the general condition of the patient.

There are some clinical features which are helpful in diagnosis. Cavitation is more common with anaerobic bacteria, staphylococci, and mycobacteria. Pneumocystis infection causes marked dyspnoea, and the chest X-ray shows bilateral infiltrates typically radiating from the hilum. The disease may however be indolent, and can cause lobar consolidation.

Table 8.1. Causes of fever and pulmonary infiltration in immunocompromised patients

Bacteria	*Streptococcus pneumoniae*
	Gram-negative organisms
	Mycobacteria
	Legionella
Fungi	Aspergillus
	Candida
	Cryptococcus
Viruses	Cytomegalovirus
	Herpes simplex
	Measles
Protozoa	Pneumocystis
Treatment	Cytotoxic drugs
	Radiation pneumonitis

Cytomegalovirus infection mainly occurs in severely immune-depressed patients, particularly during allogeneic bone-marrow transplantation. The disease may also cause myocarditis, neuropathy and ophthalmitis. The pulmonary infiltrate is usually bilateral. Candida infection can cause a wide variety of X-ray changes. There is often candida infection elsewhere. Panophthalmitis may occur and the organism can sometimes be isolated from the blood. Aspergillus infection is usually rapidly progressive in these patients. Blood cultures are usually negative and the infiltrate can be in one or both lungs.

Faced with this diagnostic uncertainty the following scheme can be adopted.

1 *In the patient without neutropenia or thrombocytopenia.* Investigate with blood cultures, sputum culture, bronchoscopic washings, transbronchial biopsy, where possible.

If blood and sputum cultures are negative, treat with broad spectrum bactericidal antibiotics (usually with an aminoglycoside, penicillin and metronidazole or equivalent combination). If pneumocystitis is a possible cause, high dose co-trimoxazole should be given. If there is no response consider acyclovir for herpes simplex infection and antifugal therapy with amphotericin or ketoconazole. Acyclovir is not effective against cytomegalovirus.

If blood or sputum culures are positive treat

as appropriate; but if there is no response consider a mixed infection.

2 *In the patient with neutropenia or thrombocytopenia.* Bronchoscopy can be carried out, but biopsy may not be possible and treatment may have to proceed along the lines indicated without full diagnostic investigation. Before and after bronchoscopy, antibiotics and platelet transfusion may be necessary.

Urinary tract infections

Infection is common in patients with obstruction to outflow, particularly from the bladder. Obstruction may be by tumour or due to an atonic bladder in a patient with cord compression. Diagnosis is made by urine culture and treatment is with antibiotics and relief of obstruction if possible.

Gastro-intestinal infections

Oral thrush (infection with *Candida albicans*) is a frequent complication of chemotherapy. It is particularly likely to occur in immunosuppressed patients, in patients on steroids and in those treated with broad spectrum antibiotics. The mouth and pharynx become very sore and white plaques of fungus are visible on an erythematous base. The infection may penetrate more deeply in some malnourished patients and extend down into the oesophagus, stomach, and bowel. Oral nystatin, amphotericin or miconazole are usually effective. The lozenges must be sucked at frequent (4-hourly) intervals. Herpes simplex cold sores are often troublesome in leucopenic patients and the lesions may become very widespread. Treatment is with acyclovir given topically for minor infections in immunosuppressed patients, and systemically for more serious infections.

Candida infection in the oesophagus requires treatment with oral nystatin suspension, but if this is ineffective treat with ketoconazole or a short course of amphotericin. Candida infections of the bowel should be treated with amphotericin.

Perianal infections are common in neutropenic patients. Preventative measures should always be employed, with scrupulous perineal hygiene and stool softeners to prevent constipation and anal tears. Spreading perineal infection can be a life-threatening event, and urgent treatment with intravenous antibiotics active against gram-negative and anaerobic bacilli is required.

Meninges

CNS infections are rare, but patients with lymphoma or leukaemia occasionally develop meningitis due to *Cryptococcus neoformans*. The onset is insidious with headache. The organism can be detected by India ink staining of the CSF. Detection of cryptococcus antigen in blood and CSF is possible in most patients. Many patients will improve with amphotericin and some will be cured.

Skin

Apart from infection introduced at infusion sites the most common skin infection is shingles (varicella-zoster). This infection, which is due to a reactivation of varicella-zoster virus in dorsal root ganglia, is a dermatomal vesicular eruption which is particularly severe in immune-compromised hosts and which may disseminate as chicken pox and cause a fatal pneumonia. Severely compromised patients, those with a progressive local eruption and widespread dissemination should be treated with acyclovir. This has been a major advance in management.

Prevention of infection in the leucopenic patient

When a patient is leucopenic it is prudent for reverse barrier nursing procedures to be instituted. How rigorous these need to be is a matter which has provoked much discussion. Many of the infections are from the patient's own bacteria rather than from staff or relatives. For short periods of granulocytopenia, disposable aprons, face masks and careful washing of hands is probably satisfactory. For more persistent leucopenia (e.g. with bone marrow transplantation) a protected environment has much to commend it. Here the air is filtered free of bacteria and a laminar air flow is established from one end of the room to the other. The patients are 'decontaminated' before entry with oral antibiotics to kill intestinal bacteria, and cutaneous antiseptic cleansing. The oral antibiotic regimen usually contains framycetin, colistin and nystatin. Protected environments can lower the infection rate but their contribution to overall reduction in mortality is small since the hazards of the disease and other effects of treatment are greater. The psychological stress and cost of isolation are other major disadvantages.

Other important preventative measures are scrupulous hygiene in the placing of intravenous drugs, perineal hygiene, and high standards of staff training. It has recently been shown that prophylactic oral acyclovir is effective in preventing varicella-zoster, and ketoconazole appears to lower the incidence of fungal infections.

CANCER CACHEXIA AND THE NUTRITIONAL SUPPORT OF THE CANCER PATIENT

Weight loss is a common symptom of cancer but profound and rapid weight loss usually indicates disseminated tumour. When cancer recurs and is widespread, loss of weight is an almost invariable accompaniment. This leads finally to the cachetic state in which the patient becomes wasted, weak and lethargic.

Occasionally, rapid weight loss and weakness may occur with a small tumour which, when removed, leads to restoration of normal health. It is more usual to find that profound cachexia is an indication of advanced malignancy and attempts to reverse it are inappropriate.

Pathogenesis of malnutrition in cancer

Anorexia is a major factor in causing weight loss in patients with cancer. The mechanism of the anorexia is poorly understood. It frequently accompanies widespread disease, in particular the presence of hepatic metastases. In the case of tumours of the gastro-intestinal tract, anorexia may be profound even when the tumour is small. Typically the patient loses all interest in food and has an altered perception of taste and smell such that the thought of eating can become repugnant.

There have been many studies on the metabolism of patients with cancer cachexia (10). A variety of abnormalities have been found (Table 8.2) but the findings are not consistent

Table 8.2 Factors contributing to weight loss and cachexia

Factor	Cause
Anorexia, nausea and vomiting	Tumour Treatment Psychological factors (pain and depression)
Loss of protein, blood and minerals	Diarrhoea Ulceration Bleeding
Malabsorbtion and intestinal obstruction	Carcinoma of pancreas and ovary
Metabolic abnormalities induced by the tumour	Increased protein breakdown, metabolic rate or fat breakdown Altered glucose metabolism due to increased lactate recycling or insulin resistance
Tumour metabolism of protein and carbohydrate	
Iatrogenic factors	Chemotherapy (nausea, vomiting and mucositis, Radiotherapy (nausea, vomiting, diarrhoea)

from patient to patient and there is no uniform abnormality which is always present in cachectic individuals. The abnormalities which have been demonstrated are:

1 An increased metabolic rate which has been demonstrated in some patients but by no means all. The mechanism is unknown.
2 An abnormality of glucose metabolism has been suggested. It is proposed that the metabolism of glucose is altered with a production of excess lactate by the tumour, which is then reutilized to form glucose—a process wasteful of energy.
3 An overall increase in protein metabolism associated with a negative nitrogen balance has been demonstrated in some patients.

It has frequently been proposed that the tumour might itself contribute towards cachexia by metabolizing essential nutrients, and that tumours continue to utilize proteins and amino-acids while other body tissues have diminished uptake.

Similarly the consumption of glucose by the tumour, at a time when there is decreased carbohydrate intake, might contribute towards the wasting seen in these patients. It has been calculated that a 1 kg tumour might consume as much as 100 g of glucose daily. The remote metabolic effects on the host might also be due to so-far unidentified products released from the tumour.

On the face of it, it seems sensible to try and reverse the cachectic process in patients with cancer. In considering nutritional support for an individual cancer patient, the objectives of treatment must be clear. First the question must be answered as to whether the cancer is curable or not. If a potentially curative treatment is being considered either with surgery, chemotherapy, or radiotherapy then there is some evidence (see later) that effective nutritional support may improve the result. Well-nourished cancer patients frequently lose weight as a result of cancer treatment, whether with surgery, chemotherapy or radiotherapy. If the effects of radical treatment are likely to persist over a week or more, and considerable weight loss can be anticipated, it is probable that nutritional supplements will decrease morbidity. If, on the other hand, there is no prospect of cure and treatment is to be palliative, then nutritional support should also be seen as a palliative procedure. Aggressive and uncomfortable means of maintaining nutrition are in this case completely inappropriate. There is no evidence at present that the malnutrition and wasting which accompany advanced and incurable cancer can be reversed by any form of feeding. If nutritional support is thought to be necessary it must be given in a form which will be effective in reversing the malnourished state, and a decision made as to whether this should be enteral or parenteral.

Nutritional support available for the cancer patient

ENTERAL FEEDING

If the patient can be fed by mouth then this is clearly the best method. At the simplest level, careful attention to diet and to the foods available to the patient is of great importance. This involves discussions with the patient about which food he fancies, careful dietary advice by a skilled dietitian and the support of members of the family in providing favourite foods which might encourage the patient to eat. A variety of nutritional supplements can be added to the patient's diet, including high calorie liquids such as 'Hycal' and more complete protein and carbohydrate mixtures (e.g. Complan or Clinifeed). Protein hydrolysates, providing small peptides and amino acid fragments, are also available (Vivonex). These dietary supplements can be taken by mouth. Their main advantage is the delivery of calories in liquid form at a time when the patient finds it difficult to eat solid food. The disadvantage is that they can cause osmotic disturbances and for many patients they are quite unpalatable.

Occasionally a patient may find it difficult to swallow or eat at all. Enteral support with liquid dietary supplements can be given by using a fine bore flexible nasogastric feeding tube. The aim is to provide about 2000–3000 kcal/24 hours. These supplements have a high osmolality. They can cause nausea and diarrhoea and

provide a large solute load for renal excretion. Large amounts of fluid are required to excrete this solute load, even in the presence of normal renal function. If fluid is not provided, osmotic diuresis may occur leading to salt and water depletion and prerenal uraemia.

TOTAL PARENTERAL NUTRITION

It is now possible to provide adequate calories intravenously for patients who cannot take food by mouth or by nasogastric tube. Access must be through a catheter placed in a deep vein, since parenteral nutritional solutions cause irritation and venous thrombosis will quickly occur in small peripheral veins. The incidence of venous thrombosis when catheters are inserted into the subclavian vein is small. With all subcutaneous catheters there is a risk of infection which is particularly likely to occur in the immune-compromised individual. A variety of synthetic total parenteral nutrition solutions are available commercially, usually consisting of amino-acid solutions with dextrose, vitamins, electrolytes and trace elements.

Several of the metabolic defects present in the malnourished patient can be reversed by total parenteral nutrition. Although it is difficult to demonstrate benefit, it is reasonable to support a patient with parenteral nutrition during intensive but potentially curative treatment. This includes patients undergoing major gastro-intestinal surgery, or chemotherapy with marrow ablation. Total parenteral nutrition is complex, expensive and potentially hazardous, and is of no proven value as a routine measure in patients undergoing cancer therapies, or in the vast majority of patients with malnutrition from cancer who have disseminated disease in whom curative treatment is out of the question.

ACUTE METABOLIC DISTURBANCES

Hypercalcaemia

A raised plasma calcium is a frequent accompaniment of cancer. In a hospital population, carcinomas of the bronchus, breast, and kidney are, together with multiple myeloma, the commonest malignant causes of hypercalcaemia. Life-threatening hypercalcaemia is usually due to cancer. Minor elevations of plasma calcium (up to 2.8 mmol/l) are not usually associated with any symptoms. As the plasma calcium rises, patients experience anorexia, nausea, abdominal pain, constipation and fatigue. There may be proximal muscle weakness, polyuria and polydypsia. With increasing hypercalcaemia, severe dehydration, confusion and finally coma may supervene.

Bone metastases are much the commonest cause of hypercalcaemia in cancer. Most patients with severe hypercalcaemia have demonstrable metastases on X-ray or on bone scanning. Bone marrow aspiration may show infiltration with tumour. Even if metastases are not detectable at presentation, they usually quickly become apparent. Metastases in bone may liberate factors which are responsible for bone dissolution. Amongst the factors which have been incriminated, are an osteoclast activating factor which has been demonstrated in myeloma (11), and prostglandins particularly in the E category. It seems unlikely that these factors are able to produce hypercalcaemia by causing bone dissolution at sites distant from metastases.

There is little doubt that hypercalcaemia can occasionally be caused by a tumour even if there are not bone metastases present. This is usually seen with squamous carcinomas of the bronchus, skin, head and neck and, in hypernephroma. In these cases hypercalcaemia may be cured by removal of the tumour, demonstrating that the circulating factor produced by the tumour is responsible for the raised serum calcium. The discovery that parathormone-like substances were present in tumour extracts prompted the suggestion that such tumours may be producing parathormone and this in turn was responsible for the hypercalcaemia. However, there has never been an unequivocal demonstration of this mechanism. Circulating parathormone levels are not elevated in these

patients and balance studies do not show the typical increase in intestinal absorption of calcium which is present in cases of primary hyperparathyroidism. Other hormonal mechanisms have been postulated (such as tumour-derived growth factors) and are under investigation.

The treatment of hypercalcaemia in cancer may be a medical emergency and this is particularly true in the elderly and in patients with myeloma. The raised plasma calcium may be accompanied by uraemia which is due to salt and water loss as a result of the effect of calcium on the distal tubule making it unresponsive to ADH. In addition to this element of prerenal uraemia, the high calcium appears to reduce glomerular filtration rate directly, by ill-understood mechanisms. Hypokalaemia may also accompany hypercalcaemia, and may in part be due to a renal loss of potassium. Elderly patients, and those with impaired renal function, are unable to withstand the effects of the raised plasma calcium, and life-threatening renal failure may quickly develop. In myeloma it is particularly likely to occur since other causes of renal failure are present (see Chapter 27).

In severe hypercalcaemia, the first line of treatment is therefore with salt and water replacement using isotonic saline. In the first 24 hours, 4–8 litres may be required. This may be sufficient to lower the plasma calcium to normal. In the elderly, care must be taken not to overload the patient with fluids. If the plasma calcium does not begin to fall within 24 hours, prednisolone given orally (30–60 mg/day) or hydrocortisone intravenously (50–100 mg 6-hourly) is often helpful in reducing the calcium but not all patients will respond. Frusemide promotes calciuresis but care must be taken with volume replacement, to avoid further salt and water depletion. If rehydration and steroids fail to control the hypercalcaemia, mithramycin may be given. The usual dose is 15–25 μg/kg and it is usually sufficient to give a single injection which is followed by a fall in serum calcium after 24–48 hours. Occasionally, it may be necessary to use mithramycin on 2 or 3 successive days. This carries a risk of thrombocytopenia. Doses of 15 μg/kg can be repeated every 4 or 5 days without serious risk of thrombocytopenia, but regular blood counts are essential especially in the presence of renal failure. Intravenous or oral phosphate therapy is seldom necessary to control the plasma calcium, but phosphate infusions (usually with serum calcium of 4 mmol/l or more) may be helpful in patients who are gravely ill. Calcitonin may produce a fall in the plasma calcium but its effect is variable and its usefulness is limited. It may be more effective combined with steroids. The usual dose is 100–200 units of salmon calcitonin subcutaneously 12-hourly.

Although it is not usually difficult to diagnose the cause of malignant hypercalcaemia, diagnostic problems can occur when hyperparathyroidism is an alternative diagnosis in cancer patients who do not have evidence of disseminated disease. The steroid suppression test will not reduce the plasma calcium in hyperparathyroidism but 75% of patients with cancer show a fall after 10 days of hydrocortisone administration. If serious doubt remains, elevation of plasma parathormone is found in 80% of patients with primary hyperparathyroidism, but not in patients with cancer. Discriminant analysis (12) is an accurate alternative if parathormone assay is not available.

Tumour lysis syndrome

An acute metabolic disturbance may occur as a result of the rapid dissolution of tumour following chemotherapy. This is particularly likely to occur in children in Burkitt's lymphoma or acute lymphoblastic leukaemia, and in non-Hodgkin's lymphomas in children, adolescents and young adults. The syndrome occurs when there is extreme sensitivity of the tumour to treatment, and is uncommon in adults with non-lymphoid neoplasms. When it occurs, tumour masses may disappear very rapidly and as the cells are killed they release products of nitrogen metabolism especially urea, urate and large amounts of phosphate.

The rapid reduction in tumour mass causes hyperuricaemia, hyperphosphataemia, hyperkalaemia and uraemia. The hyperuricaemia may result in acute urate deposition in the renal tubules (urate nephropathy) leading to acute renal failure or, less dramatically, to a reduction in glomerular filtration rate which exacerbates the hyperuricaemia. Occasionally, the syndrome can be sufficiently severe to cause an acute and prolonged uraemia. The hyperphosphataemia results in a reciprocal lowering of the plasma calcium and can result in tetany.

The syndrome is more likely to occur in children with Burkitt's lymphoma who have extensive disease, particularly if there are intra-abdominal masses, impaired renal function from tumour infiltration of the kidney, or post renal obstruction due to lymph node enlargement. The syndrome is rare in adults since the tumours are generally less sensitive to chemotherapy, and their dissolution less rapid. It may, however, occur if there is coincidental renal failure due to some other cause, ureteric obstruction, or infiltration of the kidney with tumour.

The tumour lysis syndrome is usually preventable. Before beginning chemotherapy in a high risk patient, allopurinol should be given (usually by mouth) in full dose (50–100 mg 8-hourly in children, twice this dose in adults) for 24 hours. This xanthine oxidase inhibitor partly prevents the formation of urate. Allopurinol should be continued for the first few days of treatment and discontinued when the plasma urate is in the normal range. If 6-mercaptopurine is being given the dose should be reduced to 25% since allopurinol inhibits its metabolism. At the same time the patient should be given adequate fluids usually in the form of intravenous saline to establish a good diuresis. These measures should prevent both hyperuricaemia and hyperphosphataemia. In Burkitt's lymphoma, the initial induction chemotherapy is sometimes given at reduced dose until there has been considerable tumour shrinkage and then the full dose is administered. In adults with high grade lymphoma starting treatment with intensive chemotherapy, allopurinol should be given and its use should be considered in other cases if there is any possibility of renal impairment.

If hyperuricaemia and acute renal failure develops this can usually be treated by cessation of chemotherapy, cautious administration of intravenous fluids with alkalinization of the urine to promote urate excretion, and allopurinol. If the blood urea and plasma urate continue to rise, peritoneal dialysis may be needed to tide the patient over the acute renal failure. If preventative measures are taken this should rarely be necessary.

EFFUSIONS AND ASCITES

Many patients with cancer develop a pleural or pericardial effusion or ascites during the course of their illness. These can be difficult to treat and can be a major cause of discomfort and breathlessness.

Pleural effusion

Pleural fluid must reach a volume of about 500 ml before it can be detected clinically, though lesser degrees can be radiologically apparent.

The commonest malignancy to cause pleural effusion is a primary lung cancer with involvement of pleura. This may be the first evidence of the tumour but more commonly it occurs later in the disease. Typically the effusion is substantial in volume (1–4 litres), accumulates rapidly, and may be bloodstained. It often causes dyspnoea with dry cough probably due to irritation of central mediastinal structures particularly the phrenic nerve. Although cytological demonstration of cells confirms the nature of the effusion, it is common for a malignant effusion to be repeatedly cytologically negative, in which case pleural biopsy will often be indicated if there is clinical doubt as to the diagnosis. Other important tumours causing pleural effusion include pleural metastases (sometimes from an unknown primary site), lymphoma and mesothelioma. Pleural metastases are common in cancer of the breast, bronchus and ovary.

Occasionally, patients with cancer develop a pleural effusion from a non-malignant cause and alternative explanations should always be considered if a patient with apparently controlled cancer unexpectedly develops a pleural effusion. Diagnosis is by clinical examination and chest X-ray supported by cytological examination and microscopy of the pleural fluid.

Management is rarely straightforward. Most patients require therapeutic aspiration (thoracocentesis) to improve symptoms of cough and dyspnoea, and large volumes (1–5 litres) may have to be removed for worthwhile benefit. Since aspiration of volumes above 1.5 litres can sometimes cause acute heart failure, the aspirations may have to be performed slowly over several days, or on several occasions over a week. In some patients, particularly those with secondary pleural deposits and disseminated disease elsewhere, chemotherapy or endocrine therapy will be given as well. In these patients, this systemic treatment may prove effective in preventing re-accumulation of pleural fluid. In others, where effective systemic therapy is unavailable the question of whether to instil an intrapleural sclerosant, to prevent or reduce fluid accumulation, will arise.

Treatment with simple physical or antibiotic sclerosants (talc, tetracycline or quinacrine), cytotoxic drugs (mustine, thio-Tepa, doxorubicin, bleomycin and others) or radioactive colloids are all commonly used. Each has its disadvantages and is effective only in a proportion of cases. Tetracycline can cause severe local pain, mustine and doxorubicin are painful and may be nauseating and bleomycin can cause fever and chills. There are few direct comparisons of one treatment with another and many clinicians feel that there is little to choose between them.

However, in a controlled study comparing bleomycin, doxorubicin and tetracycline, the cytoxic agents were more effective (the response to bleomycin is approximately 60%). Although intrapleural bleomycin can be effective and may at present be the treatment of choice, it requires careful preliminary drainage so that the pleural space is as dry as possible, and a subcutaneous test dose (5 mg) is advisable. The intrapleural dose is 30–60 mg. Colloidal ^{32}P or ^{198}Au have been used with success rates of the order of 50% but they are expensive, and require particular care over administration and patient position to produce maximal effect with minimal staff exposure. External beam irradiation has also been used but its value is restricted because of the wide field of irradiation which limits the total dose to the hemithorax to approximately 20 Gy (2000 rad) in 3 weeks.

If simple measures fail, thoracoscopy and tube drainage with talc insufflation and pleurodesis is often more successful than simple intrapleural drug instillation. Occasionally, pleurectomy will be required for adequate control of an effusion due to pleural secondary deposits and should be considered if the patient's general condition warrants (13).

Pericardial effusion

This is an infrequent clinical problem and in contrast to pleural effusion, pericardial effusions are less commonly due to malignancy than other causes such as infections, myxoedema, collagen disorders and rheumatoid arthritis. Although the diagnosis is often a radiological one, with 'globular' enlargement of the heart shadow, clinical signs include faintness of the heart sounds, pericardial friction rub and loss of apex beat. Tamponade may occur, with raised venous pressure, hypotension and paradoxical pulse.

The commonest causes of malignant pericardial effusions are carcinomas of breast and bronchus, and lymphoma including Hodgkin's disease. Post-mortem studies have shown that pericardial effusion is substantially underdiagnosed during life. In patients with widespread metastases, it may occur concurrently with a malignant pleural effusion. The diagnosis can be simply confirmed by echocardiography,

which also gives useful quantitative information regarding the volume of the effusion. Because pericardial aspiration is both more hazardous and technically more difficult than pleural aspiration, it should not be undertaken in asymptomatic patients where the diagnosis is almost certain.

Treatment is by means of the same agents that are used for pleural effusion including cytotoxic drugs, tetracycline, radioactive gold and external beam irradiation. There may in addition be a useful response to systemic chemotherapy or endocrine therapy in which case intrapericardial instillation should be withheld. Pericardectomy has no place in the management, but creation of a surgical 'pericardial window' into the mediastinum may be beneficial if the condition is persistent and the patient relatively fit.

Ascites

Ascites is a common clinical problem in cancer. The usual cause is widespread peritoneal seedlings which cause exudation of fluid and block lymphatic drainage. Liver metastases are often present and hypoalbuminaemia contributes to the accumulation of fluid by lowering plasma osmotic pressure. Common cancers causing ascites include carcinomas of ovary, breast, bronchus (especially small cell), large bowel, stomach, pancreas and melanoma.

Patients usually present with abdominal distension, bulging of the flanks and with peripheral oedema if there is associated hypoalbuminaemia and/or IVC obstruction. The umbilicus may be everted and some patients have a fluid thrill. Some patients with moderate ascites are unaware of the distension, taking more note of the ankle oedema. It is important not to assume a malignant diagnosis, particularly when the tumour was previously thought to be localized or controlled by treatment. Important non-malignant causes include: portal hypertension (usually from cirrhosis or portal vein thrombosis), hepatic vein thrombosis (Budd-Chiari syndrome), raised systemic venous pressure as in longstanding cardiac failure and hypoalbuminaemia from other causes.

Diagnosis is by clinical examination, abdominal X-ray, ultrasound and aspiration cytology. Plain X-ray of the abdomen often shows a 'ground-glass' appearance due to a general blurring of the bowel and other intra-abdominal images by the fluid. There may be dilatation of the bowel and fluid levels indicating partial or subacute obstruction if the ascites is accompanied by an intra-abdominal tumour such as carcinoma of the ovary or bowel. Ultrasound examination is a sensitive technique for demonstrating ascites. Malignant ascites is usually turbid and straw-coloured with a protein concentration above 25 g/l. Malignant cells may be detected cytologically though this examination is frequently negative even in cases confirmed by other means.

Treatment includes both therapeutic aspiration (paracentesis) and general measures designed to prevent recurrence. Slow drainage over several days, via a peritoneal dialysis catheter, may be necessary to give relief of symptoms. Instillation of cytoxic agents is less frequently practised and less frequently successful than in malignant pleural effusion, but intraperitoneal thiotepa, mustine, bleomycin and other agents have all been used. Systemic chemotherapy (or endocrine therapy in breast cancer) may occasionally help to control ascites and should be considered if the patient's general condition warrants it. Intraperitoneal radioactive colloids can be given via peritoneal dialysis catheter, and are reportedly effective in about half of all cases (14). External irradiation is of little value except in some cases of ovarian cancer.

In the presence of hypoalbuminaemia, treatment with diuretics can be helpful in preventing recurrence. Combination treatment with frusemide and spironolactone is often used. Surgical procedures such as peritoneo-venous shunts have been attempted if the patient is fit and suffering from repeated episodes of ascites, with a reported success rate of over 70%. The prognosis for patients with malignant ascites is poor, the majority dying within 6 months of diagnosis.

CARCINOMATOUS MENINGITIS

Malignant meningitis is increasingly recognized as a complication of cancer. It is common in acute leukaemia. The most frequently associated solid tumours are non-Hodgkin's lymphoma, breast cancer and melanoma. Management is discussed further in Chapter 11.

MANAGEMENT OF HEPATIC METASTASES

Many patients with cancer will develop hepatic metastases and when these are widespread the expectation of life is only 2–3 months. In many cases there will be widespread dissemination and the liver involvement will not be a separate medical problem. In some tumours such as small cell carcinoma of the bronchus, breast cancer or lymphoma there is a reasonable likelihood of a response to chemotherapy with symptomatic and biochemical improvement. There are however many occasions when the liver is involved with metastatic cancer for which chemotherapy is inappropriate due to primary or acquired drug resistance.

The usual symptoms are fatigue, weight loss, anorexia and right upper quadrant pain. There may be abdominal distension from ascites. Episodes of sudden severe pain may occur when there is haemorrhage into a metastasis. Later, jaundice develops with advancing cachexia. Survival is usually a few months depending on the extent of involvement and rate of progression. Metastatic carcinoid tumours may be very slow growing and in this disease hepatic metastases are compatible with survival of 3–5 years.

Almost all treatment of hepatic metastasis is palliative and the value of each approach depends on the circumstances of each patient. The main symptoms are anorexia, nausea, pain, fever and malaise. Jaundice is a late feature unless there is obstruction to the porta hepatis by a tumour or lymph node mass. Itching and steatorrhoea may then be major symptoms. The following approaches can be taken to relieve symptoms.

Pharmacological

Anorexia, fever and malaise may all be relieved for a time by corticosteroids. Prednisolone 20–30 mg/day is usually adequate but the symptoms often recur after a few weeks and muscle wasting becomes profound if this dose is continued for long. Phenothiazines or metoclopramide before meals may help a little with the nausea, and aspirin or indomethacin may also relieve fever. Pain is treated with analgesics as described in Chapter 7.

Radiotherapy

Although the liver does not tolerate large doses (above 35 Gy), radiotherapy has a useful role in palliation of pain and may also improve nausea and vomiting. With a dose of 20–35 Gy to the whole liver, over 70% of patients will experience some improvement, particularly relief of pain (15). In chemoresistant tumours the addition of chemotherapy or hypoxic cell sensitizers does not improve these results. Often a particularly painful metastasis can be treated with a local field using a few large fractions, producing quick relief of pain without adverse effects.

Chemotherapy

In the case of responsive tumours such as small cell lung cancer or breast cancer, chemotherapy may be very effective, with responses in 50–60% of patients. If the primary tumour is of a type not usually amenable to chemotherapy, it is unlikely that cytotoxic agents will be of much value. For metastatic adenocarcinoma of the bowel, 5FU has been most widely used but the objective response rate is only 10–20%. Subjectively, particularly with respect to pain, the response rate is higher. Regional perfusion with 5FU via the hepatic artery is of unproven value and is a complicated and somewhat hazardous technique although worthwhile pain relief has been claimed.

Surgical

Hepatic artery ligation or embolization can produce pain relief and shrinkage of metastases but they recur rapidly with regeneration of the blood supply. Occasionally a slowly growing solitary metastasis is worth resecting in a fit patient with, for example, a carcinoid tumour.

RADIOTHERAPEUTIC EMERGENCIES

There are two common clinical situations which require urgent consideration by the radiotherapist. These are acute spinal cord compression, and superior vena cava obstruction.

Acute spinal cord compression

This syndrome results from pressure on the cord, most commonly as a result of vertebral metastases causing crush fractures, or by extension into the extradural space. Extradural compression may develop in the absence of deposits in the spine. Very occasionally, intramedullary metastases will cause acute cord compression from within. Cord compression most commonly occurs in diseases where bony metastases (particularly spinal metastases) are frequent. Carcinomas of the breast, prostate and lung (particularly small cell carcinomas), lymphoma and myeloma are the commonest causes followed by carcinomas of the thyroid, kidney, bladder, bowel and melanoma. Lymphomas may produce cord compression by extension from paraspinal lymph nodes through the intervertebral foramina.

Characteristically, the patient complains of back pain often with a root distribution, weakness of the legs, dribbling, hesitancy and incontinence of urine and sluggish bowel action. In most cases, only one or two of these symptoms will be present, and limb weakness and bladder dysfunction are late signs. Higher cord lesions will also be accompanied by symptoms and signs in the upper limb.

The cauda equina syndrome, where the compression occurs below the lower level of the spinal cord (L1/2), is often difficult to diagnose (see p. 197). The features include leg weakness, sacral anaesthesia, retention of urine and erectile failure. Clinical diagnosis is particularly important since in this syndrome radiological studies, including myelography, often fail to demonstrate any definite abnormality. Careful neurological examination may reveal loss of sacral sensation (saddle anaesthesia) which will only be detected if perianal sensation is tested with a pin, and anal sphincter tone is assessed on rectal examination.

Spinal cord compression may occasionally occur at more than one site, giving rise to neurological signs (for example a mixture of upper and lower motor neurone weakness) which would otherwise be difficult to explain on the basis of a single lesion.

Investigation should include plain X-ray of the spine and myelography. Plain X-ray may show evidence of multiple bone metastases, a crush fracture at the site of pain, or less obvious changes such as erosion of a pedicle (Fig. 8.1). Myelography will delineate the site of block if it is above L1/2.

Treatment of cord compression is either by surgery, radiation therapy, or a combination of both (16, 17). With acute cord compression in a patient in good general health and with no other evidence of metastatic disease, decompressive laminectomy is the treatment of choice. Most neurosurgeons feel that laborious attempts to remove all of the tumour are generally fruitless, so that in the majority of cases, neurosurgical treatment will be followed by radiotherapy in an attempt to control the residual local disease. In patients with multiple metastases and with a short life expectation, radiotherapy may be used without surgery. This

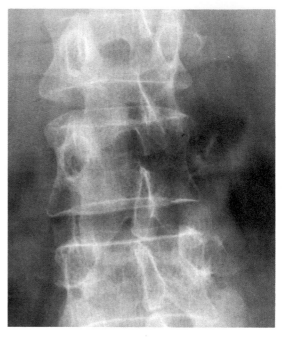

Fig. 8.1. *X-ray of lumbar vertebrae showing destruction of the left pedicle L₃.*

will of course be particularly beneficial in patients with radioresponsive tumours. In small cell carcinoma of the bronchus, it has been shown that treatment with radiotherapy alone is as beneficial as treatment by surgery and radiotherapy in combination, as judged both by recovery of power, mobility and also survival. Where radiotherapy is employed as the sole method, dexamethasone is often used routinely as a means of reducing local oedema, particularly where acute radiation hyperaemia of the cord might pose additional problems. In multiple myeloma, radiotherapy is often preferred to surgery since there may be multiple sites, and patients with cord compression from myeloma are often unfit for surgery. Myeloma deposits are very sensitive to irradiation.

The prognosis for patients with cord compression relates to the degree of neurological damage before treatment and the underlying cancer. If the patient has progressed to paraplegia before treatment, the chance that he will walk after treatment is less than 5%. Early diagnosis is essential since with less severe damage, 50% will be ambulatory. Widespread radioresistant tumour (e.g. melanoma) has a bad prognosis. Chemotherapy plays no part in the initial management of cord compression.

Superior vena caval obstruction (SVCO)

This most commonly results from a right-sided carcinoma of the bronchus (particularly small cell carcinoma). It also occurs in lymphoma (particularly Hodgkin's disease, in which mediastinal involvement occurs in about one-quarter of all patients), as well as carcinoma of the breast, kidney and other tumours which may metastasise to mediastinal nodes. Occasionally it may be a presenting feature of a primary mediastinal tumour such as a thymoma, or a germ cell tumour. It is characterized by swelling of the face, neck and arms, sometimes with a typical plethoric cyanotic facies. There is non-pulsatile engorgement of veins and large collateral veins may be visible over the surface of the shoulders, scapulae and upper chest. Retinal veins may also be engorged and there is often conjunctival oedema. The most constant physical sign is that of leashes of tiny bluish venules which occur over the chest wall, particularly in the precordial, subcostal and infrascapular regions. Patients are almost always dyspnoeic and hypoxic, and the chest X-ray usually shows a substantial right-sided mass (Fig. 8.2).

Urgent treatment with radiotherapy is the mainstay of management and is undoubtedly the treatment of choice for non-small cell carcinomas of bronchus and other tumours not amenable to chemotherapy, and where treatment must be started before the diagnosis is known. However, with the advent of effective chemotherapy for lymphoma and small cell carcinoma of the bronchus, combination chemotherapy should be considered in SVCO due to these conditions and has a number of advantages. In the first place, patients may be several miles (and an uncomfortable journey) from a radiotherapy centre, whereas chemotherapy can

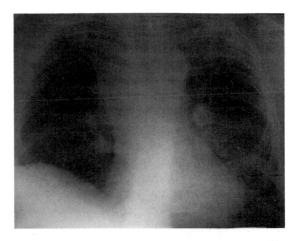

Fig. 8.2. *Typical radiological findings in superior vena cava obstruction.* The tumour is usually right-sided. In this case the diaphragm is raised because of involvement of the phrenic nerve.

be given without moving the patient; secondly, many of them will have extensive disease which would be left untreated by local irradiation; thirdly, chemotherapy is given as a single intravenous injection whereas radiotherapy has to be given daily for several days or weeks. Finally, the response to chemotherapy is often at least as quick as with radiotherapy, which can still be given if chemotherapy fails.

Radiation dosage in treatment of SVC obstruction should depend on the primary diagnosis. In small cell carcinoma of the bronchus, a total of 40 Gy (4000 rad) midline dose is given in 20 daily fractions over 4 weeks (or the equivalent over a shorter time). However, in non-small cell lung cancer, this dose is generally inadequate and treatment with radical intent will demand that at least 56 Gy (5600 rad) be given over 5–6 weeks, using a planned multifield arrangement in order to avoid over-treatment of spinal cord. As with spinal cord compression, dexamethasone is a useful addition to treatment. Although in lung cancer SVC obstruction has long been considered a serious prognostic sign. In small cell carcinoma of the bronchus, which is the commonest cause, this does not appear to be the case.

Other radiotherapy emergencies

Orbital or intraocular metastases most commonly occur in carcinoma of the breast and in malignant melanoma. They present with proptosis, oculomotor palsy or visual loss which may be acute if there is bleeding into the eye from a choroidal deposit. These metastases may be bilateral. Early treatment with radiotherapy is important since permanent visual loss or ocular palsy may occur in a patient whose life-span may be several years. Careful radiation planning is required in order to avoid treatment to the anterior half of the eyes and to the contralateral lens. A single lateral radiation field with a dose of 30 Gy (3000 rad) in 10 daily fractions over 2 weeks of treatment is usually adequate. Chemotherapy plays no part in the management of these complications.

Primary or secondary cancers at other critical sites may also lead to a necessity for urgent treatment. Impending collapse of a lung from severe bronchial narrowing may be the cause of an urgent referral from a chest physician who has been following an asymptomatic patient with known carcinoma of the bronchus for months or even years. The development of a unilateral monophonic wheeze, usually heard at its loudest over the main or lobar bronchus, is the most reliable physical sign. The sequence of chest X-rays often shows increasing shadowing and obstruction of part of the lung. Radiotherapy may well reverse this picture and relieve the patient's dyspnoea. The role of radiotherapy in carcinoma of the bronchus is more fully discussed in Chapter 12.

For the severe, localized and unremitting pain of bony metastases, radiotherapy is preeminently the treatment of choice. Palliative radiotherapy is often given as a matter of urgency in patients with severe bone pain who have not previously been treated maximally with radiotherapy to the painful site especially if a single metastatic site is evident on clinical examination, X-ray or isotope bone scan. Analgesics (usually opiates) will need to be given during the course of treatment and often after-

wards as well (see p. 115) for discussion of pain control. If an area of spinal cord is included in the field, the treatment is often fractionated over 2 weeks (30 Gy (3000 rad) in 10 daily treatments) though shorter treatment periods are certainly acceptable for patients with a short life span, and may be perfectly safe. Common regimens for the relief of bone pain include 5 fractions of 5 Gy (500 rad) calculated at depth, or 4 fractions of 6 Gy (600 rad). Single fraction treatments of 8–14 Gy (800–1400 rad) are becoming more popular and are certainly more convenient. It is not yet clear whether such treatments are as effective.

REFERENCES

1 Mitchell R. (1976) Red Cell Transfusion. *Clinics in Haematology* **5**, 33–71.
2 Petz L. D. (1983). Red Blood Cell Transfusion. *Clinics in Oncology* **2** (3), 505–527.
3 Kelton J. B. & Ali, A. M. (1983) Platelet transfusions—A critical appraisal. *Clinics in Oncology* **2** (3), 549–585.
4 Young L. S. (1983) The role of granulocyte transfusions in treating and preventing infection. *Cancer Treatment Reports* **67**, 109–111.
5 Schiffer C. A. (1983) Granulocyte transfusion therapy. *Cancer Treatment Reports* **67**, 113–119.
6 Bodey G. P., Buckley, M. & Sathje Y. S. (1966) Quantative relationship between circulating leucocytes and infection in patients with acute leukaemia. *Annals of Internal Medicine* **64**, 328.
7 Siber G. R., Weitzmann S. A., Aisenberg A. C., Weinstein H. J. & Schiffmang (1978) Impaired antibody response to pneumonococca vaccine after treatment for Hodgkin's disease. *New England Journal Medicine* **299**, 442.
8 Weitzman S. & Aisenberg A. C. (1977) Fulminant sepsis after the successful treatment of Hodgkin's disease. *American Journal of Medicine* **62**, 47.
9 Joshi J. H. & Schimoff S. C. (1983) Therapy of infection in granulocytopenia patients with cancer. *Clinics in Oncology* **2** (3) 611.
10 Calman K. C. (1982) Cancer cachexia. *British Journal of Hospital Medicine* **27**, 28–34.
11 Mundy G. R., Luben, R. A., Raisz L. G., Oppenheim J. J. & Buell D. N. (1974). Bone-resorbing activity in supernatants from lyphoid cell lines. *New England Journal of Medicine* **290**, 867.
12 Cohen L. F., Balow J. E., Magrath I. T., Poplack D. G. & Ziegler J. L. (1980) Acute tumour lysis

syndrome. A review of 37 patients with Burkitt's lymphoma. *American Journal Medicine* **67,** 486.

13 Anderson C. B., Philpott G. W. & Fergison T. B. (1974) The treatment of malignant pleural effusions. *Cancer* **33,** 916.

14 Dybecki J., Balchum D. J. & Meneely G. R. (1959). Treatment of pleural and peritoneal effusion with intracavitary colloidal radio-gold (198 Au). *Archives of International Medicine* **104,** 802.

Cloud L., Troy C. A. & Piro A. J. (1978). Palliation of hepatic metastases. *Cancer* **41,** 2013.

16 Bruckman J. E. & Bloomer W. D. (1978) Management of spinal cord compression. *Seminars in Oncology* **5,** 135.

17 Gilbert R. W., Kim J. H. & Posner J. B. (1978). Epidural spinal cord compression from metastatic tumour. Diagnosis and management. *Annals of Neurology* **3,** 40.

Chapter 9

Hormonal and Paraneoplastic Syndromes

Cancers are frequently associated with constitutional disturbances which are not due to the local effect of the tumour—Table 9.1 illustrates metabolic and paraneoplastic syndromes in non-endocrine neoplasms. For example, although cancer of the head of the pancreas will frequently cause obstructive jaundice leading to steatorrhoea and weight loss, these metabolic upsets are due to the physical presence of the tumour obstructing the common bile and pancreatic ducts. However, the tumour may occasionally give rise to remote effects such as fever, thrombophlebitis or mood change, and the mechanisms whereby these symptoms are caused are poorly understood. Such systemic metabolic effects of cancer are common and often add to the patient's symtoms. Sometimes these paraneoplastic syndromes may be the presenting feature of cancer and lead to other diagnoses being made in error, before a cancer is suspected. An awareness of these complications of cancer is therefore essential for proper management because the symptoms can often be controlled and the patient made more comfortable even when the primary tumour cannot be removed. Furthermore, the symptoms may be wrongly interpreted as being due to metastases and an opportunity for effective treatment thereby lost.

The pathogenesis and management of weight loss, cachexia, and hypercalcaemia are discussed in Chapter 8.

FEVER DUE TO MALIGNANT DISEASE (1)

Most patients with cancer who develop a fever do so because of infection. Fever is, however, a symptom of cancer itself and may be the presenting feature. The pathogenesis is obscure. Lymphomas, especially Hodgkin's disease, are often accompanied by fever and in these diseases the pyrexia usually indicates an aggressive and advanced tumour. The typical relapsing Pel-Ebstein fever is only present in a minority of patients with Hodgkin's disease. Nonspecific intermittent or remittent fever is much more common.

Hypernephroma is notorious for its tendency to cause fever and to present in this way. It may be associated with leucocytosis (often extreme) and thus mimic a pyogenic infection. Other carcinomas may present similarly especially if they are metastatic to the liver and bone marrow. Sarcomas and primary liver cancer are also frequently associated with pyrexia.

When cancer is the cause of the presenting pyrexia it can usually be diagnosed fairly easily. Isotope or ultrasound scans of the liver are often abnormal, the liver enzymes are elevated, especially alkaline phosphatase, and there are usually symptoms and signs of the primary tumour. If nothing can be done to treat the cancer itself, symptomatic relief can sometimes be obtained by aspirin, non-steroidal anti-inflammatory agents and by steroids. The control of symptoms usually lasts a few weeks or months.

Table 9.1. Metabolic and paraneoplastic syndromes in non-endocrine neoplasms.

Syndrome	Tumour	Syndrome	Tumour
Endocrine and Metabolic		Erythrocytosis	Renal carcinoma, hepatoma, uterine cancer, cerebellar haemangioblastoma
Cushing's syndrome	Small cell bronchogenic cancer, thymoma, bronchial carcinoid, medullary carcinoma of the thyroid	Red cell aplasia	Thymomas
		Disseminated intravascular coagulation	Mucinous adenocarcinomas
Inappropriate ADH secretion	Small cell bronchogenic cancer, thymoma, lymphoma, duodenal carcinoma, pancreatic carcinoma	*Neurological*	
		Peripheral neuropathy	Small cell bronchogenic carcinoma, breast, ovary, lymphoma
Gynaecomastia	Teratoma, large cell lung cancer, tumours of liver and adrenal	Cerebellar degeneration	Small cell lung cancer
		Eaton-Lambert syndrome	Small cell lung cancer
Hypoglycaemia	Retroperitoneal sarcoma and lymphoma, hepatoma	*Muscle and Joint*	
		Polyarthritis	Adenocarcinomas (gut, breast, ovary)
Hyperpigmentation	Small cell bronchogenic cancer	Dermatomyositis	Lung cancer, oesophageal cancer, adenocarcinomas
Cachexia, Anorexia, altered taste	All tumours		
Hypercalcaemia	All cancers with widespread bone metastases, squamous cancers, renal and ovarian carcinoma	*Skin* See Table 9.2	
		Renal	
		Nephrotic syndrome	Adenocarcinomas
Haematological			
Multiple thromboses	Pancreatic cancer, other adenocarcinomas		

ECTOPIC HORMONE PRODUCTION IN CANCER

Many cancers (perhaps the majority) produce hormone precursors and peptides, some of which have biological activity (2). In the formation of a hormone in an endocrine gland the precursor hormone (prohormone) is often the major storage form and is biologically inactive but is cleaved to the active hormone at the time of secretion. In the blood and tissues the hormone is degraded to the inactive carboxyl fragment and the amino fragment which may retain activity. Tumours may produce inactive pro-hormones or the active principle. They may also produce biologically active peptides such as human chorionic gonadotrophin (HCG) or variants of HCG which have a reduced carbohydrate content and which have lost activity. Similarly a biologically active glycopeptide hormone may have two chains both of which are necessary for biological activity. If only one chain is made by the tumour it will be inactive.

The mechanism of ectopic synthesis is not clear but may be due to activation of DNA as a result of malignant transformation. In this section, 'ectopic' hormone is taken to mean production of a hormone by a non-endocrine tumour. Clearly cancers of the adrenal, pancreas or endocrine cells in the gut may cause hormonal disturbances. These are discussed in the appropriate chapters.

Syndrome of inappropriate ADH secretion (SIADH)

This syndrome is characterized biochemically by a plasma sodium below 130 mmol/l with a low plasma and high urine osmolality. Clinically it usually becomes apparent only when the plasma sodium reaches 120 mmol/l or below, when the patient becomes tired, then drowsy and confused. The commonest underlying tumour is small cell bronchogenic carcinoma which is usually apparent on chest X-ray. Up to 50% of patients with this disease have impaired water handling, but only 10–20% have a plasma sodium below 130 mmol/l (4). The ADH is identical with that produced by the neurohypophysis. A low plasma sodium may be found in very ill patients regardless of cause. This has been called the 'sick cell' syndrome but is probably due to inappropriate ADH release from the posterior pituitary. This syndrome is occasionally difficult to distinguish from ectopic ADH production. In small cell lung cancer, marked hyponatraemia (assumed to be a reflection of ectopic ADH) is associated with a worse prognosis.

Treatment of the tumour with drugs and radiotherapy may improve the metabolic abnormality. While this is being done, demeclocycline (300 mg by mouth 6–8 hourly at first then 8–12 hourly) is effective in correcting the plasma sodium. It does this by rendering the distal tubule unresponsive to the ectopic ADH. This drug can impair renal function and the blood urea should be measured regularly. In severe cases water restriction may be temporarily required but this is difficult to sustain and is sometimes ineffective. In an acutely ill patient with life-threatening hyponatraemia, a 3% saline infusion combined with i.v. frusemide (to increase free water clearance) is effective emergency treatment.

Ectopic ACTH production

Excess production of ACTH is an uncommon metabolic complication of cancers which are normally neuroectodermal in origin. The commonest tumour to produce the syndrome is small cell carcinoma of the bronchus. Small carcinoid tumours in the lung, thymus and pancreas may also cause the syndrome. Raised ACTH levels have been found in half of all patients with small cell lung cancer and immunoreactive ACTH can be extracted from the majority of these tumours (5). Clinical manifestations of ectopic ACTH production are very unusual, and when they occur the clinical picture is usually different from classical Cushing's syndrome. There is generally hyperkalaemia, glucose intolerance, hypertension and muscle weakness. These patients usually have extensive disease with a poor prognosis. Estimates of the frequency of this syndrome vary depending on the criteria used to define it. Presentation with the features described above has occurred in less than 2% of over 600 patients with small cell lung cancer treated in our collaborative studies at University College Hospital, London.

The syndrome occurs rarely in squamous lung cancer, adenocarcinomas of the gut or kidney and medullary carcinoma of the thyroid. It has also been described in thymoma and ganglioneuroblastoma in childhood. Some of these tumours contain molecules of a prohormone with a higher molecular weight than normal ACTH which may not be biologically active. Other tumours can produce a corticotrophin releasing factor which acts on the pituitary.

Clinically, the syndrome caused by small cell lung cancer is rarely confused with other forms of Cushing's syndrome. The diagnosis is more difficult when the tumour is a bronchial carcinoid. In lung cancer with ectopic ACTH, high dose dexamethasone does not suppress the plasma cortisol level, in contrast to pituitary-dependent Cushing's syndrome. The plasma ACTH will be very low with an autonomous adrenal adenoma or carcinoma. In the latter, the plasma cortisol may also fail to suppress with dexamethasone.

Treatment is to the primary tumour. If this is ineffective then aminoglutethimide will block steroid synthesis. Metyrapone will also block 11-hydroxylation of corticosteroids causing a fall in plasma cortisol. This drug can be useful in seriously ill patients before definitive treatment of the tumour begins, but neither drug will produce lasting benefit in the absence of treatment of the disease.

Hypoglycaemia

Hypoglycaemia is a very uncommon complication of some cancers. It occurs with large thoracic and abdominal sarcomas especially those situated retroperitoneally and with hepatomas, adrenal carcinomas and lymphomas (6). It does not seem to be produced by insulin which cannot be found in plasma or tumour extracts. Elevated plasma levels of somatomedin-like substances have been found. These are peptides normally made in the liver as a result of stimulation by growth hormone and which have an action like insulin. These peptides have occasionally been extracted from the tumour itself. Other substances may be produced which have insulin-like activity or which bind to insulin receptors.

The hypoglycaemia attacks may be spontaneous or associated with fasting and can be very severe. Clinically the episodes are indistinguishable from those produced by islet-cell tumours, but the plasma insulin is not raised. If the tumour cannot be completely removed the hypoglycaemia may be partially controlled by frequent feeding, diazoxide, glucagon or corticosteroids.

Gynaecomastia and gonadotrophin production

Gynaecomastia is an increase in the glandular and stromal tissue of the male breast. In most instances when it complicates a non-endocrine malignancy, it is probably caused by tumour-related human chorionic gonadotrophin pro-

duction. Teratoma and seminoma may both be associated with HCG production and so may carcinoma of the bronchus of all histological types. Other HCG-producing tumours include pancreas (both exocrine and islet-cell tumours), liver, adrenal and breast. In most cases of non-germ cell neoplasms, HCG is produced in amounts too small to be clinically significant although it may occasionally be useful as a tumour marker (7). In other cases the hormone may not be glycosylated by the tumour and this results in its rapid removal from the blood. Some tumours secrete free alpha subunits which are not associated with biological activity. The increased oestrogen production which is the cause of the gynaecomastia is probably due to the action of the ectopic HCG on the testis. The correct treatment is removal of the tumour, but if this is not possible, or is incomplete, the HCG inhibitor danazol may be useful if the gynaecomastia is painful. Painful gynaecomastia can also sometimes be relieved by local irradiation of the breasts. Further details on HCG are given in Chapters 4 and 19.

Other ectopic hormones

Bronchial carcinoids may rarely produce growth hormone releasing substances over sufficient length of time to cause acromegaly. Galactorrhoea has been reported with cancer, due to hyperprolactinaemia (3). Hyperthyroidism may occur in triophoblastic tumours producing HCG. This does not appear to be due to TSH production, but the HCG may have TSH-like activity. Hypercalcaemia is discussed in Chapter 8.

HAEMATOLOGICAL SYNDROMES

Anaemia

Anaemia is an almost universal accompaniment of advanced cancer. Many factors contribute including gastro-intestinal bleeding leading to iron deficiency, and poor appetite with resulting iron and folate deficiency. Even if there are no secondary deficiency states, anaemia can still develop and can be regarded as a 'paraneoplastic' syndrome. Characteristically it is similar to the anaemia of other chronic diseases. It takes a few months to develop and the haemoglobin does not usually fall below 8 or 9 grams. The anaemia is normocytic and normochromic or slightly hypochromic. The serum iron is low but so is the total iron binding capacity (TIBC), in contrast to the anaemia of iron deficiency where the TIBC is high. The marrow shows stainable iron in macrophages. The red cell survival is often shortened to some degree without an increase in erythropoiesis sufficient to compensate for this. There also appears to be a block in release of iron from macrophages into the plasma.

Treatment of the anaemia depends on the successful treatment of the cancer. If this is impossible, and there are no secondary deficiencies of iron or folate, the anaemia can only be corrected, albeit temporarily, by blood transfusion. This can be of value when the anaemia may be contributing to fatigue and the transfusion may allow the patient a little more useful and active life.

An auto-immune haemolytic anaemia which usually responds to treatment with steroids may complicate B cell neoplasms and Hodgkin's disease.

Polycythaemia

The commonest cancer to produce this syndrome is renal carcinoma. Rarer causes include cerebellar haemangioblastoma, hepatoma, uterine leiomyosarcoma and fibroids (8). The probable explanation is the production of an erythropoietin-like substance in renal cancer though this may not be the cause with cancers from other sites. Only 2–5% of cases of renal cancer are associated with polycythaemia though excess production of erythropoietin occurs in over half of all patients. However, if the investigation of a high haematocrit confirms a true polycythaemia, an IVU should be performed to exclude renal carcinoma. The white blood count and platelet count are often raised in polycythaemia rubra vera but unless these values are greatly elevated it is not wise to rely on this alone in making the distinction from renal carcinoma.

Migratory thrombophlebitis

Carcinoma of the pancreas, especially of the body or tail, is occasionally associated with multiple thromboses often in superficial veins and migratory in nature. Other adenocarcinomas may give rise to the same syndrome. The tumours tend to be inoperable. The venous thromboses are sometimes in an unusual site such as the arm, and this may arouse the suspicion of the underlying diagnosis. Pulmonary embolism seldom occurs. These tumours are thought to liberate substances which promote clotting in veins.

Disseminated intravascular coagulation (DIC)

This is a complication of malignancy which has been described in many different types of cancer of which the commonest are adenocarcinomas (prostate, breast, pancreas, ovary) and other tumours such as metastatic carcinoid, neuroblastoma and rhabdomyosarcoma (9). It is probably due to the liberation of thromboplastin-like material from cancer cells, but some cancers secrete thrombin-like enzymes. Many patients with cancer have increased levels of fibrin degradation products in the blood but the degree of intravascular coagulation is usually mild. Problems with haemorrhage are very unusual except in acute promyelocytic leukaemia where DIC can be severe when treatment has been started. In solid tumours, where the DIC is chronic and low-grade, treatment is by removal of the cancer where possible. Occasionally the DIC can be associated with red cell fragmentation (microangiopathic haemolytic anaemia) especially in stomach cancer. This syndrome may also be accompanied by acute renal failure (the haemolytic-uraemic syndrome).

Red cell aplasia

Acquired suppression of erythropoiesis has been described in adults as an accompaniment of tumours, particularly thymomas, although in many of these cases the thymoma is benign. It occurs rarely in association with a variety of other cancers such as carcinoma of the bronchus. The anaemia, which is often severe, is normocytic and erythropoiesis is selectively absent from the marrow. An immune suppression of erythropoiesis provoked by the tumour is the postulated cause.

NEUROLOGICAL SYNDROMES

Cancers can be associated with neurological syndromes unrelated to direct compression or infiltration. While interesting and important, these syndromes are uncommon, their frequency often being overestimated by neurologists who, because of their specialty, see these complications not infrequently. From the point of view of the cancer specialist the non-metastatic neurological complications of malignancy are infrequently encountered, at least in a clinically significant form. Most neurological complications of cancer are due to metastases or compression and it is a grave error to fail to treat a cancer causing, for example, fits or spinal cord compression, because of a mistaken diagnosis of a non-metastatic manifestation of the tumour. The major clinical syndromes are discussed briefly below.

Peripheral neuropathy

The commonest variety of neuropathy seen in association with cancer is a *distal sensory and motor neuropathy* (10). Pathologically there is segmental demyelination of the nerves, usually distally, and axonal degeneration. It is possible that the neurones themselves may also be the site of the initial damage. The neuropathy varies in its severity. There is a mild form developing late in the course of the disease, and a more severe form occurring earlier, sometimes before

the tumour is manifest and occasionally following an intermittent course. The CSF shows a modest increase in protein (1–2 g/l), without excess cells.

The second form of neuropathy is carcinomatous *sensory neuropathy*. This is a slowly progressive sensory neuropathy, associated with pains and parasethesiae in the limbs, which may spread to the trunk and face (11). There is degeneration of dorsal root ganglia sometimes associated with a mononuclear cell infiltrate. Later, there is loss of the posterior columns leading to ataxia. The patient may become chair or bed-bound before the primary tumour has declared itself. Cancer of the lung (especially small cell cancer) is the commonest tumour but lymphoma and many other cancers can be associated. Removal of the tumour usually does not produce improvement and the neuropathy is progressive. Steroids may sometimes help.

An *acute ascending paralysis* of the Guillain-Barré type may also occur, and has been noted in Hodgkin's disease especially.

The diagnosis of carcinomatous neuropathy is often very difficult. Infiltration of the meninges with carcinoma and lymphoma may occasionally cause peripheral sensory and motor damage. The CSF should therefore always be examined for malignant cells. In young patients with lymphoma, where the risk of CNS involvement is high, it is usually best to treat the patient for CNS relapse if there is doubt about the diagnosis.

Carcinomatous myelopathy

This rare syndrome can present as a flaccid paraplegia of acute onset with loss of sphincter control (12). The primary tumour is usually lung cancer. There is necrosis of the cord with little inflammation. The mechanism is unknown and the damage irreversible. A less acute myelopathy can also occur, associated with loss of anterior horn cells and a slowly progressive lower motor neurone weakness. It is usually associated with lymphoma and lung cancer.

The diagnosis of carcinomatous myelopathy is difficult to make. Cord compression must be excluded and the CSF examined for malignant cells. Other diseases such as amyotrophic lateral sclerosis may cause a similar picture. The association with carcinoma may become apparent only late in the evolution of the disease.

Cerebellar degeneration

This rare syndrome is most commonly associated with carcinoma of the bronchus (13). It differs from the chronic idiopathic cerebellar degenerations of adult life by being more rapid in evolution, sometimes progressing to severe disability in a few months, even before the primary tumour is apparent. Unsteadiness of gait, truncal ataxia, vertigo and diplopia (sometimes with oscillopsia and opsoclonus) occur. Long tract signs due to spinal cord degeneration may develop. Unlike idiopathic cerebellar degeneration, the CSF may be abnormal with a raised protein and a few lymphocytes. Pathologically there is global cell loss in the cerebellar cortex and some perivascular inflammatory infiltrate. Degenerative changes may be found in the cord. Treatment of the primary tumour, although necessary, does not usually help. A CT scan is essential to exclude a cerebellar metastasis as far as possible.

Limbic encephalitis

In this exceedingly rare syndrome an underlying small cell carcinoma is likely to be responsible (14). It is characterized by the fairly rapid onset of confusion, memory disturbance and agitation. It may be associated with a cerebellar disturbance due to degeneration. There is temporal lobe degeneration with some perivascular infiltrate. A viral aetiology has been suspected but not proven. As with cerebellar degeneration, the main differential diagnosis is from intracranial metastasis.

Progressive Multifocal Leucoencephalopathy (PML)

This rare syndrome is not always associated with cancer, but lymphoma is by far the commonest associated disorder. The clinical features are aphasia and dementia leading to coma, visual field loss which may progress to blindness, fits and focal paralyses. The differential diagnosis includes metastases, lymphomatous meningitis, herpes encephalitis and cerebrovascular disease. The CSF is usually normal.

The brain shows patchy demyelination throughout the white matter with abnormal oligodendroglia, the nuclei of which contain viral inclusions. Papova viruses (JC and SV40) have been isolated from these brains (15). Antibodies to these viruses may be present in blood or CSF and may help in diagnosis. The disease may respond to intrathecal and intravenous cytosine arabinoside.

Eaton-Lambert Syndrome (16)

In this rare syndrome, which is found almost exclusively with small cell lung cancer, the patient complains of weakness, aching and fatigue in the shoulder and pelvic girdle muscles, and sometimes impotence. It resembles myasthenia except that the relationship of fatigue to repeated muscular activity is less clear-cut and the EMG shows an increase in muscle action potentials at higher rates of nerve stimulation. The ocular and bulbar muscles are usually spared. The syndrome may appear before the tumour. Unfortunately there is no response to oral anticholinesterases, but edrophonium in a small dose intravenously often produces improvement. Treatment of the tumour may help and guanidine hydrochloride may benefit patients whose tumours fail to respond to chemotherapy. This drug may act by releasing acetylcholine at the motor end-plate. The syndrome appears to be caused by an IgG-antibody, possibly produced to antigen on the tumour cells, which also binds to antigens in the region of the acetylcholine receptor.

MUSCLE AND JOINT SYNDROMES

Many patients with cancer complain of fatigue and sometimes of aching in the muscles which is occasionally out of proportion to the amount of weight loss. It has often been postulated that some of these patients have a more specific muscle disturbance. On the other hand, unequivocal myopathic syndromes are unusual. Arthritic complications of cancer are also uncommon.

Polymyositis and Dermatomyositis (17)

A syndrome which is typical of polymyositis, and which may be associated with skin changes indistinguishable from dermatomyositis, can, rarely, accompany cancer. All types of tumours have been reported in association. It is often stated that polymyositis in a middle-aged patient should lead to an extensive search for a cancer, which may at that stage be clinically inapparent. On the other hand, the likelihood of an occult, localized and remediable tumour being discovered is small, only 10–15% of cases being associated with a neoplasm, and by no means all curable. One therefore has to judge the extent to which investigation should be undertaken in each patient. A cancer is much more likely to be present in men over the age of 50 and when the syndrome is dermatomyositis. In this group bronchial carcinoma is by far the commonest associated malignancy.

The syndromes are characterized by symmetrical proximal muscle weakness which is slowly progressive. The skin changes consist of facial erythema and oedema especially over the nose and around the eyes. The chronic contractures and calcification typical of the childhood disease do not usually have time to occur. Steroids produce temporary improvement. Where possible, the underlying cancer should be treated.

Hypertrophic pulmonary osteoarthopathy

Nowadays, bronchogenic carcinoma is almost exclusively the cause of this uncommon syndrome although it can occur with lung metastases. The periosteum at the ends of the long bones (tibia, fibula, radius and ulna especially) is raised, thickened and inflamed and periosteal new bone formation is shown by a typical layer of calcification parallel to, and 2–3 mm above, the periosteal surface of the bone. The neighbouring joints may be hot and swollen and clubbing is usually present. The pathogenesis of the syndrome is unknown, but it may regress on treatment or removal of the cancer. A rare form of the syndrome may be associated with features of acromegaly, with raised growth hormone levels in the plasma.

Polyarthritis (18)

An asymmetrical polyarthritis is a rare complication of many types of cancer. The differential diagnosis is from rheumatoid arthritis, but tests for rheumatoid factor are negative and the arthritis is less erosive. The syndrome may subside with removal of the tumour. An SLE-like syndrome has also been reported in association with lymphoma.

DERMATOLOGICAL SYNDROMES

The skin manifestations of malignancy are extremely varied (Table 9.2). First, the skin may be infiltrated by primary or secondary cancer. Second, it may be indirectly affected by general metabolic consequences of cancer at other sites (e.g. due to obstructive jaundice or steatorrhoea). Third, some inherited disorders are associated with skin manifestations and an increased likelihood of developing cancer. Finally, some skin eruptions are non-specific manifestations of internal malignancy. Some of these (such as dermatomyositis and thrombophlebitis) have previously been described in this chapter. The following is a brief account of

Table 9.2. Non-metastatic dermatological manifestations of malignancy.

Syndrome	Tumour	Syndrome	Tumour
Metabolic		Thrombophlebitis	Adenocarcinomas
Hyperpigmentation	MSH-producing carcinoma (usually bronchial)	Thrombophlebitis migrans	Adenocarcinoma especially pancreas and ovary
Erythema	Carcinoid, gluagonoma	Erythroderma	Lymphomas
Fat Necrosis	Pancreatic carcinoma	Pyoderma gangrenosum	Myeloproliferative syndromes leukaemia, myeloma
Eruptions associated with cancer			
Acanthosis nigricans	Adenocarcinoma, lymphoma	Bullous eruptions	Many neoplasms
Dermatomyositis	Most cancers	*Generalized pruritus*	
Hypertrichosis	Adenocarcinomas		Lymphoma, leukaemia, polycythaemia

Inherited diseases (associated with cancer and with non-malignant skin lesions)

Gardner's syndrome: epidermal cysts and dermoids with multiple colonic polyps leading to carcinoma

Neurofibromatosis: neurofibromas, café au lait patches and other skin lesions, with sarcomatous change, medullary carcinoma of thyroid and phaeochromocytoma

Tylosis palmaris: hyperkeratosis of palms and soles with oesophageal cancer

Peutz-Jeghers syndrome: buccal, oral and digital pigmentation with multiple intestinal polyps leading uncommonly to gut carcinomas, ovarian tumours

Ataxia-telangiectasia: Telangiectases on neck, face, behind elbows and knees with cerebellar ataxia, IgA deficiency and increased incidence of lymphoma and leukaemia

Chediak-Higashi syndrome: defective skin and hair colour, recurrent infections, high incidence of lymphoma and leukaemia

Wiscott-Aldrich syndrome: eczema, purpura, pyoderma, thrombocytopenia, low IgM, leukaemia and lymphoma

Tuberose Sclerosis: adenoma sebaceum on cheeks, mental retardation and epilepsy. Hamartomas and astrocytoma

Bloom's syndrome: photosensitive light eruptions, facial erythema, dwarfism, leukaemia, squamous cell carcinoma of the skin

Adult progeria (Werner's syndrome): thickened tight skin, soft tissue calcification, growth retardation; soft tissue sarcomas

Fanconi's anaemia: patchy hyperpigmentation, skeletal abnormalities, anaemia leading to acute myelomonocytic leukaemia

some dermatological syndromes not discussed elsewhere.

Acanthosis nigricans

This is a brown/black eruption in the armpits, groins and on the trunk which has a velvety surface and multiple papillary outgrowths. A familial form occurs which is not associated with cancer, and the syndrome can develop without any underlying malignancy in middle age. However, when it occurs in adult life, a cancer is often present, usually an adenocarcinoma and often a gastric neoplasm. Lympho-

mas are also associated. The skin lesion may antedate the cancer, and when it recurs after treatment, may herald a recurrence.

Hypertrichosis (lanuginosa acquisita)

Very rarely an adenocarcinoma of the lung, breast, or gut, or a bladder carcinoma, may be associated with lanugo, which is fine downy hair on the face, trunk or limbs. The syndrome may be associated with acanthosis nigricans or ichthyosis. The hair growth does not usually regress after treatment of the primary tumour.

Erythroderma

A generalized, red, maculo-papular rash may complicate cancer and the underlying disease is nearly always a lymphoma. The condition may progress to exfoliative dermatitis. Control of the underlying lymphoma is essential in treatment. As the rash fades it becomes slightly scaly and bran-coloured. Relapses of the lymphoma may result in further skin rash.

Pyoderma gangrenosum

This is an infrequent complication of malignancy and can occur with other diseases such as ulcerative colitis. The lesions start as red nodules and then expand rapidly, breaking down in the centre to form necrotic, painful, infected ulcers with a rolled, erythematous edge. Although the condition responds to steroids, the dose needed is usually very high. An underlying lymphoma or myeloproliferative syndrome is the most commonly associated malignancy and the skin lesion may regress with successful treatment of the tumour.

Bullous eruptions

Very uncommonly, typical bullous pemphigoid and dermatitis herpetiformis are associated with underlying cancers.

Ichthyosis

Hodgkin's disease and other lymphomas are occasionally associated with thickened and flaking skin with hyperkeratosis of the palms and soles. Histologically there may be epidermal atrophy or hyperkeratosis. Tylosis palmaris is an inherited hyperkeratosis of the palms associated with oesophageal cancer.

Alopecia

Patchy alopecia occasionally accompanies lymphoma (usually Hodgkin's disease). There may be follicular mucinosis. The disorder may be self limiting.

Generalized pruritus

Occasionally patients present with a generalized itching without any rash. Although cancer is not a frequent cause of this problem, it is an important one and the itching may precede the clinical appearance of the tumour, sometimes by a few years.

Hodgkin's disease is one of the commonest cancers to be associated and the itching can, in this disease, become intolerable. Pruritus is usually worse at night, and in the case of polycythaemia, worse after a hot bath. Lung, colon, breast, stomach and prostate are other sites to bear in mind. Effective treatment of the cancer will often alleviate the condition and will certainly do so in Hodgkin's disease.

NEPHROTIC SYNDROME

The kidney may be involved by cancer in many ways but non-metastatic manifestations are unusual, apart from amyloidosis complicating mycloma (see Chapter 27). Massive proteinuria leading to nephrotic syndrome may occur as a direct result of glomerular damage (19). In the elderly especially, a small proportion of patients with membranous glomerulonephritis have an underlying cancer, removal of which results in remission of the renal lesion. The cancer is usually an adenocarcinoma (breast, colon, stomach). Hodgkin's disease is also associated although here there is usually minimal-change glomerulonephritis. In membranous lesions it is thought that complexes of tumour products and antibody are deposited in the glomeruli.

REFERENCES

1 Bodel P. (1974) Tumours and fever. *Annals of the New York Academy of Science* **230**, 6.
2 Blackman M. R., Rosen S. W. & Weintraub B. D.

(1978) Ectopic hormones. *Advances in Internal Medicine* **23**, 85.

3 Odell W. D., Wolfsen A. R. (1978) Humoral syndromes associated with cancer. *Annual Review of Medicine* **29**, 379.

4 Richardson R. L., Greco F. A., Oldham R. K. & Liddle G. W. (1978) Tumour products and potential markers in small cell lung cancer. *Seminars in Oncology* **5**, 253.

5 Hansen M., Hansen H. H., Hirsch F. R., Arends J., Christensen J. D., Christensen J. M., Hummer L. & Kühl C. (1980) Hormonal polypeptides and amine metabolites in small cell carcinoma of the lung with special reference to stage and subtypes. *Cancer* **45**, 1432.

6 Chandalia H. B. & Boshell B. R. (1972) Hypoglycaemia associated with extra-pancreatic tumors. *Archives of International Medicine* **129**, 447.

7 Muggia F. M., Rosen S. W., Weintraub B. D. & Hansen H. H. (1975) Ectopic placental proteins in nontrophoblastic tumors. Serial measurements following chemotherapy. *Cancer* **36**, 1327.

8 Hammond D. & Winnick S. (1974) Paraneoplastic erythrocytosis and ectopic erythropoiesis. *Annals of the New York Academy of Sciences* **230**, 219.

9 Colman R. W., Robboy S. J. & Minna J. D. (1979) Disseminated intravascular coagulation: a reappraisal. *Annual Review of Medicine* **30**, 359.

10 Croft P. B., Urich H. & Wilkinson M. (1967) Peripheral neuropathy of sensorimotor type associated with malignant disease. *Brain* **90**, 31.

11 Horwich M. S., Cho L., Porro P. S. & Posner J. B. (1977) Subacute sensory neuropathy: A remote effect of carcinoma. *Annals of Neurology* **1**, 7.

12 Mancall E. L. & Rosales R. K. (1964) Necrotizing myelopathy associated with visceral carcinoma. *Brain* **87**, 636.

13 Brain W. R. & Wilkinson M. H. (1965) Subacute cerebellar degeneration associated with neoplasms. *Brain* **88**, 465.

14 Corsellis J. A. N., Goldberg G. J. & Norton A. R. (1968) Limbic encephalitis and its association with carcinoma. *Brain* **91**, 481.

15 Wiener L. P., Hernden R. M., Nareayan O., Johnson R. T., Shaw K., Rubinstein J. Prezicse T. J. & Conley F. K. (1972) Virus related to SV40 in patients with progressive multifocal leucoencephalopathy. *New England Journal of Medicine* **286**, 385.

16 Lambert E. H., Eaton L. M. & Rooke E. D. (1956) Defect of neuromuscular conduction associated with malignant neoplasms. *American Journal of Physiology* **187**, 612.

17 Barnes B. E. (1976) Dermatomyositis and malignancy. A review of the literature. *Annals of Internal Medicine* **84**, 68.

18 Calabro J. (1967) Cancer and arthritis. *Arthritis and Rheumatism* **10**, 553.

19 Gagliano R. G., Costanzi J. J., Beathard G. A., Sarles H. E. & Bell J. D. (1976) The nephrotic syndrome associated with neoplasia: An unusual paraneoplastic syndrome. *American Journal of Medicine* **60**, 1026.

Chapter 10
Cancer of the Head and Neck

INTRODUCTION, AETIOLOGY AND EPIDEMIOLOGY

Carcinomas of the upper air and food passages constitute an important group of tumours both numerically and epidemiologically, quite apart from the exceptional challenges they pose in management. Together they account for approximately 4% of all carcinomas in Britain. Table 10.1 shows mortality from cancers of the commonest sites, and Fig. 10.1 shows age specific incidence rates.

Table 10.1. Annual mortality (England and Wales) from major sites of cancer of the head and neck.

Site	Males	Females
Lip	42	9
Tongue	206	141
Oral cavity	188	106
Pharynx	422	293
Nose, middle ear and sinuses	143	113
Larynx	608	149

Modified from data supplied for years 1971–78, from OPCS Monitor, DII1 80/3, 11.11.1980.

Important aetiological factors include excessive intake of tobacco either by smoking or chewing (a common practice in many parts of India and Asia) and alcohol (particularly spirits). In the past, syphilitic leukoplakia was an important predisposing factor in carcinoma of the tongue. Dental or mechanical trauma has also been incriminated, but with improvements

in oral and dental hygiene these factors are perhaps less important today. The Patterson-Kelly (Plummer-Vinson) syndrome of chronic anaemia, glossitis and an oesophageal web appears to predispose to postcricoid carcinoma, particularly in women. More recently, an unusual adenocarcinoma of the nasal fossa was first described in hardwood workers in the furniture industry, living in the High Wycombe area; further clusters have since been reported. Important racial differences have also emerged, particularly in relation to carcinoma of the nasopharynx, commonly seen in the Chinese and in particular those of the Mongolian race. In one report of 620 cancer patients admitted to the University Hospital at Hong Kong, 114 had a carcinoma of the nasopharynx, making it the second most common of all malignant tumours seen at that institution (1). In male Formosans, it is much the most common cause of death, and is seen more than three times as commonly as any other neoplasm. In head and neck cancers generally, there is a male predisposition (except possibly for postcricoid carcinomas), with a common male:female ratio of 3:1. For some sites, notably carcinoma of the larynx, the male:female ratio has been reportedly as high as 10:1. Data from the South Thames Cancer Registry (1974-6) indicate that if the heavily sex-determined laryngeal cancers are excluded, the true male:female ratio for other sites is approximately 2:1.

Improvements in dental and oral hygiene, coupled with reductions in intake of spirits and cigarette consumption have led to a falling incidence of cancers of the head and neck. In

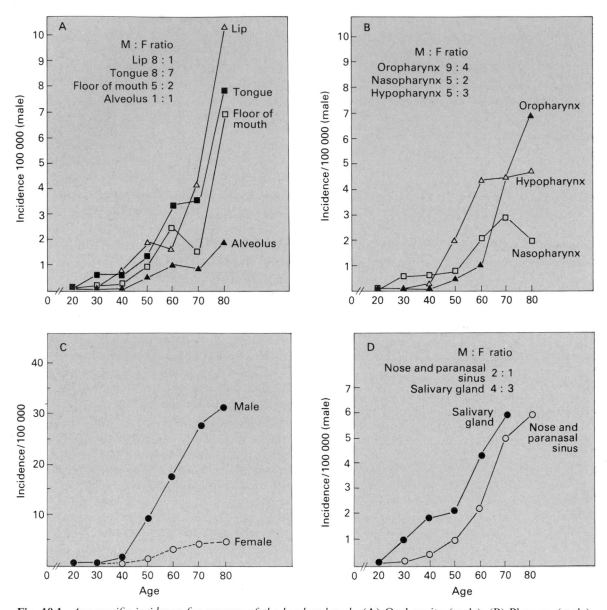

Fig. 10.1. *Age-specific incidence for cancers of the head and neck.* (A) Oral cavity (male). (B) Pharynx (male). (C) Larynx (male and female). (D) Nose and paranasal sinuses, and salivary gland (male).

1978, the number of new cases in the United States was 45 000 with an age-adjusted incidence rate of 17.2 per 100 000 for white males, and 5.6 per 100 000 for white females. Approximately 40% of these tumours prove fatal. In Britain, Scandinavia, West Germany, Japan and Israel the figure is somewhat lower, but elsewhere in North-west Europe (France, Switzerland, Italy and Scotland) the death rate is slightly higher. These survival figures may correlate with alcohol intake.

PATHOLOGY

The overwhelming majority of these tumours are squamous cell carcinomas, though the frequency of other histological types and the degree of differentiation varies markedly with site. For example, in one large series of patients with nasopharyngeal malignancy, the commonest tumours were anaplastic and squamous cell carcinomas, though lymphoepitheliomas (undifferentiated squamous cell carcinomas), malignant lymphomas, adenoid cystic carcinomas (cylindromas) and plasmacytomas, were also seen, as well as rarer tumours such as melanoma or undifferentiated sarcoma. Together these constituted a significant group of carcinomas of non-squamous origin amounting to almost 30% of all cases (2). By contrast, in a series of over 2000 cases of carcinoma of the larynx, 95% were squamous showing varying degrees of differentiation and including 97 patients with carcinoma *in situ*. Malignant lymphomas can arise anywhere within the head and neck but particularly from Waldeyer's ring. In such cases special care should be taken to establish the correct histological diagnosis since prognosis and management of lymphomas is different from epithelial carcinoma.

CLINICAL STAGING

Although no staging system is entirely satisfactory, there has been increasing agreement over the past 10 years regarding its value, both as a reminder to carry out full clinical and radiological assessment in each case, and also in order to develop logical treatment strategy and to attempt worthwhile documentation for comparison of cases. In Europe, the UICC proposals for standard TNM staging have gained wide acceptance. This has been facilitated by the adoption of the same staging notation for lymph node spread regardless of the primary head and neck site. Unfortunately this uniformity of notation has not been possible for T-staging, where some primary sites are still staged by

reference to the size of the lesion, whilst others are staged according to their spread; see Fig. 10.4 and Table 10.3 for examples.

In all cases, routine assessment and staging should include careful inspection of the primary site with measurement of its dimensions and examination for direct extension into adjacent tissues and local lymph node drainage areas. Although a reasonable attempt at clinical examination and staging can be made in the out-patient clinic, often using indirect laryngoscopy and nasopharyngoscopy with mirror techniques, most patients require an examination under anaesthetic with direct endoscopic evaluation of the upper food and air passages, before firm conclusions can be drawn. This is particularly true of nasopharyngeal carcinoma, since mirror examination of the post-nasal space can be demanding for the patient, and unreliable even in the hands of an expert. Histological confirmation must ideally be obtained in every case of head and neck cancer and this can usually be done at endoscopy though more accessible lesions, such as those in the oral cavity, can occasionally be diagnosed and staged without this examination.

Investigation

Plain, tomographic and computed tomographic (CT) radiography are of great value. In carcinomas of the larynx and hypopharynx, for example, the soft tissue lateral X-ray of the neck will often give a useful indication of the anatomical extent of the lesion, particularly when coupled with coronal or sagittal tomography, which often suggests more extensive spread than is obvious clinically. This is particularly valuable in subglottic tumours of the larynx, where extension or origin of the lesion may be difficult to assess even with direct inspection under anaesthetic. The advent of CT scanning has made a dramatic impact on the accuracy with which deep-seated lesions can now be visualized, particularly those of the nasopharynx, parotid gland, retro-orbital area, paranasal sinuses and where there is involvement of the skull

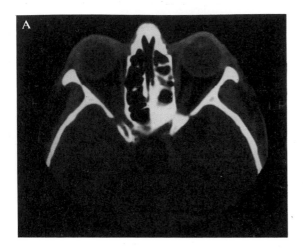

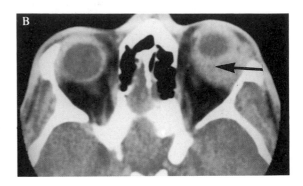

Fig. 10.2. *CT scanning in head and neck tumours.* (A) CT scan through nose and paranasal sinuses showing a large tumour of left maxilla with extensive local invasion and bone destruction (see also Fig. 4.5). (B) CT scan through orbits showing large left sided tumour (arrowed) displacing the globe forwards and downwards.

base or other evidence of bony erosion (see Fig. 10.2).

Haematogenous spread is particularly uncommon at presentation, but when it does occur the lungs are the most common site of spread. A chest X-ray should therefore always be performed and will also disclose the occasional simultaneous carcinoma of the bronchus. A routine blood count and liver function tests should also be performed.

Epithelial carcinomas of the head and neck region are best managed jointly by a surgeon and a radiotherapist with particular interest in this region, since they present technical problems of management unequalled by those at any other site. Because of the extreme variation in presentation, natural history, and response to treatment, this chapter only gives a brief outline of general principles of management; for those with a particular interest specialist texts can be recommended (3).

CARCINOMA OF THE LARYNX

Carcinomas of the larynx form the largest single group and there has been a fascinating and rapid evolution of ideas in management over the past century (4). Although the first laryngectomy for carcinoma is generally credited to Billroth in 1873, laryngofissure for tumour excision was performed 3 years before the invention and development of the laryngeal mirror. Despite the pre-eminent position of radiotherapy in the management of laryngeal carcinoma today, the first demonstration of its ability to cure this disease was as little as 60 years ago with the publication of Coutard's results (5).

The human larynx is an unusually complex organ (Fig 10.3) combining the role of a protective sphincter largely responsible for keeping the lower respiratory tract free from foreign bodies, with the highly sophisticated function of speech production. This demands extraordinary precision in the tone of the laryngeal musculature and in the approximation of the vocal cords themselves.

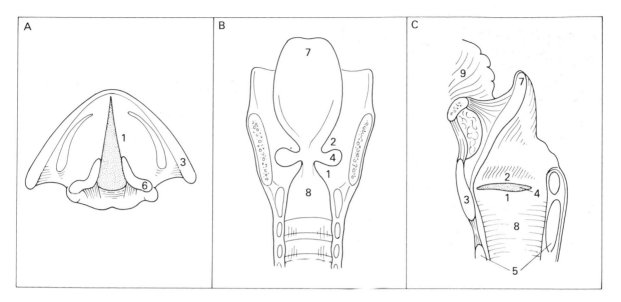

Fig. 10.3. *Anatomy of the larynx* (A) From Above. (B) Coronal plane. (C) Median sagittal plane. 1. True vocal cord. 2. False vocal cord. 3. Thyroid cartilage. 4. Laryngeal ventricle. 5. Cricoid cartilage. 6. Aryteniod. 7. Epiglottis. 8. Subglottic area. 9. Base of tongue.

Laryngeal cancer accounts for about 2–3% of all malignant disease, but the distress it causes is disproportionately high because of the severe social consequences of loss of speech. Indeed, the quality of voice and speech production is an important factor in choice of treatment (6). The larynx is sufficiently accessible to be viewed directly with ease, and comprises representative epithelial and mesodermal tissue components which lend themselves well to the study of radiation effects on both normal and abnormal tissues. For this reason, the larynx has always been of particular interest to the radiotherapist.

Of all of the aetiological factors previously mentioned, cigarette smoking is undoubtedly the most important. It almost certainly accounts for the male predominance of this disease, and there is a known correlation between precancerous laryngeal mucosal changes and the number of cigarettes smoked. The rise in incidence of laryngeal carcinoma has been shown to parallel the rising incidence of carcinoma of the bronchus, and in patients cured of early laryngeal carcinoma but continuing to smoke, carcinoma of the bronchus has become the commonest cause of death.

Hoarseness is the principal and often the only symptom, and any patient with hoarseness of more than 3 weeks duration should be referred for immediate laryngoscopy since early (T_1N_0) carcinomas can almost always be cured by radiotherapy (see below). *Dysphagia* is less common, though important in patients with supraglottic carcinoma, particularly when there is extension to the oropharynx. *Dyspnoea*, sometimes with stridor, is more often encountered with subglottic carcinomas where early obstruction is the rule and immediate tracheostomy frequently required before definitive management can be undertaken.

Carcinomas can arise from any of the three anatomical regions of the larynx, though not with equal frequency (Fig. 10.4). Lesions of the glottis are much the commonest, followed by supraglottic and finally subglottic cancers. Though early supraglottic cancer is uncommon in Britain these tumours are commoner than cancer of the glottis in some parts of Europe

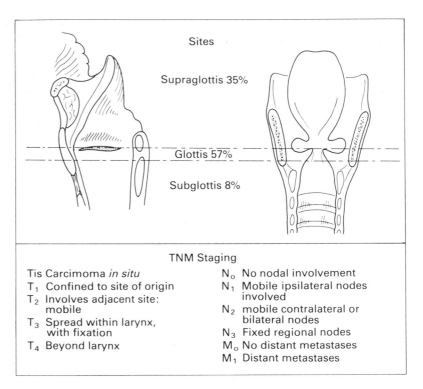

Sites

Supraglottis 35%

Glottis 57%

Subglottis 8%

TNM Staging

Tis Carcimoma *in situ*
T₁ Confined to site of origin
T₂ Involves adjacent site: mobile
T₃ Spread within larynx, with fixation
T₄ Beyond larynx

N₀ No nodal involvement
N₁ Mobile ipsilateral nodes involved
N₂ mobile contralateral or bilateral nodes
N₃ Fixed regional nodes
M₀ No distant metastases
M₁ Distant metastases

Fig. 10.4. *Relative frequency and TNM staging system in laryngeal cancer.*

including Spain, Italy and Finland. In glottic lesions, the commonest site is the anterior third of the cord, often with extension to anterior or (more rarely) the posterior commisure. The whole cord can, however, be involved. Direct spread can take place upwards via the laryngeal ventricle to the false cord and then to the remainder of the supraglottic region; or downwards directly to the subglottic area. Lymph node metastases are uncommon in early glottic carcinoma since the lymphatic drainage of the true cord is so sparse, but prognosis is highly dependent on the T stage. Most patients with T1 and T2 tumours are curable, whereas the majority of T3 and T4 lesions are not. Tumours of the epiglottis are usually advanced at presentation because there is little anatomical hindrance to direct tumour extension, particularly into the pre-epiglottic space. They do not cause hoarseness initially, and may elude diagnosis at laryngoscopy particularly if the tumour arises on the inferior surface.

Management and prognosis

Carcinoma of the glottis Radiotherapy cures at least 75% of patients where the vocal cord remains mobile (T1, over 85% and T2, 70%). Where failure occurs with radiotherapy treatment, salvage surgery is curative in over half of all cases. Total laryngectomy is usually necessary but some cases can be treated successfully by partial laryngectomy with preservation of the voice. Although conservative surgery (usually by partial vertical laryngectomy) can deal effectively with most early glottic carcinomas, the resulting voice is inferior to what can be achieved with radiotherapy. In these early cases, there are few drawbacks to radiotherapy, particularly since the field of treatment is small (often only 5 × 5 cm) with no need—at least in T1 tumours—to irradiate local lymph node areas because of the rarity of nodal involvement.

Treatment of the *advanced* case is more difficult, and always requires full discussion between surgeon and radiotherapist. Surgery may sometimes be required as an emergency procedure, particularly with subglottic extension. Many centres still employ a policy of planned radiotherapy and surgery in combination for the majority of these advanced lesions, especially if there is evidence of cartilage invasion, perichondritis, extra-laryngeal spread, or nodal metastases where the ultimate prospect for cure is so poor. In many centres, a pre-operative radiation dose of 40 Gy (4000 rad) in daily fractions over a 4 week period is followed by an attempt at surgical removal of all gross tumour about 4 weeks later. However, in other clinics, radiotherapy in combination with multi-agent chemotherapy has replaced this approach (see later). As with many tumours, adverse prognostic factors such as fixation of the primary tumour, early local invasion, extrinsic spread and lymph node metastasis are inter-related and often occur together. For the majority of these patients, even the most intensive combinations of surgery, radiotherapy and chemotherapy will fail to cure, and the ultimate 5-year survival rate for T3 lesions is about 25%.

Carcinoma of the supraglottis These tumours are more difficult to treat. They often present late because early symptoms are few. Dysphagia may not develop until ulceration and local extension takes place. Both local invasion and lymph node involvement are more common than with glottic carcinomas, and almost a quarter of supraglottic lesions extend down to the glottis. By locally invading in other directions, these tumours frequently involve the oropharynx (particularly the posterior third of the tongue) and the hypopharynx (particularly the pyriform fossa). For early lesions, a policy of radical irradiation with salvage surgery (total laryngectomy) where required (as for glottic tumours) is currently adopted in most centres, though surgery may be preferable for accessible lesions, such as those at the tip of the epiglottis. Conservative surgery is not normally undertaken for supraglottic carcinoma. An important

difference in radiotherapy technique between treatment of this region and the true glottis is that the radiation fields should routinely include the local lymph node areas, since clinical and occult lymph node metastases are common (7). For more *advanced* supraglottic lesions, the combination of total laryngectomy with pre-operative radiotherapy has traditionally been employed. Although this policy can be successful when wide field laryngectomy and a full dose of radiotherapy are routinely used, the morbidity is considerable. In expert hands, a 5-year survival rate of 60% has been achieved but at the cost of performing a number of laryngectomies only to find that on histological examination the pre-operative radiation has already produced a probable cure. For this reason it may be preferable to withhold surgery until there is evidence of recurrence or residual disease after radiation.

Carcinoma of the subglottis The outlook is even less good with these difficult tumours. In many cases there will be vocal cord fixation at the time of diagnosis, and invasion of the cricoid cartilage is common. Involvement of the thyroid gland or paratracheal lymph nodes is frequent, possibly in as many as 65% of cases, and surgical excision, if undertaken, must be radical. Such operations, which may have to include removal of the manubrium, dissection of paratracheal lymph nodes and total thyroidectomy, are performed less often nowadays, in favour of a planned combination of radiotherapy and chemotherapy, with surgery reserved for residual or recurrent disease.

Conservative surgery in laryneal cancer. Although long-term survival in patients with laryngeal cancer has remained unchanged for the past 20 years, the quality of life of survivors has improved considerably. Where surgery proves necessary in radiotherapy failures, there has been increasing interest in conservation techniques where the purpose is to ensure control of the primary lesion whilst at the same time offering the patient some chance of reasonable speech production (8). With *horizontal* supraglottic laryngectomy (Fig. 10.5), the upper part of the larynx is removed but the cords preserved. At *vertical* partial laryngectomy, the surgeon removes one vocal cord, the false cord and the vocal process of the arytenoid with part

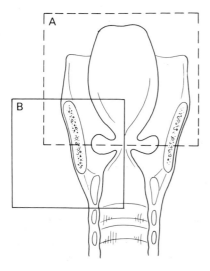

Fig. 10.5. *Conservative laryngectomy operations in laryngeal cancer.* (A) Horizontal supraglottic laryngectomy. (B) Vertical partial laryngectomy.

of the adjacent thyroid cartilage, and if necessary up to one-third of the contralateral vocal cord. Success in these procedures lies in accurate evaluation of tumour extent even though pre-operative assessment can never be completely reliable. Nonetheless the case for conservative surgery, particularly in supraglottic lesions, has been argued more strongly over the past few years (8).

Rehabilitation. Following any type of laryngectomy, and particularly after total laryngectomy, social rehabilitation is of great importance (see chapter 7, p.112, and all surgeons and radiotherapists working with these patients are aware of the immense contribution made by the speech therapist. With the appropriate training of oesophageal voice technique and stoma care, most patients who have undergone total laryngectomy can look forward to a full

and enjoyable life, usually with an adequate voice. Although this is difficult to define, the ability to speak on the telephone is often used as an important criterion.

Permanent vocal rehabilitation prostheses are being used more frequently in patients who find it difficult to develop adequate oesophageal speech. These devices contain valves which, for some patients, offer a striking improvement in voice quality. An example is the Blom-Singer valve.

CARCINOMA OF THE PHARYNX

Anatomy and patterns of metastasis

The pharynx is best considered as a passage with two distal sphincters serving the function of channelling both food and air in the right directions, namely to the digestive and respiratory passages. It is only by laryngeal constriction that the respiratory tract is effectively closed during deglutition, protecting the trachea and bronchi from inhalation of food or foreign bodies. The pharynx has three concentric coats: an internal mucus membrane, a supporting fibrous tunica and a muscular coat with a series of deficiencies for entry of vessels and nerves. These defects are important because they are the principal sites through which malignant tumours of the pharynx spread to adjacent tissues, particularly lymph nodes, in the neck.

Anatomically, the pharynx is usually described in three contiguous parts (Fig. 10.6). The *nasopharynx* is situated behind the nasal cavity and extends from the base of the skull above to the superior aspect of the soft palate below. It is bounded posteriorly by prevertebral fascia, and extends anteriorly to the junction of the hard and soft palate. The *oropharynx* is situated behind the oral cavity, extends inferiorly to the floor of the vallecula sulcus and includes the posterior third of tongue, vallecula, soft palate, uvula, faucial pillars and tonsils. The *laryngopharynx* or *hypopharynx* is situated behind the larynx, extending from the floor of the vallecula sulcus above to the level of the

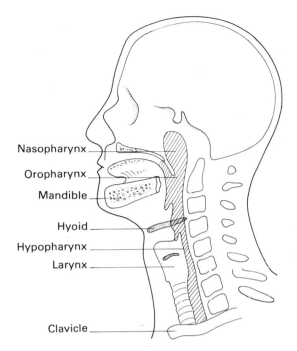

Fig. 10.6. *Anatomical divisions of the pharynx.*

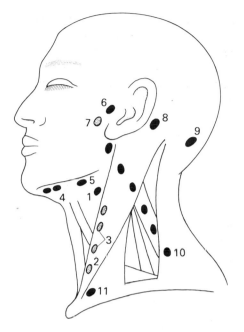

Fig. 10.7. *Lymphatic drainage of the head and neck.*
1. Jugulo-digastric. 2. Jugulo-omohyoid. 3. Deep cervical. 4. Submental. 5. Submandibular. 6. Preauricular. 7. Parotid. 8. Postauricular. 9. Occipital. 10. Posterior triangle. 11. Supraclavicular.

lower border of the cricoid cartilage below, where it joins the oesophagus. It includes the pyriform fossae, the posterior pharyngeal wall and post-cricoid area. The whole pharynx has a rich lymphatic drainage and early nodal involvement is common, with a predictable clinical pattern (Fig. 10.7). The important but inaccessible node of Rouvière is situated in the lateral retropharyngeal area, closely related to the jugular foramen and situated over the lateral masses of the atlas. Its importance lies in its critical position, making it an early site of invasion, particularly by nasopharyngeal tumours.

The relative frequency and the histological variation of neoplasms in the three pharyngeal sites, is shown in Table 10.2. Lymphomas most commonly arise in the oropharynx (particularly the tonsils) and nasopharynx. Nasopharyngeal carcinomas are more frequently anaplastic than well-differentiated, which is the reverse of the position with oropharyngeal and hypopharyngeal carcinomas. There are also important dif-

ferences in the probability of lymph node involvement at presentation. Three-quarters of all nasopharyngeal lesions present with obvious lymphadenopathy, whereas in hypopharyngeal cancer, almost half of all cases are clinically free of nodes.

Carcinoma of the nasopharynx Although uncommon in the Western world, these tumours are the commonest of all malignant tumours in many parts of China, accounting in some areas for half or more of all cancers. Even in the West, patients presenting with this tumour are often of Chinese descent. Postulated aetiological factors include diet and infective agents, possibly viral. Most patients show evidence of past or present infection with Epstein-Barr virus (EB virus). Both children and adults can be affected, and there is a male preponderance. Clinical staging is more difficult than in any other of the head and neck sites, because of the

Table 10.2. Histological classification of pharyngeal cancer.

	Nasopharynx (%)	Oropharynx (%)	Laryngopharynx (%)
Squamous cell carcinoma:			
well-differentiated	21	60	75
anaplastic	42	12	13
Lymphoma	20	15	0
Others (including unbiopsied cases)	17	13	12

Modified from Lederman and Mould (2) with permission.

inaccessibility of the lesion and its drainage routes. The clinical staging system adopted by Wang and colleagues (9) is widely used (Table 10.3).

Table 10.3. Clinical staging in nasopharyngeal carcinoma.

Stage	Description
Stage I	Tumour limited to the nasopharynx with no palpable lymph nodes or neurological signs
Stage II	Palpable cervical lymph nodes but with no other evidence of metastases
Stage III	Local invasion of the orbit, sinuses, or base of skull, and/or with neurological signs
Stage IV	Distant metastases beyond the neck

Cancers of the nasopharynx often have an insidious onset and tend to present late, often with nodal disease in the neck. Nasal obstruction, usually unilateral, and secretory otitis media are also common presenting features. Because of the close proximity of the nasopharynx to the base of the skull, many patients present with cranial nerve involvement, particularly nerves III–VI, since these pass through the cavernous sinus which the tumour frequently invades. The IX–XII nerves may also be involved by direct tumour extension where they pass through the parapharyngeal space in proximity to the lateral nasopharyngeal wall. Cranial nerve involvement usually implies bony destruction of part of the base of the skull. Other extrapharyngeal sites include the paranasal sinuses, nasal fossa, orbit and middle ear. Involvement of these regions causes pain, nasal stuffiness or discharge, unilateral deafness and ophthalmoplegia.

Treatment is by radical radiotherapy. In order to encompass the likely local extension of disease, particularly when lymph node involvement is known to be present (i.e. in the majority of cases), the irradiation volume must be large. This must be achieved without any concession in total dosage, which by common consent should be at least 60 Gy (6000 rad) delivered within 6–6½ weeks. The challenging technical difficulties include avoidance of the upper part of the spinal cord and temporal lobe of the brain (both of which have limited radiation tolerance yet are unavoidably included in the treatment portals), as well as the minimization of mucosal reaction as far as possible. The approach of Lederman (Fig. 10.8) aims at non-uniform high dose irradiation to the primary and bilateral cervical nodes, using lateral and anterior fields with appropriate shielding and field changes to avoid dangerous overtreatment of the upper cervical spinal cord without compromising the dosage to the lymph nodes. Even with this technique, a small portion (usually about 4 cm) of the spinal cord is treated to a dose of 50 Gy (5000 rad), and treatment complications will be inevitable in some cases. Other complications of treatment such as perichondritis or radionecrosis are uncommon with careful fractionation and avoidance of

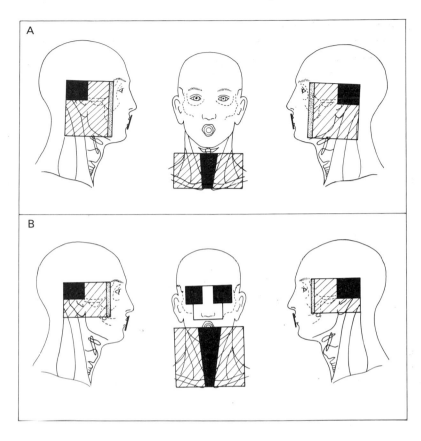

Fig. 10.8. *Radiation field arrangement for radical treatment of carcinoma of the nasopharynx.* (A) First phase of treatment (40 Gy in 4 weeks). (B) Second phase of treatment (to 60 Gy total dose in 6 weeks). (From Lederman and Mould (2), with permission.)

over-dosage. A sensible dental policy is required, and it is important to avoid removal of teeth during or shortly after treatment. Local shielding to sensitive areas such as the cornea and buccal cavity can often be safely achieved, and penumbra trimming is also important when using equipment with poorly defined beam margins (see Chapter 5). It is generally accepted that surgery has no place other than biopsy of the primary lesion, and occasionally in removal of residual lymph node disease by block dissection if the primary appears controlled.

Results of treatment are closely related to Stage (Table 10.3); median disease free 5-year survival, even in patients with Stage I disease, is less than 50%. The largest single group (Stage II) have a 5-year disease free survival of about 30%. A significant number of patients alive at 5 years will ultimately die of recurrence, and prolonged control followed by late relapse is common in this tumour. With Stage III and IV disease very few patients survive 5 years. Overall 5-year survival is better in younger people and in women (9). Recent attempts to improve results have included the use of intracavitary caesium implants to increase the dose to the primary site.

Carcinoma of the oropharynx These are more accessible, and in many ways simpler to treat. The important sites in this area include the soft palate, faucial pillars, tonsil, posterior third of tongue, and pharyngeal wall. The relative incidence of tumours of these sites is shown in Figure 10.9. TNM staging is now standard for oropharyngeal tumours and is shown in Table 10.4. The presenting symptoms include dysphagia with pain as well as aspiration of liquids. There may also be dysarthria with large tumours of the posterior tongue. The tumour is

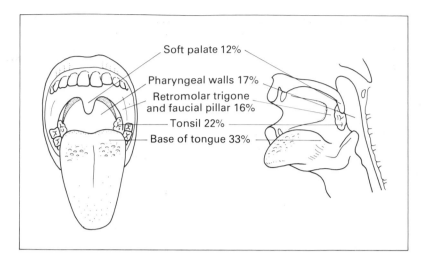

Fig. 10.9. *Carcinoma of the oropharynx: relative frequency at different sites.*

usually easily visible providing the anterior portion of the tongue is carefully retracted. There may be enlarged cervical lymph nodes. Radiological assessment can be very useful. Plain lateral views of the neck, tomography, barium contrast studies and CT scanning may all help to delineate the tumour. There are important differences in the presenting stage of tumours at different sites within the oropharynx; lesions of the tonsillar fossa are more often T3 and T4 at presentation than tumours of the retromolar trigone or anterior faucial pillar. Lymph node involvement is common, and again varies with the site. Half of all patients with soft palate, retromolar trigone and anterior faucial pillar tumours have lymph node involvement at presentation, whilst with carcinomas of the tonsil three-quarters of patients have palpable lymph nodes. About 20% of patients with positive nodes have bilateral involvement, and it is not unusual for lymph node enlargement to be the presenting sign, sometimes preceding the primary site by more than a year.

In most centres, combinations of surgery and radiotherapy are routinely used in managing these lesions though increasingly, the emphasis has been on radical radiotherapy (sometimes in combination with chemotherapy) with surgery reserved for radiotherapy failures. The radiotherapeutic technique is much simpler than with carcinoma of the nasopharynx since direct ex-

tension of tumour can usually be dealt with simply by extension of the field in the appropriate direction. The direct route of spread is via the parapharyngeal space lying between the mandible and the pharynx. More difficult problems arise when there is extension into the hard palate, mandible, tongue or larynx, and these are usually best dealt with by high dose radiation (with or without chemotherapy), or by surgery if treatment by irradiation and chemotherapy is unable to control the primary tumour. This is also true of lymphatic metastases. *En bloc* radical neck dissection may be required and can even be performed bilaterally if necessary. Despite this, most of the representative series suggest that a more aggressive surgical attack on the primary does not lead to better control or to a worthwhile improvement in recurrence-free survival (10). Surgery and radiation are probably equally effective in controlling both the primary and the node metastases though with a far better functional result in patients treated by radiotherapy. Combined surgery and radiation may be valuable in more advanced tumours, particularly those arising in the anterior faucial pillar. For tonsillar tumours, excision biopsy of the whole tonsil is usually advisable for reliable histology and may be sufficient if the resection margins are clear.

For patients with oropharyngeal cancers who relapse after radical irradiation to the primary

Table 10.4. TNM Staging for oropharyngeal and oral cavity carcinoma.

T—Primary tumour

Tis	Pre-invasive carcinoma (carcinoma *in situ*)
TO	No evidence of primary tumour
T1	Tumour 2 cm or less in its greatest dimension
T2	Tumour more than 2 cm but not more than 4 cm in its greatest dimension
T3	Tumour more than 4 cm in its greatest dimension
T4	Tumour with extension to bone, muscle, skin, antrum, neck etc.
TX	The minimum requirements to assess the primary tumour cannot be met

N—Regional lymph nodes

NO	No evidence of regional lymph node involvement
N1	Evidence of involvement of movable homolateral regional lymph nodes
N2	Evidence of involvement of movable contralateral or bilateral regional lymph nodes
N3	Evidence of involvement of fixed regional lymph nodes
NX	The minimum requirements to assess the regional lymph nodes cannot be met

M—Distant metastases

MO	No evidence of distant metastases
M1	Evidence of distant metastases
MX	The minimum requirements to assess the presence of distant metastases cannot be met

Stage grouping

Stage I	T1	NO	MO
Stage II	T2	NO	MO
Stage III	T3	NO	MO
	T1, T2, T3	N1	MO
Stage IV	T4	NO, N1	MO
	Any T	N2, N3	MO
	Any T	Any N	M1

site, surgical removal offers the only prospect of cure. These operations are complex and require careful consideration, usually demanding close co-operation between the head and neck surgeon who will undertake the radical excision and the plastic surgeon who is responsible for the reconstruction. Modern repair techniques, for example using jejunal replacement of the pharynx, are beginning to improve the functional results.

Lymphomas of the pharynx A significant proportion of nasopharyngeal and tonsillar tumours will prove histologically to be lymphomas rather than epithelial tumours. Invariably these are non-Hodgkin's lymphomas, usually lymphocytic B-cell neoplasms. It is wise to undertake full investigation as for non-Hodgkin's lymphomas at other sites, because distant spread occurs. The stomach is involved in 20% of cases at some stage but spread to the marrow and other extra-nodal sites is unusual at presentation. Nasopharyngeal lymphomas also have a tendency to spread directly to the paranasal sinuses and nasal fossae. Routine treatment of these contiguous areas is often recommended whenever a primary nasopharyngeal lymphoma is encountered. Although this represents an unusually large treatment volume, local control can usually be achieved with a more modest dose than for epithelial tumours. Generally 40 Gy (4000 rad) in 4 weeks is adequate.

Carcinoma of the laryngopharynx (*hypopharynx*) These are at least as common as those of the oropharynx, and accounted for 960 cases in Lederman's comprehensive review of 2400 carcinomas of the pharynx seen in his 30 years experience at the Royal Marsden Hospital, London (2). As with other sites, excessive cigarette and spirit consumption are the chief aetiological factors, and common symptoms include dyspnoea, dysphagia, anorexia, inanition and sometimes stridor. Most are well-differentiated squamous carcinomas. Palpable lymph nodes are present in about half the cases at diagnosis and a quarter of these have bilateral lymphadenopathy. The majority of patients have advanced lesions at presentation.

Although the prognosis in general is poor, some sites are prognostically more favourable than others. Carcinomas of the upper part of the laryngopharynx, including the aryepiglottic fold and exophytic lesions of the pharyngolaryngeal fold have a better prognosis than those of the more infiltrating or ulcerative variety, which usually arise from the pyriform fossa, cervical oesophagus and posterior pharyngeal wall. In general, these tumours have a very poor prognosis despite intensive treatment with radiotherapy, surgery and chemotherapy in patients whose general condition warrants it. In a large series of patients treated primarily with radiotherapy, Dalley (11) confirmed 5-year survival rates of 14% for tumours of the pyriform fossa, 9% for the postcricoid region and 12.5% for tumours of the lateral and posterior pharyngeal walls. A small group of tumours without direct extension or node involvement has a better prognosis, including a remarkable 5-year survival rate of 50% for early lesions of the pyriform fossa. Although good results with radiotherapy alone have occasionally been claimed for individual patients with advanced disease, it is clear that the chief use of radiotherapy lies in palliation, and the avoidance of mutilating surgery which would in all probability fail to cure. Radical surgery is, however, occasionally indicated in patients with operable lesions and in good general health; these individual decisions are best made by a surgeon and radiotherapist working jointly in a combined clinic. Most patients ultimately die of local or regional recurrence (rarely because of lymph node disease alone) though an increasing proportion have evidence of more widespread dissemination at the time of death.

Radiation technique in these tumours is complicated by the large volume which is frequently required, especially since delineation of the lower extent of spread in laryngopharyngeal tumours is often very difficult. When the disease is localized to the neck, the technique usually consists of lateral opposed field treatment with either open (direct) or wedged fields (see Chapter 5). A major technical problem arises when the tumour has extended below the thoracic inlet since easy access by lateral fields is limited by the shoulders. In this situation, a more complicated radiation field arrangement is required, and these tumours pose some of the greatest technical challenges in clinical radiotherapy. This particularly applies to postcricoid tumours. For treatment to be curative, a radical dose 60 Gy (6000 rad) in 6 weeks, or equivalent, is always necessary.

TUMOURS OF THE ORAL CAVITY

Tumours of the oral cavity include those arising from the lip, the mobile portion of the tongue (anterior to the circumvallate papillae), buccal musosa, alveolae (gingiva), floor of mouth, hard palate and retro-molar trigone. Age-specific incidence is shown in Figure 10.1. Although these tumours have become less common over the past 20 years due to better dental and oral hygiene, possibly coupled with more moderate consumption of tobacco, they are still among the commonest tumours seen in any combined head and neck oncology clinic, and are often surprisingly advanced at presentation. TNM staging is now widely used (Table 10.4), and clinical photographs are particularly valuable as a permanent and routine part of clinical staging since most of these tumours are easily visible.

Cancers of the oral cavity usually present as non-healing ulcers on the lip, tongue, cheek or floor of the mouth. Pain, though usually present, is not invariable. Cancers of the lip can arise on the upper or lower vermilion borders, or an adjacent area such as the philtrum, with direct involvement of the lip itself. The primary lesion can be raised, ulcerated, excavated, pigmented, well or poorly demarcated, painful or painless. Many oral cavity lesions are first diagnosed by a dentist and are sometimes hidden by dentures. Leucoplakia is a predisposing cause. On examination the usual findings are of a raised erythematous ulcerated lesion, often with an area of necrosis. Large tumours of the tongue may reduce mobility and interfere with speech.

Clinical examination should include careful bimanual palpation and the lesion should always be measured. Examination of the neck may reveal enlarged lymph nodes.

Investigation should include chest X-ray, full blood count and liver function tests. In patients with tumours of the floor of mouth or lower alveolus, investigation should always include radiological examination (orthopantomogram) of the lower jaw since asymptomatic involvement can occur, even when the lesion is not tender on digital palpation. Fine needle aspiration cytology of neck nodes is easily performed and may confirm a clinical suspicion of lymph node metastasis.

The clinical behaviour and probability of metastases varies with the site. For example, carcinomas at the tip of the tongue are far easier to control than tumours of its lateral margins, though cancers of the dorsum are most difficult (Fig. 10.10). In general, tumours of the floor of mouth, buccal mucosa, hard palate and alveolus show similar and relatively low metastatic rates whereas tumours of the oral portion of the tongue have a higher propensity for nodal spread.

Metastases are more frequent with poorly

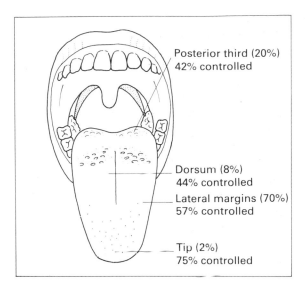

Fig. 10.10. *Relative frequency (in parentheses) and control rates in carcinoma of the tongue.* (Modified from Ash (14)).

differentiated tumours. Large oral cavity tumours (more than 4 cm in diameter) are both more difficult to control at the primary site, and more likely to be accompanied by cervical node metastases. Bilateral node involvement is common in patients with lesions of the floor of the mouth and faucial arch. The anatomical position of the abnormal nodes varies with the primary site. For carcinomas of the oral tongue and floor of mouth, the commonest sites are the jugulodigastric and submaxillary nodes, whereas palatine and retromolar trigone lesions are more frequently accompanied by lymphadenopathy at the angle of the jaw.

Management

Optimum management is best achieved in joint consultative clinics staffed by a surgeon, radiotherapist and medical oncologist. Principles of management are similar for the major sites within the oral cavity and will be considered together, except for carcinomas of the lip (see p. 167).

Small accessible tumours (T1) of the oral cavity These have an excellent cure rate with radical radiotherapy, with very good preservation of function. Most radiotherapists employ interstitial implantation techniques for intra-oral tumours (i.e. excluding those of the lip), since the treatment volume can be kept sufficiently small for a high dose to be given with safety. Implants of radium, caesium, gold, tantalum and iridium are all satisfactory. Intra-oral sites often treated by interstitial irradiation include tongue, buccal mucosa, floor of mouth, palate and lower alveolus. Very small lesions (less than 1 cm) can be treated with an interstitial implant alone, without external beam irradiation, though most radiotherapists use a combination of interstitial and external irradiation in larger tumours which are still small enough to implant (T1 and small T2 cancers). With an interstitial implant, a tumour dose of 60 Gy is usually given over 4–7 days. Where interstitial and external radiation are used together, many authorities recommend that the volume implant is taken to 50 Gy (5000 rad) in 5–7 days, followed by external beam irradiation to 30 Gy in 3 weeks (12). In some clinics, excisional surgery is preferred for small tumours of the anterior tip of the tongue.

Larger tumours of the oral cavity (T2–T4) In these tumours, external beam irradiation is the mainstay of treatment, though a dual modality approach using combined radiation and chemotherapy is increasingly being employed (see later). With external irradiation, doses of 60 Gy (6000 rad) over 6 weeks are usually considered essential for adequate control and it is known that tolerance is related to the volume irradiated. Radiation technique usually involves treatment by lateral open (direct) or wedged fields, to include both the primary tumour and the initial drainage node group since these are so commonly involved. For cancers of the tongue, floor of mouth and lower jaw, the palate can safely be excluded from treatment by means of a mouth gag which depresses the tongue.

The proper management of metastases in neck nodes remains contentious. Many clinics recommend routine radical neck dissection in patients with mobile nodes, and prophylactic node dissection in clinically node-negative patients has revealed a significant incidence of micro-metastatic tumour. In patients without evidence of neck node involvement (NO), most radiotherapists give prophylactic treatment to the neck, to a slightly lower dose (50 Gy (5000 rad) in 5 weeks or equivalent) than radical dosage, on the grounds that occult nodal spread is common and that nodal recurrence is reduced by such treatment. Most centres employ external beam irradiation, sometimes in combination with surgery, to control metastatic neck nodes, though ultimate survival rates in patients with N2 and N3 nodes is poor whatever the approach.

Patterns of recurrence and overall survival are clearly dependent on the size and stage of the tumour. Although some intra-oral sites (particularly floor of mouth) have a notorious reputation, there is little evidence that, stage for stage, this is borne out in survival figures. In one study the cumulative 3-year survival in mobile tongue/floor of mouth lesions without lymphadenopathy was 57% whereas for patients with palpable lymphadenopathy, the survival rate fell to 42% (13). Where lymph node involvement is obvious at presentation, failure at the primary site is common despite intensive radiotherapy.

Occasionally it is possible to control a limited relapse (usually the primary site) with an interstitial radioactive implant though radical surgery is usually required later since durable control is rarely achieved.

In the UK, surgery is usually undertaken if local relapse occurs after primary radiation therapy. A wide resection is invariably required, preferably with sophisticated reconstructive surgery. The advent of free flap grafting with micro-vascular anastomosis has dramatically improved the cosmetic results. The difficulty is that in general, complete surgical extirpation of the initial area at risk has to be undertaken, and often results in substantial local damage with loss of function despite the recent improvements in reconstructive surgery. A typical operation for a recurrent lesion of the floor of mouth might include a hemiglossectomy, excision of the floor of the mouth, hemimandibulectomy and neck dissection (commando procedure) with pedicle and/or microvascular free flap grafting in order to achieve adequate healing—a major undertaking in patients who are often debilitated enough to require hyperalimentation before surgery. Intensive rehabilitation and speech therapy are also critically important. Chapter 7, p. 111, provides a fuller discussion of rehabilitation of patients following this type of extensive surgery.

Chemotherapy may also be valuable in the primary or secondary management of these tumours and is further discussed in the final section of this chapter.

CARCINOMA OF THE LIP

Carcinomas of the lip constitute about one-fifth of all oral cavity lesions. These are almost always squamous cell carcinomas, often well-differentiated and presenting relatively early since the tumour is usually visible. The incidence has fallen rapidly during the past 25 years, and less than 300 new cases are now seen annually in Britain.

Metastasis is relatively uncommon, and is to local lymph nodes. About 7% of patients have involvement of local nodes at diagnosis, and the same proportion will develop metastases in local lymph node groups after primary treatment. Nodal invasion is usually directly to the submaxillary or submental nodes. Metastases to other node groups or organs is extremely unusual.

Treatment

Treatment is by surgery or radiotherapy. Most carcinomas of the lip are curable by radiation

therapy, particularly where the tumour is small (T1). External beam therapy with photons or electrons, and brachytherapy with radium moulds or interstitial iridium implants have all been used, and local recurrence is very rarely seen. Surgery also offers excellent local control, though the cosmetic result may be slightly less satisfactory, particularly where excision of a substantial portion of the lip needs to be undertaken. In larger tumours (T2), which might require reconstructive surgery, radiotherapy is generally accepted to be the better method of treatment, both cosmetically and functionally, since excision of large portions of the lip leads to poor closure of the mouth and may interfere with phonation. With large destructive cancers of the lip (T3, T4) it is difficult to achieve an adequate cosmetic and functional result by either method of treatment, and the incidence of local recurrence is higher. Fortunately, very few cancers of the lip now fall into this category. Healing may be excellent even following large doses of radiation therapy, but surgical reconstruction will often be necessary.

External beam irradiation is most commonly employed though formerly, the lip was one of the classic sites for brachytherapy with a radium mould. Superficial X-ray therapy (100–150 kV) has the advantage of adequate penetration with simple and effective protection of gums, teeth and mandible by intra-oral lead shielding which can be positioned by the radiographer for each fraction of treatment. As with treatment of skin cancer, an individually designed lead cut-out can be used to allow for treatment of any size and shape of field. Tumours larger than 3 cm are usually treated with higher energy (200–250 kV). Electron therapy has also been used and possibly offers superior cosmetic results. Treatment schedules are varied, though the best cosmetic result requires careful fractionation. Common schedules include 40 Gy (4000 rad) applied dose in 10 fractions daily over 2 weeks, 50 Gy (5000 rad) applied dose in 20 fractions over 4 weeks, 45 Gy (4500 rad) in 10 fractions given on alternate weekdays over 3.5 weeks, or, in centres preferring lengthy radical dosage, 60 Gy (6000 rad) in 30 consecutive daily fractions over 6 weeks. This latter regiment is probably the most suitable for large volumes.

In the unusual patient with nodal metastasis, radical neck dissection is the treatment of choice though radiotherapy can also be effective. With radical radiation therapy, surgery or a combination of both techniques, the results in carcinoma of the lip are excellent, and virtually all patients without lymph node involvement should be considered curable. Even in patients with lymph node metastases, the overall survival is 60–70% at 5 years. Overall, it is estimated that less than 10% of patients with carcinoma of the lip will die with uncontrolled primary tumour.

NASAL CAVITY AND PARANASAL SINUSES

These uncommon tumours, where presentation is often late and accompanied by early invasion of critical structures, are amongst the most difficult of all tumours of the head and neck region. The exposed nature of these facial cancers adds to the patient's burden, and demands great skill not only in eradicating the tumour, but also in offering acceptable reconstruction. They tend to be slow growing tumours, usually well-differentiated squamous carcinomas, in which local recurrence is the major problem. Other tumour types are occasionally encountered, with differing patterns of clinical behaviour and natural history. Melanoma of the nasal cavity is well recognized, accounting for

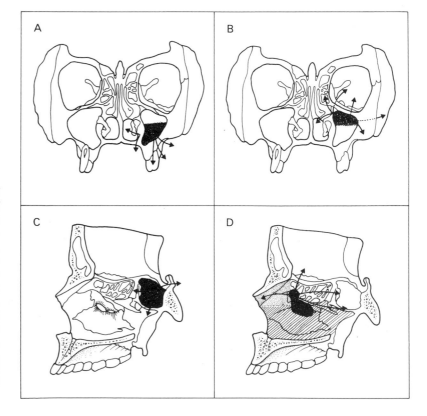

Fig. 10.11. *Pathways of local spread of tumours of the nasal cavity and paranasal sinuses.* (A) and (B) lower and upper maxillary tumours spreading to orbit, nasal fossa, palate, upper alveolus and soft tissues. (C) Sphenoid sinus tumours (lateral view) into nasopharynx, base of brain, ethmoid and nasal cavity. (D) Nasal fossa tumours (lateral view) into orbit, base of skull, sphenoid and posterior choana. (Modified from Boone *et al* (1968) *Am J. Roentgenol* **102** 627–636. With permission.)

almost 10% of nasal cavity cancers. Tumours of the nasal cavity and paranasal sinuses spread to other paranasal structures and the nasopharynx (Fig. 10.11). Although late presentation is the rule in tumours of the paranasal sinuses, those originating in the nasal cavity tend as a group to present earlier, usually with nasal obstruction, stuffiness or offensive discharge. Anatomically, the commonest tumours are those of the maxillary antrum, followed by tumours of the nasal cavity (Table 10.5).

Table 10.5. Distribution of tumours of nasal cavity and paranasal sinuses.

	% frequency
Site of primary	
Maxillary antrum	60
Nasal cavity	20
Ethmoid sinus	15
Nasal vestibule	4
Frontal and sphenoid	1
Histological type	
Squamous carcinoma	54
Anaplastic carcinoma	17
Transitional cell carcinoma	7
Adenocarcinoma	6
Melanoma	5
Lymphoma	6
Other	5

Adapted from Robin P.E. et al. (15)

Localized tumours of the maxillary antrum are usually asymptomatic; symptoms such as swelling and erythema of the cheek should raise a suspicion that the disease has extended beyond the confines of the primary site. Upward extension results in erosion of the floor of the orbit and displacement of the globe, leading to diplopia and ophthalmoplegia. Spread may also occur downwards into the oral cavity or posteriorly into the pterygoid region. Adjacent sites such as the nasal cavity, the ethmoid and sphenoidal sinuses are often involved (Fig. 10.11).

Aetiologically, little is known of the predisposing factors, though excessive alcohol intake, cigarette smoking and oral hygiene are held to be important. Adenocarcinoma of the nasal cavity is known to be commoner in hardwood furniture makers, and is presumably due to the inhalation of an occupational carcinogen. Because of difficulties in accurate assessment of the size and local extension of these tumours, staging by TNM or other conventional criteria has on the whole been disappointing. CT scanning gives far more information (Fig. 10.2) and this investigation should now be routinely performed, though simpler radiographic examinations are also of value.

Although some groups recommend either radical surgery or radical radiotherapy alone, the concept of combined modality treatment is well established. In 1933, Ohngren advocated treatment by a combination of surgery and irradiation on the grounds that this combination gave better results than either treatment alone. In general, this approach has been validated and is now standard policy, particularly for treatment of the maxillary antrum. Fortunately, surgical healing after radical doses of radiotherapy is not usually a problem at this site, and conversely there seems little prospect of reducing the extent of surgery for tumours which have usually spread beyond their primary confines at the time of diagnosis. Although no worthwhile comparative trials have been reported, many large series have demonstrated a 5-year survival of up to 40% with combined treatment. More localized cases are occasionally treated by surgery alone, but even in cases too advanced for surgery to be a realistic consideration, a 20% 5-year survival has been achieved with the use of radiotherapy alone. Modern prosthetics have allowed many of these patients to face the world with a normal appearance despite substantial anatomical deficiences.

TUMOURS OF THE MIDDLE EAR

Cancer of the middle ear is extremely unusual, and tends to occur in middle aged men with a history of chronic otitis media, often making diagnosis difficult since the symptoms may well be little more than an accentuation of the discharge which the patient has suffered for many years, with the addition of bleeding and pain. Direct local spread to mastoid air cells or external auditory canal is the rule, sometimes producing severe pain particularly when bony erosion (usually of the temporal bone), has occurred (16). The tumours are usually squamous carcinomas, presumably arising as a result of squamous metaplasia of the columnar epithelial cells normally present. Adenocarcinoma is very rarely encountered. Both radical surgical removal and radical irradiation have been advocated, but complete surgical removal is often impossible, and local control difficult to achieve. Extension beyond the temporal bone makes the prognosis very poor. Local extension to the brain may occur. Since survival rates are similar (about 25% at 5 years) whichever local method of treatment is employed, radical irradiation is usually preferred. Other rare tumours include soft tissue sarcomas and primary tumours of bone. In these cases, radical surgery is seldom possible and the mainstay of treatment is radiotherapy.

Glomus jugulare tumours arise from neuro-endocrine chemoreceptors of the jugular bulb, and should be considered with similar tumours (chemodectoma, paraganglioma) arising at other sites such as the bifurcation of the carotid artery (carotid body tumour) or posterior mediastinum. They are three times commoner in women, and may occasionally be bilateral. Although histologically benign, these tumours invade locally. Surgery is hazardous, since they are highly vascular and usually involve the middle ear and petrous temporal bone. Presentation is with deafness, cranial nerve palsies, local pain and tinnitus. Radiotherapy is the treatment of choice and modest doses (40–

50 Gy, 4000–5000 rad in 4–5 weeks) are adequate though regression may be slow.

CARCINOMA OF THE PINNA AND EXTERNAL AUDITORY CANAL

In this group of tumours, the pinna is the commonest primary site, followed by the external auditory canal. Tumours of the external auditory canal are usually squamous cell carcinomas. On the pinna, the commonest cell type in Britain is the basal cell carcinoma though squamous carcinomas are commoner in the United States. Malignant melanoma of the pinna is occasionally encountered. These tumours present either with a visible lesion of the pinna, or, in the case of tumours of the external canal, with discharge (sometimes bloodstained), crusting, or unilateral deafness. Pain is unusual. Local extension of tumours of the external canal may occur to preauricular structures, tympanic membrane, middle ear or mastoid and can be difficult to detect even with isotope bone scanning or CT scanning.

Although removal by radical surgery can be curative, it is widely accepted that treatment by radical radiotherapy is equally effective and offers a better functional result even though mucosal oedema, sterile fluid collections in the middle ear and perforation of the eardrum may occur with high radiation dose.

CHEMOTHERAPY IN SQUAMOUS CARCINOMAS OF THE HEAD AND NECK

Although both surgery and radiotherapy can be curative for localized squamous cancers of the head and neck (and even in some cases with lymph node involvement), the prognosis of patients with recurrent or disseminated disease is very poor. The first attempts at using cytotoxic chemotherapy in these patients were made at least 30 years ago, often using intra-arterial perfusion. More recently, interest has shifted from the use of single agents to combination chemotherapy, and from treatment of recurrent disease to the use of adjuvant chemotherapy in the initial management. Both of these approaches remain controversial (17).

Methotrexate was the first drug shown to be capable of producing responses, though it rapidly became apparent that with conventional doses, the response duration was short, often a matter of a few months or less. The ill health of many of these patients, coupled with the wide variety of clinical presentations and primary sites, has made it difficult to assess this drug. Treatment by the intravenous or intra-arterial route gives an overall response rate of about 50%, with no obvious advantage in favour of either method (17) though there may be a tendency to higher response rates with intensive weekly schedules. Although attempts have been made to increase the response rate by the use of high doses of methotrexate with folinic acid rescue, the evidence in favour of

this approach is limited; recent studies have demonstrated slightly higher response rates can be expected, but that duration of response and overall survival are not significantly improved. Where methotrexate has been employed concomitantly with surgery and radiotherapy, mucosal reactions have often been dose limiting. In addition, these patients are usually poorly nourished, cachectic and elderly, which makes aggressive treatment hazardous.

Newer drugs have been less adequately studied, though bleomycin has been used as a single agent in some 300 patients, with a response rate of about 30%, including a small number of complete responses. Bleomycin is now often used in combination with other drugs such as 5FU, cisplatin, vinca alkaloids and other drugs which have activity (Table 10.6). Several groups have reported results with combinations of these agents and although impressive response rates are sometimes claimed (Table 10.6(b)), the duration of response tends to be short. There is at present no definite evi-

Table 10.6. Chemotherapy in squamous carcinoma of the head and neck.

Regimen	% Total Response*
(a) Single agent response rates	
Methotrexate**	
Low dose	30–40
High dose	40–50
Bleomycin	30
Cisplatin	30
Vinblastine	25
5-Fluorouracil	15
Cyclophosphamide	35
Doxorubicin	20
Hydroxyurea	30
(b) Typical combination chemotherapy regimens	
Cisplatin and bleomycin	50
Cisplatin, bleomycin and methotrexate	60
Bleomycin, methotrexate, cyclophosphamide and 5FU	55
Vincrastine, bleomycin, methotrexate, 5FU, doxorubicin and hydrocortisone	67
Methotrexate, bleomycin and vinblastine	75

* These are approximate response rates from several studies.
** Low dose—below 80 mg/m². Considerable variability in reported response rates.

dence that multi-drug regimens are superior in survival to single agents.

A major area of controversy surrounds the use of adjuvant combination chemotherapy immediately following (or in some cases preceding) local treatment with surgery or radiotherapy. Both American and European groups have reported better local control and survival by comparison with historical controls. However, at present it is difficult to say whether the routine use of adjuvant chemotherapy offers a better chance of control and cure, or simply represents an expensive and dangerous method of seeing greater numbers of responses without any ultimate survival benefit. In Britain a randomized trial is in progress to attempt to answer this important question.

TUMOURS OF SALIVARY GLANDS

Although uncommon, accounting for about 2% of all neoplasms, salivary tumours are of great interest to pathologists and clinicians since they are of varied histology and present technical problems in management. The most common primary site is the parotid, accounting for almost 90% of all cases though the other major (submandibular and sublingual) and minor salivary glands can be affected. Occasionally, tumours of minor salivary glands can grow to a large size, mimicking cancers of the nasopharynx or palate.

Anatomy

The parotid gland is an accessible organ, overlying the styloid process and situated between mastoid and mandible, for the most part lying anterior to the pinna. Its deep aspect is in close relation to the parapharyngeal space and lateral pharyngeal wall. Superiorly, it rarely extends beyond the zygomatic arch. The gland is divided by the facial nerve and its branches into a superficial and deep lobe, and surgical excision of parotid tumour is often limited for fear of

surgical damage to this nerve. The submandibular gland lies beneath the horizontal portion of the mandible, and the sublingual gland (the smallest of the three major salivary glands) lies in the floor of the mouth, in contact with the inner surface of the mandible, often extending to the midline where it meets the contralateral gland.

Pathology

The wide variety of histological types of salivary tumour encompasses both benign and malignant disorders (Table 10.7). About three-quarters are benign, mostly pleomorphic adenomas or 'mixed salivary tumours', which is much the commonest tumour in the parotid gland and less frequently found in other sites (only 40% of tumours in minor salivary glands). About 65% of these tumours occur in women, mostly in the age group 50–65, though pleomorphic adenomas of the parotid have been reported in children and adolescents. Histologically, the tumours are very varied, with epithelial cells showing either acinar formation or arranged in clumps or sheets of cells, and situated within a stroma which is often myxoid in consistency. Several populations of cells may be present, but in general the overall pattern, though bizarre, pleomorphic and disorganised, is not one of malignancy.

Twenty-five per cent of parotid tumours are malignant. *Malignant mixed tumours* or pleomorphic adenocarcinomas, often resemble pleomorphic adenomas histologically though foci of malignant change are typically scattered throughout the specimen. These patients usually give a history of slow-growing and painless parotid swelling, often for several years, followed by a sudden change, with increased swelling and pain. This well recognized development represents one of the best examples of malignant change within an area of benign neoplasia—a most unusual phenomenon at other sites. The *adenoid cystic carcinomas* or cylindromas are rather more common (about 15% of malignant salivary tumours) and

Table 10.7. Histological types and prognosis in salivary gland tumours.

	% frequency	5-yr survival	10-yr* survival
Pleomorphic adenoma	75	96	93
Adenocarcinoma	8	50	—
Mucoepidermoid			
low grade	3	90	80
high grade	3	20	10
Adenoid cystic	4	60	38
Malignant mixed	2	55	30
Acinic cell	1	80	65
Squamous	3	25	—
All (men)			60
(women)			75

* Where available

arise not only in major salivary glands but also quite typically in the minor glands, for example in the palate. Characteristically, these tumours spread by direct extension along perineural spaces, a feature which may lead to unusual presentations of this tumour. Pain and perineural extension have been well correlated in clinicopathological studies. *Mucoepidermoid carcinomas* are now well recognized, and consist histologically of two distinct populations of cells, with both mucus secretion and typical epidermoid features. These often tend to be less malignant tumours and the lowest grade ones are clinically benign thoughout the other end of the spectrum is a high grade mucoepidermoid carcinoma which can be difficult to control and may be rapidly fatal. *Acinic cell tumours* are rare, more common in females, with a slow clinical evolution and an unusual histological picture suggesting an origin in acinic epithelial cells. *Squamous cell carcinomas* and *anaplastic carcinomas* of the salivary glands must be diagnosed with caution since there is a problem in distinguishing these from secondary deposits arising from a head and neck tumour site of more typical squamous origin. Histologically, the squamous or anaplastic element may be one component of a mixed malignant or other type of salivary tumour. True anaplastic or squamous tumours of the salivary gland are

amongst the most malignant of tumours, with a very poor prognosis. *Lymphoma* of the parotid is occasionally seen, but it is difficult to be sure if its site of origin is the parotid itself or an adjacent lymph node. *Adenolymphoma* (Warthin's tumour) is an unusual lesion, sometimes misdiagnosed as an abscess, and of doubtful origin. It is never malignant, may even be degenerative, and is characterized by large pink-staining cells surrounded by a lymphoid 'follicle'. The 'oncocytic epithelium' may enclose a centrally cystic area.

Clinical features

Benign salivary tumours usually present with a slowly growing painless mass. The onset of pain or a facial palsy is a sinister development suggestive of malignancy in a parotid tumour. The most rapidly growing tumours are anaplastic and squamous carcinomas, when the history of swelling will be shorter. Most of the other malignant salivary tumours tend to present with a more insidious onset. With adenoid cystic carcinomas, pain is a common feature due to the perineural spread which characterizes these tumours. Lymph node involvement is unusual in salivary tumours though reportedly higher in high grade mucoepidermoid carcinoma. Haematogenous spread is well recognized, particularly with anaplastic, mixed malignant tumours and cylindromas.

Management of salivary gland tumours

Surgical excision is undoubtedly the most important method of treatment for both benign and malignant salivary tumours. For benign parotid tumours, which occur most commonly in the superficial portion of the gland, superficial parotidectomy with preservation of the facial nerve is the operation of choice, giving excellent results provided that complete excision is possible. When excision is incomplete, postoperative radiotherapy is indicated since recurrence rates following this combined treatment are as low as those following complete excision. Although some surgeons recommend follow up observation after incomplete excision, this policy carries the disadvantage that a second operation may then be required, with the consequent risk of damage to the facial nerve. It would seem safer to offer routine postoperative radiotherapy to patients with incompletely excised parotid tumours. At other sites such as the submandibular and sublingual glands, experienced surgeons are often able to achieve wider excision than with parotid lesions since they are freed from the fear of facial nerve trunk damage.

The indications for routine radiotherapy in malignant tumours are: inadequate surgical excision margins; tumours of high grade (particularly squamous, anaplastic and mixed malignant lesions); when surgery has been performed for recurrent disease; and for malignant lymphoma of the parotid, where surgery plays no part in the management, other than for biopsy. Lymphomas and adenocarcinomas are generally the most radiosensitive types of salivary tumour. Occasionally, surgery is contraindicated, for example in unfit or elderly patients, or those with malignant tumours of the minor salivary glands in nasopharynx or palate. In these circumstances, long term control can sometimes be achieved with radiotherapy alone.

In summary, the usual policy for malignant parotid and other salivary tumours is one of excisional surgery followed routinely by postoperative radiotherapy. Exceptions might include low-grade malignant lesions with complete surgical excision, particularly where a capsule or pseudocapsule can be demonstrated in the specimen. The radiotherapy technique may be technically demanding since large volumes of tissue need to be uniformly irradiated and care is required to avoid overtreatment to sensitive structures—the brain stem, eye and mucous membranes. The usual arrangement is a wedged pair of fields. Particular care must be taken to avoid irradiation of the contralateral eye from the exit beam. A dose of 50–55 Gy (5000–5500 rad) in 5–5½ weeks is adequate treatment for residual benign tumours. Malignant parotid tumours need higher doses and 60–70 Gy in 6–8 weeks is often recommended if there is residual disease postoperatively. Because of the initially large treatment volume, a shrinking field technique may be necessary (see Chapter 5). Careful planning should allow treatment of the whole parotid bed as high as the zygomatic arch and inferiorly to the level of the hyoid, in order to include the jugulodigastric and upper cervical nodes. For submandibular and sublingual tumours, large treatment volumes are also required since in general, the whole gland will need to be irradiated. With adenoid cystic lesions, it is particularly important to treat widely in view of the perineural invasion; with parotid cylindromas, the mastoid should always be treated.

Opinions vary as to whether the whole of the cervical node chain should be irradiated in patients with malignant parotid tumours. Since the frequency of lymph node involvement varies with the histology, routine cervical node irradiation is only necessary in patients with squamous or anaplastic tumours, adenocarcinomas or mucoepidermoid and malignant mixed tumours of high grade. In some clinics, particularly in the United States, these patients are treated by elective lymph node dissection.

Promising preliminary results have been reported for neutron therapy (Chapter 5) as primary treatment for malignant salivary gland tumours (18), but this treatment is not generally available.

Prognosis

Prognosis in salivary gland tumours depends on the histological type (19) as well as its operability (Table 10.7). Routine use of postoperative radiotherapy has been shown to increase local control in all of the major types, but squamous, anaplastic and high-grade mucoepidermoid carcinomas carry a poor prognosis, because of both local recurrence and metastatic spread. Better results are seen with low-grade mucoepidermoid tumours and acinic cell tumours, with adenoid cystic and malignant mixed tumours carrying an intermediate prognosis. Overall, women have a better prognosis than men (10-year survival of 75% and 60% respectively).

Further surgical excision is sometimes possible for recurrent disease at the primary site, whilst for distant metastases palliative radiotherapy is sometimes useful, particularly with less aggressive slow-growing tumours. Pulmonary and other distant metastases are occasionally encountered, particularly with adenoid cystic carcinoma. Treatment with chemotherapy has no established place in management.

TUMOURS OF THE ORBIT AND EYE

Orbit

Both primary and secondary neoplasms occur in the orbit (Table 10.8). Lymphoma and rhabdomyosarcoma are the commonest primary tumours. Soft tissue sarcoma, nerve and nerve sheath tumours (including optic nerve gliomas) and meningiomas are all seen occasionally. Orbital secondary deposits are likely to be due to carcinomas of the breast, bronchus or thyroid.

Table 10.8. Tumours of the orbit (excluding globe).

Benign	Malignant
Haemangioma	Lymphoma
Lacrymal gland tumours	Rhabdomyosarcoma
Meningioma	Optic nerve glioma
Lymphangioma	Metastases
Neurofibroma	Angiosarcoma and other
Dermoid cysts	sarcomas
(Pseudotumour)	Myeloma

CLINICAL FEATURES

Because of its rigid bony structure, forward displacement of the globe (proptosis) is the cardinal physical sign. Ophthalmoplegia may also occur because of interference with the external ocular muscles or, less commonly, because of a third nerve palsy, particularly with posteriorly placed tumours. Proptosis can be extreme and disfiguring, particularly in children. Chemosis and infection are common and may lead to a misdiagnosis of cellulitis. Panophthalmitis can lead to perforation of the globe and unilateral blindness is common with advanced tumours. The rapid onset of chemosis and lid oedema suggest that the tumour is malignant. Marked proptosis with normal ocular movement usually indicates a slow growing benign tumour. Tumours within the muscle cone produce less disturbance of ocular movement but more proptosis and greater visual loss; those outside the cone produce eccentric proptosis and affect vision later.

INVESTIGATION

Plain X-rays and tomography can be extremely helpful and give good views of the orbital margins and optic canals. Even greater detail is obtained with CT scanning which gives reliable information on the site, size and degree of intra- and extra-orbital spread as well as a clear indication of bony erosion and soft tissue tumour invasion (Fig. 10.2). This is now an essential investigation. Ultrasound examination is often helpful in providing a rapid demonstration that a tumour is present. Biopsy confirmation of the diagnosis should be obtained where possible, but there may be formidable difficulties in so doing with a risk of tumour spillage, haemorrhage and blindness. If the tumour is encapsulated it is usually best to excise it entirely.

Lymphoma Malignant lymphomas of the orbit are almost always of the non-Hodgkin's variety and may be isolated or seen as part of a more generalized lymphoma (see Chapter 26). Full investigation is usually required as for any other lymphoma, since evidence of systemic disease will be found in a proportion of patients. Biopsy of these lesions is usually easy since they tend to be anteriorly placed, and treatment with radiotherapy is usually successful in eradicating all signs of disease. Even where systemic lymphoma is discovered, radiotherapy is used as an addition to systemic treatment in order to prevent local recurrence, and modest doses of the order of 30 Gy (3000 rad) over 3 weeks are usually adequate.

Orbital pseudo-tumour is a condition characterized by a mass in the orbit which consists of a well-differentiated lymphocytic lesion. It may regress spontaneously, but if the proptosis is troublesome, radiotherapy can be useful. It is sometimes considered to be a very low-grade lymphoma, and generalized disease occasionally develops.

Rhabdomyosarcoma This is usually embryonal in type, occurring chiefly in infants, young children and adolescents, and slightly more commonly in males. Local spread may involve the maxilla, paranasal sinuses, frontal bone or even the brain, via the anterior or middle cranial fossa. Haematological spread may also occur, chiefly to lung or bone, but tends to be less common than with rhabdomyosarcomas presenting at other sites. Lymph node involvement, present in about one-quarter of cases, usually involves the upper deep cervical or pre-auricular nodes. Once established,

these tumours tend to advance rapidly, leading to particularly severe proptosis with chemosis and lid oedema. Wherever possible, full staging, including bone marrow aspiration, should be performed before treatment, in order to formulate a rational treatment plan. Although surgery was formerly used for control of the primary lesion, radiotherapy has become increasingly recognized as a satisfactory alternative, with low local recurrence rates. High doses of the order of 50 Gy (5000 rad) over 5–6 weeks are required and a high proportion of these patients will preserve useful vision in the affected eye provided that the lachrymal apparatus is shielded to ensure against xerophthalmia (see later).

Routine adjuvant chemotherapy is now an established part of treatment, and combinations of cyclophosphamide, vincristine and actinomycin D or doxorubicin are recommended. Generally at least one course of combination chemotherapy is given before the orbital radiation, because of the high probability of extraocular spread and also because rapid resolution occurs which will make the child more comfortable and the radiotherapy technically easier. The chemotherapy should normally be continued for about 1 year. Local irradiation is important as a means of ensuring local control even when metastases are present. Routine use of chemotherapy has improved prognosis from a survival rate of less than 40% using surgery and radiotherapy alone to about 75% at 5 years, with a particular improvement in tumours of younger children, which were previously notorious for their high probability of dissemination (see Chapter 24).

Lachrymal gland tumours These are usually considered with orbital tumours, though they are extremely rare. Commonest in young adults, their histological spectrum is reminiscent of that of salivary gland tumours, with pleomorphic adenomas and adenoid cystic carcinomas the most frequently encountered types. There is usually a long history (longer than a year) of a slowly expanding, hard, painless mass. With more rapidly growing lesions, a biopsy is imperative and complete surgical removal of the tumour should be carried out if possible. Where total removal of the lachrymal gland cannot be performed (either for a patient with a pleomorphic adenoma or any of the malignant tumours) radiotherapy should also be given. Local recurrence is very common even after a high dose, so every effort should be made to remove these tumours. True carcinomas of the lachrymal gland are rare, and extra-orbital spread tends to occur early. Malignant lachrymal gland tumours are a miscellaneous group, difficult to treat and with a poor overall prognosis and a 5-year survival rate in the order of 20%.

Optic nerve glioma This is discussed in Chapter 22.

RADIATION TECHNIQUES FOR TUMOURS OF THE ORBIT

Although lead shielding of the cornea, lens and lachrymal sac is routinely recommended, it is impossible to arrange for homogeneous irradiation of the whole of the orbital content as well as adequate shielding of sensitive structures. A wedged pair of fields (see Chapter 5, Fig. 5.8) is the usual arrangement. Great care must be taken to avoid irradiation of the contralateral eye, even though useful vision is sometimes retained in the treated one. It is often useful to ask the patient to look directly into the beam during treatment both to fix the gaze and to avoid the inevitable build-up effect of the closed lid. With supervoltage beams, the maximal energy deposition is deep to the cornea and may even partly spare the lens. Partial or complete corneal shielding can usually be achieved with a simple cylindrical shield, and conjunctival damage is uncommon particularly as low doses of radiation are well tolerated by this part of the eye. Where shielding is impossible, painful keratitis, sometimes with iridocyclitis or even corneal ulceration may occur. Failure to shield the lachrymal gland will usually pose a greater threat to the integrity of the eye since the lachrymal apparatus has a lower tolerance, and doses of greater than 30 Gy (3000 rad) over 3 weeks will cause significant reduction of tear production with consequent dryness of the eye, requiring regular instillation of lubricant drops.

The most radiosensitive structure in the eye is the lens itself (see Chapter 5, p. 69) and cataracts can develop after doses of a few Gy though clinically important lens opacity is rarely seen with doses below 15 Gy (1500 rad). With doses above 25 Gy (2500 rad), progressive cataract is almost invariable; fortunately, these cataracts can be removed. Other parts of the eye such as the retina and the sclera have a much higher radiation tolerance closely similar to that of the central nervous system, and clinically important changes are uncommon where doses of less than 60 Gy (6000 rads) are given by carefully fractionated external beam therapy.

Tumours of the eyelid and conjunctiva

Tumours of the eyelid are not uncommon and include basal cell and squamous cell carcinomas mostly occurring in elderly patients. The lower lid and inner canthus of the eye are the commonest site. The management is discussed in Chapter 22. In the conjunctiva both melanoma and squamous cell carcinoma are occasionally encountered, and are important to diagnose early since small lesions can be effectively treated by radiation, with conservation of the eye and preservation of vision. In general, local surgical excision is advisable, followed by radiotherapy using an applicator carrying a radioactive source, often ^{90}Sr. It is important to distinguish true melanomas from precancerous ocular melanosis (a diffuse flat pigmented lesion) which can be clinically diagnosed with confidence, and should be observed without biopsy since malignant change may take years to develop. Overall prognosis of conjunctival melanoma is good (5-year survival about 75%), though patients with bulky lesions have a high risk of early fatal dissemination. Squamous carcinomas have an even better prognosis provided that adequate surgery and/or radiotherapy can be given.

Tumours of the globe

The two main tumours are retinoblastoma and uveal (choroidal) melanoma. Retinoblastoma is discussed in Chapter 24.

Malignant melanoma of the uveal tract is the commonest intra-ocular tumour of adults (6 per 1 000 000 per year). Blood-borne metastases are common, but may not become clinically apparent for many years. Only 15% arise in the ciliary body and iris. These present earlier and they are more easily visible. Choroidal melanomas (85% of the total) may cause no symptoms at first unless they are at the macula. At other sites a peripheral field defect may go unnoticed. Retinal detachment may occur.

The diagnosis is normally made on inspection. Primary choroidal melanomas must be distinguished from secondary deposits since the choroid is a known site of metastasis of cutaneous melanoma.

In the past immediate enucleation has been preferred to biopsy in the belief that biopsy was dangerous. A more conservative approach has been adopted in recent years especially in the elderly. Small melanomas can probably be watched and surgery only considered when the tumour enlarges. Treatment is then by photocoagulation, cryotherapy, local irradiation to a high dose, or surgery. In small lesions and tumours of the iris, enucleation can sometimes be avoided though it may be necessary for large lesions or where there is macular/optic nerve involvement or retinal detachment. Pain, local extension and secondary glaucoma are also indications for enucleation.

REFERENCES

1 Digby K.H., Fook W.L. & Che Y.T. (1941) Nasopharyngeal carcinoma. *British Journal of Surgery* **28**, 517.

2 Lederman M. & Mould R.F. (1968) Radiation treatment of cancer of the pharynx: with special reference to telecobalt therapy. *British Journal of Radiology* **41**, 251.

3 Suen J.Y. & Myers E.N. (1981) *Cancer of the Head and Neck*. Churchill Livingstone, Edinburgh.

4 Lederman M. (1971) Cancer of the larynx. Part I: Natural history in relation to treatment. *British Journal of Radiology* **44**, 569–78.

5 Coutard H. (1940) Present conception of the treatment of cancer of the larynx. *Radiology* **34**, 136.

6 McNeil B.J., Weichselbaum R. & Parker S. (1981) Speech and Survival. Trade-offs between quality and quantity of life in laryngeal cancer. *New England Journal of Medicine* **305**, 982.

7 Harwood A.R., Beale F.A., Cummings B.J., Keane T.J., Payne D.G., Rider W.D., Rawlinson E. & Elhakin T. (1983) Supraglottic laryngeal carcinoma: an analysis of dose-time-volume factors in 410 patients. *International Journal of Radiation Oncology Biology Physics* **9**, 311

8 British Medical Journal (1978) Conservation surgery for laryngeal cancer (leading article). *B.M.J.* **2**, 1318–9.

9 Wang C.C., Little J.B. & Schultz M.D. (1962) Cancer of the nasopharynx: Clinical and radiotherapeutic considerations. *Cancer* **15**, 921.

10 Calinas M. & Fletcher G.H. (1973) Incidence and causes of local failure of irradiation in squamous carcinoma of the faucial arch tonsillar fossa and base of tongue. *Radiology* **108**, 383.

11 Dalley, V.M. (1968) Cancer of the laryngopharynx. *Journal of Laryngology and Otology* **82**, 407.

12 Henk J.M. (1976) Neoplasms of the Head and Neck. In Hope-Stone H.F. (ed) *Radiotherapy in Modern Clinical Practice*, pp. 108–42. Crosby Lockwood Staples, London.

13 Montana G.S., Hellman S., von Essen C.F. & Kligerman M.M. (1969) Carcinoma of the tongue and floor of the mouth: Results of radical radiotherapy. *Cancer* **23**, 1284–9.

14 Ash C.L. (1962) Oral cancer: a 25 year study. *American Journal of Roentgenology* **87**, 417.

15 Robin P.E., Powell D.J. & Stansbie, J.M. (1979) Carcinoma of the nasal cavity and paranasal sinuses: incidence and presentation of different histological types. *Clinical Otolaryngology* **4**, 431.

16 Holmes K.S. The treatment of carcinoma of the middle ear by the 4MV linear accelerator (1960) *Proceedings of the Royal Society of Medicine* **53**, 242–4.

17 Hong W.K. & Bromer R. (1983) Chemotherapy

in head and neck cancer. *New England Journal of Medicine* **308,** 75.

18 Kurup P.D., Mansell J., TenHaken R.K., Hendrickson F.R., Cohen L., Awschalom M. & Rosenberg, I. (1984) Response of epidermoid and non-epidermoid cancers of the head and neck to fast neutron irradiation: the Fermilab experience. *International Journal of Radiation Oncology Biology Physics* **10,** 473.

19 Hickman R., Cawson, R.A. & Duffy S.W. (1984). The prognosis of specific types of salivary gland tumours. *Cancer* **54,** 1620–24.

Chapter 11

Tumours of the Nervous System

BRAIN TUMOURS

Brain tumours are amongst the most devastating of all malignant diseases frequently producing profound and progressive disability leading to death. In addition they may be difficult to diagnose and are invariably challenging to treat. The peak incidence is in the first decade of life and age 50–60 years. Brain tumours are one of the most important groups of childhood tumours, second in frequency only to the leukaemias and lymphomas. In Britain the incidence is approximately 6 per 100 000, with 2200 deaths each year. Almost nothing is known of the aetiology. Cerebral lymphoma occurs in chronically immunosuppressed patients, and an increase in both benign and malignant brain tumours has been noted following radiation of the scalp for benign conditions in childhood.

Over the past 25 years, refinements of both neurosurgical and radiotherapeutic techniques have resulted in changes in management and, in some instances, improvement in prognosis. More recently, medical oncologists have begun to demonstrate a possible role for cytotoxic drugs, though their contribution is not yet fully established.

Pathological classification of brain tumours

The majority of brain tumours are gliomas, thought to arise from malignant change of mature glial elements, usually with differentiation towards one particular type of glial cell.

Taken together, astrocytomas, ependymomas, oligodendrogliomas and medulloblastomas comprise over 90% of all primary brain and spinal cord tumours. In cases where the tumour is well-differentiated, there is usually no difficulty in recognizing the type of cell from which the tumour has arisen.

These tumours are classified according to the cell of origin and a widely accepted working classification is given in Table 11.1. Other more detailed classifications have been proposed by the World Health Organisation but the simpler system outlined in Table 11.1 is used in this chapter.

GLIOMAS

Astrocytomas are much the commonest variety and arise from astrocytes which are the supporting cells of the brain. They are divided into four grades (according to Kernohan) on the basis of cytomorphological characteristics. Grade I is the least malignant. Grades II–IV show progressively more malignant characteristics. The degree of malignancy is assessed according to histological features such as invasion, tumour necrosis, cellularity and mitotic activity together with cytological features including nuclear abnormality and variation in cell size and morphology. Low-grade gliomas occur most commonly in the frontal, parietal and temporal lobes and in the brain stem and cerebellum of children. Because of their relatively slow evolution, local destruction is not usually encountered, in contrast to the more high-grade gliomas, in which degeneration, nec-

Table 11.1 Classification of brain tumours.

Primary Tumours		Secondary Tumours

Gliomas
  Astrocytoma
  Glioblastoma multiforme
  Ependymoma
  Oligodendroglioma
  Medulloblastoma
	Pineal tumours
	  Pinealoblastoma
	  Pinealocytoma
	  Germinoma
	  Teratoma
		Common sites of origin
		  Lung
		  Breast
		  Melanoma

Pituitary tumours
  Pituitary adenoma
  Craniopharyngioma
  Pituitary carcinoma
	Intracranial lymphoma
	  'Histiocytic' lymphoma
	  Microglioma
	
	Acoustic neuroma
	
	Chordoma
		Less common sites of origin
		  Ovary
		  Testis
		  Gut
		  Bladder
		  Kidney
		  Pancreas
		  Liver
		  Leukaemia and lymphoma

Meningioma
  Benign
  Malignant (meningiosarcoma)
	Neuronal tumours
	  Ganglioneuroma
	  Ganglioglioma
	
	Colloid cyst
		Miscellaneous
		  Histiocytosis X

rosis, haemorrhage, infarction and local destruction are characteristically found.

As with tumours at other sites, biopsy specimens may not necessarily be representative of the whole tumour, and mixed varieties are common. Descriptive terms are sometimes used where a particular morphological feature predominates. Pathologists may use the terms fibrillary, protoplasmic, gemistocytic or pilocytic to describe relatively well-differentiated types of astrocytoma. These subdivisions are of doubtful prognostic significance. In highly malignant gliomas it may be quite impossible to recognize the initial cell of origin, and these tumours are amongst the most bizarre and undifferentiated of all, often termed gliobastoma multiforme (Fig. 11.1). They grow rapidly by direct extension, and are always much larger than suggested by pre-operative angiography or CT studies. They are rarely operable, do not as a rule respond to irradiation, and are usually fatal within a year. By contrast, grade I gliomas enlarge much more slowly and can usually be excised completely though local recurrence does sometimes occur. Oddly, gliomas at different sites appear to behave quite differently despite a similar histological appearance. For

this reason, localized gliomas of the optic nerves are often left untreated and may regress spontaneously whilst gliomas of the pons or brain stem behave much more aggressively and demand urgent attention with wide field irradiation.

Ependymal tumours comprise about 5% of all primary brain tumours and are derived from the ciliated lining cells of the CNS cavities. The tumour cells form characteristic rosettes. (Fig. 11.1C). This tumour most commonly occurs in childhood and early adult life, and just over half arise from infratentorial sites. Tumour spread occurs by direct invasion and also by seeding throughout the CNS, particularly with high grade ependymoma and where the primary tumour is infratentorial. Although tumour grading is perhaps less important than with astrocytomas there is general agreement that low grade ependymomas have a far better prognosis than the higher grades. Most aggressive of all is the ependymoblastoma.

Oligodendrogliomas are derived from other supporting cells and are usually very indolent in their growth pattern with a long history,

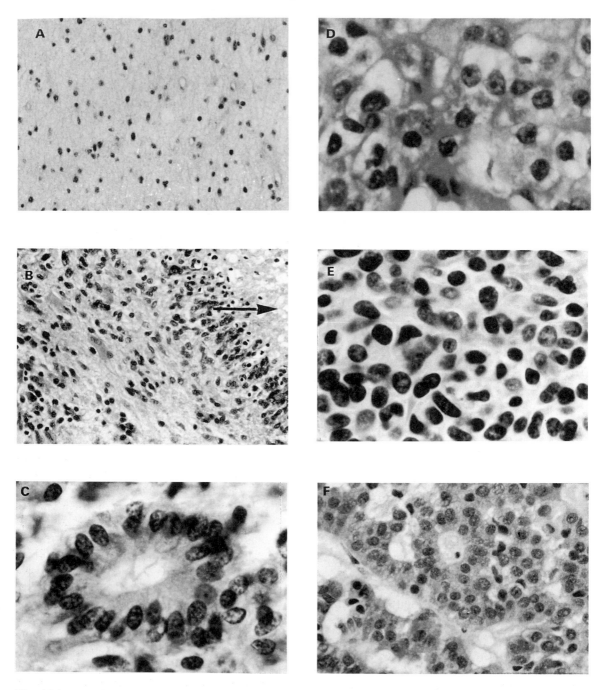

Fig. 11.1. *Histological appearance of the commoner brain tumours.* (A) Low grade glioma showing sparse cellularity with no vascular proliferation. Original magnification ×200. (B) High grade glioma showing cellular pleomorphism and necrosis (arrowed). (×200.) (C) Ependymoma. Tumour forms typical rosettes. (×400.) (D) Oligodendroglioma, showing typical 'boxed-in' cell appearance. (×400.) (E) Medulloblastoma, showing small, darkly staining, closely packed cells. (×400.) (F) Pituitary adenoma. The appearance is characteristic of endocrine tumours. (×250.)

often calcifying. The cells have a typical appearance (Fig. 11.1D) with a clear zone around the nucleus, the cells appearing 'boxed-in'. Typical sites are the frontal, parietal and temporal lobes. The commonest age range is 40–60 years.

Medulloblastoma (3% of brain tumours) is predominantly a disease of childhood and young adult life, with few cases occurring after the age of 25 years. There is a peak age incidence of 4–10 years, and the male:female ratio is over 2:1. The tumour cells form rosettes (Fig. 11.1E). Medulloblastoma chiefly arises in the posterior fossa, from the vermis, cerebellar hemispheres or the fourth ventricle. Patients usually present either with cerebellar symptoms or signs, or with raised intracranial pressure (see later). Because of close proximity to the cerebrospinal fluid (CSF) the tumour metastasises via CSF, either to the spinal cord, or elsewhere in the brain. Occasionally, distant metastases are seen outside the central nervous system, and bone metastases (mostly osteosclerotic) and marrow involvement are occasionally encountered.

PITUITARY TUMOURS

These account for about 10% of all primary intracranial neoplasms. They usually arise from the glandular epithelial cells, producing tumours which are histologically classified according to the staining characteristics of the cytoplasmic granules. In most of these, granular staining is absent (chromophobe tumours, Fig. 11.1F) but in a minority there is characteristic acidophilic or basophilic staining. Non-epithelial pituitary tumours are thought to arise from cell rests from Rathke's pouch, producing tumours of the hypothalamus or true pituitary known as craniopharyngiomas. The pituitary and hypothalamus are not uncommon as sites of secondary cancer, chiefly from breast and small cell lung cancers.

Chromophobe adenomas comprise about three-quarters of all pituitary tumours, and are most frequently encountered in adult life. They

tend to be non-functional, though ACTH, growth hormone, prolactin and other hormones are sometimes produced. They frequently attain a large size, particularly if non-functioning, and may extend upwards out of the sella, to involve the optic chiasm leading to the characteristic visual disturbance of bitemporal hemianopia (Fig. 11.2). Of the chromophil tumours, the

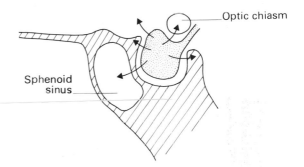

Fig. 11.2. *Local effects of pituitary tumours.* Extension commonly produces pressure on the optic chiasm, base of brain, and anterior and posterior clinoid processes. Extension occurs inferiorly and laterally, to sphenoid and cavernous sinuses.

acidophile adenomas are chiefly associated with excessive production of growth hormone, leading either to acromegaly if the tumour arises in adult life, or very rarely to gigantism when the tumour is encountered in childhood. Basophilic tumours tend to be smaller, and usually secrete ACTH and/or MSH leading to Cushing's syndrome sometimes with hyperpigmentation. These tumours are usually small and rarely involve the suprasellar area, so visual signs are unusual.

Craniopharyngiomas, unlike the other common pituitary tumours, are most frequently encountered in children. These tumours may be solid or cystic, and radiologically show characteristic calcification. They often involve suprasellar structures and can be particularly difficult to remove surgically, especially when there is heavy calcification.

MENINGIOMA

These tumours comprise about 10% of all brain tumours and arise from the meninges. There is a predilection for certain sites, particularly the parasagittal region and sphenoid ridge. They tend to compress the brain from without, and frank invasion is very uncommon except for the rare malignant meningioma, sometimes referred to as meningiosarcoma. Pressure outwards may cause bony erosion of the inner table of the skull, whilst inward displacement of the brain may lead to epilepsy as an early feature. Meningiomas may be chiefly fibrous in nature (fibroblastic meningioma) or very vascular (angioblastic meningioma), the latter having a more rapid evolution and more frequent malignant transformation.

OTHERS

Tumours of the pineal and third ventricle are now increasingly recognized, and are a diverse group arising either from the pineal itself, the third ventricle, or less commonly from ectopic sites of pineal tissue, particularly in the hypothalamus. Common types include the pinealoblastoma which histologically resembles medulloblastoma; the pinealocytoma which is a tumour of mature pineal cells; and germ cell tumours, which can be either pure seminoma (pineal germinoma) or teratoma which often contains highly differentiated mesenchymal structures. These latter tumours may produce AFP and HCG which can be measured in CSF or in blood and which can be helpful in diagnosis and management (see Chapter 4). At the anterior end of the third ventricle, the histological types are even more varied and include pituitary tumours, germinomas, meningiomas, optic nerve glioma, histiocytosis X and non-malignant granulomas which can occasionally cause diagnostic difficulty, such as tuberculosis and sarcoidosis. In proven pineal and suprasellar germinomas there is a high risk of spinal seeding (20–30%), possibly aggravated by attempts at surgical excision.

True intracerebral lymphomas are very unusual. The two chief types are the 'histiocytic' lymphoma which can occur at any site in the brain and appears more frequently in immunosuppressed patients such as renal transplant recipients; and the microglioma, a rare intracranial lymphoma not seen outside the central nervous system (see Chapter 27).

Thalamic and brainstem tumours are usually gliomas, though surgical biopsy is generally thought inadvisable. Thalamic gliomas are seen both in children (usually well-differentiated tumours) and adults (usually glioblastoma multiforme). Brainstem tumours are also chiefly encountered in children and are usually astrocytomas of variable differentiation.

Tumours of cranial nerves and nerve sheaths Acoustic neuroma is a tumour of adult life, rather more common in females, and arising from the VIII nerve, usually in its vestibular part. These tend to be slow growing tumours which present with unilateral deafness, vertigo, tinnitus, and involvement of other cranial nerves. Although strictly benign, they exert a local space occupying mass effect. Other less common neuronal tumours include the ganglio-neuroma and ganglioglioma which are also typically benign though dangerous because of local pressure effects.

Chordomas are uncommon malignant tumours, originating from the remnants of the embryonic notochord. Although occasionally encountered in children and young adults the peak age of incidence is 50—60 years and the characteristic sites are in the extremes of the spinal cord: a spheno-occipito-cervical group (40% of all cases) and a sacro-coccygeal group (equally frequent). The tumour consists of very characteristic solid cords of polygonal or mucin containing 'physalipherous' cells sometimes with a lobulated pattern. Local pressure symptoms are common, including bulbar, occipital or neck symptoms from tumours at the upper end of the spine, or constipation and low back pain from sacro-coccygeal tumours. Extensive bone destruction may occur.

Colloid cysts occur chiefly in the cerebellum and masquerade as malignant tumours because of their space occupying nature. Although these tumours are rare they can usually be diagnosed with confidence on CT scanning.

Clinical features

Brain tumours can be difficult to diagnose. The onset of symptoms may be late, particularly in tumours situated in less critical areas of the brain. In these parts of the cerebral hemispheres, they may grow to a substantial size before diagnosis, and may only produce rather subtle changes in personality, muscular power or co-ordination. In more critically sited tumours, obvious symptoms such as convulsions, ataxia or sensorimotor loss will lead to much earlier diagnosis.

In general, the symptoms can be broadly divided into four main groups. First, brain tumours can exert a mass effect and lead to raised intracranial pressure, with headache, drowsiness, nausea and vomiting as the cardinal symptoms. The headache is often worse in the morning, typically clearing by lunchtime. Vomiting may be sudden, unexpected and not preceded by nausea. Tumours situated around the fourth ventricle, in the cerebellum and around the pons are particularly likely to lead to raised intracranial pressure while tumours situated in the cerebral hemispheres may reach a large size without producing such symptoms. Papilloedema is usually present though it may be unilateral. With the advent of CT scanning, (Fig. 11.3) it is now recognized that ventricular enlargement, presumably caused by raised intracranial pressure, can be unaccompanied by papilloedema.

Secondly, there is a large group of focal symptoms caused by damage to local structures. These symptoms are determined by the site and size of the tumour. In a relatively small space, occupying lesions can cause devastating symptoms if sited in the motor cortex, Broca's area or the base of the brain. Accurate siting of tumours is often possible as a result of these specific symptoms: myoclonic seizures, development of late onset grand mal epilepsy or hemiparesis all point to lesions in the motor cortex, whereas lip smacking, hallucinations and other psychotic disturbances are typical of a temporal lobe lesion. For tumours situated more deeply, abnormalities of the visual pathways may give helpful diagnostic information since the optic nerves, chiasm, tract, radiations and visual cortex traverse the brain from front to back and

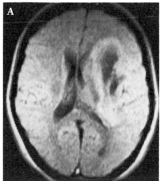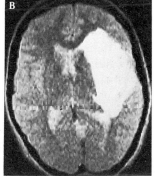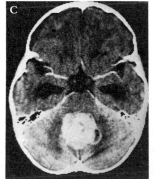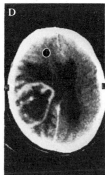

Fig. 11.3. (A) CT brain scan showing a large mass in the L hemisphere. (B) MRI scan from same case as (A). (C) CT brain scan showing large mid-line tumour of the posterior fossa. This was a medulloblastoma. (D) CT brain scan showing large parieto-occipital glioma. Note the obvious rim of contrast with oedema and ventricular dilatation.

interruption at a particular site will lead to recognizable abnormalities of the visual fields. At the base of the brain, the classical features are those of cranial nerve lesions, often multiple. In particular, tumours near the jugular foramen may cause a specific pattern of cranial nerve palsies since many of the lower cranial nerves exit at or near this point. Ataxia, nystagmus and diplopia are typical of cerebellar lesions, and are often coupled with nausea and headache due to raised intracranial pressure.

The third group of symptoms results from remote endocrine effects and occurs with tumours of the pituitary and hypothalamus. Damage to local structures is of great importance in pituitary tumours which can extend upwards to the suprasellar area and optic chiasm, inferiorly into the sphenoid sinus or laterally to the cavernous sinus or beyond, sometimes into the middle or posterior fossa (Fig. 11.2). Damage to the III, IV and VI cranial nerves may occur. Bleeding into a pituitary tumour (pituitary apoplexy) may result in sudden deterioration of vision, severe headache and hypopituitarism. Lesser degrees of pan-hypopituitarism are common in pituitary tumours though different end-organs may be variably affected. The florid syndrome includes hypothyroidism from reduction in TSH production, hypocorticism with hypotension from reduction in ACTH and hypogonadism with loss of secondary sexual characteristics, libido and amenorrhoea with infertility. In adults, lack of growth hormone results in hypoglycaemia. In children, reduction or cessation of growth is more characteristic. Sophisticated endocrinological investigations are often required to determine the full extent of the pituitary syndrome, but simple measurements of T3, T4, TSH, cortisol and gonadotrophins are usually sufficient for demonstration of the basic defects.

Finally, tumours of the central nervous system occasionally metastasise. Although this usually occurs late in the disease, patients may rarely present with symptoms caused by the metastases becoming apparent before the primary tumour itself. Although very unusual in adults, metastases are well recognized in children with medulloblastomas and poorly differentiated ependymomas. Secondary spread from these tumours is almost always through the CSF, usually presenting as spinal or meningeal deposits. Bone metastasis is also a well-recognized complication of medulloblastoma.

Diagnosis

The accurate diagnosis of brain tumours has been revolutionized by the advent of CT scanning. Previously, the only worthwhile non-invasive investigations for patients with suspected brain tumours were a chest X-ray to ensure the symptoms were not due to secondary deposits from an obvious primary carcinoma of the bronchus; a skull X-ray and tomography which rarely gave useful information but occasionally revealed erosion of the pituitary fossa or midline shift of a calcified pineal gland; and isotope brain scanning with its high incidence of false-negative results. Subsequent investigations such as carotid angiography and air ventriculography yielded important anatomical information to the neurosurgeon but were unpleasant, hazardous and occasionally fatal: not the sort of test to request if one was suspicious but uncertain of the diagnosis.

CT scanning has now all but replaced the need for these dangerous investigations, and also carries the advantage of being repeatable so that response to treatment can be easily assessed. The routine use of intravenous contrast material has increased the value of CT scanning still further (Fig. 11.3), as has the continual evolution of technological refinements which have resulted in scanners with far superior resolving power, and the ability to reconstruct the image in sagittal and other planes. CT brain scanning does however have its limitations particularly in tumours of the posterior fossa and brain stem. Pituitary tumours require high resolution since they are often small and close to bony structures. Most CT scanning machines can reliably detect lesions of greater than $1\,cm^3$ but low-grade gliomas are sometimes poorly visualized. Angiography is still indicated to exclude arteriovenous malformations and occasionally to visualize posterior fossa, deep-seated and thalamic lesions and other sites poorly visualized by CT scanning. In addition, pre-operative angiography may be helpful in defining the tumour's vascular supply. The development of nuclear magnetic resonance imaging (MRI) equipment represents a further area of brain tumour imaging research which has already been shown capable of accurate pre-operative diagnosis in areas where CT scanning is unreliable (Figs. 4.10 & 11.3).

Management of brain tumours

The approach to management depends on the histological nature of the tumour and its site. Surgical removal is desirable both for histological diagnosis and sometimes for definitive treatment. Radical excision can however be extremely hazardous and occasionally impossible. Stereotactic CT guided biopsy can be useful for histological confirmation in inoperable cases. Where hydrocephalus is present surgical decompression by ventricular drainage results in dramatic improvement. Both ventriculoperitoneal and ventriculo-atrial shunts are employed and can be permanently implanted. For deep-seated tumours (e.g. thalamic, pineal and brainstem) even a biopsy may be out of the question. Urgent reversal of acute cerebral oedema may be necessary which may include the use of intravenous urea, mannitol, or high doses of dexamethasone (see p. 195 for management details). Radiotherapy is frequently employed as an adjunct to surgery and sometimes as the definitive treatment (3). The role of chemotherapy is still debatable.

GLIOMA

Low grade (Kernohan grades I and II). For low grade astrocytomas, complete surgical excision is the rule since these lesions tend to be well localized and can often be removed from adjacent structures without causing too much damage. In most cases surgery is the sole method of treatment. However, late local recurrences may occur. Routine irradiation has been shown to be worthwhile in incompletely resected tumours. Leibel and colleagues, in a series of over 100 patients with incompletely resected low-grade astrocytomas (1) showed that the 10-year survival rate was only 11% in patients where radiotherapy was not given, compared with 35% in patients who were irradiated. At 20 years, the survival difference was more striking still: 0% compared with 23%. These results lend support to the conclusions of Bouchard and Peirce who suggested over 20 years ago that irradiation was a useful adjunct to surgery for well-differentiated astrocytomas (2). In general the radiation treatment volume

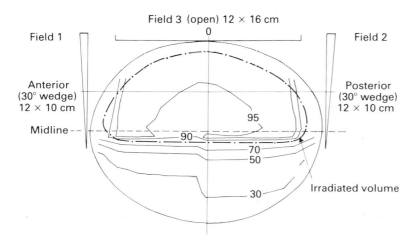

Field 3 (open) 12 × 16 cm

Field 1   Field 2

Anterior (30° wedge) 12 × 10 cm

Posterior (30° wedge) 12 × 10 cm

Midline

95

90

70

50

30

Irradiated volume

Fig. 11.4. *External beam radiation for cortical glioma.* Typical 3 field plan treating whole hemisphere. The irradiated volume is shown by the interrupted line.

can be limited since these tumours do not infiltrate widely. Doses of 45–60 Gy (4500–6000 rad) in 4–6 weeks are normally recommended.

High-grade (Kernohan grades III—IV). For these tumours radiotherapy is almost always employed as an adjunct to surgery (Fig. 11.4), first because complete surgical removal is rarely possible, and secondly because the results of surgery alone are so poor. In 1962 Taveras *et al.* (4) asked the pertinent question; 'should we treat glioblastoma multiforme?' In a study of over 400 patients, these authors showed that where patients had undergone biopsy alone or partial resection, postoperative irradiation was beneficial. Their recommendations of adequate surgical decompression with partial or gross surgical removal where possible and radiation therapy shortly after operation, are still followed. More recent studies of postoperative irradiation for glioblastoma multiforme have demonstrated that, although at 1 year there are no survivors with surgery alone, almost one-fifth of patients receiving postoperative radiation are still alive. With these high-grade tumours, large radiation volumes are required and some radiotherapists routinely treat the whole of the brain. Doses of 40–50 Gy (4000–5000 rad) in 4½–6 weeks are often used (Fig. 11.4). Although the ultimate prognosis is very poor indeed, <6% of patients with Grade IV disease survive for 5 years. For patients with Grade III tumours, the survival is better, and

over half of the surviving patients achieve an independent life (Fig. 11.5).

Attempts to improve these dismal figures have led to the use of wide field irradiation or treatment to higher dosage, since local recurrence at the initial tumour site is almost always the cause of death. Autopsy findings on patients with glioblastoma dying shortly after diagnosis have confirmed that the tumour has almost always infiltrated much more widely than is apparent even on surgical inspection. Nevertheless, even where the treatment field is increased to include the whole brain, with boosting of the primary site to a very high dose, later local recurrence is almost inevitable. A 50% 1 year survival rate has been achieved with this high dose technique in a small group of patients with Grade IV astrocytoma, without prohibitive immediate or delayed radiation complications either clinically or at autopsy (5). Although these patients relapsed later, this work does at least suggest that intensive irradiation of brain tumours is possible and that if means of increasing the dose could safely be found, better local control might yet be obtained.

Because high-grade astrocytomas recur locally and rarely disseminate, other attempts have been made to increase the biological effectiveness of local treatment. Urtasun and colleagues (6) performed a randomized trial using metronidazole an hypoxic cell sensitiser. In this small study there appeared to be a significant improvement in median survival,

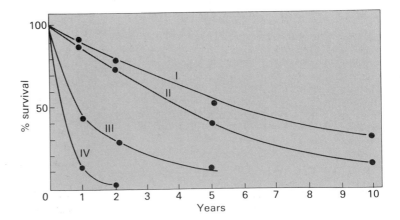

Fig. 11.5. *Survival related to grade in malignant glioma.* Note the small proportion of 10 year survivors even with low grade tumours.

and further trials are now being performed both with this agent and with misonidazole, a theoretically more effective compound but one with the disadvantage of greater toxicity including a dose related peripheral neuropathy. Unfortunately, a large randomized study by the Medical Research Council has failed to confirm these preliminary findings (7).

An alternative approach has been the use of neutrons, since the relative biological effectiveness (RBE) is much higher than for photons (see Chapter 5). Although autopsy data suggests that local recurrence may be less likely with neutrons than with photons, no clear benefit has yet been reported. This may be because the RBE for neutrons is also higher in normal brain and since initial trials employed a high neutron dose the possible benefit of improved local tumour control may have been offset by greater toxicity. In one study, microdegeneration of white matter was seen and dementia occurred in some patients.

There has been increasing interest in the use of cytotoxic agents as an adjuvant to surgery and radiotherapy for high-grade gliomas. The nitrosoureas, BCNU and CCNU have received most attention, since they are known to be lipid soluble and cross the hypothetical blood/brain barrier (see Chapter 6). Assessment of response of brain tumours to chemotherapy is difficult, but there is no doubt that some patients with recurrent disease benefit with an objective response rate of about 40% (Table 11.2). Unfortunately, most of these responses are short-lived and are seen in patients with relatively well-

Table 11.2 Response to cytotoxic drugs in gliomas.

Drug	% Responders*
BCNU	47
CCNU	44
Procarbazine	52
VM26	25
Cisplatin	30
BCNU and Vincristine	44

*Most of these are partial responses. Criteria of response vary considerably.

differentiated gliomas. Patients with grade IV tumours are very unlikely to respond. In a large prospective multicentre trial, Walker and colleagues showed that routine use of BCNU as an addition to surgery and radiotherapy prolonged the median survival by a few weeks (8). The study also confirmed that treatment by surgery and chemotherapy (but no irradiation) was much less successful. Other data also suggest that nitrosoureas do offer a small survival advantage, with a possible superiority for CCNU over BCNU.

Other agents with known activity are vincristine and procarbazine (Table 11.2). These drugs have the added advantage of being relatively non-toxic. Cisplatin and VM26 have recently been shown to have some activity.

Ependymoma. This tumour is far less common than astrocytoma and behaves rather differently. It arises from cells lining the ventricles and central canal of the spinal cord, and has a tendency to seed throughout the subarachnoid space giving rise to symptomatic spinal deposits in about 10% of patients. Spinal seeding is particularly likely in patients with high grade lesions, especially those arising from the lining cells of the fourth ventricle. For this reason, routine cranio-spinal irradiation is usually recommended in all patients with high-grade ependymomas and for ependymomas of the posterior fossa regardless of grade (see p. 191 for details of technique and toxicity). The primary site should receive a high dose (50 Gy or greater in 5–7 weeks) with full craniospinal treatment in patients with high grade tumours. There is evidence that spinal cord primaries tend to be of lower grade than intracerebral tumours, with a better survival rate.

The overall survival of ependymomas is better than with astrocytomas. At least 50% of patients live for 5 years. Several series have however confirmed the importance of radiation dose. In a report by Phillips and colleagues (9), the 5-year survival of patients given *intensive* radiotherapy was almost 90%, twice the *overall* survival rate of 40% (which included those who died postoperatively without treatment as well as patients who received inadequate irradiation dosage). From this it is clear that the approach should be intensive with full treatment to the whole cranio-spinal axis at least in patients with high-grade or infratentorial tumours.

Oligodendrogliomas. These are uncommon tumours, often relatively well-differentiated, slow growing and amenable to complete surgical removal. In such cases there is no definite indication for postoperative irradiation although treatment is usually advised where there has been incomplete surgical excision, or where there are histologically aggressive features (sometimes termed oligodendroblastoma). In a group of over 30 patients, reported by Sheline, the 5-year survival with surgery alone was 31% compared with an 85% survival rate in patients receiving postoperative irradiation (10).

Deep-seated gliomas. Gliomas situated deep to the cerebral cortex present particular problems of diagnosis and management. Important sites include the thalamus and hypothalamus, pons, brain stem, pineal region and optic nerves. The common difficulty with tumours in these areas is that histological confirmation is often not possible because any attempt at surgical intervention would be hazardous though gliomas of the pineal area are increasingly being considered suitable for surgical removal.

Their clinical behaviour varies at each of the different sites. Optic nerve gliomas which usually present with proptosis or blindness are often thought to be benign and unresponsive to radiotherapy. However, in some cases the tumours are bilateral, involve the optic chiasm or extend backwards to the ventricles, sometimes with hydrocephalus. These patients should be treated with radiotherapy. Although uncomplicated lesions may be self-limiting, radiotherapy may produce complete relief of distressing proptosis, and objective response verified on CT scanning. For thalamic tumours, radiotherapy is almost invariably indicated. Surgical attempts at excision or even histologi-

cal confirmation are particularly dangerous at this site.

The prognosis for these tumours appears to vary with age, though as expected, histological grade (usually obtained only at autopsy) is also important. The 5-year survival rate in young patients with grade III lesions is about 25%. Tumours of the pons and brain stem carry a particularly poor prognosis and often present with florid symptoms including cranial nerve palsies, ataxia or involvement of the long tracts. These are usually high-grade astrocytomas and infiltrate widely, often attaining a large volume before diagnosis. They are a challenge to the radiotherapist since they are surgically untreatable, but often present with urgent problems in management. Although the majority show some symptomatic response to radiotherapy, the ultimate survival rate (approximately 15%) is poor. A large review of patients with brain stem tumours showed an average survival of 4 years for irradiated patients compared with only 15 months if untreated (11). In patients who showed a response to treatment, the average survival was over 5 years. In general, there seems to be no point in attempting to treat these lesions with highly localized radiation fields. Large lateral opposed fields are required since the tumour has usually spread throughout the whole of the pons, brain stem and medulla and often to the upper cervical spine. Doses of 40–55 Gy in 4–5 weeks daily treatment are usually recommended although some centres employ fewer fractions, for example a total dose of 45–48 Gy in 15 daily fractions.

Medulloblastoma. Surgical treatment alone is unsuccessful, and postoperative radiotherapy has been routinely employed since the 1920s, when the marked radiosensitivity of this tumour was first noted. With increasingly accurate treatment planning, the use of supervoltage equipment and prophylactic irradiation of the whole brain and spinal cord, the 10-year survival rate has improved and is now in the order of 30–40% (12).

Many surgeons limit their operation to biopsy and decompression, recognizing that an attempt at bulk removal is bound to increase the complication rate. The operative mortality is still in the region of 10%. However, although these tumours are radiosensitive, they do recur at the primary site, and it is possible that removal of tumour bulk might reduce the rate of local recurrence. Most neurosurgeons excise as much tumour as is safely possible, and survival following 'complete' removal of the tumour is better than when the tumour has been only partially removed. It is now routine practise to irradiate the whole of the cranio-spinal axis, as soon after surgery as possible. Treatment planning must be meticulous, taking particular care to treat the base of the brain, retro-orbital area and brain stem. (Fig. 11.6). These sites can be undertreated if adult surface anatomical boundaries are used without regard to the anatomy

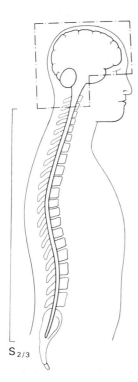

$S_{2/3}$

Fig. 11.6. *Cranio-spinal irradiation.* Schematic representation of the field arrangement for cranio-spinal irradiation in medulloblastoma and other tumours which seed through the CSF.

of the developing brain. The technique which we employ is carried out as follows.

1 Irradiation of the whole brain with large lateral opposing fields, including the midbrain and upper cervical vertebrae as far as the lower limit of C2, to a midline dose of 30 Gy in 3 weeks.

2 Boosting of the posterior fossa and midbrain as far anteriorly as the anterior clinoid process, to 45 Gy at the same rate.

3 At the same time as the posterior fossa boost is commenced, spinal irradiation is begun, from the lower border of the cerebral fields to the lower border of vertebra S2 so that the entire spinal cord including the conus medullaris and cauda equina are treated. A dose of not less than 30 Gy is given to the spine over 4–5 weeks.

4 For the final part of treatment, the posterior fossa is boosted to a still higher dose. The final brain doses are as follows: posterior fossa 50–55 Gy in 6–7 weeks, midbrain 45 Gy in 5–6 weeks, cerebral hemispheres and anterior part of brain 35 Gy in 4 weeks, spinal cord 30 Gy minimum dose in 4–5 weeks.

It is important to monitor the blood count during treatment of the spine, but with this technique and dose rate the treatment rarely has to be discontinued, though the white blood count frequently falls to about 2×10^9/l by the end of treatment.

Irradiation of the whole neuraxis carries a number of drawbacks. Fortunately, skull growth is usually almost complete by the time of treatment, so that permanent reduction in skull volume is very rarely seen. Nonetheless, some degree of shortness of stature (particularly sitting height) must be expected from irradiation of the whole spine coupled with pituitary irradiation (see Chapter 5). In addition, midline organs such as the thyroid, larynx, oesophagus, thymus and heart are directly in the path of the exit beam, and the kidneys and female gonads are also likely to receive a significant amount of scattered irradiation despite the most careful planning. The need for whole spine irradiation has therefore been questioned, especially as only 1 in 10 children will develop spinal cord metastases. However, current practise favours more extensive surgery even though there is a theoretical risk of spinal seeding because of shedding of tumour cells during the operation.

Despite these hazards and the possible added problem of cognitive and learning defects, over three-quarters of surviving children with medulloblastoma lead independent and active lives and at least one study has shown that intellectual achievement in these children is not impaired (13). In the context of possible curative treatment for children with medulloblastoma, there seems no doubt that the possible hazards of treatment have to be accepted.

Chemotherapy has mainly been used for treatment of recurrent disease. Lipid soluble agents have been used both singly and in combination. The approximate response rates are shown in Table 11.3. The responses are usually short-lived and combination chemotherapy may be difficult if relapse follows soon after cranio-spinal irradiation because of the volume of bone marrow which has been irradiated. Methotrexate, which may be of some value, may be hazardous within 6 months of irradiation as it can cause a severe leucoencephalopathy.

Since there is some responsiveness to drugs

Table 11.3. Chemotherapy of recurrent medulloblastoma.

Drug	Response Rate
Single Agent	
Vincristine	probably 50%
CCNU	probably 50%
High dose Methotrexate	uncertain 0–60%
Combinations	
Procarbazine	
Vincristine	60%
CCNU	
Mustine	
Vincristine	
Procarbazine	approximately 50%
Prednisolone	

and radiotherapy is often not curative, there has been interest recently in using cytotoxic drugs as an adjuvant to surgery and radiotherapy. The International Society for Paediatric Oncology has undertaken a large trial to assess the role of adjuvant chemotherapy with vincristine and CCNU, given both during the radiotherapy treatment and as maintenance for 2 years afterwards. In a series of over 330 cases, a number of preliminary points have begun to emerge. The main beneficiaries of adjuvant chemotherapy appear to be the groups where the tumour was incompletely removed, with brain stem spread and below the age of 3 years.

It is often possible to obtain symptomatic improvement in patients with recurrence by further radiotherapy.

PITUITARY TUMOURS

Pituitary tumours are usually treated surgically, both in order to make the diagnosis and in many cases to provide definitive therapy. For small tumours without suprasellar extension, many surgeons now favour the trans-sphenoidal route, which avoids the complications of craniotomy, although infection and CSF rhinorrhoea are occasionally encountered. However, for larger tumours and particularly for those with extension outside the pituitary fossa, a craniotomy is necessary. In children with craniopharyngioma, surgery can be particularly difficult because the chalky calcific material which is often encountered can be impossible to remove completely.

The routine addition of postoperative irradiation for patients with pituitary tumours decreases the likelihood of local recurrence. Chromophobe pituitary adenomas are probably more radiosensitive than chromophil tumours. In patients with acromegaly (almost always due to a chromophil tumour) arrest or reversal of the syndrome can be achieved with surgery and postoperative irradiation in 75% of cases. Craniopharyngioma requires a high local dose for eradication (50–60 Gy in 5–7 weeks).

Careful tumour localization, multifield planning and attention to detail are essential for successful radiation treatment. A three field plan is normally employed, with particular care to avoid over-treatment of the eyes and optic chiasm. For most tumours the field size can be limited, though chromophobe pituitary adenomas can reach a very large size. In some centres a rotational plan is used. The radiation technique is the same regardless of whether the patient is treated postoperatively as an adjuvant to surgery, or later for recurrence—though in the latter instance, the treatment volume may have to be larger.

Alternatives to the use of conventional external beam irradiation include interstitial Yttrium seeds or heavy particles (proton or alpha particle) irradiation. The use of bromocriptine has been advocated in recent years as an alternative to surgery and/or radiotherapy treatment for pituitary adenomas. This agent is particularly useful for small tumours producing prolactin only (prolactinomas). Although widely used, patients on bromocriptine do sometimes develop frank recurrence; it also uncertain how long the drug needs to be continued. If bromocriptine fails, prolactinomas may have to be removed surgically.

MENINGIOMAS

Meningiomas should be surgically excised. If they arise at an inaccessible site they can be difficult to remove and in such cases, postoperative irradiation may reduce the incidence of local recurrence. As these tumours are not very sensitive to radiation, high doses are required. For patients with 'malignant' meningioma, radiotherapy is always required though the overall prognosis in these cases is very poor.

PINEAL TUMOURS

These present particular problems of management since they are often not biopsied by the surgeon for fear of causing irreparable damage. Many pineal tumours are sensitive to radiotherapy and in patients without histological

verification of the type of pineal tumours a trial of radiotherapy is always justified. Pineal germinomas and pinealoblastomas are the most radiosensitive of pineal tumours, and repeat CT scanning after as little as 2 weeks treatment often shows dramatic reduction in the size of the primary tumour. In these cases, it can reasonably be assumed that the diagnosis is either pineal germinoma or pinealoblastoma since other pineal tumours (particularly pineal teratoma and pinealocytoma) are less radiosensitive. Although radiotherapy is appropriate for pineal tumours in general, the technique varies with different types of tumour. With the radiosensitive group, there is a tendency for involvement of the whole CNS and full craniospinal irradiation should be employed. This is not required with other pineal tumours, though they require a high local radiation dose. Neurosurgeons are increasingly prepared to attempt biopsy or even total removal of pineal tumours, so an accurate histological diagnosis is now more frequently available. For the less radiosensitive group, total surgical removal is likely to be of particular benefit. Pineal teratomas like teratomas at other sites can produce alpha fetoprotein and human chorionic gonadotrophin which can be measured in CSF and also in the blood. Chemotherapy may have a part to play in management and is certainly effective in recurrent disease, using conventional teratoma regimens (see Chapter 19).

INTRACRANIAL LYMPHOMA

Microgliomas and histiocytic lymphomas are also radiosensitive. The surgical approach depends on the site of the lesion and surgery is sometimes complete. Nonetheless, radiotherapy should be offered in all cases and a remarkable degree of radiosensitivity is sometimes encountered although durability of response is often disappointing (see Chapter 26). In general, the best results have been obtained with high dosage, and full cranio-spinal irradiation is generally advocated since these tumours can spread throughout the nervous system.

CHORDOMA

Surgical removal is essential though often difficult because of the anatomy of the tumour. These tumours often have a 'dumbell' appearance with an intraspinal component, making total removal impossible. Post-operative radiotherapy is therefore usually necessary though these lesions are rather insensitive. High radiation dose is particularly difficult to achieve in the cervical spine, though sacral chordomas can often be treated to a high dose since there is no danger of damage to the spinal cord. Despite the marginal radiosensitivity of chordomas, long survival has occasionally been documented in patients treated by subtotal surgical removal and radical postoperative radiotherapy.

OTHER TUMOURS

Acoustic neuromas, and other neuronal tumours, are best treated surgically and are minimally radiosensitive. Nonetheless, postoperative radiotherapy should be considered where surgery has been incomplete.

Treatment on relapse

For recurrent brain tumours, the question of retreatment radiotherapy often arises. When the disease-free interval has been short, as with high-grade gliomas, there is little value in retreatment since only a modest radiation dose can be safely achieved and is of doubtful benefit where more intensive radiotherapy has already failed. However, in patients with low-grade glioma of any type, or those with medulloblastoma, late recurrences are common. The feasibility of retreatment radiation therapy increases according to the time interval from first treatment, and if a sufficient time has elapsed (10 years or more), a complete retreatment dose can be contemplated. With medulloblastoma particularly, widespread late primary, cerebral and spinal metastases can develop, with continued responsiveness to repeated courses of radiotherapy. Dexamethasone often provides valu-

able symptomatic relief. Chemotherapy may produce transient responses and is discussed above.

Prognosis of brain tumours

For malignant gliomas, the prognosis is heavily dependent on tumour grade. Although there are four pathological (Kernohan) grades, patients with malignant glioma fall chiefly into two prognostic groups since those with grades I and II tumours have a relatively good prognosis and 5 and 10 year survival rates of approximately 65 and 35%, whereas those with grade III and IV tumours have a 5-year survival rate of under 10% (Fig. 11.5), with a worse prognosis in the grade IV category. In all grades incomplete removal is associated with a worse prognosis.

In medulloblastoma, a variety of factors are thought to contribute to prognosis. Patients undergoing total surgical excision undoubtedly do better though this may be as much a result of tumour size as the contribution of surgery *per se*. Age at diagnosis is also important and children over 15 years of age have a better prognosis. Children with spinal metastases at presentation are rarely cured. The adequacy of the irradiation, both in technique and dose, is crucial, with evidence emerging that 5-year survival rates of over 40% should now be expected with modern techniques.

In ependymoma, overall prognosis depends on tumour grade and the median survival following surgery in low-grade ependymoma is approximately 10 years. When recurrences occur, they are frequently of a higher histological grade, and median overall survival in high-grade ependymoma is no better than 2–3 years.

Both pituitary tumours and meningiomas have an excellent prognosis following surgical removal and, where appropriate, postoperative radiotherapy. Few large series of pineal tumours have been reported. Survival is very variable, reflecting the heterogeneity of tumours at this site, but in pineal germinoma, 5-year survival rates of up to 70% have been reported in patients undergoing radical radiation therapy. In chordoma, the prognosis is poor since these tumours are not usually entirely resectable or fully radiosensitive.

SECONDARY DEPOSITS

Cerebral metastases are common and account for about a third of all brain tumours. The commonest primary sites include carcinoma of the breast and bronchus and melanoma. In each of these tumours, autopsy series confirm that the probability of dissemination to the brain is very much greater than the frequency of pre-mortem diagnosis. About 60% of all patients with small cell lung cancer have demonstrable brain metastases at autopsy, and in melanoma about three-quarters of patients who die from disseminated disease have brain metastases. Many other tumours can metastasise to the brain, though at a much lower frequency (Table 11.1).

Metastases may be either single or multiple and diagnostically may be difficult to distinguish from primary brain tumours, particularly when, as occasionally occurs, there is no known primary. Small cell lung cancer and melanoma are particularly likely to give rise to multiple intracerebral deposits.

About half of all brain metastases are found in the distribution of the middle cerebral artery and are characteristically cortical deposits. Any other site may be involved and cerebellar, thalamic and pituitary deposits are all encountered. As with primary brain tumours, the characteristic symptoms are those of raised intracranial pressure, focal neurological damage or convulsions. The diagnosis is usually suggested by isotope or CT brain scanning which may show single or multiple abnormal areas of increased uptake of isotope or a typically spherical lesions often with obvious contrast enhancement on CT scanning (Fig. 11.3). Although local oedema is often present, this is usually less than that seen with high-grade primary brain tumours. In patients with known cancer, parti-

cularly lung or breast cancer or malignant melanoma, further investigation is not usually indicated, especially where the primary diagnosis has been made within the previous 5 years, although alternative diagnoses should always be considered. With apparently solid metastases, the most important differential diagnosis is from benign brain tumour, particularly meningioma (especially of course if the tumour is anatomically located at a common meningioma site). In case of multiple metastases, the presumed diagnosis is almost always correct, though occasional confusion with intracerebral abscesses may occur.

Occasionally patients with a known primary cancer develop headache, mental confusion or focal signs suggestive of cerebral metastases, yet the CT scan fails to show an abnormality. Such patients may well have cerebral secondaries and a trial of dexamethasone may be indicated. A good response usually implies that the diagnosis is correct and that radiotherapy to the brain should be considered.

TREATMENT OF SECONDARY DEPOSITS IN THE BRAIN

Reversal of oedema. Treatment with dexamethasone, often at high dosage (6 mg every 6 hours, initially by intramuscular or intravenous administration) is often valuable to provide rapid reduction of intracranial pressure and relief of cerebral oedema. Response to this powerful agent is a useful indicator that an intracerebral tumour is present, and is often thought to be a helpful determinant of the likelihood of response to radiotherapy. The important clinical point about dexamethasone treatment is that it exerts its effect rapidly, and can often be quickly reduced in dosage. It is a great mistake to allow patients to remain on dexamethasone for too long, because of the inevitability of steroid complications, particularly proximal myopathy and facial swelling. In general, we usually recommend gradual discontinuation of dexamethasone after 4–6 weeks, though this policy occasionally results in patients developing symptoms and signs of raised intracranial pressure because of too rapid reduction. In these cases, the dose can easily be increased again, and patients almost always respond quickly. There is considerable variation in the rapidity with which patients can be weaned off dexamethasone. In patients where dexamethasone is ill-advised or dangerous (e.g. where there is a history of bleeding peptic ulcer or severe hypertension or diabetes) it is sometimes possible to achieve the desired reduction in cerebral oedema by the use of intravenous urea (1 g/kg, in dextrose solution), mannitol (2 g/kg as a 20% solution) or oral glycerine which can be made palatable by making it up in a 50% mixture with lemonade. Most patients dislike this latter treatment because it rapidly induces diarrhoea, but it can be a highly effective means of improving symptoms of raised intracranial pressure.

Radiotherapy. Radiotherapy is indicated in a large proportion of patients with secondary brain deposits, though the decision to treat requires careful thought. Patients likely to benefit include those with known radiosensitive tumours (particularly small cell carcinoma of the bronchus and to a lesser extent carcinoma of the breast), those where there has been a good response to dexamethasone, where the patient's general condition is good (particularly if there is no other evidence of distant metastases) and in patients with multiple intracerebral deposits in whom there can be no question of surgery.

The choice of fractionation and dosage remains contentious. A recent large multicentre study has suggested that there is no advantage to prolonged fractionation and that a total dosage of 20 Gy (2000 rad) in 5 daily fractions, or 30 Gy (3000 rad) in 10 daily fractions over 2 weeks, are as effective as much more prolonged treatment regimens (14). In patients with less radiosensitive tumours (adenocarcinomas, melanoma and others) higher doses may be required, particularly in the case of single metastatic deposits where the relatively limited volume can be treated to a higher dose.

Surgery. Neurosurgical removal of metastases is occasionally performed in the mistaken supposition that the surgeon is dealing with a primary brain tumour. In these cases, where there has been complete macroscopic removal, it is not clear whether treatment with postoperative radiotherapy is of benefit. Deliberate surgical removal of metastases is valuable in a small proportion of patients. Relative indications for surgery include: young fit patients with a solitary brain metastasis and with no evidence of disease elsewhere; where there has been a long treatment-free interval (this is often the case in patients with breast cancer); and where the single metastasis is unlikely to be radiosensitive (as for example in adenocarcinoma of the bronchus or thyroid). In this selected group of patients, surgical removal can be the treatment of choice.

Chemotherapy. This is not an established treatment, though there is some evidence that in chemosensitive tumours such as small cell carcinoma of the bronchus or testicular teratoma, chemotherapy may be effective. In general, chemotherapy is not a useful modality of treatment, though the long held concept of a blood/brain barrier, making intravenous chemotherapy invariably inappropriate, may well be erroneous. Intrathecal chemotherapy is of no value for intracerebral metastases.

Patients with intracerebral metastases have a very poor survival, particularly where the primary diagnosis is a small cell lung cancer or melanoma. In other cases such as breast cancer and adenocarcinoma from other sites, survival may be more prolonged, particularly where neurosurgical removal of a solitary metastasis has been successfully accomplished.

Lymphomatous or carcinomatous meningitis is increasingly recognized in a variety of tumours, particularly acute leukaemia, non-Hodgkin's lymphoma, breast cancer, lung cancer, melanoma and ovarian cancer. It typically presents with the symptoms and signs of headache, clouding of consciousness, ataxia and focal cranial nerve palsies particularly of the

III, IV, VI and VII cranial nerves. Although an extremely grave site for metastasis, it may temporarily be responsive to treatment both with whole brain irradiation and also with intrathecal chemotherapy. In patients with breast cancer (much the commonest primary site in patients with carcinomatous meningitis), we employ whole brain irradiation to 30–40 Gy (3000–4000 rad) in daily fractions over 2–3 weeks, initially coupled with twice weekly intrathecal methotrexate 10–12.5 mg. If there has been a good response to treatment during the first 3 weeks, it is best to continue with regular, less frequent intrathecal chemotherapy, for a prolonged period. Insertion of an Ommaya or Rickham intraventricular reservoir makes drug administration easy, avoiding repeated lumbar punctures, and should be considered in patients where obvious response to the initial treatment justifies continued CSF treatment.

TUMOURS OF THE SPINAL CORD

Primary tumours of the spinal cord are very uncommon though secondary deposits involving the cord are frequently encountered. Table 11.4 shows the main types of spinal cord tumour. Ependymoma is the commonest glioma to arise from the spinal cord, astrocytoma being much less frequently seen. Schwannomas, vascular tumours and meningiomas are the other relatively common types. Secondary deposits may be intramedullary but are more often extramedullary (usually extradural), frequently resulting from direct spread from the adjacent involved vertebral body. Management of acute cord compression is also dealt with in Chapter 8.

Table 11.4. Classification of tumours of spinal cord (with % frequency).

Intradural (55%)	Extradural (45%)
Extramedullary	Metastases (25%)
Meningioma (15%)	Myeloma (6%)
Neurofibroma (10%)	Lymphoma (5%)
Congenital and others (7%)	Sarcomas (5%)
	Others (4%)
Intramedullary	
Ependymoma (5%)	
Astrocytoma (5%)	
Angiomas (6%)	
Others (6%)	

Symptoms

Pain is the usual presenting symptom and is generally felt directly over the cord lesion, though the site of pain can be misleading. More laterally situated tumours (often involving the nerve roots as well) may cause more specific and focally sited pain than centrally placed tumours, for example fusiform intramedullary lesions which can extend in a clinically silent way throughout several segments. Tenderness on palpation of the overlying vertebra is often found though the bone may have to be pressed firmly or even struck, to elicit this sign. Sensorimotor loss is also frequently present, with defects of both power and sensation at and below the level of involvement. At the site of the lesion, there may be an obvious sensory loss (especially evident in lesions of the dorsal and lumbar spine involving loss of sensation over the trunk). Muscular weakness in the upper limbs is a feature of lesions of the cervical spine. Below the affected area of an incomplete cord compression there may be partial preservation of function with less obvious neurological abnormalities and only patchy sensory loss. When the cord compression is complete a severe paraparesis results. Complete loss of sphincter function is a late sign with a poor prognosis (see Chapter 8), but lesser degrees occur earlier and their significance is often missed.

Tumours situated below the lower end of the spinal cord (vertebral level L1/2) may produce a typical cauda equina syndrome with sacral anaesthesia, sciatic pain (often bilateral), gluteal weakness and wasting, impotence and bladder dysfunction with retention and overflow incontinence. However, most cases of cauda equina compression are far less symptomatically clear-cut and in practice the diagnosis is often very difficult to establish. Even in proven cauda equina compression the myelogram may be normal and cannot therefore reliably exclude the diagnosis. Ependymomas constitute the largest single group of primary tumours at the lower end of the cord (conus medullaris and filum terminale). Lateral compression of the spinal cord may cause a complete or partial Brown–Séquard syndrome with ipsilateral spastic weakness, reduced vibration sense and proprioception together with contralateral insensitivity to pain and temperature change. Tumour progression causes an increasingly florid clinical picture with weakness, sensory loss, hyperreflexia and autonomic dysfunction (Table 11.5).

In general, the clinical picture depends on the site of the tumour rather than its origin, though destructive secondary deposits, which more often involve the vertebral column than the spinal cord, produce more local pain and tenderness than some of the less common primary cord lesions. Common primary sites of vertebral or cord metastases include carcinoma of the bronchus (particularly small cell), carcinoma of

Table 11.5. Syndromes of spinal cord compression.

Complete Compression
Sensory level just below level of lesion
Loss of all modalities of sensation—variable
 in degree at first
Bilateral upper motor neurone weakness below
 lesion
Bladder and bowel dysfunction

Anterior Compression
Partial loss of pain and temperature below lesion
Bilateral upper motor neurone weakness below
 lesion
Bladder and bowel dysfunction

Lateral Compression (*Brown Séquard*)
Contralateral loss of pain and temperature (touch
 much less affected)
Ipsilateral loss of proprioception and vibration
Ipsilateral upper motor neurone weakness

Posterior Compression
Loss of vibration and position below lesion
Pain, temperature and touch relatively spared
Painful segmental paraesthesia at level of lesion.

---

the breast and myeloma. Less common primary tumours include carcinomas of the thyroid, large bowel and kidney and also malignant melanoma.

Differential diagnosis

Although the clinical syndrome of spinal cord compression usually implies a malignant aetiology, a few non-malignant lesions can produce a similar clinical picture. These include inflammatory cord lesions (particularly transverse myelitis, infectious polyneuropathy or Guillain–Barré syndrome), anterior spinal artery occlusion, abscess of the cord, syringomyelia and haemorrhage into the cord (haematomyelia). Very occasionally an acutely prolapsed intervertebral disc may produce symptoms of cord compression.

Investigation

Radiological investigation is always required. Plain X-rays of the spine may show an obvious lytic secondary deposit in the vertebra(e) at the level of compression, but X-ray changes may be very subtle, with loss of the pedicle of the spine but no other significant features. Myelography either by the lumbar or cisternal route, gives good anatomical demonstration of the spinal cord lesion and will show whether the block is partial or complete (Fig. 11.7). With complete block, it is difficult to be certain of the upper extent of the abnormality and occasionally a cisternal myelogram will also need to be performed if full anatomical definition is considered important for therapy. For oncologists, myodil myelography has the advantage that patients can easily be re-examined since the myodil remains in the spinal sac for months or even years. The more recent introduction of metrizamide gives better definition of root pathology but, being water-soluble, is rapidly cleared so that re-examinations require a further lumbar puncture. In tumours with doubtful or difficult physical signs, CT scanning can be invaluable. This investigation can be

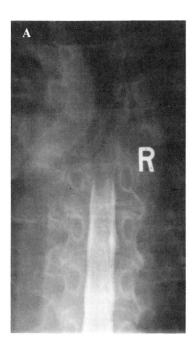 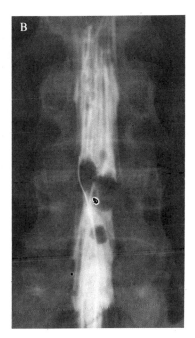

Fig. 11.7. *Radiological changes in spinal cord compression.* (A) Complete cord compression. (B) Partial cord compression due to multiple deposits from an ependymoma.

even more informative when combined with metrizamide myelography.

Management

For primary tumours of the spinal cord, surgical removal is the treatment of choice where possible. Technical difficulties are often encountered and intramedullary tumours are almost always unresectable. At surgery the tumour should be totally removed where possible, reduced in bulk by subtotal excision, or at least biopsied. Surgical decompression is invaluable even where the tumour cannot be removed, and this is generally achieved by laminectomy often encompassing several segments. Occasionally, spinal neoplasms may extend over a considerable length of the cord. Such tumours are usually low-grade gliomas and even these can sometimes be totally excised. Many benign or extramedullary and intradural tumours of borderline malignancy can be totally removed without need for further treatment. This group includes meningiomas, low-grade gliomas, neurofibromas and tumours of the coverings of the cord (angiomas, fibromas and lipomas).

For more malignant tumours and in patients with secondary deposits involving the spinal cord, surgical decompression followed by postoperative radiotherapy is usually the treatment of choice. If rapid transfer to a neurosurgical centre is difficult or if the patient is unfit or unsuitable for surgery (perhaps because of widespread malignant disease), intensive radiotherapy can often provide excellent palliation, particularly if the cord lesion is a secondary deposit of a radiosensitive tumour such as small cell carcinoma of the bronchus or lymphoma. In malignant primary cord tumours such as high-grade gliomas, total surgical removal is usually impossible and postoperative radiotherapy mandatory. A high radiation dose will be required since these tumours are not usually very radiosensitive, and most radiotherapists would treat the spinal cord to its tolerance dose (see later). Very careful judgement of anatomical details, field length, fractionation and total dose are always required.

High doses of dexamethasone are invaluable in reducing cord oedema making intensive radiotherapy safer. The role of chemotherapy is not established and has no routine place in the management of spinal cord tumours. The detailed management of cord compression was further dealt with in Chapter 8.

TUMOURS OF THE PERIPHERAL NERVES

These are rare tumours, more often benign than malignant. Multiple neurofibromatosis (von Recklinghausen's disease), the commonest peripheral nerve tumour, is most frequently encountered. In 5–10% of cases, sarcomatous change takes places (neurofibrosarcoma). Tumours of the nerve sheath (Schwannomas) can occur in both cranial and peripheral nerves, particularly the acoustic nerve, spinal nerve roots, peripheral nerves and occasionally the V, IX, or X cranial nerves. These may occasionally undergo malignant change. *Neuroepithelioma* is an exceedingly rare malignant tumour of peripheral nerve, sometimes occurring in conjunction with von Recklinghausen's disease. The histological appearance suggests a neural crest origin, and metastases are frequent.

Treatment of peripheral nerve tumours is by surgical excision where the tumour is producing troublesome pressure symptoms or where there is any suspicion of malignant change. Routine surgical excision of neurofibromas in patients with von Recklinghausen's disease should be discouraged unless there is a sudden increase in size of one of the peripheral lesions. Management of sarcomatous tumours is dealt with in Chapter 23.

RADIATION DAMAGE IN THE BRAIN AND SPINAL CORD

With radical radiotherapy, particularly of midline tumours, the treatment volume may include the spinal cord. For example, in lung cancer a portion of the cord is usually irradiated. The radiation tolerance of the brain and spinal cord is of great clinical importance since it frequently sets the dose limit. Both acute and late damage

may occur, the latter being of much greater importance. In the brain, the early effects include headache, nausea, vomiting and lassitude from raised intracranial pressure, both as a result of the tumour itself and also from acute cerebral oedema produced by the radiotherapy. Drowsiness and irritability have been described as side-effects of whole brain irradiation in children (somnolence syndrome) but is transient and self-limiting. An early syndrome of demyelination may develop but is extremely rare. Late changes include haemorrhage, gliosis, demyelination and necrosis of the brain. These complications are especially likely to occur in the cerebral hemispheres and when retreatment has been undertaken. The usual clinical features are those of progressive focal or generalized neurological damage, occurring months or even years after radiation. Damage to the optic chiasm is well recognized in patients treated for pituitary tumours and is clearly dose related with minimal risk when daily fraction size is kept between 1.8–2.0 Gy. Radiation tolerance of the brainstem is generally thought to be rather lower than that of the cerebral hemispheres.

Early radiation damage to the spinal cord is frequently encountered and is usually transient. The commonest feature is Lhermitte's syndrome, characterized by 'electric shock' sensations in the extremities (usually the feet), and is particularly marked on flexion of the neck. It usually occurs a few weeks after the treatment, but may develop several months afterwards. It is usually self limiting and without long-term effect.

In late radiation damage to the cord, myelopathy can cause progressive motor and sensory changes at the irradiated site, leading to paraparesis, anaesthesia and in severe cases, a paraplegia with physiological transection of the cord. If less than the total width of the cord has been irradiated, a Brown–Séquard syndrome may result. These changes are due to direct damage to neurological tissue with loss of anterior horn cells, other neurones and oligodendroglia as well as direct vascular damage leading to infarction of the cord. Progressive and chronic radiation myelopathy is usually irreversible and leads to spastic paraplegia with sphincter disturbance. This is fatal in over 50% of cases, particularly where the lesion is in the cervical or upper dorsal cord.

Radiation tolerance of the cord is inversely related to the length of cord irradiated. It is generally accepted that for a 10 cm length of cord, a dose of 40 Gy (4000 rad) in daily fractions over 4 weeks is safe, though this dose may have to be exceeded in patients with relatively insensitive lesions which cannot be completely excised, for example a chordoma. Fraction size is clearly important since treatment to 50 Gy (5000 rads) in daily fractions over 5 weeks is usually safe, whereas many cases of cord damage have been documented following treatment to a dose of 40 Gy (4000 rad) in daily fractions over 3 weeks (15).

REFERENCES

1 Leibel S. A., Sheline G. E., Wara W. M., Baldrey E. B. & Nielsen S. L. (1975) The role of radiation therapy in the treatment of astrocytomas. *Cancer* **35** 1551–7.
2 Bouchard J. & Peirce C. B. (1960) Radiation therapy in the management of neoplasms of the central nervous system, with a special note with regard to children: 20 years experience 1939–1958.
3 Sheline G. E. (1986) Radiotherapy of brain tumours: The Edelstein memorial lecture. *Clinical Radiology* (in press).
4 Taveras J. M., Thompson H. G. & Pool J. L. (1962) Should we treat glioblastome multiforme. *American Journal of Roentgenology* **87**, 473.
5 Salazar O. M., Rubin P., McDonald J. V. & Feldstein M. L. (1976) High dose radiation therapy in the treatment of glioblastoma multiforme: a preliminary report. *International Journal of Radiation Oncology Biology Physics* **1**, 717–27.
6 Urtasun R., Band P., Chapman J. D., Feldstein M. L., Mielke B. & Fryer C. (1976) Radiation and high dose metronidazole in supratentorial glioblastomas. *New England Journal of Medicine* **294**, 1364–7.
7 Bleehan N. M., Wiltshire, C. R., Plowman P. N., Watson J. V., Gleave J. R. W., Holmes A. E., Lewin W. S., Treip C. S. & Hawkins T. D. (1981) A randomized study of misonidazole and radiotherapy for grade III and IV cerebral astrocytoma. *British Journal of Cancer* **43**, 436–42.
8 Walker M. D., Green S. B., Byar D. P. et al (1980) Randomized comparisons of radiotherapy and nitrosoureas for the treatment of malignant glioma after surgery. *New England Journal of Medicine* **303**, 1323.
9 Phillips T. L., Sheline G. E. & Boldrey E. (1964) Therapeutic considerations in tumours affecting the central nervous system: ependyomomas. *Radiology* **83**, 98–105.
10 Sheline G. E., Boldrey E. B., Karlsberg P. & Phillips T. L. (1964) Therapeutic considerations in tumours affecting the central nervous system: oligodendrogliomas. *Radiology* **82**, 84.
11 Panitch H. S. & Berg B. O. (1970). Brain stem tumours of childhood and adolescence. *American Journal of Diseases of Children* **119**, 465–72.
12 Bloom H. J. G., Wallace E. N. K. & Henk J. M. (1969) The treatment and prognosis of medulloblastoma in children: a study of 82 verified cases. *American Journal of Roengenology* **105**, 43–62.
13 Broadbent V. A., Barnes N. D. & Wheeler T. K. (1981) Medulloblastoma in childhood: long-term results of treatment. *Cancer* **48**, 26–30.
14 Borgelt B., Gelber R., Kramer S., Brady L. W., Chang C. H., Davis L. W., Perez C. A. of Hendrickson F. R. (1980) The palliation of brain metastases: final results of the first two studies by the Radiation Therapy Oncology Group. *International Journal of Radiation Oncology Biology Physics* **6**, 1–9.
15 Wara W. M., Phillips T. L., Sheline G. E. & Schwade J. G. (1975) Radiation tolerance of the spinal cord. *Cancer* **35**, 1558–62.

Chapter 12

Tumours of the Lung and Mediastinum

CARCINOMA OF THE BRONCHUS

Introduction and aetiology

Carcinoma of the bronchus is by far the commonest cancer in the Western world, having increased steadily in incidence since the 1930s. It had an overall incidence in Britain of 112 per 100 000 males and 27 per 100 000 females in 1978. The incidence is strongly related to age (Fig. 12.1). As a result of the increasing prevalence of cigarette smoking since the First World War, carcinoma of the bronchus has become the leading cause of cancer death in males over

the past 50 years. In recent years, more women have become cigarette smokers with the result that lung cancer has become increasingly common in women, and continues to rise (1). In 1952, the male:female ratio for lung cancer incidence was 13:1; in 1984 the figure stood at 4:1. Although several aetiological factors have been implicated, including exposure to radioactivity and possible environmental hazards, these pale into insignificance beside the highly carcinogenic effect of prolonged exposure to cigarette smoke. Recent studies have shown that even a smoky atmosphere may be dangerous, and that non-smokers married to life-long smokers are at double the expected risk for developing lung cancer.

A great deal of political debate has followed the demonstration of an incontravertible link between cigarette smoking and lung cancer, in which health education, cost of treatment, possible loss of tax revenue, reduction in productivity resulting from ill-health and freedom of choice have been the principal points for discussion. At an international level, there has been a wide variety of approaches towards the restriction of smoking, stemming from the differing philosophies of different countries. In many Scandinavian countries, for example, it is now almost socially unacceptable to smoke in public places and cigarettes have become extremely expensive with the result that smoking related illnesses are beginning to decline. In Britain cigarettes are now relatively cheaper than they were 25 years ago, and restriction of smoking in public areas has been a protracted and uphill battle. There is now a clear inverse rela-

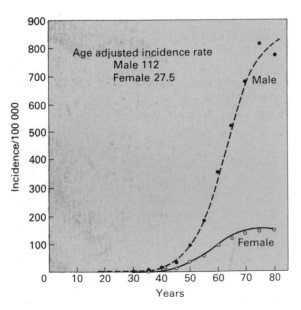

Fig. 12.1. *Cancer of the lung.* Age-specific incidence rates for men and women.

tionship both in Britain and the United States between socioeconomic status and incidence of lung cancer. The death-rate from this disease is disproportionately high in comparison to incidence because of the low cure rates currently achieved (less than 10% at 5 years overall). At present the British Health Education Council has an annual budget of about half a million pounds per annum to spend on its anti-smoking campaign, compared with an estimated seventy

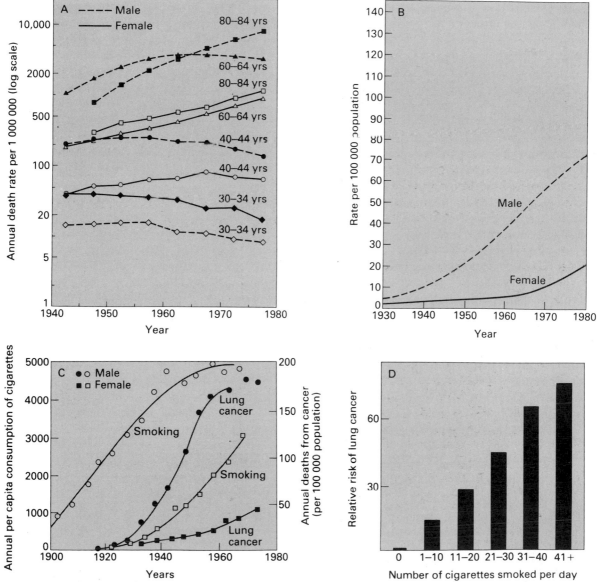

Fig. 12.2. *Smoking and Lung cancer.* (A) Trends in lung cancer mortality for men and women of different ages (England and Wales). (Modified from Doll R. *Harveian Oration* (1982). Royal College of Physicians. With Permission.) (B) Age-adjusted lung cancer mortality rates (United States). (C) Smoking prevalence and lung cancer mortality in men and women (England and Wales). (From Cairns J. Smoking Prevalance and Lung Cancer. Copyright © (1975) by Scientific American, Inc. All rights reserved.) (D) Relative risk of lung cancer according to daily cigarette consumption.

million pounds spent on advertising by the tobacco industry. So far, attempts at screening even in high-risk groups, have met with very little success. In the Third World, cigarette consumption is rapidly rising and high-tar brands which are no longer popular in this country are widely advertised. Despite overwhelming evidence of the dangers of cigarette smoking, major tobacco companies are urging Third World farmers to change from production of staple arable crops to growing tobacco.

Fortunately, the carcinogenic effects of cigarette smoke are to some extent reversible. In their classic study of the smoking habits of British doctors, Doll and Hill (2) were able to demonstrate a gradual reduction in mortality of British doctors who gave up smoking in the 1960s and 1970s. After 12 years of total abstinence from cigarette smoking, the risk of developing lung cancer is almost as low as in non-smokers, except for heavy smokers (more than 20/day), in whom the risk never falls to that of the non-smoker. In the lower age groups (30–45 years), there is at least some evidence for a slight fall in death rate over the past 15 years (Fig. 12.2). Since there has been little decrease in the number of cigarettes smoked in Britain, this reduction may possibly be due to the wider use of low-tar brands. Nonetheless, insufficient time has elapsed since the intro-

duction of these brands for us to be confident that the risk is indeed lower.

Other aetiological factors, thought or known to have a role, include asbestos exposure, industrial pollution, ionizing radiation, occupational hazards and others (see Chapter 2 and Table 12.1). Of these, asbestos exposure is probably the most critical, both for lung cancer and also mesothelioma (see p. 222). This is particularly important when combined with cigarette smoking: in smokers with occupational exposure to asbestos, the risk of lung cancer is 45 times above that of the normal population.

Pathology of lung cancer

HISTOLOGICAL TYPES

Lung cancer is only rarely a tumour of the true lung parenchyma, arising far more frequently in large and medium-sized bronchi. There are many histological types of lung cancer. It is however, convenient to consider the commonest varieties in four major groups although there is substantial histological variation within each of these (Table 12.2). There has been considerable debate as to whether the cell of origin is different in the different histological types. There is however a great deal of circumstantial evidence to suggest that the cancers arise from

Table 12.1. Aetiological factors in lung cancer.

Cigarette smoking	Air pollution	Occupational
Particulate phase	Coal and tar fumes	Asbestos
Benzyprene	Nickel	Radioactivity (uranium mines, radon)
Benzofluoranthenes	Zinc	Metal workers (nickel, chromium, iron oxide)
Dibenzanthracene	Benzpyrene	Arsenicals (sheep-dip workers)
Nicotine		
Catechol		
Nickel and Cadmium		
Vapour phase		
Nitrogen oxides		
Formaldehyde		
Hydrazine		
Urethan		

Table 12.2. Histological classification of lung cancer*

Squamous carcinoma

Small cell carcinoma

Adenocarcinoma
 Bronchogenic; acinar
 Bronchioloalveolar

Large cell carcinoma
 With or without mucin, giant cell
  and clear cell variants

Mixed squamous and adenocarcinoma

Other tumours
 Carcinoid, cylindroma,
  sarcoma and mixed histological types

---

* Adapted from WHO classification.

a common precursor cell which has the capacity to differentiate into a variety of histological types.

Squamous cell carcinoma This is the commonest histological type and is characterized by the presence of keratinization and/or intercellular bridging, and is often subdivided on the basis of differentiation. Most of these tumours arise proximally in large bronchi (though they may also arise peripherally), and tend to be polypoid or infiltrating, often with distinct borders. Since the bronchi at this level are not normally lined by squamous epithelium, it is likely that neoplastic change at this site is preceded by squamous metaplasia, though studies of carcinoma *in-situ* have suggested that this may not always occur.

Small cell (oat cell) carcinoma is characterized by a diffuse growth of small cells with fine granular nuclei, inconspicuous nucleoli, and scanty cytoplasm. The cells tend to be tightly packed or moulded, with little evidence of supportive tissue. Occasionally, combinations of small cell and squamous cell carcinomas are seen, though many pathologists think that such tumours should be classified as poorly differentiated squamous cell carcinoma. Neurosecretory gran-

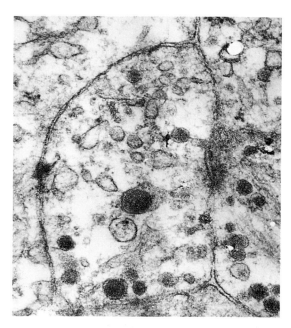

Fig. 12.3. *Electron microscopy appearances in small cell carcinoma.* Dense neurosecretory granules are shown in cell processes. (× 52250)

ules are typically seen on electron microscopy (Fig. 12.3). These may be the site of origin of the variety of hormones such as ACTH, ADH and calcitonin which are sometimes produced and give rise to ectopic hormone syndromes which may be clinically significant (see Chapter 9). It is possible that small cell carcinomas are derived from APUD (amine precursor uptake and decarboxylase) cells which contain neurosecretory granules. Tumours of APUD cells at other sites give rise to multiple endocrine syndromes (see Chapter 15 p. 272). Small cell carcinomas also arise typically from proximal large bronchi and are characterized by extensive local invasion associated with early blood-borne and lymphatic metastases, making them almost invariably unsuitable for surgery. Indeed, a significant proportion of these tumours are diagnosed by biopsy of palpable supraclavicular or cervical lymph nodes.

Adenocarcinomas show the typical features of neoplastic cells derived from glandular epithelium, with formation of acini, papillae and mucus. Many adenocarcinomas are peripheral in site of origin, frequently invading the pleura. These cancers sometimes arise in scar tissue, and may occur in fibrotic lung disease. Adenocarcinoma is less clearly related to cigarette smoking than either squamous or small cell carcinoma, and was the predominant cell type before the advent of cigarette smoking. Unlike other forms of lung cancer it is slightly commoner in females. There is some evidence that it is increasing in frequency. The very unusual bronchiolo-alveolar carcinoma sometimes presents as a multicentric tumour with alveoli lined by neoplastic columnar cells.

Large cell carcinoma refers to undifferentiated tumours with a variety of appearances. The cells are large, often with featureless cytoplasm and show little tendency towards keratinization or acinar formation. In a proportion of these tumours, there is evidence of mucus production, and there may also be other ultrastructural characteristics which are reminiscent of adenocarcinoma. The tumour borders are generally well-defined, and the tumour itself may arise from a sub-segmental or more distal bronchus.

PATHOLOGICAL DIAGNOSIS

In over 80% of patients with lung cancer, malignant cells are found in the sputum, using standard exfoliative cytology techniques. The likelihood of a positive sputum diagnosis increases from 58% with a single specimen, to 78% when four specimens are obtained. This proportion is also increased when specimens are obtained at bronchoscopy either from trap, brush or lavage specimens. The four major categories can be distinguished with an accuracy of 80% by either cytological or histological methods. Occasionally a mixture of cell types is seen, for example mixed small and large cell carcinoma or adeno-squamous tumours. About one-quarter of autopsy cases show mixed histologies, although this high proportion may be related to a treatment-induced change in the histology (3). Cases with mixed histology are one line of evidence suggesting that these carcinomas do not arise from different cells, but that the cancer-inducing event results in cells which can differentiate along more than one pathway.

The clinical distinction between primary adenocarcinoma of the bronchus and secondary pulmonary deposits from primary adenocarcinomas at other sites may be a difficult one, especially if no endobronchial lesion is seen at bronchoscopy. Similarly the clear-cell carcinoma variant of large cell carcinoma can be mistaken for metastatic hypernephroma. One important clinical feature of squamous cell carcinomas is that they frequently cause cavitation and may therefore be confused with a lung abscess.

Patterns of local invasion and metastasis

Carcinoma of the bronchus spreads by local invasion and by lymphatic and haematogenous routes (Fig. 12.4). Locally, the tumour may spread into the mediastinum or through the bronchial wall, lung parenchyma and to the pleural space and chest wall. There may be erosion of overlying ribs. Apical tumours typically spread from the apex of the lung to involve the brachial plexus with erosion of upper thoracic ribs and local nerves such as the thoraco-cervical sympathetic chain (Pancoast's tumour). At the hilum of the lung the tumour may damage the phrenic or left recurrent laryngeal nerve. It may also erode posteriorly into the oesophagus or vertebrae.

Lymphatic spread within the chest is chiefly to hilar and mediastinal, sub-carinal, tracheobronchial and paratracheal nodes. Beyond the chest, involvement of supraclavicular, cervical and axillary nodes may occur. Lymphatic involvement below the diaphragm is frequent in small cell carcinoma, especially to upper para-aortic nodes.

Blood-borne spread is especially frequent in small cell carcinoma and typically occurs earlier than with other lung cancers. The skeleton is

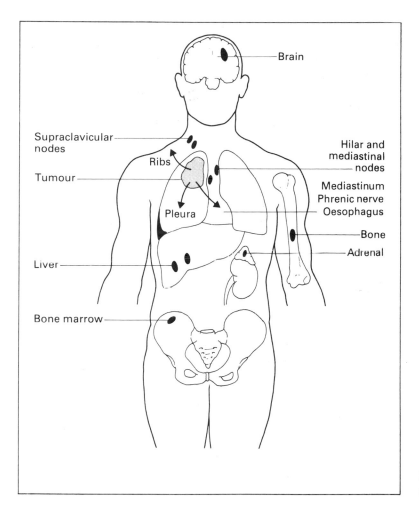

Labels in figure: Brain, Supraclavicular nodes, Ribs, Tumour, Pleura, Liver, Bone marrow, Hilar and mediastinal nodes, Mediastinum, Phrenic nerve, Oesophagus, Bone, Adrenal

Fig. 12.4. *Local and metastatic spread in lung cancer.*

frequently involved, particularly vertebrae, ribs and pelvis and widespread infiltration into bone marrow occurs, especially in small cell carcinoma where estimates of frequency vary from 5–30%, depending on the number of marrow aspirations and the extent of the tumour. Other common sites include the brain (65% of autopsies in small cell carcinoma), liver and adrenals, but secondary deposits can be found in any organ. Early and rapid dissemination is particularly characteristic of small cell carcinoma, which also has the most rapid volume doubling time of any of these tumours.

CLINICAL FEATURES

Most patients with lung cancer present with symptoms directly related to the tumour such as haemophysis, cough, dyspnoea or chest pain. Since many of these patients are smokers, some of these symptoms (particularly a cough) will already be familiar to them as a result of chronic bronchitis and emphysema. This may well delay them from seeking advice, though a substantial number are sufficiently aware of the increased intensity of their symptoms to give up smoking; often after a life-time of being unable to do so. The cough is often persistent, nocturnal and may be productive. Sputum may be blood-streaked or persistently discoloured as a result of infection which cannot clear due to atelectasis beyond an obstructing endobronchial tumour. Haemoptyses, though intermittent, usually become increasingly severe. Pain, usually aching, is present in over 50% of patients. It seems to be commoner in patients with mediastinal involvement or at electasis, and is much commoner than the typical 'sharper' pain of bone metastases.

More peripheral tumours often present rather late, when already of significant size. They may well cause pain in the chest wall by direct extension to the pleura or periosteum of the ribs, often trapping or invading intercostal nerves. Direct tumour invasion of the left recurrent laryngeal nerve may result in hoarseness of the voice, which is a frequent presenting symptom. Pleural effusion, phrenic nerve palsy, and lobar or total lung collapse may all contribute to increasing dyspnoea. Pneumonias that fail to clear should be regarded as suspicious. Dysphagia may result from enlarged mediastinal lymph nodes which compress the oesophagus, usually at its mid or lower third, or by direct invasion. Wheeze and stridor are important signs of obstruction of large airways, generally due to proximal tumours.

Tumours at specific sites may produce typical syndromes. Pancoast's tumour, situated at the apex of the lung, causes severe pain in the shoulder, chest wall and arm as a result of relentless local invasion which destroys ribs and infiltrates the brachial plexus. Weakness of the small muscles of the hand may occur, with parasthesiae on the inner aspect of the arm, due to C8/T1 motor loss. Tumours of the right main or right upper lobe bronchus (often with associated right paratracheal node enlargement) may compress the great veins leading to superior vena cava (SVC) obstruction. Producing a typical clinical syndrome comprising swelling of the face, neck, and upper arms, plethora or cyanosis and rapid development of a visible collateral circulation over the scapula and upper chest wall. In severe cases, conjunctival oedema and chemosis are also seen. The majority of cases of SVC obstruction are caused by small cell carcinomas and prompt treatment may produce a gratifying resolution of these symptoms (see Chapter 8).

Some patients notice a 'mass' in the neck due to lymph node enlargement. In other patients the presenting symptoms are caused by secondary deposits, especially in small cell cancer. Pain in the back may be due to vertebral collapse, and is particularly important since cord compression with paraplegia may develop with great rapidity unless the diagnosis is made and treatment started promptly. Other typical metastatic presentations include neurological symptoms and signs (focal lesions, raised intracranial pressure, cerebellar syndromes) and weight loss and nausea from hepatic involvement.

Constitutional symptoms are also common and most patients with lung cancer complain of anorexia, weight loss, weakness and fatigue. Although many patients do not notice clubbing of the fingers, this is a common manifestation particularly associated with squamous cell carcinoma and rare in small cell carcinoma. Pain in the limbs may result from hypertrophic pulmonary osteoarthropathy which can be severe.

A wide variety of paraneoplastic non-metastatic syndromes have been described in association with lung cancer. These are discussed in Chapter 9. Many of these syndromes are uncommon. Hypercalcaemia (without obvious bone metastases) is most frequently found in squamous cell cancer, and the syndromes of inappropriate antidiuretic hormone secretion (SIADH) and ectopic ACTH production are both commoner in small cell carcinoma. The symptoms and management of hypercalcaemia are discussed in Chapter 8 and of ectopic hormone production in Chapter 9.

TNM staging notation

Although complex, the TNM staging system is becoming increasingly used in non-small cell lung cancer. A staging system based on TNM definitions has been proposed (Table 12.3) and has been shown to be useful prognostically,

Table 12.3. TNM staging system for non-small cell lung cancer.

T-Primary tumour

TO	Primary tumour not demonstrable.
TX	Positive cytology but tumour not demonstrable.
Tis	Carcinoma *in-situ*
T1	Tumour less than 3 cm diameter, no proximal invasion.
T2	More than 3 cm, or invading pleura or with atelectasis, more than 2 cm from carina.
T3	Tumour any size with invasion of chest wall; or less than 2 cm from carina; or causing lung collapse or effusion.

N-Regional lymph nodes

NO	Nodes negative
N1	Ipsilateral hilar nodes
N2	Mediastinal nodes

M-Distant metastases

MO	No metastases
M1	Metastases present

Stage grouping

Stage 1	T1	NO	MO
	T1	N1	MO
	T2	NO	MO
Stage 2	T2	N1	MO
Stage 3	Any T3		
	Any N2		
	Any M1		

except in the case of small cell carcinomas, in which the prognosis is so poor that staging systems have little prognostic relevance.

Investigation and staging

Staging of *non-small cell lung cancer* is important since a crucial distinction between operable and inoperable tumours has to be made. To the surgeon, the most important criteria are the site of tumour, absence of metastases and the general fitness of the patient. Before any consideration of surgery, the maximum amount of information must therefore be obtained. Chest X-ray may indicate that the tumour is inoperable. Findings indicating inoperability include large central primary tumours particularly extending across the midline; widening of the su-

perior mediastinum due to enlargement of paratracheal nodes; intrapulmonary, rib or other bony metastases; pleural effusion; bilateral tumours. Further assessment is often needed; bronchoscopic evaluation is usually required to make the diagnosis and is essential to assess operability.

Most patients with suspected lung cancer are first seen by a chest physician and the diagnosis made by fibreoptic bronchoscopy. This instrument has the advantage of permitting good access to lobar and segmental bronchi and is especially helpful in evaluating upper lobe tumours out of biopsy range of the rigid bronchoscope. The rigid instrument is, however, sometimes preferable since it may give a better view of proximal bronchi and allows a larger biopsy in doubtful cases.

At bronchoscopy some tumours can be shown to be inoperable. Features indicating inoperability are: endobronchial tumour within 2 cm of the main carina, extrinsic compression and widening of the angle of the main carina indicating mediastinal spread and paralysis of the left vocal cord resulting from recurrent laryngeal nerve palsy.

With very few exceptions mediastinal involvement is a definite contraindication to surgery. Assessment of the mediastinum is therefore essential in any patient being considered for operation. Clinical evidence of involvement includes a hoarse voice with a typical 'bovine' cough, resulting from recurrent laryngeal palsy, Horner's syndrome from involvement of the cervical sympathetic chain, pain in the shoulder, SVC obstruction, cardiac dysrhythmia and dysphagia. Further assessment can be made by tomographic views of the mediastinum, and by barium swallow which may show enlarged mediastinal nodes causing extrinsic oesophageal compression. CT scanning is a useful aid in the pre-operative assessment of tumour extent, sometimes demonstrating unexpected lymph node involvement or direct invasion of other structures (Fig. 12.5). Chest wall involvement, for example, usually indicates inoperability. It is, however, important not to

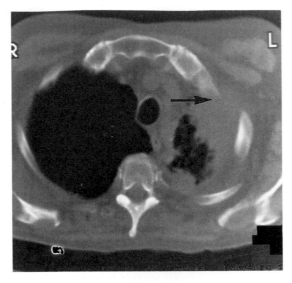

Fig. 12.5. *CT scan of thorax, at level of manubrium, in a patient with squamous carcinoma of the lung.* The tumour is shown extending through the pleural space into the chest wall, eroding the ribs (arrowed).

no neurological symptoms or signs, isotope liver or brain scan will seldom be positive and are therefore not routinely indicated. A bone scan may however show unsuspected metastases.

Finally, the surgeon needs to know whether his patient is likely to withstand a surgical operation. Routine exercise testing, spirometry and other lung function tests such as ventilation/perfusion scanning can all be valuable. Patients with poor pulmonary reserve may have to be excluded from surgery even though their tumours are operable by other criteria. As a rough guide, patients with FEV_1 (forced expiratory volume/second), less than 1.2 litre do not withstand pneumonectomy but this also depends on age, sex, size and especially height. Patients over 70 years of age also tolerate pneumonectomy poorly (particularly right-sided).

For patients with *small cell lung cancer*, the rationale for staging is altogether different. The

rule out surgery on the basis of an equivocal CT scan since not all lymph node enlargement will prove to be neoplastic at thoracotomy.

The mediastinum can be directly visualized by mediastinoscopy (Fig. 12.6). In this procedure the surgeon makes a small incision in the suprasternal notch and the mediastinum is inspected through a mediastinoscope. Biopsies of the nodes are taken where possible. For left-sided tumours an additional mediastinotomy may be necessary, and it is generally performed through the bed of the second intercostal cartilage. In patients whose mediastinoscopy is negative the resectability rate is at least 85% and in over 50% of cases the nodes will not be involved at thoracotomy. In a further 30% the stage will be N_1 only (Table 12.3). Clearly, if the diagnosis has been made from supraclavicular node biopsy or biopsy of metastatic lesions, these patients are unsuitable for surgery. Other evidence of obvious distant spread, such as abnormal liver function tests combined with an abnormal liver scan or hepatic ultrasound, are also obvious contraindications to operation. If the liver function tests are normal and there are

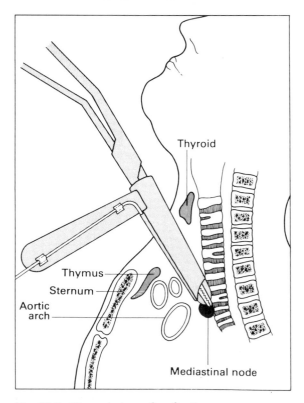

Fig. 12.6. *The technique of mediastinoscopy.*

characteristic early and widespread dissemination of this tumour makes surgical intervention inappropriate in the large majority of cases, though the occasional instance of 'surgically resectable' small cell lung cancer is encountered (less than 3% in our experience of over 800 unselected cases).

In some instances, determination of the degree of spread in small cell lung cancer is both logical and necessary. For example, although radiotherapy alone is no longer considered to be the best treatment for this disease (see later), it is sometimes used, for example in elderly or unfit patients, or those otherwise considered unsuitable for chemotherapy. Alternatively in patients undergoing treatment with chemotherapy, radiotherapy is sometimes reserved for those with 'limited' disease in whom no metastases can be demonstrated and disease is confined to one hemithorax. If the proposed treatment is only with cytotoxic drugs, irrespective of extent of disease, then routine staging is unnecessary although investigation of specific symptoms is sometimes indicated on clinical grounds.

If staging in small cell lung cancer is to be undertaken, the most useful investigations include liver function tests (including measurement of serum albumin), plasma electrolytes and calcium determination, full blood count, bone marrow aspiration (bearing in mind that aspiration from two sites doubles the yield), isotope bone scanning and liver scanning in patients with abnormal liver function tests. CT scanning of the brain in asymptomatic patients is seldom abnormal and not performed as a routine.

Treatment

The principles of treatment of non-small cell and small cell lung cancer are very different. Small cell lung cancer is seldom surgically resectable, usually widespread at presentation and is both more chemosensitive and radiosensitive. For these reasons their management is considered separately.

SURGERY FOR NON-SMALL CELL LUNG CANCER

For non-small cell cancer, surgical resection offers the best hope of cure. The percentage of operable cases varies with the philosophy of the surgeon, but the criteria for operability are not usually met in more than about 30% of cases. Approximately 50% of tumours are obviously unresectable by chest X-ray or bronchoscopic criteria. Physiological evaluation, biochemical testing and mediastinoscopy raises the unresectability rate still further (see previously).

For patients in whom surgery is possible, the choice of operation depends on the location of the tumour and the patient's respiratory capacity. If the tumour is peripheral with no evidence of local extension, a wedge or segmental resection may occasionally be sufficient, particularly in patients whose pulmonary reserve is poor. In patients with more centrally located tumours contained within a single lobe, lobectomy is the usual procedure, provided the hilar nodes are clear. An adequate margin of normal looking lung should be removed where possible. Pneumonectomy is necessary for tumours originating within the main stem bronchus, where the primary tumour involves more than one lobe, or where the hilum is involved. Clearly, these patients should undergo particularly careful measurement of respiratory function before such an operation can be contemplated.

Although patients with evidence of local spread are usually considered to have inoperable lesions, many surgeons are prepared to undertake an operation in Pancoast's tumour since cancers at this site (superior sulcus) may be biologically more favourable. Despite local invasion of pleura and ribs, they can sometimes be removed surgically, and regional lymphatic metastases appear to be unusual.

The mortality (5%) and morbidity associated with pneumonectomy are of course greater than with a lesser operation such as a lobectomy (2% mortality); many surgeons do not operate in patients over the age of 70 years, since mortality rises steeply with advancing age.

Results of surgical treatment. The results of surgical treatment depend largely on the degree of patient selection; surgeons using the most stringent criteria for operability will have the best results. A large retrospective survey by Mountain of over 800 patients undergoing thoracotomy (4) showed that histological type and stage of the tumour were important prognostic criteria. Patients with squamous cell carcinoma had the best survival, 37% of all patients surviving 5 years (Fig. 12.7). Patients with adenocarcinoma or large cell carcinoma did less well, and the 5-year survival was 27%. The importance of tumour stage is shown in Figure 12.8. For patients with Stage 1 disease, the 5-year survival rate was over 50% for all histologies (but approaching 80% for T_1 squamous carcinomas), suggesting that in non-small cell lung cancer tumour stage is more important than histology in determining survival. One additional finding was that in patients with squamous cell carcinoma, the presence of local nodal involvement did not necessarily imply early death from blood-borne metastases. In

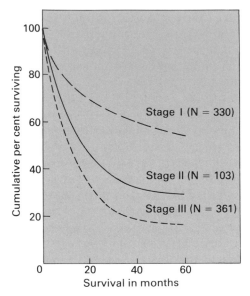

Fig. 12.8. *Tumour stage and survival after curative resection for lung cancer.* (Modified from Mountain C.F. (1977) *Annals of Thoracic Surgery* **24**, 365–73. With permission.)

these patients, radical surgery, in the absence of other effective curative measures, seemed the most fruitful approach if the mediastinal node involvement was limited. This is why some surgeons feel that early mediastinal nodal involvement should not be regarded as an absolute contraindication to surgery, although in general, the presence of mediastinal involvement is an unquestionably adverse feature. In this series, the effectiveness of surgery for local control was further emphasized by the finding that approximately three-quarters of patients who developed recurrent disease first recurred outside the initial site of the tumour (usually brain, bone or contralateral lung). Nonetheless, despite modern operative techniques and more careful case selection, the data shown in Figures 12.8 and 12.9 are only slightly better than those obtained in the 1950s (5).

RADIOTHERAPY IN NON-SMALL CELL LUNG CANCER

Although patients with non-small cell lung cancer have always formed a large part of the

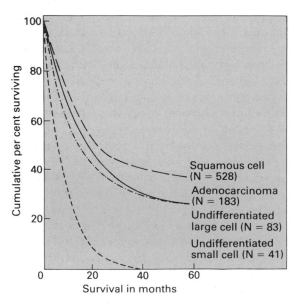

Fig. 12.7. *Prognosis in relation to histology after curative resection for lung cancer.* (Modified from Mountain C.F. (1977) *Annals of Thoracic Surgery* **24**, 365–73. With permission.)

radiotherapist's work there is continued debate regarding the indications for its use. In judging which patients are suitable for treatment, the radiotherapist has to decide whether his intention is radical or palliative. In the majority of cases, palliation is the only realistic expectation though long-term survival is occasionally seen in patients irradiated only with palliative intent.

Palliative radiotherapy. The majority of patients referred to the radiotherapist have inoperable disease. For most of these patients, radical radiotherapy with curative intent is inappropriate and the decision facing the radiotherapist is whether and when to treat. Over half of these patients are clearly inoperable on bronchoscopic grounds, though a significant minority will have come to thoracotomy, the tumour having initially been thought to be resectable. Although criteria for treatment are difficult to define, palliative radiotherapy is often recommended for patients with loco-regional disease considered unsuitable for surgery but without evidence of distant metastases. Such patients include those with tumours of the main stem bronchus within 1 cm of the carina, those with invasion of important mediastinal structures such as the recurrent laryngeal or phrenic nerves, and those with troublesome symptoms including haemoptysis, obstruction of a major bronchus, severe cough and pain. In this latter group, radiotherapy produces clinical benefit in the majority of cases. Finally, in patients in whom obstruction to a bronchus is imminent or where SVC obstruction is present, radiotherapy is indicated whether the patient is symptomatic or not.

Relative contraindications to treatment with radiotherapy include metastases beyond the loco-regional nodes, multiple lesions, bronchial fistula, supraclavicular node involvement, or a large tumour mass. Even under these circumstances, palliative treatment may still offer benefit, if the patient's symptoms demand it. If the patient is symptomatic, treatment should be given as soon as possible.

When should treatment be used in asymptomatic patients with inoperable disease? A study from Oxford has addressed this question (6). In this trial, Durrant and colleagues employed radiotherapy, chemotherapy or a combination of both in the treatment of inoperable lung cancers. In a further group, no treatment at all was recommended. Survival was the same in all groups (approximately $8\frac{1}{2}$ months), and careful measurement of palliation showed no advantage for treatment unless specific symptoms were present. The best palliation of all occurred in patients in whom no initial treatment was given, delaying radiotherapy until the onset of a specific symptom. This not infrequently allowed a patient 4 or 5 months before treatment proved necessary, and this group of patients had the best palliation of all. Many radiotherapists therefore with-hold palliative treatment until such time as symptoms demand it.

Radical radiotherapy. Occasionally, patients with operable lung cancer are referred to a radiotherapist either because of refusal to undergo an operation, or because of coexistent medical conditions which would make surgery hazardous. In these technically operable cases where the tumour is often small and easily encompassed by the radiation fields, radiotherapists often treat the patient radically with the intention of cure if possible. There are however very few data on the dose required or the proportion of long term survivors. In one study in which surgery and radiotherapy were directly compared, the results of surgery for squamous cancer were unequivocally better (7). Even in carefully selected patients the 5-year survival following radiotherapy alone is probably no greater than 10%.

From this rather minimal information, it seems likely that radiotherapy can occasionally cure patients with carcinoma of the bronchus, particularly in patients with small, technically operable tumours. In these patients, a radical approach should be employed if for any reason surgery is refused or considered inappropriate. This involves treatment to a higher dose than is generally employed for palliation of symptoms, in the region of 50–60 Gy (5000–6000 rad) over 5–6 weeks in daily fractions or equivalent (see Chapter 5, Fig. 5.8). Such treatment is frequently accompanied by side-effects which include dysphagia, pericarditis and skin reactions. In addition, irradiation of the spinal cord is unavoidable even with the most sophisticated planning techniques. However, with careful tumour imaging and the use of multifield techniques this problem can almost always be avoided. Radiation damage to the spinal cord is discussed on pp. 68 & 200.

There is no place for routine pre-operative radiotherapy in operable lung cancer. Occasionally a patient with Stage 3 disease, with mediastinal involvement, may show a rapid and striking clinical regression with a relatively low dose of radiotherapy. However, even in such cases, it is exceptional for surgery to become a practical proposition. Combined treatment with surgery and pre-operative radiotherapy is often recommended for Pancoast's tumour (see previously), but overall the results are not dramatically better than those of surgery alone.

CHEMOTHERAPY OF NON-SMALL CELL LUNG CANCER

A variety of single agents has been shown to have some activity in non-small cell lung cancer (Table 12.4). The response rates are low and no survival advantage has been shown for any of these drugs used as a single agent. Attempts have therefore been made to try and improve response rates by using drugs in combination. Typical combinations are shown in Table 12.4. The response rate even to these combinations of drugs is low, moreover the durability of response is also disappointing. Although it is true that patients who achieve a complete response live longer than those who do not, it is also the case that patients who have better performance status and who do not have adverse prognostic features are more likely to achieve a complete response. The prognosis in these patients is therefore likely to be intrinsically better even without chemotherapy.

Table 12.4. Chemotherapy in non-small cell lung cancer.

Agent	% Response
Single agents	
Nitrogen mustard	10–15
Cyclophosphamide	5–10
Ifosphamide	30
Doxorubicin	15
Vincristine	5
Vindesine	17
Cisplatin	12
Bleomycin	5
Etoposide	15–20
Methotrexate	5–15
Combination therapy	
Cisplatin, vindesine	40
Cisplatin, doxorubicin cyclophosphamide	23–35
Methotrexate, doxorubicin CCNU, cyclophosphamide	35–45
Bleomycin, doxorubicin cyclophosphamide, vincristine, CCNU	20

The platinum-based combination chemotherapy introduced by Gralla *et al* (8) appears to be associated with a higher response rate but complete responses are only seen in about 10% of patients. There are as yet very few randomized prospective studies of combination chemotherapy against symptomatic palliative treatment on which judgement of the overall benefit of chemotherapy in non-small cell lung cancer can be based. At present it seems wise to reserve combination chemotherapy only for patients who are anxious for treatment and in whom there are no adverse prognostic factors. It is also preferable to treat these patients in the context of a clinical trial in which evidence of the effectiveness of the chemotherapy can be gathered. If chemotherapy is started in patients with non-small cell lung cancer, it should not be continued if there is no response, or in the face of severe toxicity.

Treatment of small cell lung cancer

The majority (two-thirds) of patients present with extensive disease. That is, thoracic disease involving more than one hemithorax or with metastatic spread. In these patients radiotherapy has a palliative role only and even with modern chemotherapy the prognosis is very poor. In patients with limited disease (confined to one hemithorax) chemotherapy is the mainstay of treatment and the value of additional thoracic irradiation is as yet undecided.

RADIOTHERAPY IN SMALL CELL LUNG CANCER

Small cell lung cancer is much the most radiosensitive histological type, and complete radiological response of the primary tumour is seen in over 80% of cases. Even large primary lesions associated with massive hilar and mediastinal lymphadenopathy may regress completely, following moderate doses of radiotherapy, 40–50 Gy (4–5000 rad) over 4–5 weeks. In one of the earliest comparative cancer trials, the Medical Research Council demonstrated that in 'operable' cases of small cell lung cancer, radiotherapy produced better long-term results than surgery with a mean survival time of 7 months and a small number of long-term survivors (9). Only half of the cases assigned to surgery proved to be technically resectable. In highly selected cases there may still be a place for surgery combined with radiotherapy as the sole treatment for small cell lung cancer, but such cases are very unusual.

Although the initial response to radiotherapy is usually gratifying, recurrence in the irradiated area is frequent and long-term local control of the disease is not always achieved. As might be expected, there is evidence that more durable local control may be obtained by higher radiation dosage although at the cost of greater toxicity, particularly if chemotherapy is also used.

Radiotherapy is of great palliative value in small cell lung cancer, and is the treatment of choice for painful bony metastases, and for brain metastases. Clinical evidence of brain metastases occurs in 25% of patients with small cell lung cancer and is demonstrable in about two-thirds of patients at autopsy. Treatment with radiotherapy to the whole brain to a total dose of 20 Gy (2000 rad) in 5 fractions in a week is often effective and well tolerated; there seems to be no advantage for more prolonged regimens. Similar fractionation is usually satisfactory for painful bony deposits.

Because symptomatic brain metastases are frequent many groups now routinely offer treatment with prophylactic cranial irradiation (PCI) in small cell lung cancer. Routine use of PCI has decreased the clinical frequency of brain metastases from 25% to less than 10%, and the autopsy frequency from 65% to 25% (10), though it does not increase survival. Our policy is to offer PCI only to patients who have had a good response to chemotherapy, thereby avoiding unnecessary cerebral irradiation in non-responding patients whose survival time will be short. Attempts at prolonging survival by prophylactic irradiation at other sites (liver, adrenal and para-aortic nodes) has so far proved unsuccessful.

In view of the radiosensitivity of small cell carcinoma, coupled with the relatively disappointing results with aggressive combination chemotherapy (see later), several groups have investigated the use of 'systemic' irradiation in small cell lung cancer, using either total body or hemi-body radiation. The results so far have not been encouraging, particularly where low doses have been given. Total body irradiation dose is necessarily limited unless marrow grafting is employed, and no large series of marrow-grafted patients has yet been reported. Hemi-body irradiation appears more promising, and in one study, seemed to be as effective as combination chemotherapy in patients with limited disease (11).

CHEMOTHERAPY OF SMALL CELL LUNG CANCER

It has long been apparent that small cell lung cancer is a rapidly dividing tumour, usually metastatic at the time of presentation. For this reason a systemic approach to treatment is essential. Many studies have shown that small cell lung cancer is relatively sensitive to cytotoxic agents and chemotherapy has become the mainstay of treatment. The Medical Research Council carried out a randomized prospective study comparing radiation alone versus radiation and combination chemotherapy (12). This study showed a clear short-term survival advantage for the patients treated with both chemotherapy and radiation compared with radiation alone, although the toxicity was greater in the chemotherapy treated patients. The long term results remained disappointing, with very few patients alive at 3 years.

Many single agents have been shown to have activity. Cyclophosphamide is the single most useful alkylating agent. Many other drugs such as etoposide, methotrexate, nitrosoureas, vinca alkaloids, cisplatin and anthracyclines are effective in treatment of the disease (Table 12.5).

Table 12.5. Single agent chemotherapy in small cell lung cancer.

Agent	% Response
Cyclophosphamide	35
Ifosfamide	35
Vincristine	15
Methotrexate	20
Etoposide	40
Cisplatin	35
CCNU	10
Doxorubicin	30

However, it has become apparent that single agent chemotherapy rarely produces complete radiological resolution of the tumour, and single-agent chemotherapy has largely been discarded except under special circumstances which are discussed below.

The effectiveness of combination chemotherapy in Hodgkin's disease and in acute leukaemia led to this approach being applied in other tumours including small cell lung cancer. In the past 15 years numerous trials of combination chemotherapy have been carried out, using a wide variety of regimens and schedules. In a series of studies from the National Cancer Institute and elsewhere it has been shown that increasing the intensity of chemotherapy increases the response rate and median survival (13). Using combination chemotherapy the median survival in extensive disease is about 9–12 months, and in limited disease 12–18 months.

Combination chemotherapy schedules vary both in the drugs which are used and in the timing of their administration. Typical examples of some schedules and results are shown in Table 12.6. There is some evidence that more intensive chemotherapy produces a higher response rate and better median survival.

Table 12.6. Combination chemotherapy in small cell lung cancer.

Regimens	Response rates (%)	Survival* (weeks)
Cyclophosphamide, methotrexate, CCNU	78	42
Vincristine, doxorubicin, cyclophosphamide	88	40
Cyclophosphamide, methotrexate CCNU, alternating with vincristine, doxorubicin, procarbazine	90	42
Cisplatin, doxorubicin, etoposide	86	60
Doxorubicin, cyclophosphamide, etoposide	87	50

* Includes patients with both limited and extensive disease

There have been several attempts to induce more complete and durable responses by use of so-called 'non cross-resistant' combinations. It is a moot point whether there is such a thing as non-cross-resistance between one schedule and another (see Chapter 6). What is usually meant is the use of a regimen which contains drugs of a different class from those which have been used initially. The consensus of opinion at the present time is that alternating schedules of drugs have not significantly improved median survival; nor has chemotherapy on relapse.

In the last few years an attempt has been

made to increase the response rate and duration in small cell lung cancer by using very high dose chemotherapy. There is some evidence that the dose-response relationship for alkylating agents is steep and that a ten or fifteen fold increase in dosage might be associated with a great increase in tumour destruction (see Chapter 6). Very intensive chemotherapy may require the use of autologous bone marrow transplantation in which marrow is extracted from the patient under a general anaesthetic from multiple puncture sites, and then re-infused after very high dose chemotherapy has been given. High dose chemotherapy has improved remission rates in carefully selected patients but its contribution to management is still speculative and much more work needs to be done before it could be regarded as superior to conventional treatment.

The toxicity of chemotherapy is considerable and the gains in survival are as yet modest. With limited disease it is now possible to achieve survival of 2 or 3 years in 15–20% of patients but it is not yet clear how many of these patients will be cured. Even though there is a chance of long survival and possibly cure with chemotherapy, the morbidity of treatment is sufficient to raise serious doubts about the advisability of chemotherapy in every case. Much more information is needed about the

Table 12.7. Adverse prognostic factors in small cell lung cancer.

Poor performance status
Extensive disease
Low plasma albumin and sodium
Abnormal liver function tests
Brain metastases
Marrow infiltration or anaemia

---

quality of life in patients receiving chemotherapy. There are certain factors which are known to be associated with a poor prognosis in small cell carcinoma, and these are listed in Table 12.7. Of these, the most important are extensive disease, poor performance status, low plasma albumin and sodium, and abnormal

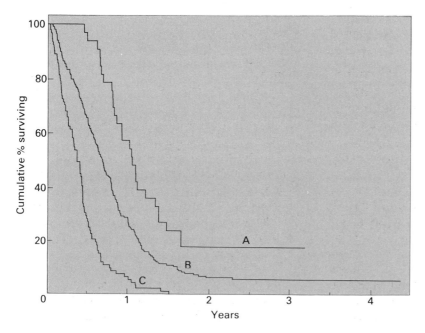

Fig. 12.9. *Prognostic factors in small cell lung cancer.* In A all patients had good performance status and normal biochemistry (see Table 12.7). In C patients had poor performance status and more than two biochemical abnormalities. Group B is by exclusion. (From Souhami R. L. *et al* (1985) *Cancer Research* **45**, 2878. With permission.)

liver function tests (Fig. 12.9). In elderly patients, in whom these poor prognostic factors are often present, it is unwise to persist with chemotherapy beyond the first two or three cycles unless there is a clear improvement in the tumour and in the patients' well-being. For younger patients with limited disease and in whom there are no adverse prognostic features, intensive combination chemotherapy offers the best chance of long-term survival. There will be many patients who fall between these two extremes and here the physician must decide individually what appears to be the best policy.

COMBINATIONS OF CHEMOTHERAPY AND RADIOTHERAPY IN SMALL CELL LUNG CANCER

Combination chemotherapy has now become so widely used that an important question now being asked in several centres is whether radiotherapy has any useful role as an additional local treatment in patients treated with combination chemotherapy (14). Several randomized trials have examined this problem and to date the conclusion has been that whilst local recurrence may be reduced, there appears to be no improvement in median survival in patients treated with chemotherapy and radiotherapy compared with chemotherapy alone (15). It is, however, possible that long term survival is more likely if radiotherapy is part of the treatment. Radiotherapy has been used traditionally in patients presenting with superior vena cava obstruction (see Chapter 8). Even in this situation patients undergoing treatment with combination chemotherapy appear to have the same overall survival as those treated with radiotherapy in addition (16).

In summary, the place of routine thoracic irradiation in small cell lung cancer is still not determined. Its use should be considered under the following circumstances:
1 In patients with limited disease, where there is an incomplete response to chemotherapy but no evidence of distant disease.

2 In patients with limited disease who have completed chemotherapy and are in complete remission. These patients may have a better chance of cure when radiation is employed.
3 In patients with extensive disease who have had a complete response with chemotherapy.
4 For local recurrence.
5 For superior vena caval obstruction unresponsive to chemotherapy.

Immunotherapy of lung cancer

There have been several attempts at 'immunotherapy' in both small cell and non-small cell lung cancer but, as yet, none have shown any benefit. McKneally (17) instilled BCG intrapleurally following resection of localized carcinomas of the bronchus, and reported a prolonged disease-free interval at 2 years, but not after 4 years of follow-up, compared with controls. This result was not confirmed when the trial was repeated, and the toxicity of intrapleural BCG was considerable. BCG vaccination and intravenous *Corynebacterium parvum* have both been used in small cell and non-small cell lung cancer, and conflicting claims for their effectiveness have been made. An objective view of the literature fails to support their use, and both methods of treatment are associated with toxicity. The same is true for both levamisole and interferon. As with most cancers, there is little to justify these methods as part of current treatment.

TUMOURS OF THE MEDIASTINUM

The mediastinum lies at the centre of the chest and is bordered by the thoracic inlet superiorly, the diaphragm inferiorly, the vertebral column posteriorly, the sternum anteriorly and the pleural reflections laterally (Fig. 12.10). A great variety of tumours can arise in the mediastinum and tend to occur at different sites within it.

The *anterosuperior compartment* of the mediastinum is bounded inferiorly by the diaphragm, anteriorly by the sternum and posteriorly by the vertebral column down to the

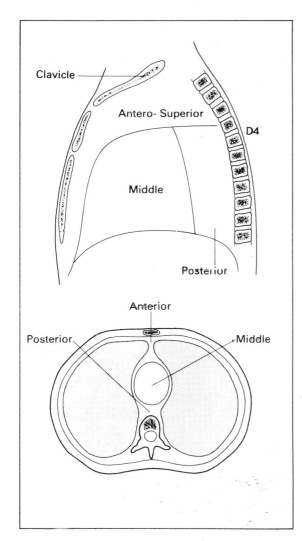

Fig. 12.10. *Anatomy of the mediastinum.*

4th thoracic vertebra, and then by the anterior pericardium. It contains the upper trachea and oesophagus, the aortic arch and the thymus and may also include a retrosternal portion of a normal thyroid gland, with parathyroid structures and embryonic cell rests. The *middle compartment* of the mediastinum is bounded anteriorly by the anterior pericardium and posteriorly by the oesophagus, and extends downwards to the diaphragm. It contains the heart, ascending aorta, main bronchi, hila and carina, and the subcarinal and other closely related tracheobronchial lymph nodes. The *posterior mediastinum* lies between the vertebral column and posterior pericardium and contains the oesophagus, the descending thoracic aorta and the sympathetic nerve chains. The pattern of tumours arising in the mediastinum reflects these anatomical divisions (Table 12.8).

Table 12.8. Tumours of the mediastinum.

Antero-superior
Thymoma
Teratoma
Thyroid and parathyroid tumours
Sarcoma (haemangiosarcoma,
    haemangiopericytoma)
Mesothelioma
Lipomas

Middle
Malignant lymphoma
Tumours of the heart
Secondary lymph node involvement
Pericardial tumours

Posterior
Neurofibroma, neurilemmoma, Schwannoma
Neuroblastoma
Neurofibrosarcoma
Phaeochromocytoma
Chordoma
Paraganglioma

ANTEROSUPERIOR MEDIASTINUM

The commonest malignant tumours are thymomas and germ cell tumours including teratomas of various types and also seminomas. In addition, thyroid and parathyroid adenomas occur at this site and can cause diagnostic difficulties, and carcinomas of the thyroid may occasionally arise from the retrosternal portion of the gland. Symptoms from superior mediastinal tumours are usually caused by pressure on local structures such as the oesophagus, trachea and laryngeal or phrenic nerves. Dysphagia, dyspnoea, stridor, cough and superior vena caval obstruction are relatively common, and vocal cord palsy and/or diaphragmatic paralysis are sometimes seen. These symptoms occur less frequently with slowly growing tumours (such as retrosternal goitre and some thymomas).

Thymoma. Thymic tumours form a mixed histological picture often including more than one population of cells. Lymphocytes, epithelial cells and spindle cells tend to predominate and 'typical' thymomas may contain lymphocytic and epithelial components as apparently distinct populations. Unfortunately, thymic tumour histology is a poor predictor of the behaviour of the tumour, though the macroscopic appearance is more valuable. Some thymic tumours grow very slowly over many years. Others grow more rapidly with local invasion and pleural spread. The criteria for malignancy are difficult to define in thymomas, and most authorities divide the tumours into invasive and non-invasive. Distant metastases are rare. Occasionally, Hodgkin's disease can arise from thymic tissue, without evidence of lymphadenopathy elsewhere. In these cases surgical excision is less important than with other types of thymic tumour.

A variety of clinical syndromes are associated with thymomas. The commonest is *myasthenia gravis* which occurs in 50% of patients. Myasthenia may be the presenting feature of the tumour which is benign or malignant. Myasthenia gravis is associated with antibodies to acetylcholine receptors but its relationship to the tumour is not well understood. Removal of the thymoma results in remission of the myasthenia in approximately 30% of cases. *Red cell aplasia* occurs in 4% and may be associated with leucopenia and/or thrombocytopenia. A spindle cell thymic tumour is the commonest pathology. The red cell aplasia may be due to an antibody to red cell precursors in the bone marrow. Occasionally the aplasia recovers after removal of the tumour. Other syndromes include hypogammaglobulinaemia, connective tissues diseases, pernicious anaemia and autoimmune thyroiditis.

Investigation includes chest X-ray and CT scan of the chest which may show pleural metastases (Fig. 12.11). Treatment is by surgical removal whenever possible. Complete removal is usually achieved if the tumour is encapsulated and in such cases local recurrence is un-

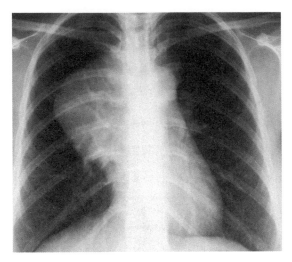

Fig. 12.11. *Typical PA chest X-ray appearance in a thymic tumour*. There is a well demarcated tumour mass and the lung fields are clear.

usual. Capsular invasion, direct extension to the pleura or pericardium or incomplete resection are all indications for postoperative radiotherapy which reduces the local recurrence rate. A dose of 35–45 Gy (3500–4500 rad) in 3–5 weeks is commonly employed. More distant spread of recurrence after radiotherapy is sometimes treated by chemotherapy although experience is limited and the results are often poor. The most widely used drugs are doxorubicin, cyclophosphamide and cisplatin.

Encapsulated thymomas have an excellent prognosis and 60% of patients are alive 20 years later. Invasive thymomas have a much worse prognosis, and only 50% of patients are alive at 5 years.

Carcinoid of the thymus occurs occasionally and probably develops from APUD cells within the thymus (see Chapter 15). These rare tumours may give rise to Cushing's syndrome by producing ACTH and causing adrenal hyperplasia. They are occasionally malignant.

Germ cell tumours. Primary germ cell tumours of the mediastinum are now increasingly recognized. Although teratomas and mixed tumours are the commonest, pure seminoma is also described. The tumours may secrete β-HCG and AFP as do testicular tumours (see Chapter 19). As with thymomas, the usual clinical presentation is with local pressure symptoms, chiefly dyspnoea, cough and dysphagia. Occasionally, gynaecomastia is the presenting feature. Haematogenous metastasis is unusual, lung and brain being the commonest sites. Local lymphatic invasion may occur. Any young male with an unexplained superior mediastinal tumour of uncertain origin should have plasma tumour markers (AFP and β-HCG) measured since histological interpretation can be difficult even in experienced hands and these tumours can be misdiagnosed as adenocarcinoma.

Plain chest X-ray, tomography and CT scanning are essential to delineate the tumour and for following progress after treatment. CT lung scanning will occasionally reveal unsuspected metastases. The principles of management are essentially as for testicular germ cell tumours (see Chapter 19). Primary treatment is with combination chemotherapy (currently using combinations including cisplatin, bleomycin, vinblastine and etoposide), except possibly for pure seminomas, which are in some cases curable by local radiotherapy; 40 Gy (4000 rad) in 20 daily fractions over 4 weeks is adequate.

In mediastinal teratomas, the role of radiation for residual disease is uncertain. Surgical removal of suspicious residual masses should always be considered, ideally when tumour markers have returned to normal. Previous treatment with large doses of bleomycin may lead to pulmonary toxicity with stiff lungs and poor lung compliance, which may make the post-thoracotomy period particularly hazardous. Recent reports of combined chemotherapy and surgical treatment have been encouraging, with several long term survivors, probable cures, by contrast to earlier reports in which cure was rare.

MIDDLE MEDIASTINUM

In the middle compartment of the mediastinum, lymphomas are the commonest malignant tumours, and both Hodgkin's disease and non-Hodgkin's lymphomas occur. The differential diagnosis includes an important group of non-malignant conditions—pericardial and bronchogenic cysts, mediastinal lipoma, tuberculosis, sarcoidosis and infectious or malignant causes of hilar and/or mediastinal lymphadenopathy. In the absence of palpable lymphadenopathy in an accessible site, the diagnosis is usually made by mediastinoscopy or limited thoracotomy. Tissue diagnosis is essential and examination of fresh (unfixed) tissue is valuable for the histopathologist since the use of immunocytochemical stains can help distinguish difficult lymphomas from each other and from anaplastic carcinomas (see Chapter 3).

Staging and management of mediastinal lymphomas follows similar principles to those at other sites (see Chapter 26). Surgical excision has no place in the routine management of these tumours which are sensitive both to chemotherapy and radiotherapy. Occasionally, mediastinal lymphoma causes severe superior vena caval obstruction which requires emergency treatment (see Chapter 8).

A particularly characteristic non-Hodgkin's mediastinal lymphoma occurs. This is a T cell convoluted, lymphoblastic, diffuse lymphoma (previously termed Sternberg's sarcoma). It is seen predominantly in adolescent males. Hodgkin's disease of the mediastinum, usually in association with obvious lymphadenopathy in the neck and/or axilla, occurs in about 30% of all supradiaphragmatic cases, but the mediastinum may occasionally be the sole site of involvement.

POSTERIOR MEDIASTINUM

Tumours of the posterior mediastinum are chiefly neurogenic in origin, and usually arise from the thoracic sympathetic chain or intercostal nerves Table 12.8. They are frequently asymptomatic but may cause back pain, dysphagia or ptosis due to Horner's syndrome. Neurofibromas are the commonest, and can usually be removed surgically. They can arise sporadically or in patients with Von Reckling-hausen's disease. Other neurogenic tumours include Schwannomas (both benign and malignant) and neurofibrosarcoma. These neurogenic tumours may extend through the intervertebral foramina (dumb-bell tumours) and cause cord compression. This is suggested by vertebral erosion on lateral chest X-ray. Ganglioneuromas are probably the commonest of the sympathetic nerve tumours and are generally well-differentiated, encapsulated and surgical resectable. In some cases, urinary VMA may be raised and can be useful for monitoring progress. A less well-differentiated form (gangioneuroblastoma) is also encountered, and has a worse prognosis because of local recurrence and metastases. Phaeochromocytoma, another hormonally active tumour, frequently presents with symptoms of catecholamine excess rather than with pressure symptoms, such as paroxysmal hypertension, headache, palpitation, chest pain and excessive sweating. They should be surgically excised where possible. In children, neuroblastoma is a common cause of posterior mediastinal tumour accounting for about one-fifth of all childhood neuroblastomas. The management of neuroblastoma is discussed in Chapter 24.

Of the rare tumours, chordoma occasionally presents as a posterior mediastinal tumour and its management is discussed in Chapter 11. Paraganglioma (chemodectoma) is rare and may be locally invasive, usually involving the great vessels.

Diagnosis of posterior mediastinal tumours requires careful radiological assessment (sometimes with contrast studies such as aortography or contrast CT scanning) as well as precise tissue diagnosis, which usually requires thoracotomy. Management is by surgical removal of the tumour wherever possible. For incompletely excised malignant tumours, postoperative radiotherapy is usually recommended.

MESOTHELIOMA

This relentless malignant tumour arises from the surface of the pleura, occasionally remaining well localized at the primary site but more often spreading diffusely and involving a substantial area of the pleura including the inner surface of the visceral pleura, thereby encroaching onto the pericardium. Pleural effusion is common, and the disease is occasionally bilateral. Primary peritoneal mesothelioma, without pleural involvement, is well described and peritoneal disease occasionally develops in patients in whom the pleura is the main or primary site of disease. Most patients with mesothelioma give a history of asbestos exposure though there is characteristically a delay of 20 years or so before the disease becomes apparent. The incidence of mesothelioma is apparently rising, presumably because of the widespread use of asbestos products. However, the past 10 years have seen increasingly stringent constraints on the use of asbestos, and we are probably now at the 'peak' of asbestos-related lung disease. Crocidolite is thought to be the most carcinogenic fibre.

PATHOLOGY

Pathologically the tumours appear sarcomatous, often with both fibrous and epithelial elements which may be so anaplastic as to be almost indistinguishable from a poorly-differentiated carcinoma. The degree of anaplastic change correlates poorly with clinical behaviour. Direct extension is characteristic and mesotheliomas typically invade ribs and chest wall. Early and widespread involvement of intercostal bundles probably accounts for the severe pain so typical of this tumour. In addition, extension through the diaphragm, invasion of local lymph nodes and distant blood-borne metastases are all commonly found.

CLINICAL FEATURES

Patients typically complain of increasing chest pain, which can be very severe, coupled with

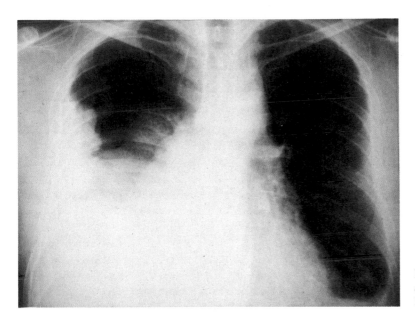

Fig. 12.12. *Chest X-ray appearances in mesothelioma.* Note the large pleural masses on the right.

shortness of breath on exertion. The dyspnoea tends to be progressive and unremitting, often leading to severe incapacity even at rest. On examination there are signs of diminished chest movement and pleural effusion. Radiologically the most typical feature of asbestos exposure is the pleural plaque, often multiple, and usually associated with pleural effusion (Fig. 12.12). In mesothelioma there is extensive pleural infiltration extending into the mediastinum and causing 'crowding' of the ribs on the affected side because of contracture caused by the tumour.

DIAGNOSIS

The diagnosis can usually be confirmed by pleural biopsy. In cases with such widespread involvement that surgical resection is impossible, diagnostic thoracotomy should be avoided, particularly since tumour seeding of thoracotomy scars is common and can produce additional severe pain. CT scanning is of great importance for definition of the tumour anatomy, particularly with respect to the juxta-pericardial reflection of the pleura, and the adjacent pericardium, which are often poorly visualized by plain X-ray of the chest.

TREATMENT

Treatment of mesothelioma is highly unsatisfactory. Surgery is possible only in a very small minority of cases with localized involvement, though surgical cures are well documented. Local recurrence is common, and most surgeons favour wide excision where possible, including sacrifice of part of the chest wall, diaphragm, pericardium and adjacent lobe of lung where necessary.

Radiotherapy is of very little value, though pain relief and apparent reduction in the rate of tumour growth occasionally occur. Adequate irradiation of the whole pleural surface is technically difficult because of the proximity of the lung, but new methods of tangential arc irradiation may allow this technique to be explored further. A wide variety of chemotherapeutic agents has been used in mesothelioma but with no long-term success although responses to doxorubicin, cisplatin and other agents are occasionally reported. Intrapleural chemotherapy is occasionally attempted for control of the malignant pleural effusion, but the results are discouraging. The very poor results of treatment argue strongly for rigid control of the use of asbestos products, and patients with mesothelioma and a clear history of industrial asbestos exposure are usually considered by independent tribunals to be strong candidates for compensation

REFERENCES

1 Loeb L. A., Ernster V. L., Warner K. E., Abbotts J. & Laszlo J. (1984) Smoking and lung cancer: an overview. *Cancer Research* **44**, 5940–58.

2 Doll R. & Hill A. B. (1964) Mortality in relation to smoking: ten years' observation on British doctors. *British Medical Journal* **1**, 1399–410, 1460–7.

3 Abeloff M. D., Eggleston J. C., Mendelsohn G., Ettinger D. S. & Baylin S. B. (1979) Changes in morphologic and biochemical characteristics in small cell carcinoma of the lung. A clinico-pathologic study. *American Journal of Medicine* **66**, 757.

4 Mountain C. F. (1976) The relationship of prognosis to morphology and the anatomic extent of disease. In Israel L. & Chahinian A. P. (eds) *Lung Cancer* pp. 108–41. Academic Press, New York.

5 Spjut H. J. (1958) Results in the treatment of bronchogenic carcinoma: an analysis of 1008 cases. *Journal of Thoracic Surgery* **36**, 316.

6 Durrant K. R., Berry R. J., Ellis F. Ridehalgh F. R., Black J. M. & Hamilton W. S. (1971) Comparison of treatment policies in inoperable bronchial carcinoma. *Lancet* **i**, 715–9.

7 Morrison R., Deeley T. J. & Cleland W. P. (1963) The treatment of carcinoma of the bronchus. *Lancet* **1**, 683.

8 Gralla R. J., Cvitkovic E. & Golby R. B. (1979) Cisdichlorodiammine-platinum (II) in non-small cell carcinoma of the lung. *Cancer Treatment Reports* **63**, 1585–8.

9 Fox W. & Scadding J. G. (1975) Medical Research Council comparative trial of surgery and radiotherapy for primary treatment of small cell or oat celled carcinoma of bronchus. Ten year follow-up. *Lancet* **ii**, 63–5.

10 Bunn P. A., Nugent J. L. & Matthews M. J. (1978) Central nervous system metastases in small cell bronchogenic carcinoma. *Seminars in Oncology* **5**, 314.

11 Urtasun R. C., Belch A. R., McKinnon S., Higgins E., Saunders W. & Feldstein M. (1982) Small cell lung cancer: initial treatment with sequential hemi-body irradiation vs. 3-drug systemic chemotherapy. *British Journal of Cancer* **46**, 228–35.

12 Medical Research Council Lung Cancer Working Party (1981) Radiotherapy alone or with chemotherapy in the treatment of small-cell carcinoma of the lung: the results at 36 months. *British Journal of Cancer* **44**, 611–7.

13 Cohen M. H., Creaven P. J., Fossieck B. E., Broder L. E., Selawry O. S., Johnston A., Williams C. L. & Minna J. D. (1977) Intensive chemotherapy of small cell bronchogenic carcinoma. *Cancer Treatment Reports* **61**, 349.

14 Bleehen N., Bunn F. A. & Cox J. D. (1983) Role of radiation therapy in small cell anaplastic carcinoma of the lung. *Cancer Treatment Reports* **67**, 11–9.

15 Souhami R. L., Geddes D. M., Spiro S. G., Harper P. G., Tobias J. S., Mantell B. S., Fearon F. & Bradbury I. (1984) A controlled trial of radiotherapy in small cell lung cancer treated by combination chemotherapy. *British Medical Journal* **288**, 1643–6.

16 Spiro S. G., Shah S., Harper P. G., Tobias J. S., Geddes D. M. & Souhami R. L. (1983) Treatment of obstruction of the superior vena cava by combination chemotherapy with and without irradiation in small-cell carcinoma of the bronchus. *Thorax* **38**, 501–5.

17 McKneally M. F., Maver C. M. & Kansel H. W. (1977) Intrapleural BCG-immunisation in lung cancer. *Lancet* **i**, 593.

Chapter 13

Breast Cancer

INCIDENCE, AETIOLOGY AND EPIDEMIOLOGY

Breast cancer is the commonest of all malignant diseases in women, with an incidence of 21 000 new cases annually in England and Wales and 100 000 new cases in the United States. The age-related incidence is shown in Figure 13.1. One in 14 women will develop breast cancer during their lifetime, making it the leading cause of death from malignant disease in Western women. Incidence rates vary markedly in different parts of the world, with a world average of 65 per 100 000. There is a very high incidence in North America and Northern Europe, and a low incidence in Asia and parts of Africa.

There are a number of known aetiological factors (1). Women with a first degree relative with breast cancer have a three-fold increase in risk. Women bearing their first child over the age of 30 are three times more likely to develop breast cancer than those who are less than 20 years and there is an increased risk in patients who have a history of benign breast disease. Follow-up of victims of Hiroshima has shown a late increase in incidence of breast cancer. It seems likely that demographical differences are due more to diet, cultural or geographical differences than to racial characteristics, since Japanese or Hawaiian women who settle in the United States have daughters and grand-daughters whose likelihood of developing breast cancer follows the American pattern after as little as two generations. Finally, in the UK the overall incidence of breast cancer appears to be

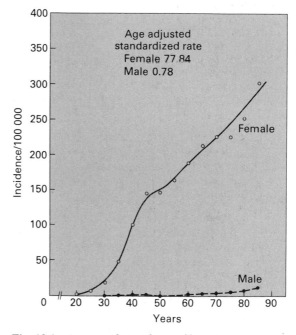

Fig. 13.1. *Age-specific incidence of breast cancer.*

rising slowly, with an 11% increase in the years 1968–78. In the United States a similar increase has been noted.

PATHOLOGY AND MODE OF SPREAD

Almost all breast cancers arise from the glandular epithelium lining the lactiferous ducts and ductules, and are therefore typical adenocarcinomas. Although true intraduct carcinomas are sometimes encountered, most primary breast cancers have invaded into the stroma of the breast by the time of diagnosis. The great majority of these present as breast lumps, though a small number have eroded through the skin of the breast by the time they are first seen, presenting as fungating tumours. Lesser degrees of skin involvement lead to skin dimpling or tethering, and *peau d'orange*, in which skin infiltration leads to local lymphatic obstruction.

The wide variability in histological appearance has led to a number of attempts at classifying these tumours according to their microscopic characteristics (recently with the help of histochemical stains). Descriptive terms are often used, and include: *polygonal* cell carcinoma, *scirrhous* carcinoma (in which there is a marked fibrous stromal reaction), *comedo* carcinoma (with macroscopic appearance suggestive of a small skin papule or blackhead), and *mucinous* (or colloid) carcinoma (with pronounced mucus formation). These terms are generally unhelpful since they have little bearing on prognosis. Important exceptions are firstly *inflammatory* carcinoma of the breast, which has a distinct microscopic and clinical appearance. In these tumours the subdermal lymphatics are infiltrated with undifferentiated cancer cells. Clinically there is erythema of the whole breast often with a little tenderness. This is a particularly aggressive form of the disease, with early local invasion and lymphatic involvement. Secondly, *medullary* carcinoma; this is generally a slow growing tumour with marked lymphocytic infiltration and a good prognosis. *Lobular* carcinoma arises from small ductules and is usually non-invasive. *Paget's disease of the breast* (nipple) causes an eczematous irradiating superficial eruption with intraduct carcinoma invading the nipple.

Far more important is the histological grade of the tumour, since this appears to reflect the aggressiveness of the neoplastic process and is an important determinant of the ultimate outcome. Although the concept of tumour grade is difficult to define, low-grade carcinomas tend to resemble their cell of origin more closely, whereas higher grade tumours appear increasingly bizarre under the microscope. Increase in cell size, degree of pleomorphism, nuclear-cytoplasmic ratio and cellular pyknosis are all indications of a more malignant tumour. These characteristics may differ in various parts of the tumour and for this reason the validity of grading has been questioned. There has also been criticism on the grounds of subjectivity in histopathological interpretation. However, several independent groups have shown that grade significantly affects prognosis. Other features, such as a marked lymphocytic and histiocytic cell reaction to the tumour, may indicate a better prognosis.

Modes of spread in breast cancer (Fig. 13.2) have been the subject of great controversy. Local dissemination may occur, either to underlying chest wall and related structures including the ribs, pleura and brachial plexus, or to overlying skin. Lymphatic spread is to axillary lymph nodes and to the supraclavicular, internal mammary or contralateral groups. Blood-borne metastasis occurs particularly to bone (especially the axial skeleton) liver, lung, skin and central nervous system (both brain and spinal cord). Intra-abdominal and pelvic metastases, including ovarian and adrenal deposits, are common. Many patients manifest particular patterns of spread and it is not unusual to encounter patients with widespread bone disease but without any evidence of soft tissue disease. Some patients develop relentless local recurrence of disease, cancer *en cuirasse*, without evidence of distant metastasis but with a deep fungating ulcer which may involve a substantial part of the chest wall. The reasons behind these patterns are unclear and they are unrelated to histological characteristics or pathological grade.

Haematogenous spread is of particular importance since patients die from distant metastases rather than uncontrolled local disease. The likelihood of axillary lymph node metastases correlates closely with the size of the primary tumour. The presence of nodal deposits increases the likelihood of blood-borne metastases, as evidenced by the importance of axillary involvement as a predictor of 5-year survival. There is a quantitative relationship

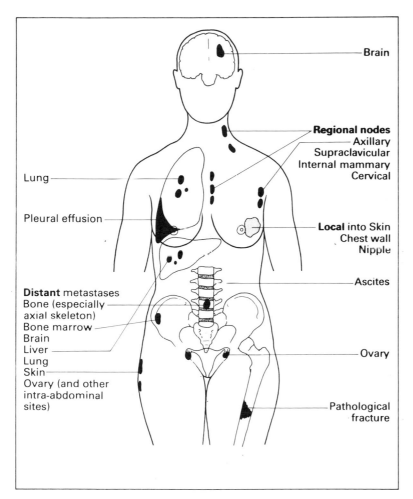

Fig. 13.2. *Local, nodal and distant spread in breast cancer.*

between the number of metastatic lymph nodes and survival (2), see also Figs. 4.2 & 13.9. Internal mammary node involvement is an important early site of spread of medially placed tumours. Indeed, such tumours are often considered unsuitable for mastectomy. The finding of supraclavicular lymphadenopathy at diagnosis is a particularly adverse clinical sign.

CLINICAL FEATURES

Most women with breast cancer present to their GP with a lump in the breast. Most breast lumps are benign and the commonest causes are cysts, fibroadenomas or areas of fibroad-

enosis. Although a skilled surgeon can often give a correct clinical diagnosis, all breast lumps should be regarded as potentially malignant and firm histological diagnosis is nearly always necessary.

Not all women with breast cancer present with a lump; pain in the breast, discharge or bleeding from the nipple, and pain or swelling in the axilla are also quite frequently encountered.

Signs which indicate that a breast lump is likely to be malignant include: a large mass, tethering to skin and/or chest wall, axillary or supraclavicular lymph node enlargement, *peau d'orange*, nipple inversion and skin infiltration. Although cancers are typically firm or indurated, this may also be true of a simple cyst. Although women are now presenting more often with relatively early disease, the lump is sometimes deliberately ignored, and can even be present for years before the patient finally presents with a fungating mass of tumour. Alternatively, the patient may present with symptoms from a secondary deposit, for example in the spine or brain. The symptoms may include pain in the back, due to vertebral metastasis leading to vertebral collapse and/or spinal cord compression (see p. 135). Focal neurological signs and raised intracranial pressure are frequent findings in patients with cerebral metastases. General symptoms such as lassitude and anorexia may reflect advanced and widespread disease, particularly liver involvement.

CONFIRMING THE DIAGNOSIS

There are several methods of confirming the diagnosis. Aspiration cytology of cysts is easy and frequently performed. The finding of a cyst with typical greenish fluid and disappearance of the lump after aspiration makes the diagnosis of cancer extremely unlikely. More recently, aspiration cytology from solid lesions has been gaining ground as a useful and accurate technique. If there is real doubt, a much larger piece of tissue can be obtained by drill biopsy with a 'Tru-cut' or other percutaneous biopsy needle, which usually yields an adequate core of tissue. If the diagnosis has not been obtained in this way, excision biopsy will be necessary. Many surgeons now feel that it is unjustifiable to proceed to mastectomy without giving their patients an opportunity to consider both the implications of the diagnosis and the alternative approaches for primary control of the tumour.

Mammography, either using conventional X-rays or xeroradiographic techniques, is widely used in diagnosis. Although not entirely reliable, carcinomas have a characteristic mammographic appearance, with fine calcification and areas of irregularity; fixation of deep lesions either to chest wall or skin can some-

times be seen. Mammographic examinations should be kept to a minimum to avoid unnecessary radiation exposure—a problem which has limited the more widespread use of mammography as a screening tool (see later).

Pre-operative investigation

Before mastectomy is contemplated, several screening procedures are usually performed in order to ensure that no patient with obvious metastatic disease is needlessly subjected to an operation. A good deal of controversy has surrounded the question of which investigations are helpful in influencing management. In some centres patients are extensively investigated with isotope scans of bone, liver and brain, skeletal X-rays, tumour marker analyses and estimations of urinary hydroxyproline. However, the general view at present is that the most valuable tests are a chest X-ray, full blood count and simple assessment of liver function. The contribution of isotope bone scanning is not entirely clear, since false positives are sometimes encountered as a result of previous trauma, arthritis and other conditions. However, this is a valuable investigation sometimes revealing widespread but asymptomatic bony metastases. In the absence of neurological symptoms or signs, isotope and CT brain scanning have a very low diagnostic yield. The same is true for isotope liver scanning in patients with normal liver function tests.

Staging notation

There have been a number of attempts to devise a simple staging system to describe the degree of advancement of the tumour. Most of these classifications depend on the size of the primary tumour, the presence or absence of axillary node metastases by palpation (and subsequently at operation), and the presence of distant metastases. The Manchester classification (Table 13.1) was successful to the extent that it classified patients into three groups which could be shown to have significantly different prog-

Table 13.1 Staging systems in breast cancer.

Stage	Description
Manchester Staging System	
Stage 1	Breast alone involved +/− overlying skin
Stage 2	Breast as for stage 1 and axillary nodes involved, but mobile
Stage 3	Skin invaded, fixed or ulcerated, or tumour fixed to underlying muscle or pectoral fascia
Stage 4	Fixed axillary lymphadenopathy, supraclavicular involvement and/or distant metastases
TNM Staging Notation for Breast Cancer	
T1*	Tumour less than 2 cm in diameter
T2*	Tumour 2–5 cm in diameter
T3*	Tumour >5 cm
T4	Tumour of any size with direct extension to chest wall or skin
N0	No palpable node involvement
N1	Mobile ipsilateral nodes
N2	Fixed ipsilateral nodes
N3	Supraclavicular or infraclavicular nodes or oedema of arm
M0	No distant metastases
M1	Distant metastases

*T1, T2 and T3 tumours further divide into (a) no fixation and (b) with fixation to underlying pectoral fascia or muscle.

noses. However, this classification is proving increasingly limited because more detailed information has now been obtained concerning the prognostic importance of variables such as the size of the primary tumour and the number of involved axillary lymph nodes (see p. 243). The TNM staging system proposed by the International Union against cancer has become widely accepted for classifying tumours more precisely (Table 13.1). Further modifications are likely, in order to take account of more detailed information regarding the pathological grade of the tumour, and its endocrine receptor status.

Hormone receptors in breast cancer

It is now well recognized that a proportion of breast cancers carry cellular receptors for oestrogen and other steroid hormones (including progestogen) both in their cell nuclei and also the cytoplasm (3). These receptors are present in 65% of cancers in postmenopausal women but only 30% of those premenopausal. Hormone dependence of some breast cancers can be demonstrated clinically by alteration of the hormonal environment (see p. 237). It is now established that the presence of an oestrogen receptor (ER) in a breast cancer cell correlates with the probability of hormone dependence in an individual tumour, making it possible to predict response to hormonal treatments. This has considerable clinical implications. Oophorectomy, for example, can be avoided in patients who are known not to have an ER positive tumour.

It is not entirely clear whether ER status is the reflection of a genuine and fundamental difference between 'negative' and 'positive' breast cancers or whether there is a continuous distribution from ER rich tumours to those with no detectable ERs whatever. The evidence at present favours the latter view, and ER 'positivity' is normally used to describe tumours in which the level of ER is greater than a certain defined figure, usually 5 fmole/mg cytoplasmic protein, or 25 fmole/mg nuclear DNA (see Chapter 6).

It seems that ER positivity is associated with well-differentiated tumours (particularly tubular, lobular or papillary types) and with microscopic elastosis in the tumour. Clinically it is apparent that slow-growing tumours tend to be ER positive. Both primary tumours and metastases show similar ER content, though ER negative metastases are sometimes encountered from an ER positive primary tumour. The reverse is rarely true.

How successful have ER measurements been in the prediction of hormone responsiveness? It is now clear that at most 5–7% of ER negative tumours will respond to hormone manipulation. Conversely, 55% of ER positive tumours will respond, so ER positivity, although useful, is not entirely reliable. There is however a detectable semi-quantitative response; tumours very rich in ERs are clinically hormone dependent in 90% of cases. A probable explanation for the failure of ER positive tumours to respond to hormone manipulation lies in the observation that the receptor although present, may not induce a change in cellular growth or metabolism. One result of ER activity is an increase in concentration of progesterone receptors (PR) within the cell. For this reason tumours rich in PRs are usually clinically hormone responsive (more than 80% of cases).

Screening for breast cancer

The general principles of cancer screening are discussed in Chapter 2. At first sight, breast cancer would appear to be an ideal tumour for a screening programme. First, it is relatively common (1 case per 1000 women per year) and secondly, it is relatively accessible to clinical examination by doctors, nurses, paramedical staff and by the patient herself. In addition, mammography often demonstrates a breast cancer before it is clinically evident. Furthermore, there are known groups of patients at relatively high risk: those with a strong family history of breast cancer, those with late first pregnancies or with a history of benign breast disease.

However, unselected mass clinical and mammographic screening has not yet been justified by the results. Apart from the substantial cost, it is not clear if the cure rate would be appreciably higher as a result of the earlier detection though at least one study has suggested an impressive reduction in mortality in patients over 50 years (4), possibly resulting from detection of the cancer at an earlier stage. However even low-dose mammography may not be entirely safe, though the radiation dose of this investigation has fallen sharply in recent years. Screening of selected high risk patients may however be more worthwhile. Breast self-examination (BSE) is perhaps more appropriate since it is cheap and can be repeated frequently. It has been shown that patients who practise BSE and who then develop breast cancer have a lower T stage than others.

MANAGEMENT OF THE PRIMARY TUMOUR

Surgical operations for breast cancer

A good deal of controversy surrounds the choice of operation in patients with 'early' breast cancer. The classical operation of radical mastectomy, introduced by Halsted over 80 years ago, was designed to ensure local control by removing the breast and, as far as possible, all of the primary lymphatic routes of spread — an entirely logical approach at a time when lymphatic spread was thought to be of critical importance and dissemination via the blood stream largely unrecognized.

In this procedure (Fig. 13.3) the whole breast is removed, with division of the pectoralis major and minor muscles and complete dissection of the axillary contents. In order to achieve a total clearance, the surgical incision is a large one, and the loss of contour very considerable since far more soft tissues than the breast itself are routinely removed.

There is no doubt that excellent results, in terms of freedom from local recurrence, are achieved by radical mastectomy even in patients with axillary node involvement. In such patients the additional use of postoperative radiotherapy will reduce the local recurrence rate still further but only by a small degree and at the cost of a much increased risk of arm swelling (lymphoedema). This disabling and often untreatable complication of treatment, which is due to lymphatic and venous obstruction, is much less frequent with simple mastectomy, or when postoperative radiotherapy is withheld.

With increased understanding that patients with breast cancer die not from uncontrolled local disease but from distant blood-borne metastases, there has been an increasing tendency

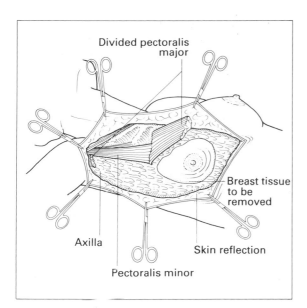

Divided pectoralis
major

Breast tissue
to be
removed

Axilla

Skin reflection

Pectoralis minor

Fig. 13.3. *Radical Mastectomy*. In this operation a large oblique incision is usually made, the pectoralis major is divided and often removed. The axillary contents are dissected and removed together with all breast tissue. Modifications of this operation have been devised in which the pectoral muscles are preserved, and/or the axillary nodes sampled, but not fully removed. Less radical procedures also include quandrantectomy or local excision.

to offer less mutilating procedures though the radical operation (Fig. 13.3) still has many proponents. Indeed, radical mastectomy has once again been advocated during the past two decades as a means of obtaining detailed information as to the degree of local invasion and axillary lymph node involvement.

Although a high survival rate from radical operations has been claimed for patients with small tumours without axillary node involvement, many British surgeons now favour a more conservative approach, using the 'total mastectomy' (essentially a simple mastectomy plus axillary dissection with removal of the pectoralis minor but preservation of the pectoralis major) which was described by Patey. The advantage of this operation is that there is less surgical mutilation with better preservation of contour and often better mobility of the shoulder. More conservative still was the

approach favoured by McWhirter in Edinburgh, in which simple mastectomy without full axillary dissection was followed by postoperative radiotherapy to local nodal drainage areas (5). All of these procedures give comparable 5-year survival rates (Table 13.2). There is little, if any, evidence that survival depends on the extent of the operation itself, provided that local control is ensured. Inflammatory carcinoma should never be treated by mastectomy alone, because of its locally advanced nature and poor prognosis.

Table 13.2. 5-year survival rates in operable breast cancer*.

Operation	5-year survival rate (%)
Extended mastectomy (Urban)	67
Radical mastectomy (Halsted)	69
Total mastectomy (Patey)	67
Simple mastectomy and radiotherapy (McWhirter)	66
Radical radiotherapy with local excision of tumour (Calle)	74

* modified from (27).

Surgical reconstruction of the breast has advanced considerably over the past 10 years and there are a variety of techniques now available. Most commonly used are silicone implants and myocutaneous flap reconstruction. Some women find that the improved contour is valuable and helps their confidence and self-image. However, the cosmetic result is mediocre by comparison with the best results from radical irradiation and reconstruction of the nipple is not generally performed, which is a further drawback.

Combinations of surgery and radiotherapy

Patients with positive axillary nodes confirmed at mastectomy are known to be at risk both of local recurrence and also of distant spread. In these patients, postoperative chest wall and local nodal irradiation has often been advo-

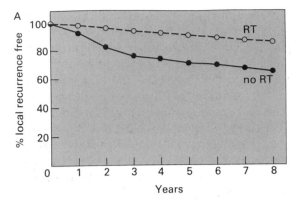

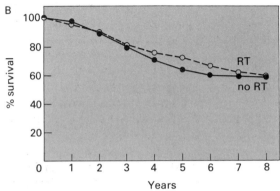

Fig. 13.4. Local recurrence and survival following simple mastectomy with or without irradiation. (A) The probability of local recurrence. Local recurrence is much more frequent in those not receiving radiotherapy (no RT). (B) The probability of survival. There is no difference between the two groups. (Reproduced from Cancer Research Campaign Working Party (1980) *Lancet* **ii**, 55. With permission.)

cated. Unfortunately, most comparative studies have shown no survival benefit from the routine use of radiotherapy in axillary node-positive cases. These trials have generally been retrospective or uncontrolled. The most important exception is the large Cancer Research Campaign King's/Cambridge study which compared simple mastectomy with simple mastectomy plus local irradiation in patients with early breast cancer who were prospectively randomized to receive one of the two treatment alternatives (6). This study now has a 10 year follow-up and the clear result is that local recurrence is indeed reduced by radiotherapy (from 30% to 11% at 10 years) but that survival

is unchanged (Fig. 13.4). This sort of study can of course be interpreted in a variety of ways. One extreme view would be that despite the improvement in local control, radiotherapy should not be routinely applied since survival is not improved. This approach implies a considerable reliance on radiotherapy as a therapeutic procedure in patients who later develop local recurrence (of whom there would be a substantial number, approaching one-third of all women treated by simple mastectomy alone). The other view would be to advocate routine radiotherapy in all these cases on the grounds that local recurrence is unpleasant, largely preventable and may even be fatal in patients in whom radiotherapy for overt local recurrent disease is unable to deal effectively with the problem. Where simple mastectomy has been performed, it is usual practice to offer postoperative irradiation in the axillary node-positive group, particularly in high-grade or large tumours where the risk of local recurrence is particularly high. However the increasing use of adjuvant hormone therapy and chemotherapy may, by reducing the incidence of local recurrence, make postoperative irradiation unnecessary. This point remains unresolved.

Views on the desirability of routine postoperative radiotherapy have altered with changing surgical attitudes. Halsted radical mastectomy, with formal axillary clearance, yielded a very low local recurrence rate, of the order of 4%. However, fewer and fewer surgeons now practice these radical procedures, and in this country the commonest operation is now the simple mastectomy with partial axillary clearance, in which there is no attempt at radical axillary dissection. The proportion of patients referred for radiotherapy is therefore rising, since such an operation cannot be expected to yield the low local recurrence rates achieved by radical mastectomy. Indeed it is the increased confidence that irradiation can produce sterilization of local disease which has led to the greater acceptance of less radical surgical procedures.

Techniques of postoperative irradiation vary

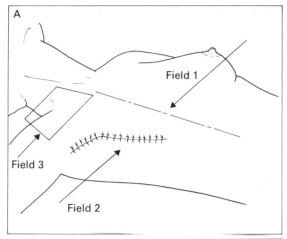

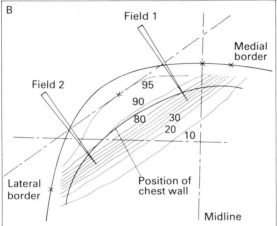

Fig. 13.5. *Postoperative irradiation following mastectomy.* (A) Use of two wedged fields tangentally applied to irradiate chest wall, axilla and internal mammary nodes. Field 3 irradiates the supraclavicular and lower cervical nodes using a directly applied radiation beam. Many other field arrangements are in common use. (B) Transverse view showing isodose distribution from the two tangential fields (1 and 2) in relation to the breast and chest wall.

widely. For example, some authorities omit regional node irradiation entirely (unless there is histological evidence of axillary disease), treating only the chest wall. An example of a field arrangement with dose distribution is shown in Figure 13.5.

To date, there have been two important prospective studies comparing radical mastectomy with a lesser surgical procedure plus routine ir-

radiation of the breast. In the first, patients at Guy's Hospital, London, were prospectively randomized either to undergo radical mastectomy followed by radiotherapy to the chest wall and nodal drainage sites, or to undergo wide excision, followed by the same radiotherapy (7). Although patients with Stage I breast cancer did equally well whichever method of treatment was given, those with more advanced disease (Stage II) did substantially worse if surgery was restricted to a wide excision rather than the radical mastectomy (Fig. 13.6). Although this study is frequently quoted, most radiotherapists feel that the trial design was seriously flawed by the very low dosage of radiotherapy given: a maximum of 38 Gy (3800 rad) in 3 weeks to the breast and only 27 Gy (2700 rad) to the axilla. This is likely to be the explanation for the relatively poor results in the group who underwent the conservative operation. Certainly these doses are far lower than those currently employed, and are now considered inadequate.

A more recent study, from Veronesi and colleagues in Milan, has prospectively allocated patients with small cancers of the upper outer

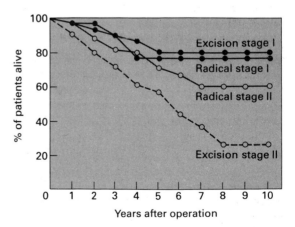

Fig. 13.6. Survival according to surgical treatment by radical mastectomy or wide local excision. Both groups received postoperative irradiation to a modest dose. These data (from Guy's Hospital, London) suggest that in stage 1 disease there is no advantage for radical surgery but that for stage 2 disease local treatment may influence survival. However the results in stage 2 disease treated by radical surgery were much better than in most other series.

quadrant and no evidence of axillary involvement ('low-risk' patients) to treatment by radical mastectomy alone or by 'quadrantectomy', in which the affected quadrant of the breast is excised, leading to a cosmetically acceptable though far from perfect result (8). Full axillary dissection and local irradiation are performed in all cases. So far, after 10 year follow-up, there has been no difference in survival or local control. The major treatment-related difference has been a much lower incidence of lymphoedema in the group treated more conservatively.

The role of radical radiotherapy

Can mastectomy be replaced altogether by radical irradiation? Although this approach has been considered unorthodox and even hazardous, primary radiotherapy has been used in breast cancer for well over 50 years. In 1937 Keynes (9) published the results of treatment in 250 patients in whom he had used interstitial implants of radium since 1924. The results were comparable to those obtained with mastectomy. Keynes (himself a surgeon) was clearly aware of the psychological morbidity and fear of mastectomy which led so many women to take no action if they discovered a lump in the breast. Sadly, his work was interrupted by the Second World War, though a follow-up report confirmed that the long-term results were as good as those obtained with any form of mastectomy.

This intriguing problem has become a dominant issue in cancer medicine over the past decade. Impressive results have been claimed, particularly from centres in France and the United States, using sophisticated techniques (Fig. 13.7) whereby the breast itself, the chest wall and all local nodal drainage sites are irradiated to a high dose (10). The bulk of information comes from Calle at the Fondation Curie in Paris, where over a thousand cases of operable breast cancer have now been treated, not by mastectomy, but by a combination of radical external beam radiation therapy, given as the sole method of treatment for large primary tumours (>3 cm) or combined with excision biopsy of the primary tumour in smaller lesions.

Calle's results at 5 and 10 years are certainly within the range achieved by more conventional surgical approaches, and his detailed analysis of the 10 year results gives survival figures remarkably comparable to those obtained by radical surgical techniques (Table 13.2). As a

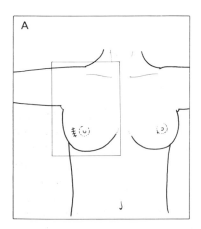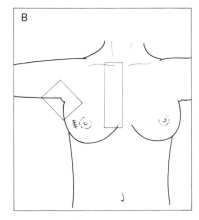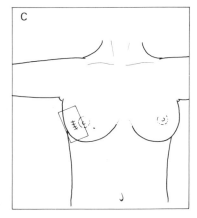

Fig. 13.7. *Combined external and interstitial irradiation (Pierquin) for patients undergoing local excision or biopsy alone.* (A) Treatment of breast, chest wall and local lymph nodes using ^{60}Co to 45 Gy. (B) Boost with electrons to upper internal mammary chain and axilla, to additional 24 Gy. (C) ^{192}Ir—wire implant to tumour bed (25–27 Gy). Comparable results can probably be achieved using external irradiation alone. (From Pierquin *et al* (11), with permission.)

result, the large majority of these women retain their breast, though a small number develop a local recurrence for which mastectomy has then to be performed. Others have pointed out that this does at least offer a 'double strategy', whereby women are allowed the opportunity of keeping the breast, with mastectomy held in reserve should it prove to be necessary. One interesting aspect of this approach is that about half of these patients who later require mastectomy, do subsequently prove to be long survivors (5 years or more), suggesting that local recurrence following 'adequate' initial treatment may not necessarily be accompanied by widespread metastases. There is however considerable difficulty in assessment of the breast, particularly where a high radiation dose has been given to a large volume. A number of patients, subjected to mastectomy for what was judged to be local recurrence, proved not to have disease on histological examination. The presumed recurrence (usually a palpable mass) may be no more than radiation-induced fibrosis of the breast.

Other groups rely not only on excision biopsy and external beam irradiation but also on interstitial implantation using ^{192}Irridium wires treating the tumour bed to a high radiation dose (Fig. 13.7). Complete 10-year follow-up data are not yet available, but at 5 years the survival and local control rates are both impressively high. In one series 93% of all women with T1 tumours surviving 5 years needed no further surgery (11).

An important American study on the role of breast-conserving primary treatment has just been published by the NSABP (National Surgical Adjuvant Breast Project, 12). Although preliminary, this 5-year follow-up report has given strong support for the concept of breast preservation. Over 1800 patients were randomized to undergo treatment either with simple mastectomy alone, or local excision ('lumpectomy') with or without postoperative radiotherapy. All patients underwent full axillary node dissection and those with node-positive disease were given adjuvant chemotherapy.

Disease-free survival after local excision plus radiotherapy was better than following simple mastectomy; furthermore, overall survival with local excision was if anything slightly better than following mastectomy. Ninety-eight per cent of patients with axillary node-positive disease, treated by local excision, axillary dissection, radiotherapy and adjuvant chemotherapy remained free of local recurrence, compared with 64% of patients not undergoing radiotherapy.

It is highly probable that the conventional approach for management of early breast cancer will change in favour of these more conservative treatments, even though this would lead to a tremendous extra burden on radiotherapy departments. The results from France, the USA and elsewhere suggest that the cosmetic result of radical irradiation of the breast is highly satisfactory in the majority of cases, and is unlikely to be equalled by surgical implant techniques. Now the psychological and sexual implications of mastectomy are beginning to be better understood (13), it is likely that the demand for radiotherapy as an alternative to mastectomy will rapidly increase.

Adjuvant hormone and cytotoxic therapy is discussed on p. 241.

RADIOTHERAPY FOR LOCALLY ADVANCED BREAST CANCER

For patients with locally advanced disease (T3, T4 and the majority of patients with N1b or N2 disease) the results of mastectomy have been disappointing and radiotherapy has usually been preferred. Even before the advent of wide-field treatment with supervoltage beams, implantation with radium needles could achieve a surprising degree of local control (9). With modern techniques, treatment to a high dose has led to a local control rate of 90% at 5 years, though the overall survival is only 20–25%. The probability of local control is inversely related to the size of the primary tumour, and other features such as fixation to the chest wall, fixed axillary lymphadenopathy or involvement of supraclavicular lymph nodes all contribute to inoperability and a higher probability of local recurrence. For radiotherapy to be successful a high local dose is essential. In one recent series, treatment to a dose of 60 Gy or more resulted in a local control rate of 78% whereas a lower dose achieved local control in only 39%; all these patients had stage III disease (13). The addition of chemotherapy reduced these local recurrence rates still further.

Complications of local treatment

Swelling of the arm. This complication (sometimes called lymphoedema) is due to lymphatic and venous obstruction. It is a frequent (about 10%) and troublesome sequel to treatment for breast cancer, particularly likely to occur when both radical surgery and radiotherapy have been used, and less common after more conservative procedures. Other factors which contribute to its development include infection and recurrent or persistent disease. If arm swelling appears years after primary treatment, a local recurrence should be suspected. Apart from the disfigurement, the swelling can be very uncomfortable, and can also be a focus for spreading subcutaneous infection (cellulitis).

The management of the swollen arm is difficult and often unsuccessful. The patient should be instructed in isometric exercises with the arm elevated, in an attempt to improve the muscle pump. Avoidance of infection is essential, and the patient must take care not to damage the skin of the affected arm, and to wear gloves for tasks such as gardening. Cellulitis must be treated promptly with antibiotics. If a local recurrence of tumour is confirmed it is usually better treated with systemic treatment rather than further radiotherapy, in order to avoid additional radiation damage. Air-driven compression sleeves are sometimes helpful in massaging fluid out of the limb but they often need to be used for several hours to be effective. Nocturnal elevation of the arm (for example by

a roller towel arrangement or by resting on pillows) is often recommended if the patient can tolerate it.

Stiff or frozen shoulder. Every patient undergoing mastectomy should be given a programme of graded exercises postoperatively. These will increase shoulder mobility, prevent stiffness and help to prevent lymphoedema. The movements should begin 3 or 4 days after operation and increase in degree as the wound heals. The aim is to develop normal elevation and rotation in the shoulder joint. Abduction and elevation of the arm are most important. If a frozen shoulder has developed, physiotherapy and short-wave diatherm are helpful.

Restoring a normal breast contour. Most women adapt well to an external prosthesis. For those who do not, breast reconstruction or an internal implant should be considered.

Psychological disturbance. Any form of mastectomy is mutilating, especially radical mastectomy. The incidence of depression and psychosexual disorders is about 25% during the first year (14). These problems are more severe in women who place particular emphasis on their body-image, and this risk constitutes a relative contraindication to mastectomy. Patients can be helped by pre- and postoperative counselling, and the role of patient support and counselling groups is discussed in Chapter 7.

TREATMENT OF METASTATIC DISEASE

In most patients with apparently localized breast cancer it is probable that the disease is in fact systemic or generalized at presentation and that metastatic disease will inevitably develop. This view is supported both by the common occurrence of widespread metastases, often many years after mastectomy has been undertaken, and also by long-term studies of cohorts of patients with breast cancer followed

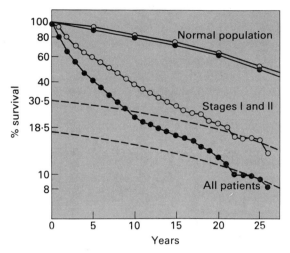

Fig. 13.8. *25-year survival of patients with breast cancer.* Dotted lines are an extrapolation parallel to the normal population to indicate proportion 'cured' at 25 years. (From Brinkley & Haybittle (15), with permission.)

up for periods of 25 years or more (Fig. 13.8). In one large study by Brinkley and Haybittle, the overall survival was only 20% after 25 years (15). Even in women deemed suitable for mastectomy (i.e. the 'early' operable group), the survival was only 30%. The clinical appearance of widespread metastases usually results in the patient's death within 3 years, though many women who respond to treatment live longer. The likelihood of dissemination is strongly linked to the presence or absence of histologically positive axillary lymph nodes at the time of operation, and a quantitative relationship between the number of positive axillary lymph nodes and the probability of metastatic disease has been established (see p. 243).

Hormonal manipulation in breast cancer (See Chapter 6)

Following the first therapeutic oophorectomy by Beatson in 1896 (16), it has become clear that about one-third of all patients with advanced breast cancer obtain symptomatic benefit from hormonal manipulation. A wide variety of procedures has been used, including oophorectomy, ovarian irradiation (sometimes termed

'artificial menopause'), treatment with oestrogens, antioestrogens, anabolic steroids, glucocorticoids and progesterones, surgical treatment by adrenalectomy or hypophysectomy and 'medical adrenalectomy' with aminoglutethimide. The conventional approach is largely based on the menstrual status of the patient. In most premenopausal and perimenopausal patients, surgical or radiation-induced ovarian ablation is first employed if metastatic disease develops. In postmenopausal patients treatment with additional oestrogen has long been recommended, though more recently, tamoxifen, which probably acts as an antioestrogen, has been increasingly preferred because of the relative lack of side-effects and in particular its freedom from severe cardiovascular and thrombotic complications. The response rate for postmenopausal patients is as good as that obtained with conventional oestrogen therapy. The dose is 10–20 mg daily by mouth. The drug is slowly cumulative, and side-effects, though very uncommon, include flushing, nausea, hypercalcaemia, a disease 'flare', thrombocytopenia, fluid retention and menstrual disturbances.

Until recently it was not possible to predict with any certainty which patients with metastatic disease were likely to respond to hormonal manipulation. However, it is now clear that patients with ER positive tumours are very much more likely to demonstrate a significant response to hormonal manipulation (3); patients with ER negative tumours rarely respond to such procedures. This test can be used as a means of identifying patients who are likely to benefit from such treatment. However the ER status is often unknown at the time when the patient presents with metastases and a trial of hormone treatment is then made without this information. Patients who are ER positive probably have a different natural history from those who are ER negative with a longer disease-free interval and overall survival (17). The fact that 35% of women whose tumours are ER positive do not respond to hormone therapy may in part be due to a blockage of the

Table 13.3. Response to endocrine therapy.

Receptor status		% response
ER−	PR−	10
ER−	PR+	40
ER+	PR−	35
ER+	PR+	70

pathway of activation induced by oestrogen despite the tumour retaining the ER protein. For this reason attempts are being made to relate response to a manifestation of ER *activity*. One such marker is the progesterone receptor (PR) whose synthesis is enhanced by oestrogen activity. Simultaneous measurements of ER and PR appear to give a better determination of the likelihood of response to hormone manipulation than measurement of ER alone (Table 13.3).

The presence of PR is also correlated with a longer disease-free interval. The site of metastatic disease may well influence responsiveness to hormonal treatment. A particular advantage with hormone manipulation is that patients with bony metastases are relatively likely to respond, although the ultimate outcome for such patients is poor, with a mean survival time from confirmation of bone metastases, of only about 12–15 months.

It is unwise to be dogmatic in making recommendations for the correct sequence of hormonal therapies in patients with recurrent disease. In general, most premenopausal patients are treated either by oophorectomy or by radiation-induced menopause in the first instance, whereas postmenopausal patients are more usually treated either with tamoxifen or additional oestrogens (often ethinyl oestradiol). In each case 30% of patients can be expected to respond, and the exogenous hormone should be continued indefinitely whilst the patient's response persists. Further hormone therapy should generally be reserved for those patients who responded to the initial hormonal procedure. In patients who have had a worthwhile response to oophorectomy, bilateral adrenalec-

tomy was formerly often employed, though it carried the hazard of life-long steroid replacement. Aminoglutethimide has supplanted adrenalectomy in recent years. This drug, which blocks the formation of oestrogen precursors in the adrenal, and their conversion to oestrogen in peripheral tissues (p. 106) appears to produce responses about as frequently as the operation. Apart from weakness and skin rashes, the drug is generally well tolerated, though lethargy, dizziness and nausea have also been reported. The chemical adrenalectomy may be enhanced by the additional use of glucocorticoid replacement which depresses ACTH output. Glucocorticoids are also medically necessary because of the adrenal suppression caused by aminoglutethimide, though low doses (without additional glucocorticoids) have also been shown to be effective. A common initial dose regimen is aminoglutethimide 250 mg 2–4 times a day with cortisone acetate 37.5 mg/day. Aminoglutethimide is best employed in postmenopausal patients since suppression of oestrogen production in premenopausal women is only partial.

When relapse occurs following these initial measures, other useful agents include anabolic steroids, progestogens and glucocorticoids. Anabolic steroids are more effective in postmenopausal women and seem to be particularly helpful with bone metastases. Twenty per cent of untreated patients will respond but side-effects of virilization can be troublesome. A convenient preparation is nandrolone decanoate (Deca-Durabolin) 50–100 mgm given intramuscularly, every 3 weeks. Progestational agents can be used if there has been a previous hormone response. The most commonly used drug is medroxyprogesterone acetate (MPA, Provera) which is often given at a dose of 100 mgm three times daily by mouth, though higher parenteral doses are also sometimes employed. Recent reports suggest that higher doses may be more effective though excessive weight gain may limit the tolerability of this approach.

The use of aminoglutethimide has led to a

reduction in the number of patients undergoing surgical adrenalectomy, and there are now few, if any, indications for this major procedure. Hypophysectomy however is a much easier operation for the patient and can be carried out by the trans-sphenoidal route. It is sometimes of benefit for relief of bone pain in patients who have become refractory to medical hormonal manipulation.

The question of whether hormone manipulation should still be preferred to cytotoxic chemotherapeutic treatment of first relapse has been widely debated. Although in numerical terms, the choice lies between hormonal manipulation which has a 30% likelihood of response and combination chemotherapy with a response rate of double this figure, this is an over-simplification of what is in fact a very complex decision. Hormone-induced responses tend to be more durable and are usually accompanied by minimal toxicity to the patient. Chemotherapy-induced responses tend to be of shorter duration and are accompanied by a wide spectrum of physical and psychological difficulties. In Britain there is no doubt that most clinicians prefer to employ hormone manipulation first, and this approach is likely to be further refined when oestrogen receptor assay techniques become more widely available.

Chemotherapy

Chemotherapy in breast cancer has become established as one of the major therapeutic modalities. Although introduced much more recently than other treatments, chemotherapy has assumed increasing importance, particularly in the management of patients with metastatic disease.

A wide variety of drugs has been investigated, and responses have been documented to many classes of drug, including alkylating agents, antimetabolites, spindle poisons, antitumour antibiotics and several others (Table 13.4). It may be difficult to measure a tumour response with accuracy. However, the likelihood of objective tumour response coupled

Table 13.4. Responses to cytotoxic drugs in breast cancer.

Drug	Approximate response rate (%)
Alkylating agents	
Melphalan	25
Cyclophosphamide	25
Anthracyclines	
Methotrexate	30
5-fluorouracil	20
Antitumour antibiotics	
Doxorubicin	40–50
Mitozantrone	30–40
Vinca alkaloids	
Vincristine ⎫	
Vindesine ⎭	20

with frequent improvement in subjective well-being, make these agents well worth considering in the management of metastatic disease. In general, skin, lymph node, and soft tissue metastases respond more readily than deposits in the liver or lung, which in turn are more likely to respond than bony metastases. Previous responsiveness to hormone therapy does not appear to predict the probability of response to chemotherapy.

Following successes with combination chemotherapy in Hodgkin's disease and acute leukaemia, it is now increasingly common to employ cytotoxic drugs in combination in breast cancer, rather than as single agents. Early work using a five-drug regimen of vincristine, methotrexate, cyclophosphamide, prednisolone and 5-fluorouracil, suggested that very high response rates could be obtained, but greater experience showed that the response rate was nearer 50%. Since that time a variety of different combination regimens has been used and some of these are shown in Table 13.5.

The most effective combination of drugs is certainly not yet established but it seems likely that combinations of three or four drugs probably offer similar response rates, with more acceptable toxicity, than more complicated combinations. Many of the newer combinations

Table 13.5. Responses to some combination chemotherapy regimens in advanced breast cancer.

Regimens	Dose and route	Response rate
CMF		
Cyclophosphamide	100 mg/m² p.o. days 1–14	53%
Methotrexate	40 mg/m² i.v. days 1+8	
5FU	600 mg/m² i.v. days 1+8 (repeated every 28 days)	
VAP		
Vincristine	2 mg i.v. days 1+8	60%
Doxorubicin	40–50 mg/m² day 1	
Prednisolone	30 mg/day for 7 days (repeated every 21 days)	
AC		
Cyclophosphamide	1 g/m² i.v. day 1	60%
Doxorubicin	40 mg/m² i.v. day 1 (repeated every 21 days)	
M–M–M		
Melphalan	10 mg p.o./day for 3 days	
Methotrexate	50 mg i.v. bolus day 1 (every 21 days)	
Mitomycin-C	15 mg i.v. bolus (given every alternate course, i.e. every 6th week)	

include doxorubicin, which is probably the most active single agent for breast cancer. Treatment with intermittent combination chemotherapy has now largely replaced low dose continuous administration. As with most regimens it is imperative to perform a full blood count before each course of treatment. Toxicity is largely predictable, but is usually no worse than would be expected from the additive use of the single agents chosen. For CMF, for example, the major problems are nausea, stomatitis and cystitis, and for VAP the commonest side-effects are neuropathy and alopecia.

Despite impressive response rates, the expected life span for patients with metastatic breast cancer has changed little, if at all, as a result of the more widespread use of these drugs (18). Although patients who respond live longer than patients who do not, and complete responders have a better prognosis than partial responders, the adverse effects in the non-responders must be weighed against these benefits. This may be one reason for the failure of combination chemotherapy to improve overall survival times. Other reasons are that the responses are often short-lived (sometimes only a few months), and that responders are perhaps more likely to be patients with an intrinsically better prognosis than non-responders. A central problem, as with so many areas of cancer chemotherapy, is to select those patients who are likely to respond well, and at the same time avoid overtreating patients who are unlikely to be helped. A worthwhile chemotherapy response is more likely to be achieved in patients who are fit, who have soft tissue rather than bone metastases, a small number of metastatic sites, who have received no previous chemotherapy, and possibly with a short disease-free interval. ER status probably has no predictive value for chemotherapy response.

Radiotherapy in metastatic and locally recurrent breast cancer

For decades radiotherapy has been widely used in patients with painful bone metastases, offering relief of symptoms in over three-quarters of all cases, though objective radiological evidence of recalcification is much less common. There is no evidence that the particular site of the bone metastasis influences the outcome of treatment though obviously some sites are particularly problematic, such as large cortical deposits in the femur or other weight-bearing bones. In such cases it is often useful to combine radiotherapy with internal orthopaedic fixation before a fracture occurs. Sternal metastases should be treated promptly since, if left untreated, the thoracic cage is unstable leading to a mid-dorsal vertebral fracture which can be life threatening.

Brain metastases are important in breast cancer since some 15% of all patients develop clinical evidence of spread to the brain. Radiotherapy is beneficial in approximately two-thirds of these cases, often with permanent control of symptoms until the patient's death. Spinal cord compression is also common, and its treatment is discussed in Chapter 8.

Pelvic irradiation to a relatively modest dose leads to complete and lasting amenorrhoea in premenopausal patients, and radiation-induced menopause has therefore been used as an alternative to oophorectomy—particularly in patients whose general condition makes surgery inappropriate. The probability of total amenorrhoea is dose dependent and fractionated treatment (12–15 Gy/5 fractions/1 week) is usually given. Radiation-induced menopause appears as successful as oophorectomy for relief of symptoms. Clinical problems from metastases at other sites, such as skin, lymph node, pelvic or painful hepatic deposits can often be alleviated by local radiotherapy even when systemic treatments have failed.

Following treatment by surgery alone, local recurrence of disease in the chest wall, ipsilateral regional lymph nodes or residual breast occurs with a frequency of 7–30%. It is more common with large tumours (above 5 cm) and when axillary nodes are involved. In patients with disease of an equivalent stage it is much less common after radical mastectomy than after simple mastectomy. However postoperative radiotherapy greatly reduces the frequency of local recurrence (see p. 232).

When local recurrence does occur in previously unirradiated patients, radiotherapy is undoubtedly the treatment of choice. However local recurrence often occurs in the context of systemic metastases, and if after investigation there is evidence of more widespread disease, a systemic treatment may be more appropriate.

Even under these circumstances radiotherapy may be the best treatment for a troublesome local recurrence.

If postoperative radiotherapy has previously been given it may be difficult to give further treatment because of the radiation tolerance of local structures such as skin and lung. Treatment by electron beam irradiation can be helpful in this difficult situation.

ADJUVANT CHEMOTHERAPY AND HORMONE THERAPY

Since it is clear that patients with breast cancer die from disseminated disease resulting from undetectable micrometastases which were present at the time of initial treatment, increasing attention has been paid to the concept of adjuvant systemic therapy following mastectomy, with the aim of eradicating these deposits before they become clinically apparent. This approach is supported by animal data suggesting that small metastases are more chemosensitive than large tumour masses.

Adjuvant hormone therapy

Following the demonstration that oophorectomy caused regression of advanced breast cancer, several studies of the effect of ovarian ablation as an adjuvant to mastectomy have been performed. Its effect in randomized comparisons has not been convincingly demonstrated but most of these studies were performed before ER status could be determined. In one large study (19) the combination of postoperative ovarian irradiation and oral low-dose prednisone produced in perimenopausal women a prolonged disease-free interval and increased survival time by comparison with mastectomy alone. However, the majority of women (ie those who were clearly pre- or postmenopausal) did not benefit. More recently, a large randomized study of adjuvant tamoxifen appears to have shown a prolonged disease-free interval (and possibly survival) in the treated group (20). If this finding is confirmed it will represent an important advance, particularly in view of the lack of toxicity of this form of adjuvant treatment.

Adjuvant chemotherapy

The earliest study, that of Nissen-Meyer at the Oslo Cancer Institute (21), suggested that cyclophosphamide given immediately after surgery has improved survival at 10 years.

Both the unpredictable nature of breast cancer and the need for lengthy follow-up have made early interpretation of more recent studies extremely difficult. The trial by Fisher and his colleagues (22) in which melphalan was the agent used has shown a modest improvement in disease-free survival in treated patients (compared with placebo) in premenopausal women only. There was a slight but insignificant improvement in overall survival at 5 years. Further studies from this and many other collaborative groups are in progress (Table 13.6).

Unfortunately several of the studies have been designed without an untreated control group which will make future interpretation difficult. This situation has arisen because of an excess of enthusiasm aroused by the preliminary results of the studies of Fisher and of Bonadonna (23) who compared adjuvant CMF (Table 13.6) with a control group and showed improved survival in the treated group, an effect which was most marked in premenopausal women with more than three axillary nodes involved. This study was flawed by defective randomization and at present, although there is a suggestion that premenopausal women may benefit from such chemotherapy, more information is needed from other trials. Most of the more recent studies are not showing a survival benefit from chemotherapy, though a summation of recent randomized trials has suggested a small survival advantage for patients treated with chemotherapy (see below). The effect on *disease-free survival* in premenopausal women may be due to chemotherapy-induced ovarian failure (24). The difficulty in assessment of the validity of early results of adjuvant therapy is discussed more fully in Chapter 2.

Not only is the effectiveness of adjuvant chemotherapy uncertain, but in addition the dose, duration of therapy and choice of drugs remains unclear. Bonadonna and colleagues have attempted, retrospectively, to relate the dose of drug received to relapse-free survival and claimed greater effect in patients receiving a greater dose of drugs. They have also sug-

Table 13.6. Results of large scale randomized prospective trials of adjuvant chemotherapy in operable breast cancer.

Source	Drugs	Comments
Nissen-Meyer (1978) (Oslo)	Short course (6 days) cyclophosphamide *vs* control	Improved disease-free and actual survival (10%) at 10–15 years in pre- and postmenopausal groups.
NSABP (1980) (National Surgical Adjuvant Breast Project)	Thiotepa *vs* control	10-year survival difference (not significant) in premenopausal women with 4+ nodes.
	Melphalan *vs* control	No survival difference at 5 years. Improved disease-free survival in premenopausal women.
Bonadonna (1981) (Milan)	CMF *vs* control	4% increase in survival at 5+ years survival in premenopausal women only.
Rubens (1983) (Guy's)	Melphalan *vs* control	No survival difference.
Cancer Research Campaign (1982)	Melphalan and methotrexate *vs* control	No survival differences at 5 years.

gested that the lack of effect of chemotherapy in postmenopausal women is due to the smaller amount of chemotherapy which these older women received. Such analyses are fraught with methodological artefacts. For example, if a patient relapses early, chemotherapy will be stopped so that patients who relapse quickly will have received less chemotherapy than those whoe relapse later. The mistaken conclusion may then be drawn that relapse occurred *because* the total dose was low.

In conclusion, we feel that it is at present impossible to give an unqualified answer to the question, 'Is adjuvant chemotherapy of benefit in patients with breast cancer?' The benefits arc probably confined to sub-groups of patients, and may not be substantially greater than those obtained with adjuvant hormone therapy, a much less toxic form of treatment. The toxicity of combination chemotherapy is considerable and this is one important area of cancer medicine where a possible benefit must be weighed against the quality of the patient's life (see Chapter 7). Despite these reservations, a recently performed compilation of prospectively randomized trials of adjuvant chemotherapy has shown an undoubted survival benefit in premenopausal node-positive patients (25). Whether this benefit will be equalled by the use of alternative, less toxic, forms of adjuvant treatment (for example, using tamoxifen) remains uncertain.

Until recently, current practice in the UK did not generally favour the routine use of adjuvant chemotherapy, even in premenopausal patients with node-positive breast cancer. By contrast, in the United States current recommendations include the use of adjuvant chemotherapy for Stage II disease.

PROGNOSIS OF BREAST CANCER

Very few studies have followed patients with breast cancer for prolonged periods, but there is general agreement that 5 and 10-year survival rates do not give a true picture since relapses

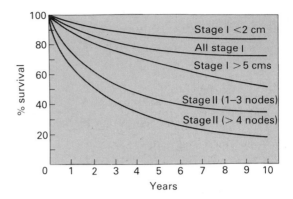

Fig. 13.9. *Survival in stage I and II operable breast cancer.* In stage I disease tumour size is an important prognostic determinant, as is degree of involvement of axillary nodes in stage II.

may occur well beyond this point (Fig. 13.8). There may even be a few additional deaths from relapse beyond 25 years. Prognosis is dependent on stage of tumour, size of the primary (Fig. 13.9) and tumour grade but probably independent of the extent of initial surgery (see also Fig. 4.2). Axillary lymph node involvement is particularly important: of patients with stage I disease (T1–2 N0) 75% are alive at 10 years whereas with stage II disease (N1–3 M0) the 10-year survival is only 35%. The significance of the age of the patient at diagnosis is uncertain though breast cancer diagnosed during pregnancy has a particularly poor prognosis. Subsequent pregnancy in patients with breast cancer does not appear to have any adverse effect. It has recently been suggested that personality factors may have a bearing on outcome (26).

Cancer of the male breast

Breast cancer in men is one hundred times less common than in women (Fig. 13.1). Little is known of the aetiology though a few family clusters have been reported, and it is possibly more common in patients who have had bilharzia with consequent liver damage and hyperoestrogenism. It has also been reported in patients with Kinefelter's syndrome, in which gonadotrophin levels are characteristically elevated, and in patients with gynaecomastia.

Most patients present with a tender indurated nipple, often with crusting or discharge, sometimes bloodstained. The disease involves the chest wall early. Routes of spread are similar to the disease in women, as is the pattern of metastasis. Most of the tumours are ER positive.

Treatment is usually by mastectomy. Many surgeons prefer radical mastectomy because of the paucity of breast tissue in males and the possibility of early direct invasion, coupled with the lesser mutilation of this operation in men. Local irradiation should be given when axillary lymph nodes are involved.

For recurrent disease orchidectomy is generally considered the treatment of choice, with responses in 60% of cases. The value of other endocrine manoeuvres is uncertain but treatment with tamoxifen, progestogens, cyproterone or hypophysectomy have all been employed. There have been few trials of chemotherapy but it is often used when hormone treatments have failed and responses may be seen.

REFERENCES

1 McMahon B., Cole P. & Brown J. (1973) Aetiology of human breast cancer: a review. *Journal National Cancer Institute* **50,** 21.

2 Fisher E. R., Redmond C. & Fisher B. (1980) Pathologic findings from the National Surgical Adjuvant Breast Project VI. Discriminants for 5-year treatment failure. *Cancer* **46,** 908.

3 McGuire W. L. (1978) Hormone receptors, their role in predicting prognosis and response to endocrine therapy. *Seminars in Oncology* **5,** 428.

4 Collette D. J. A., Day N. E., Rombach J. J. & de Waard F. (1984) Evaluation of screening for breast cancer in a non-randomized study (the Dom project) by means of a case-control study. *Lancet* **i,** 1224.

5 McWhirter R. (1955) Simple mastectomy and radiotherapy in the treatment of breast cancer. *British Journal of Radiology* **28,** 128.

6 Cancer Research Campaign (King's/Cambridge) Trial for early breast cancer. (1980) A detailed update at the tenth year. *Lancet* **ii,** 55.

7 Atkins H., Hayward J. L., Klugman D. J. & Wayte A. B. (1972) Treatment for early breast cancer: A report after ten years of a clinical trial. *British Medical Journal* **ii,** 423.

8 Veronesi U., Saccozzi R., Del Vecchio, M., *et al* (1981) Comparing radical mastectomy with quadrantectomy, axillary dissection and radiotherapy in patients with small cancers of the breast. *New England Journal of Medicine* **305,** 6.

9 Keynes G. (1937) Conservative treatment of cancer of the breast. *British Medical Journal* **ii,** 643-7.

10 Calle R., Pilleron J. P., Schlienger P. & Vilcoq J. R. (1978) Conservative management of operable breast cancer. Ten years' experience at the Foundation Curie. *Cancer* **42,** 2045.

11 Pierquin B., Owen R., Maylin C. *et al* (1980) Radical radiation therapy of breast cancer. *International Journal of Radiation Oncology Biology Physics* **6,** 17-24.

12 Fisher B., Bauer M., Margolese R., *et al* (1985) Five years' results of a randomized clinical trial comparing total mastectomy and segmental mastectomy with or without radiation in the treatment of breast cancer. *New England Journal of Medicine* **312,** 665.

13 Macguire G. P., Lee E. G., Bevington D. J., Kuchemann C. S., Crabtree R. J. & Cornell C. E. (1978) Psychiatric problems in the first year after mastectomy. *British Medical Journal* **i,** 963.

14 Harris J. R., Levene M. B. & Hellman S. (1978) The role of radiation therapy in the primary treatment of carcinoma of the breast. *Seminars in Oncology* **5,** 403-16.

15 Brinkley D. & Haybittle J. L. (1975) The curability of breast cancer. *Lancet* **ii,** 95-7.

16 Beatson G. T. (1896). On the treatment of inoperable cases of carcinoma of the mamma. Suggestions for a new method of treatment with illustrative cases. *Lancet* **ii,** 104.

17 DeSombre E. R. (1982) Breast cancer: hormone receptors, prognosis and therapy. In Furr B. J. A. (ed.) *Hormone Therapy. Clinics in Oncology,* **1**(1) 191. Saunders, London.

18 Powles T. J., Coombes R. C., Smith I. E., Jones J. M., Ford H. T. & Gazet J–C. (1980) Failure of chemotherapy to prolong survival in a group of patients with metastatic breast cancer. *Lancet* **i,** 580-2.

19 Meakin J. W., Allt W. E. C., Belae F. A., Brown T. C., Bush R. S. *et al* (1977) Ovarian irradiation and prednisone following surgery for carcinoma of the breast. In Salmon S. E. & Jones S. E. (eds) *Adjuvant Therapy of Cancer,* pp. 95-9. North-Holland Publishing Co, Oxford.

20 Baum M., Brinkley D. M., Dossett J. A., McPher-

son K., Patterson J. R., Rubens R. D. *et al* (1983) Improved survival amongst patients treated with adjuvant tamoxifen after mastectomy for early breast cancer. *Lancet* **ii,** 450.

21 Nissen-Meyer R., Kjellgren K., Malmio K., *et al* (1978) Surgical adjuvant chemotherapy. Results with one short course with cyclophosphamide after mastectomy for breast cancer. *Cancer* **41,** 2088.

22 Fisher B., Redmond C., Fisher E. R. and participating NSABP investigations (1980) The contribution of recent NSABP clinical trials of primary breast cancer therapy to an understanding of tumour biology—an overview of findings. *Cancer* **46,** 1009–25.

23 Bonadonna G., Brusamolino M., Valagussa P. *et al* (1976) Combination chemotherapy as an adjuvant treatment in operable breast cancer. *New England Journal of Medicine* **294,** 405.

24 Howell A., Bush H., George W. D. *et al* (1984) Controlled trial of adjuvant chemotherapy with cyclophosphamide, methotrexate and 5-fluorouracil for breast cancer. *Lancet* **ii,** 307.

25 Peto R. (1985) The breast cancer trials review meeting. Washington, USA, Sept. 1985. (*In press*).

26 Dilman V. M. (1981) Psychophysiological factors and the progress of breast cancer. In Stoll B. A. (ed.) *Systemic control of breast cancer*, p. 124. Heinemann, London.

27 Pierquin B., Baillet F. & Wilson J. F. (1976) Radiation therapy in the management of primary breast cancer. *American Journal of Roentgenology* **127,** 645.

Chapter 14
Cancer of the Oesophagus and Stomach

CARCINOMA OF THE OESOPHAGUS

Incidence and aetiology

Oesophageal cancer is commoner in males, with a male:female incidence of about 2:1 and a peak incidence in the age group 60–80 years (Fig. 14.1). In the UK it has increased in incid-

ence by 30% in the last 10 years. In some Scandinavian countries carcinoma of the oesophagus is as common in women as in men. There are marked geographical variations in incidence with a very high incidence near the Caspian Sea, Central Asia and Far East (Fig. 14.2). The

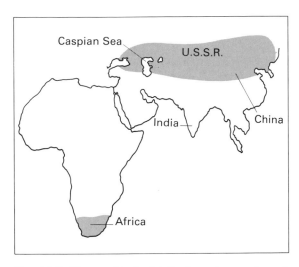

Fig. 14.2. *Geographical distribution of oesophageal cancer.* The hatched area indicates the regions of high incidence. The high-risk belt stretches from the Caspian Sea across Mongolia and Northern China.

incidence is rising in the Transkei (S. Africa) and the disease is commoner in France and Switzerland than in Britain. In the United States it is commoner in the lower socio-economic groups and three times as common in blacks as in whites. Aetiological factors include cigarette smoking, excessive alcohol intake and malnutrition. Repeated oral infection, development of benign oesophageal stricture or achal-

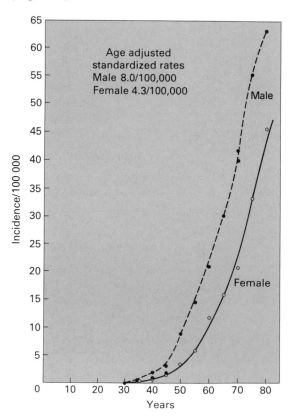

Fig. 14.1 *Age-specific incidence of carcinoma of the oesophagus.*

246

asia, and a history of syphilis, are also thought to be contributory. The Plummer–Vinson (Patterson Kelly) syndrome of a congenital web in the upper oesophagus, with glossitis and iron deficiency anaemia, is a known predisposing factor, and is more common in women. There is a 7% incidence of oesophageal carcinoma in long-standing achalasia. The rare inherited disorder of tylosis palmaris (see Chapter 3, Table 3). is also associated with oesophageal cancer.

Pathology

The oesophagus can be conveniently divided into three sections, the cervical oesophagus (distal limit 18 cm from upper incisors), mid third (distal limit 30–31 cm from incisors) and lower third (distal 10 cm of oesophagus). The most frequent sites for oesophageal cancer are the narrowed areas in the cricopharyngeal region, adjacent to the bifurcation of the trachea, and

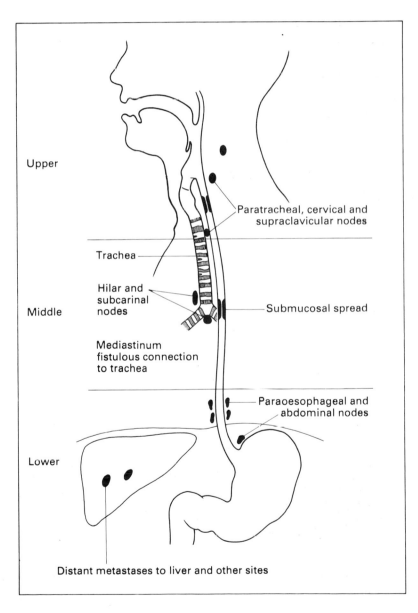

Fig. 14.3. *Local and distant spread of oesophageal cancer.*

in the lowest part of the oesophagus near the sphincter. The lower third lesions are commonest (40–45%), followed by mid third (35–40%) and cervical oesophageal cancers (10–15%). Both squamous carcinomas and adenocarcinomas occur, the histology varying with the level in the oesophagus. Cervical oesophageal and upper third lesions are always squamous cell in origin. Though adenocarcinomas are very occasionally seen in the mid third and are increasingly common in the lower third, 'true' adenocarcinoma of the oesophagus probably accounts for no more than 2% of tumours, many of the lower oesophageal adenocarcinomas being gastric cancers. Other tumour types are very rare and include melanoma and leiomyosarcoma.

Tumour spread (Fig. 14.3) occurs chiefly by direct extension and by lymphatic metastases. Direct extension occurs early in this disease, with rapid invasion within the oesophagus, both in cranio-caudal directions and also circumferentially. Insidious submucosal spread is almost universal and carries important implications for treatment. Direct mediastinal involvement occurs, usually later in the disease, by penetration of the muscular coat. The pattern of muscular involvement varies with the level of primary tumour. Fistulous connection to the trachea may occur.

Cancers of the upper or cervical oesophagus chiefly drain to the deep cervical nodes either directly or via paratracheal or retropharyngeal lymphatics. Mid and lower third lesions drain to the posterior mediastinal nodes and abdominal nodes, sometimes traversing the diaphragm. Haematogenous spread characteristically occurs later, though unexpected hepatic metastases may be encountered at laparotomy in cases thought to be suitable for radical surgery. The liver is much the commonest site of haematogenous spread, though bone, lung and brain deposits also occur.

Clinical features

Dysphagia is the commonest symptom, and is almost always accompanied by weight loss, often amounting to 10% or more of body weight. The dysphagia is more pronounced for solids than liquids, and patients have often discovered for themselves that a soft or liquidized diet is the only means of securing a regular intake of food. Typically the dysphagia becomes more severe and some patients progress to complete dysphagia with inability even to swallow their own saliva, before seeking medical advice. Although a few patients are able to point to the site at which the food lodges, a better guide to the level of obstruction is given by the interval between swallowing and the sensation of food sticking. In other patients, dyspepsia, regurgitation or acid reflux are more prominent clinical features. Pain is a late symptom of oesophageal cancer and is usually felt retrosternally. Spillover of oesophageal contents into the larynx or lung may cause cough, and involvement of the recurrent laryngeal nerve may lead to hoarseness. Haematemesis and melaena are unusual.

On examination there may be no abnormality apart from evidence of recent weight loss and malnourishment. Occasionally, patients present with metastatic symptoms—usually from liver metastases—with only minimal dysphagia. Evidence of metastases may be found on examination with enlarged supraclavicular nodes or an enlarged liver.

Investigation and staging

Patients with dysphagia should be investigated with a barium swallow and meal. Characteristically, patients with carcinoma of the oesophagus will have an obvious area of irregular narrowing well visualized by contrast radiography (Fig. 14.4). Unlike patients with achalasia of the cardia, there is usually rather minimal dilatation of the proximal oesophagus, presumably since little time has intervened for dilatation to take place. The narrowed segment may be surprisingly long and characteristically there is an irregular 'shoulder' although this may be absent. Patients with severe dysphagia may be

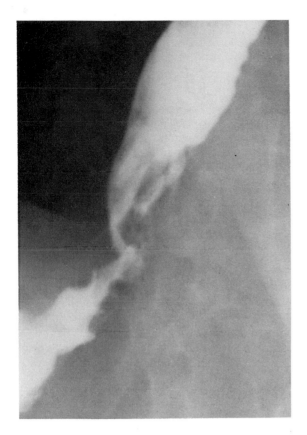

Fig. 14.4. *Barium swallow showing carcinoma of distal oesophagus.* A long irregular stricture is shown.

difficult to investigate because of the danger of aspiration of contrast material into the lungs. A chest X-ray is important since paratracheal or other mediastinal node enlargement occurs commonly, and is an absolute contraindication to radical surgery. The chest X-ray may also demonstrate that the cause of the dysphagia is secondary mediastinal lymphadenopathy from a radiologically obvious but clinically silent carcinoma of the bronchus, or that intrapulmonary metastases have occurred.

Direct oesophagoscopy and biopsy are essential in all patients who are fit enough to undergo the procedure. At the same time the surgeon may also be able to dilate a malignant stricture or insert a prosthetic tube for palliation of the dysphagia. Oesophagoscopy and biopsy carries a risk of oesophageal perforation, with mediastinitis and surgical emphysema which is usually fatal.

STAGING

No satisfactory staging system has been developed, possibly because of the inaccessibility of this tumour and difficulty in assessing the regional node involvement. The extent of the primary tumour may be impossible to determine even under direct vision and it may sometimes be difficult or dangerous to pass the endoscope so that the lower border may be inaccurately determined. CT scanning has been useful in demonstrating early mediastinal node involvement in patients with a normal chest X-ray. Since at least two-thirds of patients have lymphatic involvement at the time of diagnosis, careful assessment is required in any patient in whom surgery is contemplated.

Treatment

It is generally agreed that adenocarcinoma of the oesophagus (almost always lower third lesions) are best dealt with by surgery. In most other cases, particularly those of the upper third and cervical oesophagus, radiotherapy is the treatment of choice. Before embarking on local treatment, the surgeon or radiotherapist must be clear as to whether the philosophy of treatment is radical or palliative.

RADICAL TREATMENT

When radical treatment is contemplated in patients who are generally fit and with no evidence of distant disease, it is important to determine the extent of the lesion before definitive surgery is attempted. Exploratory laparotomy is often advocated in these cases, and in any event is a routine part of many operations when reconstruction is to be achieved by colonic transposition, creating a viable conduit between pharynx and stomach. Radical removal of the oesophagus, first attempted over 100 years ago by Czerny, is nowadays usually performed as a single stage procedure with oesophago-gastric anastomosis or colonic interposition. Formerly, operations were performed in which a permanent feeding gastrostomy was left as the means of providing nutrition.

Only a minority of patients with oesophageal cancer are suitable for radical surgery and the commonest indication is a mid or lower third lesion, particularly where the histology is adenocarcinoma, in a fit patient with no demonstrable evidence of metastases.

In patients with carcinoma of the *upper third of the oesophagus*, radiotherapy is usually considered to be the treatment of choice, though surgical treatment is preferred by some. Radiotherapy has several advantages, including wider applicability (most patients are elderly and poorly nourished), significant palliation of dysphagia in most patients, with cures in 5-10% of patients who are able to tolerate high doses:

55-60 Gy (5500-6000 rad) in daily fractions over 5-6 weeks. In addition, surgical treatment by colonic interposition (Fig. 14.5) carries a mortality of at least 10% and, unlike radiotherapy, is inappropriate in patients with locoregional spread of disease. Despite poor overall results, surgery has the advantage that palliation is often excellent and that it may sometimes be curative.

The upper third of the oesophagus is technically a difficult area to irradiate, because of the length of the treatment field coupled with the proximity of spinal cord. It is widely accepted that radiation fields should ideally extend for at least 5 cm above and below the known limits of disease, in order to treat adequately the presumed submucosal extension. Sophisticated planning techniques are often required, involving the use of twisted, wedged, oblique, multiple fields, often with compensators, and careful radiation planning at 2 or 3 levels so that a cylinder of tissue is irradiated to a

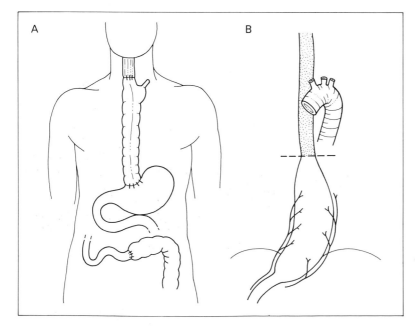

Fig. 14.5. Surgery for oesophageal cancer. (A) Colonic interposition following total oesophagectomy; (B) gastric mobilization and pull-through for carcinoma of the lower one-third.

uniform high dose without over-irradiation of the adjacent spinal cord (Fig. 14.6). A similar field arrangement is often employed in post-cricoid carcinoma.

For tumours of the *mid third of the oesophagus*, surgery is more frequently performed, using mobilized stomach as the commonest means of reconstruction (Fig. 14.5). The operation is always extensive and carries a substantial mortality. Radiotherapy has been used as definitive treatment, or in combination with surgery; some surgeons feel that the operation is easier and the long-term results better, when pre-operative irradiation is given. For pre-operative or radical radiotherapy of tumours of the middle third of the oesophagus, treatment is technically simpler than with tumours of the upper third. A planned multifield approach will still be necessary in order to deliver a high dose to the tumour and local mediastinal lymph nodes, while at the same time avoiding over-dosage of the spinal cord.

For cancer of the *lower third of the oesophagus*, surgery is preferable and reconstruction, usually employing mobilized stomach (Fig.

14.5), is less difficult. With cancer of the lower third of the oesophagus there is a risk that the stomach will be involved with tumour, making it unsuitable for reconstruction. Radiotherapy can be useful for inoperable tumours.

At all sites, complications of treatment can be severe, both for radiotherapy and surgery. Radical radiotherapy is always accompanied by radiation oesophagitis, requiring measures such as oral administration of local anaesthetic with alkali ('Mucaine') or aspirin-containing suspensions to act locally on the oesophageal mucosa. Later complications include radiation damage to spinal cord (see Chapter 11) or lung, leading to radiation pneumonitis and occasionally dyspnoea, cough and reduction in respiratory capacity. Still commoner is the development of oesophageal fibrosis and scarring, which can lead to stricturing of the oesophagus which may require regular dilatation to retain oesophageal patency.

Surgical complications include oesophageal stricture, and anastomotic leak, resulting in mediastinitis, pneumonitis and septicaemia which can be fatal.

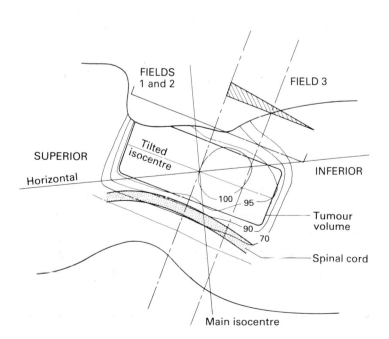

Fig. 14.6. *Radical radiotherapy for carcinoma of the cervical oesophagus.* The irregular anatomy necessitates a complex multifield treatment plan.

PALLIATIVE TREATMENT

Palliative treatment can be very valuable in oesophageal cancer. Palliation can be achieved either by passage of a Celestin or other indwelling prosthesis, by radiotherapy or by bypass surgery in which no attempt is made to resect the primary site, but an alternative conduit is created. Patients unsuitable for radical surgery or radiotherapy should always be considered for palliative treatment, particularly if the dysphagia is severe. Modest doses of radiation can result in impressive clinical improvements. In experienced hands, passage of a Celestin endo-oesophageal tube is relatively safe and effective, and can be combined with radiation therapy. Common problems associated with tube insertion include migration of the tube, gastro-oesophageal reflux (sometimes associated with lung aspiration of gastric contents) and retrosternal pain or discomfort. Complications from palliative irradiation should be minimal since dosage is low: treatment to a dose of 30 Gy (3000 rad) in daily fractions over a 2-week period is usually beneficial, provided the dysphagia is not total, and high doses are rarely warranted.

Prognosis

Results of treatment for oesophageal cancer are very poor (Table 14.1). In at least one series

Table 14.1. Survival in oesophageal cancer.*

Results of Surgery
58% of all patients were considered operable
39% of total were resectable
29% resection mortality
18% lived 1 year
9% lived 2 years
4% lived 5 years

Results of Radiotherapy
51% of all patients offered palliative radiotherapy
18% lived 1 year
8% lived 2 years
6% lived 5 years

---

* Modified from Earlam (3)

pre-operative irradiation followed by surgical resection appeared to improve the prognosis (1). Although remarkable figures were claimed by Pearson (2), who treated 123 patients with radiotherapy alone, with a 21% 5-year survival rate, no other author has produced survival figures as good as this and with the generally dismal survival statistics, there is an urgent need for careful comparison of current methods of treatment. Earlam (3) has reviewed the results of treatment in 90 000 patients with carcinoma of the oesophagus and arrived at a overall 5-year survival rate of 6% for radiotherapy and 4% for surgery. However the case selection for surgery and radiotherapy differs and the true advantage of radiotherapy may be greater, since, in general, fitter patients with more localized lesions are likely to have been treated surgically. A randomized prospective trial of surgery versus radiotherapy for localized middle and lower one-third oesophageal cancer would be needed to answer this question.

CARCINOMA OF THE STOMACH

Incidence and aetiology

Cancer of the stomach is declining in incidence but still remains an important cause of mortality. The age-specific incidence is shown in Fig. 14.7. The overall incidence in Britain is 29 per 100 000 for men and 19 per 100 000 for women. In England, as in the United States, there has been a gradual reduction of death rate in the last 20 years. In other countries the incidence is far higher, for example 80 per 100 000 in Japan and 70 per 100 000 in Chile (Fig. 14.8). Environmental causes are suggested by the fact that Japanese migrants to the United States show a reduction in incidence of the tumour but still retain a higher risk than the indigenous population. The likelihood of developing gastric cancer is also related to social class, the disease being twice as common in social classes 4 and 5 as in classes 1 and 2 (Fig. 14.9).

The causes of carcinoma of the stomach are unknown, but genetic, environmental and pre-

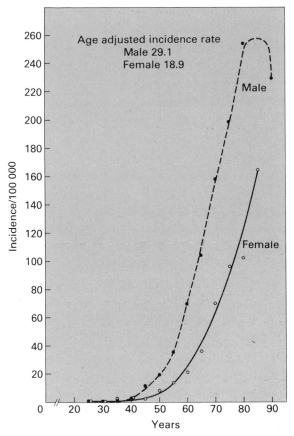

Fig. 14.7. *Age-specific incidence of carcinoma of the stomach* (England).

malignant factors have been implicated. Gastric carcinoma is three to six times commoner in pernicious anaemia which is itself an inherited disorder. The cancer is more common in persons who have blood group A than in the general population, and possibly in patients who have had a Polya partial gastrectomy. Patients with inherited hypogammaglobulinaemia have a greatly increased risk of gastric cancer. Many stomachs resected for gastric cancer show areas of metaplastic change where the stomach epithelium has been replaced by intestinal epithelium. This is associated with well-differentiated tumours and does not generally occur with poorly differentiated carcinomas. The cause of the intestinal metaplasia is not known but dietary factors are possibly important.

There appears to be an increased incidence of carcinoma of the stomach in patients with chronic atrophic gastritis. The increased risk in patients with pernicious anaemia and atrophic gastritis is approximately three-fold, but gastric cancer is most common in the elderly population, many of whom show areas of atrophic gastritis in the absence of carcinoma. The association is therefore tenuous. Gastric atrophy may be followed by intestinal metaplasia and it has been postulated that dietary carcinogens might provoke this change. An hypothesis (4) for the stepwise causation of gastric carcinoma is shown in Fig. 14.10.

In this process it is postulated that gastric atrophy leads to a rise in pH in the stomach and subsequent bacterial colonization which cannot occur at very low pH. The cause of the gastric atrophy is unknown, but it might be related to malnutrition in some countries where there is a high risk of gastric cancer. Bacterial colonization of the stomach is much more common below 50 years of age in these regions. Pernicious anaemia is accompanied by gastric atrophy, and hypoacidity may occur following Polya partial gastrectomy—both being situations where the risk of gastric cancer may be increased.

The result of bacterial colonization may be to reduce dietary nitrates (present in water, vegetables and cured meats) to nitrites, which in turn react with amino-acids to form N-nitroso compounds. These are carcinogens in animals (causing intestinal metaplasia of the gastric mucosa in rats), and may be so in man. If this hypothesis is true, blocking the formation of these compounds in patients at risk may lower the incidence of gastric carcinoma. This might be achieved by ascorbic acid, anti-oxidants (which are often added to foods) or by α tocopherol.

The association with gastric ulcer is uncertain. Much of the apparent association comes from a mistaken diagnosis of benign ulcer in an ulcerating neoplasm. In series where patients with benign gastric ulcer have been followed for several years the incidence of gastric carcinoma

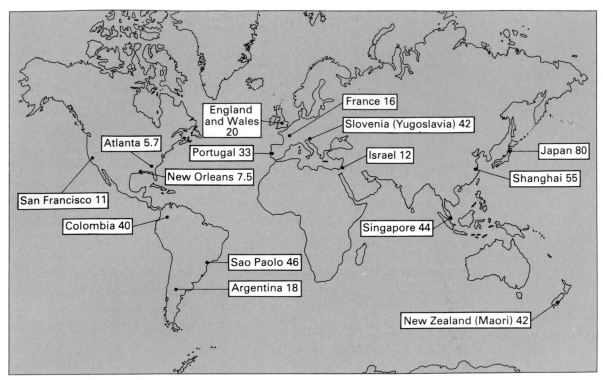

Fig. 14.8. *Geographical incidence of stomach cancer*. Figures indicate incidence per 100 000 male population. USA figures are for whites only; rates are approximately double in blacks.

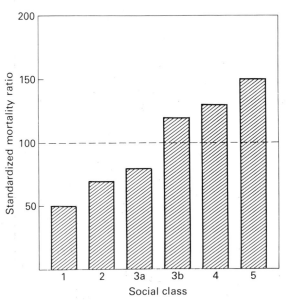

Fig. 14.9. *Gastric cancer mortality related to social class*. Figures are for men aged 15–64 for the years 1970–72 in England and Wales. (Figures from OPCS data 1978.) Values for each social class are in proportion to 100 which represents all social classes combined.

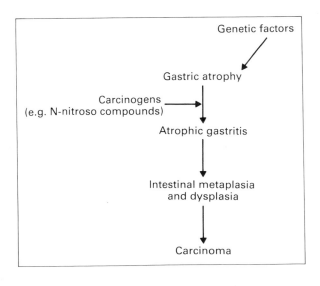

Fig. 14.10. *An hypothesis for the causation of gastric cancer*.

appears to be low, though possibly above that in the normal population. The relationship between gastric polyps and malignancy is also contentious. Gastric polyps are relatively common and 10% of them show evidence of carcimona *in situ*. This change has doubtful prognostic significance, and the lesion which seems most likely to be premalignant is the villous adenoma (5).

Pathology

Over 90% of gastric carcinomas are adenocarcinoma. Carcinoid tumours make up the remainder.

The gross pathology takes on different forms. The commonest is a diffuse infiltrating carcinoma which varies in size from 1 cm to a tumour which may occupy most of the stomach. Typically, it has a rolled thickened edge and an ulcerated central portion, and invades

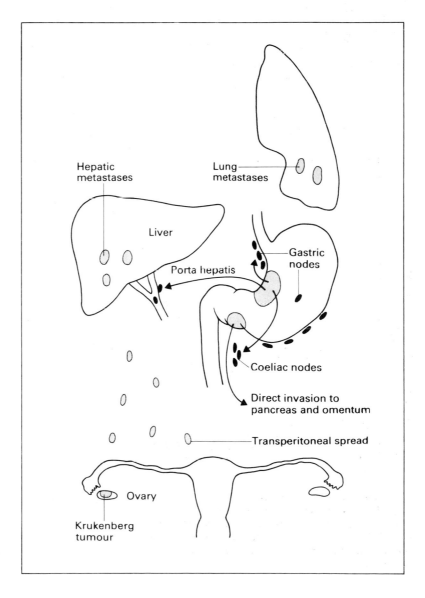

Fig. 14.11. *Common paths of spread in gastric cancer.*

the thickness of the stomach wall spreading into the pancreas and omentum. It metastasises to regional lymph nodes, to the liver and peritoneal cavity. Some tumours exhibit a polypoid growth in which a large fungating tumour projects into the lumen of the stomach, initially growing inside but later invading the stomach wall and adjacent tissues. A less usual type of carcinoma is one which spreads superficially through the mucosa, which does not tend to involve regional lymph nodes until late in the disease and which has a better prognosis. Some cancers of the stomach exhibit a diffuse sclerosis involving the whole of the stomach wall (*linitis plastica*). The stomach is small and contracted and will not distend. This tumour has a very bad prognosis. Cancers tends to arise in the antrum or lower third of the stomach and are more common on the lesser curvature. Some of the tumours are multicentric.

Microscopically the most useful division is made between those carcinomas where the cells resemble intestinal cells and there is intestinal metaplasia surrounding the tumour (intestinal type) and those which tend to infiltrate the gastric wall and are surrounded by normal mucosa (diffuse type). Tumours of the intestinal type are associated with a better survival, tend to occur in older patients and are more likely to be preceded by atrophic gastritis. In high risk populations (such as Japan) most tumours are of this type. The diffuse carcinomas occur more frequently in women, are associated with blood group A, and have a worse overall survival. Infiltrative tumours of the *linitis plastica* type are diffuse carcinomas.

In Japan, screening programmes have resulted in many tumours being diagnosed early, and the term 'early gastric cancer' has been introduced for tumours limited to the mucosa or submucosa. These can be of the intestinal or diffuse types with varying degrees of differentiation. At this stage the prognosis is excellent.

Lymphatic spread of the tumour (Fig. 14.11) is via the superficial lymphatic networks into nodes in the left gastric chain and the splenic and hepatic chains along the lines of major vascular supply to the stomach. Spread is then to nodes in the coeliac plexus, the splenic chain and into the hepatic chain around the porta hepatis. There is sometimes enlargment of nodes in the left supraclavicular region deep to the sternomastoid insertion (Virchow's node). Cancer of the stomach also spreads locally through the stomach wall into the omentum, liver and pancreas. Portions of tumour can break off and seed widely through the peritoneal space causing malignant ascites and Krukenberg tumours on the surface of the ovary. Blood-borne metastases are particularly common in the liver but pulmonary metastases also occur. Bone metastases are uncommon and central nervous system metastases are rare.

Clinical features

One of the great difficulties in diagnosis of carcinoma of the stomach lies in the fact that the initial symptoms are often mild and indefinite. Anorexia, nausea and vague upper abdominal pain are the most notable symptoms, but many patients are only diagnosed at a time when a large epigastric mass is palpable, or when there is malignant ascites making curative resection clearly impossible. Other symptoms include dysphagia, particularly when the tumour involves the cardio-oesophageal junction, and vomiting if there is outflow obstruction from involvement of the antrum. Massive gastro-intestinal bleeding does occur but is unusual. Low-grade bleeding is common and presentation with iron deficiency anaemia not infrequent. Non-metastatic manifestations of malignancy are unusual, but carcinoma of the stomach is one of the commoner causes of acanthosis nigricans (see Chapter 9).

The signs of carcinoma of the stomach are minimal except in the late stages. The patient will usually appear to have lost weight and may be anaemic. Virchow's node may be palpable in the left supraclavicular region and there may be an epigastric mass or hepatomegaly from metastases. Tumour masses may be felt on abdominal or pelvic examination and ascites may be present. All of these signs indicate advanced cancer which is inoperable and incurable.

Diagnosis

The standard diagnostic investigation has been the barium meal examination, and its accuracy has been greatly improved by double contrast techniques. Typically the malignant gastric ulcer shows elevated irregular borders with a poorly circumscribed ulcer crater (Fig. 14.12). In contrast a benign ulcer has sharply defined borders. The mucosal folds are abnormal being fused or tapered next to the carcinoma. Polypoid lesions have a coarse irregular mucosal surface. In antral lesions the volume of resting juice may be large and in *linitis plastica* the stomach appears small and contracted. Infiltrating lesions give the stomach areas of rigidity which can be seen on screening during the examination. The difficulty with barium meal examination is that it is sometimes difficult to distinguish benign from malignant ulceration and that some small carcinomas are missed.

Endoscopy has led to a great improvement in accuracy of diagnosis. Since the introduction of this technique it has become apparent that 10–30% of carcinomas may be missed in their early stages on barium meal examination. For this reason, if the diagnosis is suspected in a patient with persistent anorexia and weight loss, endoscopy should be performed in addition to the barium meal. At endoscopy, cytological washings are taken and multiple biopsies from the ulcer or tumour. A positive biopsy or cytology is obtained in over 90% of patients, except in the infiltrative forms of gastric carcinoma where the diagnosis can be missed both on endoscopic appearance and on cytological examination. In addition to these investigations liver function tests, full blood count and chest X-ray should be carried out, and hepatic ultrasound may be helpful in the detection of hepatic metastases. Serum tumour markers have not been helpful in gastric carcinomas. Carcinoembryonic antigen (CEA) is sometimes elevated but the relationship to tumour mass is too in-

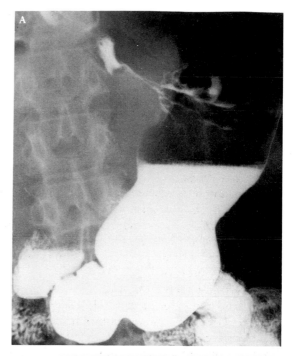

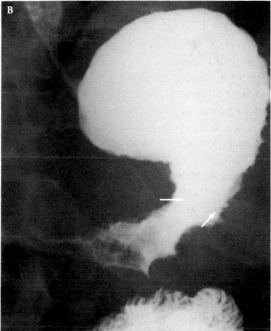

Fig. 14.12. *Barium meal appearances in carcinoma of the stomach.* (A) Carcinoma at cardio-oesophageal junction showing tumour infiltration with mucosal irregularity; (B) *Linitis plastica*. The tumour infiltrates extensively (arrows).

definite to be helpful either in diagnosis or in monitoring therapy.

A TNM staging system has been developed and is shown in Table 14.2.

Table 14.2. TNM Staging system for gastric carcinoma.

T stage
1   Limited to mucosa or submucosa
2   Extension to serosa
3   Extension through serosa
4   Invasion of local structures

N stage
0   No nodes
1   Local node involvement within 3 cm.
2   Node involvement more than 3 cm., but resectable
3   Distant node involvement

M stage
0   No metastases
1   Distant metastases

EARLY DIAGNOSIS OF GASTRIC CARCINOMA

Because so many patients present with inoperable disease, programmes have been devised for screening for the disease in countries such as Japan where there is a very high incidence. In Japan, screening with double contrast radiology in asymptomatic patients has led to a detection rate of only 1:1000. A high incidence (31%) of early carcinomas has been found with an excellent survival following surgery. It is not clear if early gastric cancer will always develop into advanced disease but it is reasonable to assume that this will usually occur. Prompt diagnosis is therefore desirable. Screening asymptomatic populations, especially in low-risk countries, has not proved cost-effective. Screening of patients with upper abdominal symptoms has been suggested as a compromise since 50% of cases of early gastric cancer diagnosed by screening had such symptoms. In countries such as the United Kingdom, such an approach is the only practical possibility in view of the declining incidence of the tumour. However at the

present time it is not even possible to define high-risk groups in whom screening should be undertaken.

Treatment

TREATMENT OF GASTRIC CARCINOMA

Surgical resection is the only curative treatment for gastric carcinoma. A variety of surgical procedures can be performed, depending on the localization of the tumour and the degree of local extension. The most radical surgery involves total gastrectomy, with removal of the entire stomach, part of the duodenum and occasionally even part of the transverse colon if it is involved by local infiltration (Fig. 14.13). For

A

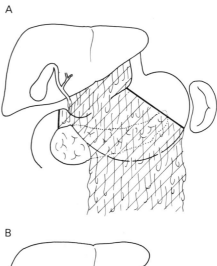

B

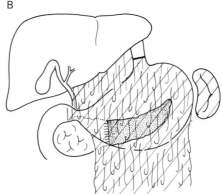

Fig. 14.13. *Operations for gastric carcinoma.* (A) Radical sub-total gastrectomy; (B) extended total gastrectomy.

most localized tumours a partial gastrectomy can be performed. At the present time some form of subtotal gastrectomy is the most generally employed surgical procedure. Total gastrectomy involves removal of the entire stomach, the greater omentum, usually removal of the spleen and occasionally of the lower portion of the oesophagus if the tumour is proximal. In a radical subtotal gastrectomy 80% of the stomach is removed with the omentum and part of the duodenum. The spleen is not usually removed unless the lesion is relatively proximal. The morbidity of total gastrectomy is considerable. There is difficulty in maintaining body weight; the necessity to eat small, frequent meals, and, if the patient survives, the inevitable production of iron and B12 deficient anaemia which requires life-long treatment.

Patients presenting with a large intra-abdominal mass are nearly always inoperable. Other indications of inoperability are malignant ascites, demonstrable nodal deposits or liver metastases. If the tumour is fixed and immobile on barium meal examination it is also likely to be inoperable. Often a decision about the operability can be made only at laparotomy. In inoperable cases bypass procedures are usually unrewarding.

The results of surgery are poor. In European studies only 60% of patients undergoing surgery prove to have resectable tumours. Of these only 20-25% will be alive at 5 years. This gives an overall 5-year survival rate of 10-15% in all operated cases. In Japan the results are much better, with a higher resectability rate (70-75%). Of those resected 55% are alive at 5 years and the overall 5-year survival rate of all operated cases is about 30%. In Japanese studies 15% of cases have early gastric cancer compared with 2.5% in the West.

RADIATION TREATMENT

Palliation of some of the symptoms of gastric carcinoma can occasionally be achieved with radiation. Treatment is difficult since there are numerous radiosensitive organs in the upper abdomen, namely the small intestine, liver, spinal cord and kidneys. A dose of 40 Gy (4000 rad) can usually be administered safely in 4-5 weeks. Anorexia and nausea are frequent and patients usually lose weight during the procedure. The intention is palliative although occasional long term survival has been noted.

CHEMOTHERAPY OF CANCER OF THE STOMACH

Cancer of the stomach is the gastrointestinal carcinoma which is most sensitive to cytotoxic drugs. Some drugs are able to produce response rates of greater than 30% (Table 14.3). Most of these responses are partial and usually last for only a few months. There is no evidence that survival is prolonged by the use of chemotherapy either as single agents or in combination, even though responders will live longer than non-responders as in most other tumours.

The single most effective agent appears to be doxorubicin and the usual dose is $60 \, mg/m^2$ every 3 weeks. 5-Fluorouracil has been widely used but the response rate is relatively low. There has been extensive experience with mitomycin C in Japan, and some trials from that country have reported response rates of 40% though the more general experience has been that the response is less than this. Nitrosoureas and alkylating agents are less useful.

Table 14.3 Response to cytotoxic agents in gastric carcinoma.

Drug	% Response
Single Agents	
Doxorubicin	15-25
5FU	15-20
Mitomycin C	25-30
Nitrosoureas	15
Alkylating agents	10-15
Combination Chemotherapy	
5FU, doxorubicin & mitomycin (FAM)	40-45
5FU, nitrosourea & doxorubicin	25-45
5FU, mitomycin, doxorubicin & nitrosourea	30

Several combination chemotherapy regimes have been used and some of these are shown in Table 14.3. One of the most widely used has been the combination of 5FU, doxorubicin and mitomycin (FAM) with a response rate of about 40% (6). There is no evidence that patients are ever cured by chemotherapy, but useful responses are sometimes seen and effective palliation can sometimes be achieved (7).

Adjuvant chemotherapy. There has been recent interest in the use of chemotherapy as an adjuvant to surgical removal of the tumour. So far most studies have failed to show an improved survival in the chemotherapy treated group compared with surgery alone. At the present time, therefore, adjuvant chemotherapy is not offered as a routine to patients undergoing gastrectomy.

REFERENCES

1 Nakayama K., Oritata H. & Yamaguchi Y. (1967) Surgical treatment combined with preoperative concentrated irradiation for oesophageal cancer. *Cancer* **20**, 778.
2 Pearson J. G. (1966) Radiotherapy of carcinoma of the oesophagus and post cricoid region in S.E. Scotland. *Clinical Radiology* **17**, 242.
3 Earlam R. & Cunha-Melo J. R. (1980) Oesophageal squamous cell carcinoma: I. A critical review of surgery. II. A critical review of radiotherapy. *British Journal of Surgery* **67**, 381, 457.
4 Correa P., Haenszel W., Cuello C. Tannerbaum S. & Archer M. (1975) A model for gastric cancer epidemiology. *Lancet* **ii**, 58–60.
5 Ming S. C. & Goldman H. (1965) Gastric polyps: a histogenetic classification and its relation to carcinoma. *Cancer* **18**, 721.
6 MacDonald J. S., Schein P. S., Woolley P. V. *et al* (1980) 5 Fluorouracil, mitomycin C and adriamycin (FAM): A new combination chemotherapy program for advanced gastric carcinoma. Annals Internal Medicine **93**, 533.
7 Earl H. M., Coombes R. C. & Schein P. S. (1984) Cytotoxic Chemotherapy for Cancer of the Stomach. *Clinics in Oncology* **3** (2), 351.

Chapter 15

Cancer of the Liver, Biliary Tract and Pancreas

PRIMARY LIVER CANCER

There are four types of primary carcinoma which arise in the liver. The most frequent is hepatocellular carcinoma which, in Britain, is about ten times more common than cholangio-carcinoma of the intra hepatic bile ducts which in turn is ten times more frequent than malignant haemangioendothelioma. Hepatoblastoma is a rare tumour of childhood. The importance of hepatocellular carcinoma is disproportionate to its incidence in the west, because there are now many clues about its aetiology and pathogenesis.

Hepatocellular carcinoma (hepatoma)

INCIDENCE

In Britain and the United States the incidence is approximately 1.8 per 100 000 for men and 0.7 for women (Fig. 15.1). The tumour can arise in childhood. Worldwide the incidence (per 100 000) varies greatly—104 in Mozambique, 29 in S Africa, 12 in Nigeria.

AETIOLOGY

In the West, most cases of hepatocellular carcinoma arise in cirrhotic livers. When the disease arises in a non-cirrhotic liver the patient is usually younger than when there is associated cirrhosis. The causes of cirrhosis with the highest risk of developing a hepatoma are chronic hepatitis associated with hepatitis B, and haemochromatosis. Hepatoma is much more common in alcoholic cirrhosis where there is evi-

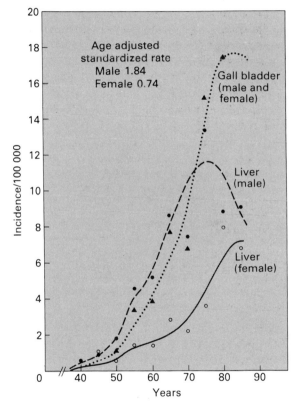

Fig. 15.1. *Age-specific incidence of cancer of the liver and gall bladder—UK figures.*

dence of previous hepatitis B infection, and is infrequent in patients who have not been infected. Patients with primary biliary cirrhosis and HbsAg negative chronic active hepatitis are less at risk (although more likely to develop the cancer than the non-cirrhotic population). The carcinoma is much more likely to develop in men (M:F 11:1) and in patients with long standing cirrhosis over the age of 50. The association

261

with cirrhosis is found in both high and low incidence areas. The duration of the cirrhosis is more important than the aetiology. The risk of development of hepatocellular carcinoma in a cirrhotic liver after 20 years is about 5% in women and 20% in men.

In Britain, 15-20% of cases are HbsAg +ve and studies in the Far East have shown a risk of 230:1 in HbsAg +ve individuals (1). Viral DNA sequences have been demonstrated in the genome of liver cells of HbsAg positive individuals and in hepatocellular carcinoma cells (2), but a direct causal link with the virus is not proven. It may be that virus infection is a predisposing, but not sufficient, cause of the disease. Epidemiological evidence has also implicated the *Aspergillus flavus* mould which grows on stored grain and which produces aflatoxin. This toxin may be one of many factors which act as promotors in tumour formation.

PATHOLOGY

In 60% of cases the liver contains multiple nodules of cancer. In 30% of cases there is a large single mass of cancer often with surrounding lesions, and, in the remaining cases, the liver is diffusely infiltrated. In 80% of cases the surrounding liver is cirrhotic. In the group of patients where it is not, the sex ratio is equal and the average age is lower. In a small subgroup of the patients without cirrhosis, the tumour forms cords with collagen strands (fibrolamellar carcinoma). In cholangiocarcinoma of the intrahepatic ducts the tumour cells form a tubular pattern usually with extensive fibrosis.

CLINICAL FEATURES

In a cirrhotic patient the development of hepatocellular carcinoma is often accompanied by a rapid deterioration in liver function. Usually the cirrhosis is advanced and long standing. Presentation is, therefore, with liver failure, jaundice, right upper quadrant pain and ascites. Ascites may be due to cirrhosis, or to the sudden onset of the Budd-Chiari syndrome due to hepatic vein occlusion. In the non-cirrhotic patient the presentation is typically with abdominal pain and a right upper quadrant mass.

On examination the patient is usually gravely ill with evidence of cirrhosis and liver failure. The liver is enlarged with a palpable mass over which there may be a bruit. There may also be a moderate fever.

DIAGNOSIS

Liver function tests have no diagnostic pattern or value but are always abnormal. The tumour may produce erythropoietin and secondary polycythaemia may therefore be present. Hypercalcaemia may occur, in most cases due to bone metastases, but in other cases it is postulated that the tumour produces parathormone-like substances. Other non-metastatic manifestations include hypoglycaemia, gonadotrophin production, ectopic ACTH and elevated plasma calcitonin (see also Chapter 9).

The malignant hepatocytes in most hepatomas produce alphafeto protein (AFP) which can be detected in the serum (3). With sensitive methods the serum AFP can be of diagnostic help. Levels below 10 ng/ml make the diagnosis very unlikely in a cirrhotic patient, although over half of non-cirrhotic patients do not have an elevated serum AFP. Levels from 10–500 ng/ml make the diagnosis probable but cirrhosis due to chronic hepatitis may be associated with levels of this magnitude (as may metastases from the gastrointestinal tract). In the West, levels above 500 ng/ml in a cirrhotic patient make the diagnosis of hepatocellular carcinoma almost certain.

Isotope and ultrasound liver scans may show a large filling defect or multiple defects, but in the presence of cirrhosis the appearances may not be diagnostic and care must be taken in interpretation. Angiography may show a tumour circulation but is usually only carried out if there is a possibility of surgical resection of the tumour or if intra-arterial chemotherapy or embolization is considered.

A biopsy of the lesion will help in diagnosis

but may not be possible if liver function has deteriorated. If the prothrombin time is prolonged by more than 4 seconds, the procedure is unsafe since the tumours are vascular. Even with a biopsy, the histological distinction from metastatic tumours (such as hypernephroma) may be difficult.

TREATMENT

Resection of the tumour offers a chance of cure. It must be considered particularly in a non-cirrhotic patient because the liver will regenerate even if three-quarters of the organ is removed. In a cirrhotic patient resection will usually precipitate a deterioration of liver function. Resection is therefore applicable to less than 5% of patients.

Embolization or ligation of the hepatic artery has been used, but these procedures also cause deterioration of function in the cirrhotic patient. Selective hepatic artery embolization may be attempted in a cirrhotic, if the tumour is localized. The value of this technique has not been adequately assessed, but pain may be relieved.

Chemotherapy may produce tumour regression, and the single most useful agent is doxorubicin (Table 15.1). This is usually given at 50–70 mg/m² every 3 weeks, but the dose should

Table 15.1. Chemotherapy of hepatocellular carcinoma.

Drug	Approximate response rate%
Doxorubicin	20
5FU	15
5FU, doxorubicin	20
5FU, nitrosurea	15

be halved if the bilirubin is twice normal since the drug is detoxified by the liver. The response to chemotherapy can be assessed by pain, AFP levels, and ultrasound or CT scan. No advantage for combination chemotherapy has been demonstrated.

RADIOTHERAPY

The liver does not tolerate radiotherapy to a high dose since radiation-induced hepatitis occurs with increasing frequency above 25–30 Gy. Fatal hepatic damage occurs when the dose to the whole liver is above 38 Gy. The value of radiotherapy in hepatoma is uncertain since for most patients the prognosis is poor. Regression of the tumour and relief of pain was reported in 50% of cases treated with a total dose of 30 Gy (4).

PROGNOSIS

When a hepatoma arises in a cirrhotic liver the prognosis is very bad, and 50% of all patients are dead in 3 months with no survivors at 12 months. Without cirrhosis only 10% will be alive at 2 years. The prognosis is better in patients who have a complete surgical resection or who show a complete response to chemotherapy.

Angiosarcoma (malignant haemangioendothelioma)

These malignant vascular tumours arise in normal livers. They are rare, but of interest since they are known to occur in workers who have had chronic exposure to polyvinylchloride (PVC). The tumours develop 15–20 years after exposure to PVC. They have also been reported in patients who have received thorotrast (a radioactive contrast agent used diagnostically in 1930–1950). The presentation is of a painful hepatic mass, and diagnosis is made by biopsy. Surgical resection may be possible.

Hepatoblastoma

This rare tumour occurs in childhood. The tumour is associated with anomalies such as hemihypertrophy, and with storage diseases and the Fanconi syndrome. The pathological features are of immature hepatic epithelial cells or a mixture of these cells with mesenchymal elements. It usually arises in the right lobe and presents with a visible asymptomatic mass which later causes pain and weight loss. Like hepatocellular carcinoma (which can also occur in children over 5 years of age) the tumour produces AFP. It can be demonstrated by isotopic ultrasound and CT scanning but arteriography gives the best localization and is essential if resection is to be attempted.

The tissue diagnosis is usually made at operation when an attempt at resection is made. It does not appear possible to cure these children without complete surgical excision. Up to 75% of the liver can be removed but haemorrhage can be severe and great skill is necessary.

Postoperative chemotherapy is usually given. Doxorubicin is the most effective agent but responses are also reported to alkylating agents and nitrosources (5). Occasionally, unresectable cases can be made to respond to chemotherapy so that surgery can be performed, and there is growing interest in pre-operative chemotherapy in this disease. Serum AFP can be used to assess response.

Carcinoid tumours

The curious name of these tumours was coined in 1907 to emphasize the benign course which they follow, although they are usually malignant or become so with time.

PATHOLOGY

Localized intestinal carcinoids are present in 0.5% of autopsies, usually near the appendix or along the small bowel or descending colon. There are, however, many other sites at which carcinoids may occur—bronchus, thymus, pancreas as well as any part of the gastrointestinal tract, ovary and testis (6).

Appendiceal carcinoids are usually near the tip. The tendency to metastasize is related to size; tumours less than 1 cm in size are rarely associated with metastases while 80% of those greater than 3 cms have metastasized. Metas-tases are much more common with small bowel carcinoids than with appendiceal tumours.

Macroscopically carcinoid tumours are often yellow or orange in colour. Microscopically they consist of densely packed epithelial cells which stain with silver nitrate (argentaffinomas). They are often regarded as being part of the APUD series of cells (see p. 272) and contain a variety of substances which, when secreted give rise to the carcinoid syndrome. The development of this clinical syndrome is related to tumour size, the presence of metastases, and the site of origin (the syndrome being rare with distal colon tumours). Both primary and secondary tumours are usually slow growing. The commonest metastatic site is the liver. Lung and bone are less frequently involved.

CLINICAL FEATURES

Local symptoms. The patient may present with local symptoms due to metastases. Pain in the right upper quadrant, due to distension of the liver by metastases, is a frequent symptom and later, weight loss, anorexia and malaise occur as liver function deteriorates. Primary intestinal carcinoids are seldom diagnosed during life unless they cause obstruction, intussusception or pain in the right iliac fossa leading to appendicectomy.

The malignant carcinoid syndrome. This syndrome occurs in about 50% of all patients with hepatic metastases from carcinoid tumours. A variety of chemicals is produced by the tumour and their release is accompanied by symptoms which may dominate the clinical picture (7). The syndrome is particularly likely to occur with bronchial carcinoid even without hepatic metastases, since the venous drainage is into the systemic circulation and not via the liver which metabolises the pharmacological mediators liberated by intestinal carcinoids.

5-hydroxytryptamine(5HT) is produced from tryptophan. A metabolite of 5HT, 5-hydroxyindoleacetic acid (5HIAA), is excreted in the urine. When present in excess it confirms the diagnosis. 5HT is quickly inactivated in the lungs and liver, so large quantities must be produced to cause symptoms. The release of 5HT is probably responsible for diarrhoea. The diarrhoea is typically episodic, watery and may be explosive leading to incontinence. It is often accompanied by noisy abdominal gurgles and cramping pains. Excess 5HT is probably responsible for endocardial fibrosis which can lead to tricuspid incompetence, which in turn may cause right-sided heart failure with ascites, and deep cyanosis in the flushed face. Bradykinin is produced by some tumours and may be partly responsible for the flushing which is characteristic of the syndrome. The flush is at first intermittent, often being precipitated by emotion and alcohol. The face and neck become red and the patient may perspire. It lasts a few minutes and is reminiscent of the flushing of menopausal women. Later the flushing becomes more frequent and some patients become almost permanently flushed. Telangiectases occur on the face, and skin may be come thickened. Prostaglandins are liberated from some tumours and may contribute to both the flushing and the diarrhoea. Bronchospasm occurs and has been variously attributed to histamine, bradykinin and prostaglandins. It is episodic at first but permanent wheezing dyspnoea may develop. Episodes of hypotension are sometimes seen and are thought to be caused by 5HT.

Other clinical features. The tumours are slow growing and the diagnosis is often missed or delayed for months or years. If all the symptoms are present the diagnosis is easy to think of, but if the complaint is of diarrhoea alone, numerous negative investigations for colon cancer or malabsorption may lead to the patient being labelled neurotic or having 'irritable bowel syndrome'. Similarly, late onset asthma may be diagnosed before the rest of the clinical picture becomes apparent. Bronchial carcinoids usually present with unilateral airways obstructions and haemoptyses. Carcinoids in the bronchus, thymus and pancreas occasionally cause Cushing's syndrome, since in some cases production of ACTH by the tumour leads to bilateral adrenal hyperplasia. The primary tumour may be small and only detectable by CT scanning of the thorax or abdomen.

DIAGNOSIS

In the patients without the carcinoid syndrome the diagnosis is made by the primary tumour in the bowel causing abdominal symptoms leading to laparotomy or, in the lung, symptoms of a bronchial adenoma leading to bronchoscopy or thoracotomy. Secondary deposits in the liver are usually diagnosed by liver biopsy.

In patients with the carcinoid syndrome the 24 hour urinary 5HIAA is usually elevated. False-positive results can be obtained with 5HT containing foods (bananas contain 4 mg of 5HT). In some patients the urinary 5HIAA excretion may vary from day to day and this leads to false-negative results and makes 5HIAA excretion an unreliable guide to treatment. Foregut carcinoids may produce 5-hydroxytryptophan and not 5HIAA.

MANAGEMENT

Localized intestinal, bronchial or foregut carcinoids should be removed surgically. In metastatic carcinoid surgery should be considered if liver secondaries are found which are well localized and which are resectable. This may relieve symptoms for months or years because the tumour is slow growing. Another means of reducing the tumour mass is hepatic artery ligation or embolization. All of these surgical approaches may result in a sudden release of large quantities of pharmacologically active agents resulting in hypotension and bronchospasm. Intravenous methysergide may be used to treat bronchospasm during surgery, and methoxamine to treat hypotension. Complications of surgery and embolization include necrosis of the gall bladder and *Clostridium welchii* infections in necrotic tumour.

In patients with metastatic disease with the carcinoid syndrome which cannot be treated surgically, the usual approach is to attempt to block the pharmacological effects of the tumours in the first instance. However, this is usually only partially successful since each symptom may be produced by more than one agent and pharmacological antagonists are partially effective against some tumour products and do not exist for others.

Diarrhoea. This may be mitigated by simple measures such as codeine phosphate, diphenoxylate or loperamide. The 5HT antagonist methysergide is sometimes effective. Methysergide may itself cause abdominal cramp and nausea, and prolonged administration carries the risk of mediastinal and retroperitoneal fibrosis. Cyproheptadine antagonizes 5HT and also blocks the histamine (H_1) receptor. It may be effective in controlling diarrhoea, and interestingly, may occasionally cause tumour regression. The drug may cause dry mouth and drowsiness. Methyldopa inhibits 5HT synthesis but the results in carcinoid are disappointing.

Parachlorophenylalanine (PCPA) inhibits any enzyme (tryptophan 5-hydroxylase) which is involved in 5HT synthesis. It will reduce urinary 5HIAA and control diarrhoea. It is toxic causing lethargy, headache, mental changes and allergic eosinophilia, the latter occurring in 50% of patients necessitating cessation of treatment.

Flushing. Bradykinin may be partially antagonized by phenothiazines and, since catecholamines can provoke bradykinin release, alpha adrenergic blockage with phentolamine may also have some effect. Prostaglandin effects may occasionally be partly alleviated by indomethacin.

Bronchospasm. Agents that block histamine (cyproheptadine) bradykinin (phenothiazines) can be tried as can conventional bronchodilators but the results are often disappointing. Isoprenaline may help.

Cytotoxic chemotherapy is usually ineffective. It is the only direct treatment for widespread liver metastases and may be indicated if the carcinoid syndrome is uncontrollable by other means. In this situation sudden destruction of the tumour may lead to release of tumour products with severe asthma, diarrhoea and flushing.

The agents with activity are streptozotocin, 5FU, cyclophosphamide and doxorubicin. Streptozotocin is probably the most effective drug. Responses to the other agents are infrequent (10–20%) but combinations of doxorubicin, 5FU and cyclophosphamide will produce temporary responses in about 30% of patients. Infusions of 5FU into the hepatic artery may reduce pain and tumour bulk. It is not known if this is more effective than full doses of the drug intravenously. There is no evidence that these regimens prolong survival since the tumour grows slowly if left untreated. They may however produce symptomatic benefit. Tumour regression has also been observed with cyproheptadine.

CANCER OF THE GALL BLADDER AND BILIARY TRACT

Incidence and aetiology

Cancer of the gall bladder and biliary tract has an equal incidence in men and women, most cases occurring after the age of 65 (Fig. 15.1) when it is commoner than hepatocellular carcinoma. Gall-stones are a predisposing cause but the incidence of gall bladder cancer in patients with untreated cholelithiasis is probably not more than 2%, which does not justify surgery for asymptomatic gall-stones. Worldwide, liver flukes are the major predisposing cause (*Clonorchis sinensis*, *Opisthorcis felineus*). These flukes produce a chronic sclerosing cholangitis which appears to be premalignant. Bile duct cancer is also associated with ulcerative colitis, occurring in approximately 0.5% of cases (8).

Pathology

Carcinoma of the gall bladder, which is the commonest cancer of the biliary system, usually arises in the body and only rarely in the cystic duct (4% of cases). The tumours are usually adenocarcinomas (85%) but anaplastic (6%) and squamous (4%) histologies occur.

Half of all bile duct cancers develop in the distal common duct, with carcinoma of the ampulla of Vater being the second commonest biliary cancer. The cancers arise in the proximal duct in 30% of cases and proximal to the porta hepatis in a further 20%. They are almost always adenocarcinomas, usually well-differentiated and sometimes with a fibrous stroma.

All these tumours spread locally and to regional lymph nodes and there may be multiple primary bile duct tumours. From these nodes, lymphatic spread is to the coeliac and aortic nodes. Hepatic metastases are common. Gall bladder cancer may seed into the peritoneum and both types of cancer may directly invade the liver. Carcinoma of the ampulla is usually slow growing and causes obstructive jaundice early before it has spread widely. The tumour often ulcerates and sometimes bleeds and the jaundice may fluctuate if the tumour sloughs. This form of biliary tract cancer has the best prognosis.

Clinical features

Cancer of the gall bladder usually presents with right upper quadrant pain, later with nausea, vomiting, weight loss and obstructive jaundice. Because of pre-existing gall-stones the symptoms may be attributed to this cause at first and the diagnosis delayed.

Cancer of the biliary tree presents similarly but usually causes obstructive jaundice. At this stage the tumour is often advanced. The gall bladder may be enlarged and palpable if the distal duct is obstructed.

Diagnosis

The diagnosis of early gall bladder carcinoma is difficult because the symptoms suggest gall-stone disease. By the time a mass is palpable surgical resection may be impossible. A chole-

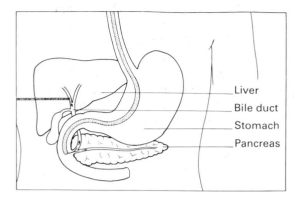

Fig. 15.2. *Percutaneous cholangiography and Endoscopic Retrograde Cholangio-Pancreatography (ERCP).*

cystogram is often unhelpful, because the gall bladder is non-functioning. Ultrasound and CT scan may show a mass, but in the majority of cases the diagnosis is only made at a laparotomy for presumed gall-stone disease. In carcinoma of the extrahepatic bile ducts, obstructive jaundice leads to investigation. Percutaneous transhepatic cholangiograms may give an outline of the proximal ducts, and endoscopic retrograde cholangiopancreatography (ERCP) may demonstrate the lower end of the block and provide material for cytological examination (Fig. 15.2). The transhepatic route may allow a catheter to be placed past the lesion with relief of jaundice either pre-operatively or as a palliative procedure.

Treatment

SURGERY

When a gall bladder carcinoma is found at laparotomy the surgeon must decide if it can be resected. The experience of the surgeon is an important factor in this decision. The results of simple cholecystectomy are not good since the tumour may be locally extensive. Portions of the liver may have to be removed for complete excision. Distant lymph node spread may have occurred and surgical excision deemed unwise, and a palliative procedure is then undertaken, if possible with biliary decompression.

A Radical pancreaticoduodenectomy

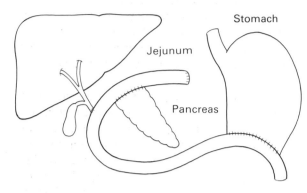

B Total pancreatectomy

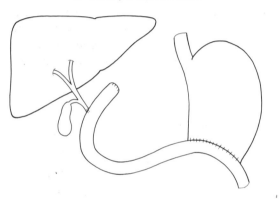

Fig. 15.3. *Surgical operations for cancer of the bile ducts and pancreas.*

In the surgical management of bile duct cancer it is of great value to have the extent of the tumour defined pre-operatively by radiographic means. Diffuse intraductal spread cannot be resected. Spread into the intrahepatic ducts, invasion of blood vessels and distant lymph nodes and peritoneal and hepatic metastases are also indications of unresectability. Microscopic examination of bile duct carcinomas often reveals intramural spread. In spite of formidable surgical difficulties, tumours at the junction of the right and left hepatic ducts can sometimes be removed as can mid and distal duct tumours, the latter by radical pancreaticoduodenectomy (Fig. 15.3).

In all, only 15% of bile duct cancers will be operable and major resections have a high mortality (10–15%). Palliative relief of obstruction may be obtained by bypass operation but internal bile duct drainage by non-surgical procedures is now becoming a preferred method of palliation. Carcinoma of the ampulla has the most favourable prognosis with a 5-year survival of 25–30% after radical pancreaticoduodenectomy.

RADIOTHERAPY

Many patients with biliary tract cancer have a localized but unresectable tumour. In these cases effective control can for a time be achieved with radiotherapy. The dose is usually 40–50 Gy in daily fractions, but the treatment details depend on the volume and site of the irradiation. Relief of pain and obstructive jaundice may be achieved.

CHEMOTHERAPY

There has been little systematic study of the role of chemotherapy in biliary tract cancer. Responses have been reported with 5FU, mitomycin and doxorubicin, but are usually short-lived.

CANCER OF THE EXOCRINE PANCREAS

Incidence and aetiology

The incidence of carcinoma of the pancreas is slowly rising. At present it is 15 per 100 000 in men and 13 per 100 000 in women (Fig. 15.4). The condition has a high mortality, less than 1% of patients surviving 5 years. The disease is twice as common in diabetes mellitus. There is possibly an increased incidence in patients with calcific pancreatitis which is, in turn, associated with excess alcohol consumption.

Pathology

The great majority of histologically verified tumours are adenocarcinomas (Table 15.2),

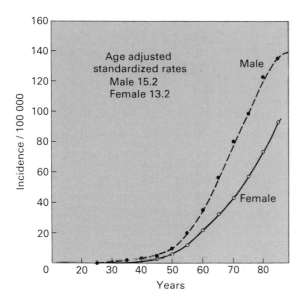

Fig. 15.4. *Age-specific incidence of cancer of the exocrine pancreas—UK figures.*

though in many patients, a histological diagnosis is never established. The adenocarcinomas are thought to arise from the ductular epithelium and those arising in large ducts tend to be more often mucin-producing than those originating in ductules. An intense fibrotic reaction often accompanies the tumour. Cystadenocarcinoma (1%) has a particularly good prognosis. Acinar cell tumours constitute 5% of

Table 15.2. Pancreatic tumours.

Tumours of exocrine pancreas

Adenocarcinoma
Acinar cell tumour
Sarcoma

Tumours of endocrine pancreas	*% malignant*
Islet cell tumours	20
Gastrinoma	70
Glucagonoma	60
VIPoma	90
Carcinoids	not known
Somatostatinoma	90

the total. Sarcoma of the pancreas is a rare disease, usually occurring in childhood.

The exocrine pancreas has an extensive lymphatic drainage along blood vessels. Spread to local nodes has usually occurred by the time of presentation in tumours of both the body and tail.

The head of the pancreas is the site of the tumour in 65% of cases, body and tail in 30% and tail alone in 5%. Local spread occurs and accounts for many of the clinical features (Fig. 15.5). Tumours in the head spread into the duodenum, obstruct the bile duct, spread back into the retroperitoneal space and forward into the lesser sac and peritoneal cavity. The portal vein may be infiltrated and tumours of the body and tail may occlude the splenic vein and extend into the transverse colon and spleen. Metastatic spread to the peritoneum, liver and lung are frequent.

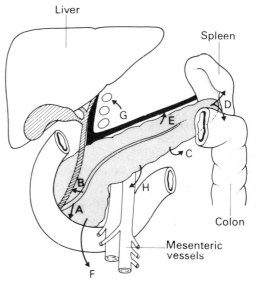

Fig. 15.5. *Sites of spread and production of symptoms in adenocarcinoma of the pancreas.* (A) To duodenum: pain, vomiting, obstruction; (B) to bile duct and pancreas: jaundice, pancreatitis; (C) to retroperitoneum: back pain; (D) to spleen and colon: left upper quadrant pain; (E) to portal and splenic vein: varices, splenomegaly, hepatic disorders; (F) to peritoneal cavity: ascites; (G) to lymph nodes: obstructive jaundice; (H) to blood stream: distant metastases.

Clinical features

Pain and weight loss are the most frequent symptoms (9). With tumours of the head the pain is usually epigastric, and with the tail it may be in the left upper quadrant. The pain gradually becomes severe and unremitting, is often nocturnal and extends into the back as retroperitoneal structures are invaded. The patient may get relief by bending forwards. Acute exacerbations may be due to episodes of pancreatitis. Left-sided abdominal pain and altered bowel habit may be caused by infiltration of the colon by tumours of the body or tail. Mental depression is said to be common but it is not clear if this is more marked in pancreatic cancer than in other causes of serious illness. Acinar cell carcinoma may be accompanied by a syndrome of patchy inflammation and necrosis of subcutaneous fat with polyarthralgia and eosinophilia. There are high levels of lipase in serum. The syndrome resembles relapsing panniculitis (Weber-Christian disease). Another non-metastatic manifestation of pancreatic carcinoma is superficial migratory thrombophlebitis (see Chapter 9). Oesophageal varices may develop if the portal vein is occluded and may lead to gastro-intestinal bleeding. Diabetes mellitus may be the presenting feature and carcinoma of the pancreas must be kept in mind in elderly patients developing glycosuria.

Obstructive jaundice is frequent and eventually occurs in 90% of patients with tumours of the head. It is usually progressive, although fluctuations may occur if the tumour sloughs. It is much less common in tumours of the body and tail. Fever may occur due to cholangitis. The gall bladder is not usually palpable—unlike a bile duct or ampullary carcinoma. Peritoneal dissemination leads to malignant ascites which is present in 15% of cases at diagnosis.

Investigation and diagnosis

It is difficult to diagnose early pancreatic carcinoma at the stage before obstruction of the bile duct or infiltration of the duodenum. It should be considered in any patient with unexplained continued upper abdominal pain. Barium examinations are usually helpful only when the tumour is large. There may be enlargement of the duodenal loop and displacement of the gastric antrum and posterior wall. The tumour may have infiltrated the duodenal and gastric mucosa and this may be seen as an abnormal pattern on the barium meal.

In recent years diagnosis of smaller tumours and tumours of the body and tail, has become somewhat easier with the use of ultrasound and CT scanning. Ultrasound examination of the pancreas is, however, a procedure requiring considerable experience on the part of the radiologist and false-negative results are not infrequent. CT scanning may show a pancreatic mass or extension of the pancreas into the fat space surrounding it and there may also be evidence of metastatic spread to adjacent nodes and the liver (Fig. 15.5). If a mass is found, fine-needle aspiration may give a cytological diagnosis. Selective coeliac and superior mesenteric artery angiograms may be of diagnostic value but are seldom performed since the advent of CT scanning.

When the disease presents with obstructive jaundice, transhepatic cholangiography (10) and endoscopic retrograde cholangiopancreatography (ERCP) will usually be performed (Fig. 15.2). The transhepatic approach will show the proximal site of obstruction and help to distinguish the tumour from carcinoma of the gall bladder, ampulla or bile ducts. ERCP may show stenosis of the main pancreatic duct or compression of the common bile duct by tumour. Specimens for cytology can be taken from the pancreatic duct. ERCP has a high diagnostic accuracy (75-85%), but early diagnosis, before biliary obstruction has occurred remains the clinical problem because symptoms are often late or non-specific. Carcinoembryonic antigen (CEA) is present in the serum of most patients but is also found in other gastro-intestinal diseases and in acute pancreatitis. A pancreatic oncofetal antigen has been described, but, like CEA, is not specific for the disease.

Treatment

SURGERY

Radical surgical resection offers the only hope of cure. Radical pancreaticoduodenectomy and total pancreatectomy are formidable surgical procedures (Fig. 15.3). Preservation of part of the pancreas is desirable but there are considerable problems with fistula formation at the anastomotic site. Total pancreatectomy leads to major problems with diabetes and lack of exocrine function.

Few patients are suitable for surgery, because at the time of diagnosis there is often nodal or distant metastases or a large infiltrating mass which is clearly inoperable. Careful definition of the extent of the tumour pre-operatively is essential. In general only tumours involving the body or tail will prove to be operable. In operable cases the mortality is 15–20% and 5-year survival not greater than 15%.

If the tumour cannot be removed, the obstruction can be relieved by a biliary bypass procedure. This is usually performed surgically, but recently it has become possible to place catheters in the biliary tree by the percutaneous transhepatic route or via the ampulla of Vater.

RADIOTHERAPY

Palliation, especially of pain, can be achieved by radiotherapy. With external beam irradiation the dose required is high (50–60 Gy). Several recent reports (11) have suggested that a few patients may achieve long term remission and occasionally cure. Intestitial radiation using I^{125} implants has also been used, sometimes supplemented with external beam irradiation. Ultrasound and CT imaging are of great help in planning treatment.

CHEMOTHERAPY

Few cytotoxic drugs are effective in pancreatic cancer (Table 15.3). Responses are sometimes seen with 5FU, nitrosoureas, mitomycin C and

Table 15.3. Chemotherapy of Pancreatic Cancer.

	Approximate response rate%
Single Agents	
5 Fluorouracil	25
Alkylating agents	?20
Streptozotocin	25
Mitomycin	25
Doxorubicin	10
Nitrosureas	10
Drug Combinations	
5FU, mitomycin, doxorubicin	40
5FU, streptozotoxin, mitomycin	35
5FU, BCNU	30

alkylating agents. The criteria for response differ in the various studies and most responses are small in degree and short in duration. Combination chemotherapy has improved the response rate a little (12) but complete responses are rare and the patients are never cured. The toxicity of treatment makes chemotherapy unsuitable for the majority of patients because of ill health and advanced disease at presentation.

PALLIATIVE TREATMENT

Pain may be relieved by analgesics, but radiotherapy may be helpful in preventing the need for opiates for several months. Chemical block using alcohol into the coeliac plexus is difficult but sometimes very helpful in relieving pain. Percutaneous drainage of the biliary tree may relieve itching and steatorrhoea due to obstructive jaundice. Steroids may help improve appetite for a while.

ENDOCRINE TUMOURS OF THE PANCREAS

A variety of endocrine tumours may develop in the pancreas (Table 15.2). Although they are uncommon, they are of importance both because they present with symptoms due to the excess hormone production and can therefore be difficult to diagnose, and because they shed light on the normal function of the endocrine pancreas. In recent years it has been proposed that these tumours originate in a single system of cells.

The APUD System

It has been postulated that there is a system of cells derived from neural crest or neuroectoderm which have particular biochemical characteristics characterized by uptake and decarboxylation of amines such as dopa and 5-hydroxytryptophan. The Amine Precursors Uptake and Decarboxylation (APUD) system is proposed as the cell of origin in medullary carcinoma of the thyroid, carcinoid tumours, small cell lung cancer, endocrine tumours of the pancreas, phaeochromocytoma, neuroblastoma and others. The concept of the APUD system has been put forward by Pearse (13) in particular but there is debate as to whether the concept can be used to account for the origin of these tumours. The hypothesis does however help to explain the syndromes of multiple endocrine neoplasms.

Multiple endocrine neoplasms (MEN)

Three syndromes are recognized:
1 *MEN 1 (Wermer syndrome)* This consists of hyperplasia or adenomas of parathyroids and tumours of islet cells, pituitary, adrenal cortex and thyroid (in order of frequency). Patients usually present with hypercalcaemia. Hypoglycaemia or pituitary tumour are less common. The pancreatic islet cell tumour may be malignant. It is usually an insulinoma but gastrinoma, glucagonoma or VIPoma may occur (see below). The condition is inherited as an autosomal dominant, and usually presents age 20–60 years.
2 *MEN II (Sipple syndrome)* This consists of medullary carcinoma of the thyroid phaeochromocytoma and parathyroid hyperplasia. The phaeochromocytoma is often bilateral. About 10% of all cases of medullary carcinoma

of the thyroid are part of the MEN II or MEN III syndrome. The syndrome usually presents with symptoms of a phaeochromocytoma or with a lump in the neck. It can occur at any age. The plasma calcitonin is elevated if medullary carcinoma of the thyroid is present and since C-cell hyperplasia precedes the development of malignancy, siblings of patients should have the plasma calcitonin measured. Treatment of these tumours is discussed in Chapter 20. The condition is also autosomal dominant.
3 *MEN III (mucosal neuroma syndrome)* In this condition phaechromocytoma and medullary carcinoma of the thyroid also occur (as in MEN II) but the patients also have neuromas of the lips, tongue, mouth and entire gut. There may be hypextensible joints, per cavus and soft tissue prognathism. The management is of the thyroid carcinoma and phaeochromocytoma as in MEN II. Parathyroid hyperplasia is less frequent than in MEN II.

Insuloma

PATHOLOGY

These are tumours of the beta cells of the islets. They produce proinsulin which is converted to insulin. The insulin is secreted with its connecting C peptide (which joins the 2 chains). The tumours are often small and arise with equal frequency in head, body and tail, and 20% are multiple and an equal number malignant. About 5% are associated with MEN I syndrome. The diagnosis of malignancy is difficult histologically but metastases occur to liver and adjacent nodes in about 10% of cases.

CLINICAL FEATURES

The patient presents with symptoms of excess insulin production: loss of consciousness, dizziness, episodic mental confusion and weakness. As the condition progresses the mental confusion is present most of the time and irreversible dementia may occur. It usually presents in middle life but can occur at any age. Other symptoms of MEN I may be present. The vagueness of the presentation often leads to considerable diagnostic delay.

DIAGNOSIS

A fasting blood sugar of below 2.8 mmol/l is the characteristic finding. The fasting test must be carefully controlled, and blood is taken for both sugar and insulin measurements. In a normal person, fasting lowers the blood sugar (but seldom less than 2.8 mmol/l) but the plasma insulin then falls. By contrast, with insulinoma the plasma insulin is either very high or inappropriately raised or maintained while the blood sugar falls. The main differential diagnosis is from self-induced (factitious) hypoglycaemia which should be suspected particularly in medical staff. Exogenous insulin is however associated with a low C peptide level while insulinoma is not. Surreptitious taking of a sulphonylurea can also cause diagnostic difficulty.

Selective arteriography is helpful in determining whether the lesions are single or multiple. CT and ultrasound scanning are sometimes useful.

TREATMENT

After localization a partial pancreatectomy is performed leaving the head of the pancreas wherever possible. When the tumour has not been localized pre-operatively, it may nonetheless be palpable at operation. The plasma insulin is monitored during the operation. If no tumour is found, a subtotal pancreatectomy is usually performed.

Metastases are uncommon but if they occur they may respond to streptozotocin, 5FU or doxorubicin. A combination of all three has also been used with response rates of 50–60%. Diazoxide can be used to treat hypoglycaemia. Glucagon is of little value.

Gastrinoma (Zollinger-Ellison Syndrome)

INCIDENCE AND PATHOLOGY

These tumours are uncommon. They probably arise from the delta or D cells of the islets and are often malignant (14). They usually present at the age of 20–45 years and probably account for 0.1% of all peptic ulcer disease. Ninety percent occur in the pancreas, 5% in the duodenum and others occur in the stomach and, very rarely, in adenomas of the thyroid and ovary. They may be single or multiple and vary greatly in size (less than 5 mm to 15 cms). Gastrinomas are most common in the body or tail and microscopically resemble carcinoids. This resemblance and the fact that occasionally other peptide hormones are produced (ACTH, VIP, glucagon) lending weight to the hypothesis that their origin is from APUD cells. In 60% of patients metastases have occurred at diagnosis usually to adjacent nodes and liver, but more distant spread is not uncommon.

Most of the gastrin produced in the tumour is a 17 amino acid peptide (G-17) but a larger molecule (G-34) is also formed. Circulating gastrin is mainly G-34. The constant stimulation of the gastric parietal cells leads to a great increase in their mass. In some patients other features of the MEN I syndrome are present— usually hyperparathyroidism.

CLINICAL FEATURES (15)

The dominant symptom is peptic ulceration. Usually the ulcer is in the first part of the duodenum or in the stomach. Occasionally there are multiple ulcers which extend down in the proximal duodenum. Recurrence soon after medical treatment, perforation and haemorrhage all occur. The symptoms of ulceration are severe and response to medical treatment is limited although H2 receptor antagonists are effective for a while.

Diarrhoea occurs in 30–50% of cases, due to the large volume of acid produced by the stomach. Pancreatic lipase is inactivated at low pH leading to steatorrhoea. The low pH also interferes with bile salt function and with the activity of intrinsic factor.

INVESTIGATION AND DIAGNOSIS

The history of recurrent severe peptic ulceration with diarrhoea in a young person should point to the possible diagnosis. There is occasionally a family history of endocrine neoplasia. Acid output is raised, but not necessarily to levels above that found in some patients with duodenal ulcer. The diagnosis is confirmed by finding an elevated plasma gastrin level. Most radioimmunoassay antibodies will detect all types of gastrin molecule produced by gastrinomas.

When the diagnosis has been made, attempts are usually made to locate tumour. CT scanning and ultrasound may be helpful in showing metastases but usually fail to demonstrate the primary, and angiography is little better. Laparotomy is usually required to assess operability.

MANAGEMENT

Pancreatectomy is seldom practicable. The tumours are often multifocal and have frequently metastasized. Histamine antagonists have greatly improved medical management. Before their introduction total gastrectomy was the preferred treatment for intractable ulceration. Death is more a consequence of the complications of ulceration than of malignancy though this may change with the use of cimetidine. About 60% of patients are alive 5 years after diagnosis.

Vipoma (Verner-Morrison syndrome)

This rare syndrome of profuse watery diarrhoea, facial flushing, hypokalaemia, hypochlorhydria and hypertension is caused by the secretion of Vasoactive Intestinal Polypeptide (VIP) by tumours of the pancreatic islets (16). VIP (and the syndrome) can be produced by phaeochromocytomas, ganglioneuroblastomas and bronchogenic (small cell) carcinoma. Hyperglycaemia and hypercalaemia may also occur and can be caused by VIP.

The tumours are usually solitary and can sometimes be shown angiographically. Treatment is by surgical removal. There is a high risk of malignancy.

Glucagonoma

These are tumours of the pancreatic alpha cell and usually affect postmenopausal women (17). The clinical syndrome is characterized by a severe skin eruption with migratory erythema, bullous ulceration and scabbing on the legs, trunk, genital area and face (migratory necrolytic erythema). In addition there is normochromic anaemia, stomatitis, diarrhoea and hypokalaemia. Most of the tumours are in the body and tail and are often malignant (60%) but with a slow growth rate. Metastasis is usually to the liver.

The diagnosis is made by the typical rash and the raised plasma glucagon levels. Glucagon causes gluconeogenesis and glycogenolysis, elevating the blood sugar. The mechanism of production of the skin rash is not known. Treatment is by surgical removal wherever possible.

Somatostatinoma (18)

These rare islet cell tumours are usually malignant. The syndrome consists of steatorrhoea and diarrhoea due to suppressed pancreatic exocrine function, gall-stones due to decreased gall bladder contractility, diabetes from suppression of insulin, and hypochlorhydria from suppression of gastrin.

Plasma somatostatin and calcitonin are elevated. Diagnosis is late because the symptoms are not specific. The tumours should be removed if metastases have not yet occurred.

REFERENCES

1 Beasley R. P., Hwang L-Y, Lin C-C, & Chien C-S. (1981) Hepatocellular carcinoma and hepatitis B virus. A prospective study of 22 707 men in Taiwan. *Lancet* **ii,** 1129.

2 Sharfitz D. A., Shouval D., Sherman H., Hadziyannis S. J. & Kew M. L. (1981) Integration of hepatitis B virus into the genome of liver cells in chronic liver disease and hepatocellular carcinoma. *New England Journal of Medicine* **305,** 1067.

3 Chen D. S. & Jung J. L. (1979) Serum alpha fetoprotein in hepatocellular carcinoma. *Cancer* **409,** 779.

4 Philips R. & Murikanin K. (1960) Primary neoplasms of the liver: results of radiation therapy. *Cancer* **13,** 714.

5 Senzer N. N., Terrell W. & Pratt C. B. (1978) Evaluation of a chemotherapeutic regimen for primary liver cancer in children. *Cancer Treatment Report* **62,** 1403.

6 Godwin J. D. (1975). Carcinoid tumours; an analysis of 2837 cases. *Cancer* **36,** 560.

7 Grahame-Smith D. G. (1974) Natural history and diagnosis of the carcinoid syndrome. *Clinics in Gastroenterology* **3,** 575.

8 Levin B., Riddell R. H. & Kirsner J. B. (1976) Management of precancerous lesions of the gastrointestinal tract. *Clinics in Gastroenterology* **5,** 827.

9 Wutsofides T., McDonald J. & Shibata H. R. (1977) Carcinoma of the pancreas and periampullary region: a 41 year experience. *Annals of Surgery* **196,** 730.

10 Pereiras R., Chiprut R. O. & Greenwald R. A. (1977) Percutaneous transhepatic cholangiography with the 'skinny' needle. *Annals of Internal Medicine* **86,** 562.

11 Doblebower R. A. (1979). The radiotherapy of pancreatic cancer. *Seminars in Oncology* **6,** 378.

12 Smith F. P. & Schein P. S. (1978) Chemotherapy of pancreatic cancer. *Seminars in Oncology* **6,** 368.

13 Pearse A. G. E. (1968) Common cytochemical and ultrastructural characteristics of cells producing polypeptide hormones (the apud series) and their relevance to thyroid and ultimo-branchial C cells and calcitonin. *Proceedings of the Royal Society,* (Series B) **170,** 71.

14 Martin, E. D. & Potet F. (1974). Pathology of endocrine tumours of the GI tract. *Clinics in Gastroenterology* **3,** 511.

15 Regan P. T. & Malagelada J. R. (1978). A reappraisal of the clinical, roentgenographic and endoscopic features of the Zollinger-Ellison syndrome. *Mayo Clinic Proceedings* **53,** 19.

16 Verner J. V. & Morrison A. B. (1976) Non-beta islet cell tumours and the syndrome of watery diarrhoea hypokalaemia and hypochorhydria. *Clinics in Gastroenterology* **3,** 595.

17 Mallinson C. N., Bloom S. R., Warin A. P., Salmon P. R. & Cox B. (1974) A glucagonoma syndrome. *Lancet* **ii,** 1.

18 Larsson L. I., Hirsch M. A., Holst J. J., Ingemansson S., Kühl C., Jenson S. L., Lunqvist G., Rehfeld J. F. & Schwartz T. W. (1977) Pancreatic somatostainoma. Clinical features and pathological implications. *Lancet* **i,** 666.

Chapter 16

Tumours of the Small and Large Bowel

CANCER OF THE SMALL BOWEL

INCIDENCE AND AETIOLOGY

Small bowel tumours represent less than 5% of all gastro-intestinal tumours and about half of these will prove malignant. Their low frequency seems particularly surprising since the small bowel comprises about three-quarters the length of the alimentary tract. Although malignant lesions occur most frequently in the duodenum and jejunum, benign lesions such as polyps, adenomas and fibromas occur more frequently in the ileum. The incidence is approximately 1 in 100 000 (Fig. 16.1) and adenocarcinomas are more common in patients with familial polyposis, Peutz-Jeghers syndrome, Crohn's disease, and Gardner's syndrome. These tumours are more common over the age of 60. Long standing coeliac disease predisposes to the development of small bowel lymphoma (see Chapter 26).

PATHOLOGY

There are four major types of malignant small bowel tumours. The commonest are adenocarcinomas (45%), carcinoid tumours (30%), lymphomas (10%) and sarcomas (mostly leiomyosarcomas). Metastatic deposits (most frequently from the ovary and pancreas) are at least as common as primary tumours.

Adenocarcinoma of the small bowel metastases to the liver and regional nodes. Histologically these are typical mucin secreting adenocarcinomas. The characteristic appearance is of an ulcerating neoplasm. Small bowel lymphomas are usually diffuse and poorly differentiated. The small bowel is an important site of non-Hodgkin's lymphoma in childhood. The management of small bowel lymphoma is discussed in Chapter 26.

Carcinoid tumours arise principally in the ileum, caecum, appendix and duodenum. They appear as small yellowish nodules in the bowel wall, arising from the chromaffin cells which probably belong to the APUD (amine precursor uptake and decarboxylase) system which secrete small polypeptide hormones and amine. The management of the carcinoid syndrome is discussed in Chapter 15.

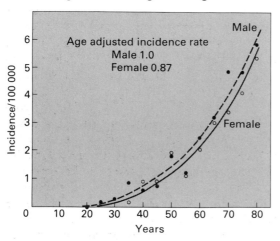

Fig. 16.1. *Age-specific incidence of malignant tumours of the small bowel.*

CLINICAL FEATURES

Clinical diagnosis is difficult and is not usually achieved before surgery. Patients often present with symptoms of obstruction or intermittent abdominal pain and a history of melaena is sometimes obtained. Intussusception is often the cause of the obstruction and pain.

Chronic anaemia may occur, from gradual blood loss. Weight loss is frequent and diarrhoea and steatorrhoea are occasionally present, particularly with lymphomas. A palpable abdominal mass may also be found, and abdominal distension if there is intestinal obstruction. Commonly, there are no abnormal physical signs. Perforation is rare with adenocarcinoma, but common with lymphoma.

DIAGNOSIS

Contrast X-rays studies are essential in diagnosis, but not always helpful. In proximal tumours, a barium follow-through is required whereas in distal lesions causing ileocolic intussusception, the barium enema is usually more useful. Hypotonic duodenography may give better visualization of duodenal lesions and small bowel enemas are helpful with lower tumours. Occasionally an ultrasound or CT scan is helpful to delineate a mass. Duodenal lesions can usually be seen endoscopically, and biopsy and cytological specimens can be obtained.

TREATMENT

In the management of small bowel neoplasms, surgical removal is the most important method of treatment. Although benign tumours can usually be removed by simple resection, adenocarcinomas require a wider excision including, if possible, removal of the lymph node drainage area since lymphatic invasion is common. Only 70% of tumours are resectable. For duodenal cancers, pancreaticoduodenectomy may be required. At the other end of the small bowel, lesions of the terminal ileum are often best treated by hemicolectomy, since better resection of regional lymphatics can be achieved in this way. With leiomyosarcomas, regional node involvement is less frequent and removal of the

lymph node drainage area may not be necessary.

For lymphomas of the small bowel, a particularly careful search of the abdomen is mandatory since involvement of local lymph nodes, liver or spleen is common. Wide resection of the involved area is necessary, with removal of adjacent nodes. Following resection, treatment with chemotherapy or radiotherapy may be necessary (see Chapter 26).

In resecting small bowel carcinoids, the site and size of the tumour are helpful guides. Carcinoid tumours of the appendix are unlikely to metastasize, and simple appendicectomy is probably sufficient. In any lesion larger than 2 cms a more widespread excision seems justified because of the risk of spread beyond the primary site.

PROGNOSIS

The survival rate for small bowel adenocarcinomas is poor, only 20% of patients surviving 5 years. For localized carcinoid tumours, 5-year survival rates of up to 90% have been reported. The prognosis for metastatic disease is discussed in Chapter 15.

Tumours of the appendix

These are uncommon, and 90% of them are carcinoids which are treated by local resection. The remainder are either adenocarcinomas of mucocoeles which contain a gelatinoid mucoid material and can undergo malignant change to become papillary mucinous cystadenocarcinomas. Rupture of these lesions leads to the condition of *pseudomyxoma peritonei*, a gelatinous, ascitic implanting tumour which can coat the entire peritoneal surface resulting in progressive abdominal enlargement, and sometimes mimicking ovarian carcinoma. Treatment of pseudomyxoma involves surgical evacuation, though repeated operations are usually required. Both whole abdominal irradiation and intraperitoneal or systemic chemotherapy have been advocated, though their effectiveness is uncertain.

TUMOURS OF THE LARGE BOWEL

AETIOLOGY AND INCIDENCE

Cancers of the large bowel (colon and rectum) are amongst the commonest of malignant tumours and represent the second largest cause of death from cancer in the Western World. Cancers of the colon outnumber rectal carcinomas by 3:2 (Fig. 16.2), and the two sites together constitute 10–15% of all cancers. The disease is uncommon in Africa, Asia and South America, suggesting a possible dietary aetiology. In the USA, the incidence rate amongst blacks increased by half between 1947 and 1969, which may reflect an increasingly 'Westernized' diet in this group. A good deal of additional epidemiological data supports this view. Western diets, containing high proportions of meat and animal fats, but little fibre, are quite unlike the typical African diet. Africans have a more rapid stool transit time, which may lead to a reduced exposure to any carcinogen passing down the alimentary canal. Japanese immigrants to the USA show an increasing incidence of colorectal cancer in succeeding generations (1). Close relatives of patients with carcinoma of the colon have a slightly higher incidence of the disease, possibly suggesting a common dietary factor. The Western diet, with a high meat and fat content favours a gut bacterial population which produces enzymes capable of converting sterols to carcinogens in the bowel. The enzyme 7-alpha-dehydroxylase converts bile acids to deoxycholic and lithocolic acid. It is known that in animal models some bile acids act as promoters of carcinogenesis in tumours initiated by carcinogens such as dimethylhydrazine.

A number of conditions are known to predispose to the development of large bowel cancers. In patients with ulcerative colitis, the risk is greater in patients with a long history and extensive bowel involvement. Patients diagnosed young are at special risk, particularly since modern treatment usually ensures lengthy survival. In the past some physicians recommended total colectomy in patients in whom the disease had been active for more than 10 years, a recommendation which was supported by the fact that these patients tend to develop multicentric and poorly differentiated carcinomas (2). More recent studies have indicated that a careful 'watch' policy is satisfactory. In some patients with ulcerative colitis, dysplastic mucosal changes appear to precede the development of malignancy. Familial polyposis coli also predisposes to malignant change. The distal colon tends to be most severely involved and the similarity of symptoms of polyposis coli and true carcinoma makes diagnosis of the development of malignancy extremely difficult. Many surgeons recommend total colectomy and ileorectal anastomosis in all patients with polyposis coli. Experience supports the view that this procedure is safe since less than 5% of patients later develop cancer in the rectal stump. In patients with this disease who already have rectal polyps, resection of the rectum with permanent ileostomy may be safer since the risk of carcinomatous change in the rectal stump is probably higher, particularly in patients with multiple rectal polyps at the time of operation. Patients with Gardner's syndrome, (multiple colonic polyps with tumours of the mandible,

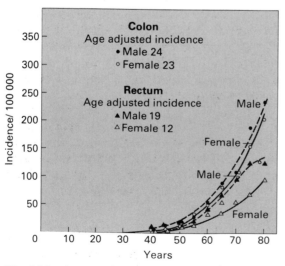

Fig. 16.2. *Age-specific incidence of carcinoma of the large bowel.*

skull vault and skin) are also at increased risk of carcinomatous change, and total colectomy is advisable.

It is still unclear whether non-familial (sporadic) adenomatous polyps are premalignant. Such lesions are found increasingly with age, and in a small percentage of patients with bowel cancer, residual evidence of an adenomatous polyp can sometimes be found. The risk of malignant change increases greatly with increasing size of the polyp (3). However, the majority of polyps do not show evidence of malignant change. Many surgeons advocate routine removal of polyps found at sigmoidoscopy, particularly since two-thirds of large bowel cancers are found in the rectum and sigmoid colon (see below). Finally, villous adenomas of the rectum and sigmoid are now generally considered premalignant. They present with diarrhoea, rectal bleeding or a characteristic picture of fluid and electrolyte loss, often with severe hypokalaemia. The incidence of malignant change is at least 15% and possibly higher, and these lesions should always be removed even if this necessitates an extensive operation.

PATHOLOGY AND SURGICAL STAGING

The distal part of the large bowel is the commonest site of malignancy: over 20% of all large bowel tumours occur in the sigmoid colon and 40% in the rectum (Fig. 16.3).

The typical lesion is either polypoid with a fleshy protuberance on a narrow base, or sessile, with a broader base and a generally flatter appearance. The most characteristic form is a well demarcated polypoid mass with ulceration in its centre, involving part or all of the bowel circumference. The tumour may have reached the full thickness of the bowel wall although lateral spread beyond 3 cm is unusual. Local lymphatic invasion is common and about one-third of these patients have evidence of nodal metastases at presentation. Blood-borne metastases are usually via the portal vein and the liver is much the commonest site of distant

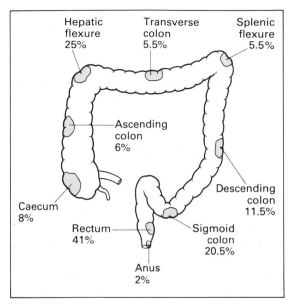

Fig. 16.3. *Cancer of the large bowel: proportion of all cases arising at each site.*

spread. Systemic haematogenous dissemination to the lung, brain and skeleton occurs less frequently. Local recurrence can be a major problem with these tumours often leading to intestinal or ureteric obstruction, or fistula formation.

Surgical staging is of great importance since there is no better guide to prognosis. Although well localized tumours carry a high probability of surgical cure, over half of all large bowel cancers ultimately prove fatal. The Dukes staging system is widely employed and is easy to apply. It is a valuable predictor of survival in both colonic and rectal lesions (Table 16.1) and extensive regional node involvement has a particularly adverse prognosis. Tumour grade and depth of penetration are also important. Some of these factors are interdependent since the higher the tumour grade, the more likely the risk of local nodal metastasis.

CLINICAL FEATURES AND DIAGNOSIS

The symptoms of colorectal cancer vary with the site of the tumour (Fig. 16.4). In the caecum and right side of the colon, the main complaint

Table 16.1. Dukes staging system for rectal cancer (with 5-year survival).

Stage	Description
A	Confined to mucosa and submucosa (80%)
B	Invasion through the musculature with no lymph node involvement (50%)
C	Metastases to regional lymph nodes
C1	Lymph nodes not involved up to point of vascular ligation (40%)
C2	Nodes involved up to level of vascular ligation (12%)

is of ill-defined abdominal pain which may be mistaken for gall-bladder or peptic ulcer disease. Chronic iron deficiency anaemia from occult blood loss is common and may be the

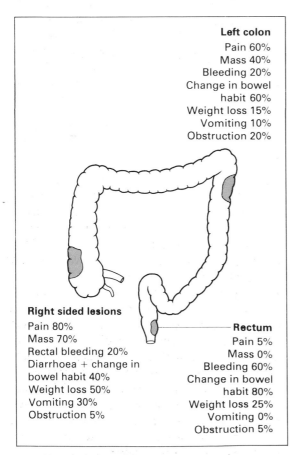

Left colon
Pain 60%
Mass 40%
Bleeding 20%
Change in bowel habit 60%
Weight loss 15%
Vomiting 10%
Obstruction 20%

Right sided lesions
Pain 80%
Mass 70%
Rectal bleeding 20%
Diarrhoea + change in bowel habit 40%
Weight loss 50%
Vomiting 30%
Obstruction 5%

Rectum
Pain 5%
Mass 0%
Bleeding 60%
Change in bowel habit 80%
Weight loss 25%
Vomiting 0%
Obstruction 5%

Fig. 16.4. *Symptoms of colorectal cancer according to site.*

presenting feature. Frank melaena may occur, and episodes of diarrhoea are not uncommon. An abdominal mass may sometimes be felt.

In left-sided colonic lesions the pain is usually cramping and suggestive of intestinal obstruction. Abdominal distension may be present. Constipation, occasionally alternating with diarrhoea, is a frequent complaint and symptomatic rectal bleeding occurs in 20% of patients. Rectal carcinoma is often accompanied by passage of bright red blood. However, this is a common symptom in the normal population since haemorrhoids are very frequent. Change in bowel habit with tenderness and constipation are later symptoms.

Rectal examination is the most important single procedure for diagnosing large bowel tumours. Three-quarters of all rectal lesions are within reach and sigmoidoscopy will usually visualize these lesions without difficulty provided care is taken with the details of the examination. Sigmoidoscopy allows examination of up to the distal 25 cm of large bowel and the majority of rectal tumours can be diagnosed in this way. The introduction of flexible sigmoidoscopy and colonoscopy into more general use has led to accurate pre-operative diagnosis of the majority of large bowel cancers, though their use is not yet routine since barium enema examinations are easier, less expensive, more widely available, and relatively efficient as a routine method of diagnosis. The double contrast enema has improved diagnostic accuracy, giving better resolution of small tumours. Radiologically the tumour may appear as a narrowed or strictured segment or as a mass indenting the contrast medium (Fig. 16.5). On the right side of the colon, the tumour is more easily missed, particularly in the caecum, which may be poorly demonstrated by the examination. In doubtful cases, the investigation should be repeated or colonoscopy performed.

In 1965, Gold and his colleagues demonstrated that colonic and rectal cancers sometimes produced a tumour marker, carcinoembryonic antigen (CEA). Unfortunately, this marker has not proved sufficiently specific to be

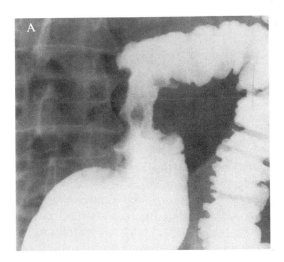

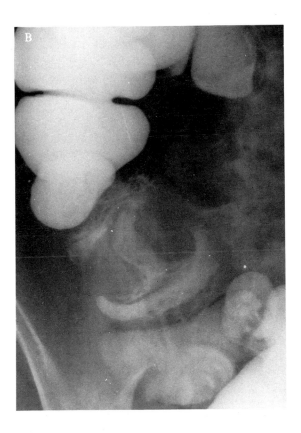

Fig. 16.5. *Barium enema appearances in large bowel cancer.* (A) Carcinoma of recto-sigmoid. (B) Carcinoma of caecum.

a reliable indicator of disease in patients with large bowel cancers since it can also be elevated in pancreatitis, inflammatory bowel diseases, and in normal people who are heavy smokers or have a high ingestion of alcohol. It can however, be useful in monitoring disease in certain patients with bowel tumours who have a raised CEA which is known to have fallen following successful surgery. In these patients, a rise in CEA may be the first sign of recurrence. The question of what to do when recurrence is suggested by a rise in CEA has not yet been answered clinically since a postoperative rise is likely to be due to unresectable metastasis (4).

The differential diagnosis of large bowel cancer includes other large bowel disorders such as diverticulitis, ulcerative colitis, ischaemic colitis and irritable bowel syndrome. Other causes of rectal bleeding, such as haemorrhoids and polyps, may cause diagnostic difficulty. Abdominal pain may suggest biliary tract or peptic ulceration. Radiologically, there may be difficulty in distinguishing left-sided neoplasms from diverticulitis, and benign tumours such as lipomas and neurofibromas may occur at any site.

MANAGEMENT

Surgery remains the cornerstone of treatment. Radical surgical resection is usually preferred to simple excision, because of the risk of unsuspected node metastases as well as the possibility of multicentric tumours. Wide removal of the involved segment should include resection of the local lymphatic drainage area (Fig. 16.6). Even in patients with evidence of hepatic or peritoneal metastases, surgical tumour removal may offer the best means of palliation. Some surgeons even recommend radical bowel resection in patients with a solitary hepatic metastasis, since hepatic resection can sometimes be accomplished at the same operation. The operative procedure should rest firmly on a knowledge of the anatomy of the vascular supply and lymphatic drainage of the affected bowel segment, and care must be taken to avoid tumour implantation into the operative field at the time of surgical excision. Anastomotic recurrences are however not uncommon.

In rectal cancer the type and extent of the excision depends on the site of the tumour. For lower and middle rectal lesions, the classic abdomino-perineal resection introduced by Miles is widely performed (Fig. 16.6). In recent years, new techniques for lower rectal resection with primary anastomosis have been introduced, preserving the sphincter and avoiding the need for permanent colostomy. Local resection is sometimes performed for small, mobile polypoid lesions of favourable histological grade. Patients who are unwell through obstruction, cachexia or perforation may benefit from an initial defunctioning colostomy before tumour removal is attempted. Even in totally unresectable lesions, a colostomy should generally be performed since this will at least allow a reasonable quality of life and makes high-dose radiotherapy for the primary tumour a feasible proposition (see below).

Surgical mortality has rapidly diminished in recent years and is now 4–8% in experienced hands. Complications include anastomotic leaks, postoperative infection and urinary dysfunction, particularly if extensive ureteric dissection has been performed. Despite radical segmental bowel excision, the incidence of local recurrence is about 10%. High grade rectal lesions are particularly likely to recur locally, particularly where regional node metastases have been demonstrated.

RADIOTHERAPY

Although many surgeons feel that radiotherapy has no established place in the primary management of carcinoma of the large bowel, there is increasing evidence to suggest that it might eventually find a role. Since the advent of megavoltage equipment capable of adequate treatment to deep seated tumours, it has become clear that radiotherapy can be useful for inoperable or recurrent cancers. In the majority of patients, troublesome symptoms of pain or rectal bleeding can be palliated and a small number have achieved long survival without further treatment. As a result of this experience, studies of pre-operative irradiation, usually to modest doses, have been carried out, though with conflicting results. A satisfactory prospective study of pre-operative radiotherapy using high dosage with modern equipment has yet to be performed. As with other abdominopelvic tumours, there seems little doubt that local lymph node involvement is less common in surgical specimens obtained from pre-operatively irradiated patients, suggesting that radiation therapy is sometimes capable of producing

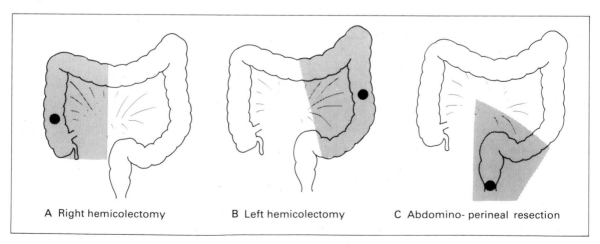

A Right hemicolectomy   B Left hemicolectomy   C Abdomino- perineal resection

Fig. 16.6 *Surgical resection of large bowel cancer*

histological resolution of lymph node involvement. In patients with obvious recurrent disease, particularly at the primary sites, radiotherapy can offer gratifying symptomatic improvement. Perineal, anastomotic or wound recurrences can be extremely painful particularly if ulceration occurs. In such cases, and indeed when the surgeon is unable to achieve complete operative removal of the primary lesion, radiotherapy is likely to be the most effective treatment. Doses in the range of 40–50 Gy in 4–5 weeks are usually recommended.

In mobile cancers of the lower rectum, Papillon (5) has developed elegant endocavitary techniques using high dosage radiation therapy to a limited volume, avoiding the need for surgery. In a carefully selected group of 133 patients, he demonstrated a 78% 5-year survival rate, often in patients whose general condition was poor.

Although it is not possible to recommend pre-operative irradiation routinely, a large prospectively randomized trial by the Veterans Administration Surgical Adjuvant group has provided some evidence in favour of its use (6). Patients were treated either by abdominoperineal excision, or by surgery preceded by modest irradiation 20–25 Gy over a 2-week period. At 5 years, the survival of the group receiving pre-operative irradiation was 40% compared with 28% for patients treated by surgery alone.

A more recent study, from the Gastrointestinal Tumour Study Group, has analysed the role of *postoperative* radiotherapy (with or without chemotherapy) for patients with Dukes' Stages B$_2$ and C rectal carcinoma (7). At 5-years after treatment, with a median follow-up of survivors of 6½ years, the recurrence rate was highest among control patients (55%) and lowest in patients given adjuvant radiotherapy and chemotherapy using 5-Fluorouracil and methyl-CCNU (33%). Time to tumour recurrence was also significantly prolonged, but overall survival was not improved though there was a trend towards a lower death rate in the chemotherapy-radiotherapy group (44% vs 64% of controls).

THE ROLE OF CHEMOTHERAPY

5-fluorouracil has been widely used in patients with *recurrent or metastatic* large bowel cancers for almost 20 years. Despite the occasional impressive symptomatic improvement, objective responses are usually incomplete and transient, and occur in not more than 20% of all patients. There is certainly no evidence as yet to suggest that such treatment prolongs survival in the whole group, though prolongation of life has been claimed in responding patients. A well tolerated drug, 5-fluorouracil can be given in a variety of ways (see Chapter 6), though increasingly, intermittent intravenous therapy is preferred. Other agents, though active, are either less effective or have greater toxicity (Table 16.2). Nitrosoureas (BCNU, CCNU and methyl CCNU) and mitomycin C have been extensively tested and produce objective responses in about 10–20% of patients (7).

Various combinations of these and other agents have been employed but with very limited success. An increased response rate has been reported using a combination of 5-fluorouracil, BCNU, DTIC and vincristine, but at the cost of considerable toxicity. The combination is slightly, though not significantly more effective than 5-fluorouracil alone. Other studies have shown a similar slight increase in responsiveness to combination chemotherapy. Despite a significant improvement in response rate for patients receiving combination chemo-

Table 16.2. Large bowel cancer—response to chemotherapy.

	Response Rate (%)
Single Agents	
5-Fluorouracil (5FU)	20
Nitrosoureas	10
Mithromycin	20
Combination	
5-FU, methyl CCNU	15–20
5-FU, methyl CCNU, vincristine	25

therapy, there is unfortunately no survival benefit. Although 5-FU/nitrosourea combinations are marginally more effective in producing responses than single agent therapy, treatment related toxity is undoubtedly greater, myelosuppression can be severe and prolonged, and survival is not improved (8).

Treatment with 5-FU has been recommended postoperatively as a *surgical adjuvant*, though no survival benefit has yet been demonstrated. Although it might be tempting to offer adjuvant chemotherapy in patients with Dukes stage C lesions, such treatment is at present unjustified though controlled adjuvant chemotherapy studies are in progress. Hepatic metastases from colorectal cancer are sometimes treated by infusion of 5FU into the hepatic artery. Pain may be relieved and regressions do occur but there is little demonstrable advantage over the intravenous route. Treatment of hepatic metastases is discussed further in Chapter 8.

PROGNOSIS

The following factors adversely affect prognosis: Dukes stage B and C particularly C2 lesions; age below 40; undifferentiated tumours; heavy mucus secretion with 'signet ring' cells scirrhous carcinoma of the distal large bowel; invasion of lymphatic channels or veins; inadequate resection margins; presentation with large bowel obstruction. Five-year survival figures are given in Table 16.1.

LIVING WITH A COLOSTOMY

Patients faced with the prospect of a permanent colostomy need sympathetic support. Quite apart from worrying about its appearance and the possibility of spillage and smell, most patients are concerned that they will find it impossible to manage the colostomy themselves without skilled help. They may need reassurance that the presence of the colostomy does not imply the residual cancer has been left behind and also that it will be possible to return to a normal active life. Despite enthusiastic help, many patients will develop depressive

symptoms and in a proportion, agoraphobia or fear of social contact may become a disability. The value of a skilled stoma therapist cannot be overestimated, and the same is true of the well informed self-help groups such as the *Colostomy Welfare Association*.

It is often valuable for the patient with cancer of the large bowel to meet a colostomy patient before the definitive surgery is performed. In many instances this has been crucial in persuading a hesitant patient to undergo what subsequently proves to be curative surgery.

SCREENING

Secondary prevention (the identification of high risk groups and early detection of the disease) has been the subject of much investigation. The three methods used have been plasma CEA, sigmoidoscopy and occult faecal blood testing. CEA has proved an insensitive test for early cancer and is no longer used. Studies using sigmoidoscopy have suggested a higher survival rate for those thus diagnosed, and flexible sigmoidoscopes may make the procedure more acceptable to patients. Occult blood testing of stools (using the guaiac test which turns blue with red cell pseudoperoxidase) has also been used in controlled trials (9). In one study the rate of positive slide tests was 2.4%, and of those who were then investigated 9% had cancer of the colon or rectum, 80% of which were Dukes' A or B. The effect of occult blood testing in the general population on the mortality from colorectal cancer is still uncertain, and a longer follow-up period is needed. In the high risk groups, such as patients with a family history of polyposis coli, yearly screening with flexible sigmoidoscopy and faecal occult blood testing is recommended.

CARCINOMA OF THE ANUS

PATHOLOGY AND CLINICAL FEATURES

Fortunately these tumours are rare, accounting for about 2% of all large bowel cancers. They are slightly more common in women and may occur in association with carcinoma of the cervix or vulva. Carcinoma of the anus is reportedly more common in male homosexuals and may be one of the AIDS-related malignancies (10). The tumours present as small firm nodules which may be confused with haemorrhoids, the true nature of the lesion becoming apparent only after histological review of the surgical specimen. Rectal bleeding and pain are common symptoms. The diagnosis is often delayed since the symptoms are attributed to haemorrhoids or fissure-in-ano. Other lesions producing occasional diagnostic confusion include leukoplakia, Bowen's disease, or Paget's disease of the anus. Local invasion of the anal sphincter and rectal wall is not uncommon, and more advanced local spread may also occur, to involve the prostate, bladder or cervix. Although mostly squamous carcinomas, other histological types occur including basal cell carcinoma and melanoma. It is important, if possible, to distinguish tumours above the pectinate line from those below since the latter tend to have a better prognosis.

TREATMENT

Surgical treatment is often successful, particularly in small perianal lesions, and in cases of *in situ* carcinoma or localized perianal leukoplakia. Low rectal and anal canal lesions usually require abdominoperineal resection with excision of local lymphatics as for other large bowel tumours.

In low anal lesions, lymphatic drainage is usually to the inguinal nodes, which should be carefully evaluated before considering surgical treatment. Both high and low lesions may however spread upwards to mesenteric and pelvic nodes. Although some surgeons recommend wide excision even in cases with obvious inguinal node involvement, radiotherapy is often preferred, as the prognosis in these cases is much worse and surgery is more difficult to justify. In cases initially treated by surgery and subsequently developing inguinal node metastases, block dissection of the nodes is usually preferable to radiotherapy as a means of ensuring local control, though additional postoperative irradiation can be useful if the dissection is incomplete. Prophylatic block dissection of the inguinal nodes is not usually recommended.

Radiotherapy has been successfully used as an alternative to surgery for primary treatment of anal cancer. Care must be taken to avoid treating the whole of the anal sphincter in order to avoid extensive fibrosis which might make defaecation impossible. Radiation treatment is usually employed for large unresectable tumours, and can offer useful palliation. However, where surgeons are prepared to refer more favourable tumours, excellent results have been obtained, particularly with the use of interstitial implants as described by Papillon (11).

PROGNOSIS

Prognosis in carcinoma of the anus depends on the location and tumour grade. The 5-year survival rate in patients undergoing abdominoperineal resection is 30–50%. For tumours of the anal verge, the 5-year survival rate is of the order of 60%. If inguinal nodes are involved at diagnosis, 5-year survival falls to 15%.

REFERENCES

1 Haenszel W. & Correa P. (1971) Cancer of the colon and rectum and adenomatous polyps. A review of epidemiologic findings. *Cancer* **28**, 14.
2 Lennard-Jones J. W., Morson B. C., Ritchie J. K. Shone D. C. & Williams C. B. (1977), Cancer in colitis: Assessment of the individual risk by clinical and histological criteria. *Gastroenterology* **73**, 1280.
3 Muto T., Bussey H. J. R. & Morson B. C. (1975) The evolution of cancer of the colon and rectum. *Cancer* **26**, 225.
4 Minton J. P. & Martin E. W. Jr (1978) The use of serial CEA determinations to predict recurrence of colon cancer and when to do a second-look operation. *Cancer* **42**, 1422.
5 Papillon J. (1975) Intracavitary irradiation of early rectal cancer for cure. *Cancer* **36**, 696–701.

6 Roswitt B., Higgins G.A. & Keehn X. (1975) Preoperative irradiation for carcinoma of the rectum and rectosigmoid colon. *Cancer* **35,** 1597.

7 Moertel C.G. (1978) Chemotherapy of gastrointestinal cancer. *New England Journal of Medicine* **299,** 1049.

8 Gastrointestinal Tumour Study Group (1985) Prolongation of the disease-free interval in surgically treated rectal carcinoma. *New England Journal of Medicine* **312,** 1465.

9 Winawer S.J. (1982) Current status of fecal occult blood testing in screening for colorectal cancer. *Cancer* **32,** 100.

10 Papillon J. (1974) Radiotherapy in the management of epidermoid carcinoma of the anal region. *Diseases of the Colon and Rectum* **17,** 181.

Chapter 17
Gynaecological Cancer

INTRODUCTION

Gynaecological cancers account for approximately one-quarter of all malignant disease in women, though there are striking geographical and age differences in incidence for each of the major primary sites (Figs 17.1 and 17.2). After carcinoma of the breast, carcinoma of the cervix is the commonest cancer in women. It has been estimated that about 3% of all women will develop cervical cancer (including cases of carcinoma *in situ*) with an annual incidence rate of about 24 per 100 000. Tumours of the female genital tract are important not only because of their high incidence, but also because many can be diagnosed whilst still relatively localized. Management of these cases often involves the combined skills of surgeons, radiotherapists and medical oncologists and many women with these diseases are best treated with a combination of these approaches.

The overall incidence rates of carcinomas of cervix, corpus uteri and ovary are approximately equal, but because curative treatment is much less likely in ovarian carcinoma, the mortality from this disease now exceeds the combined death rate from carcinomas of the cervix and corpus. There are a number of known aetiological factors for gynaecological cancer. Important clues have been obtained from epidemiological studies which have shown, for example, that the low incidence of carcinoma of the ovary in Japanese women rapidly rises within a generation or two when they emigrate to the United States—a six-fold increase which strongly suggests environmental factors pre-

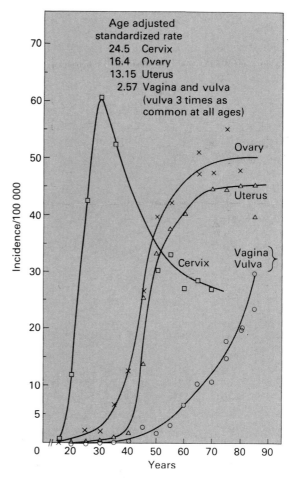

Fig. 17.1. *Age-specific incidence of gynaecological cancers.* The high incidence of carcinoma of the cervix below the age of 40 is chiefly due to *in situ* cases.

dominating over genetic ones. As the aetiology of these malignant diseases becomes better understood, it is clear that the social behaviour of

287

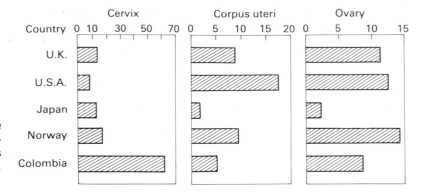

Fig. 17.2. *Geographic variation in gynaecological cancer incidence (per 100 000).* Note: figures for cervix exclude *in situ* cases.

the individual is of considerable importance as a risk factor: good examples would include the relatively high risk of ovarian cancer amongst nulliparous or subfertile women and the close relationship between carcinoma of the cervix and early sexual experience. It is encouraging that screening programmes have already helped reduce the frequency of frankly invasive carcinomas of the cervix (2).

CARCINOMA OF THE CERVIX

Incidence and aetiology

The aetiology of carcinoma of the cervix has been a subject of great interest over the past 20 years. The disease is extremely rare in nuns, and seems clearly related to sexual intercourse. More women with carcinoma of the cervix have had sexual experience before the age of 20 than groups of matched controls. There is also a suggestion of a correlation with the frequency of sexual activity and with the number of partners. Race and social class also seem important, but may not be independent factors since sexual behaviour may differ in these groups. For example, in New York city, the incidence per 100 000 women was 97.6 for Puerto Ricans, 47.8 for Blacks, 13.5 for white non-Jewish women and 3.6 for Jewish women. It has frequently been suggested that the low incidence of carcinoma of the cervix amongst Jewesses may be the result of male circumcision. However, at least one study has suggested that cir-

cumcision of the male partner may be a less important factor than was previously thought (3). Many other related aspects of hygiene could be more relevant and it is also likely that such women also start intercourse later in life and have fewer partners.

There is some evidence that the peak age of onset is falling, possibly because of changes in social habits (see below). In recent years there has been a significant reduction in invasive carcinoma of the cervix, coupled with an increase in micro-invasive or *in situ* disease. Data from the Second (1947) and Third (1969) USA National Cancer Surveys showed a decrease in the annual rate of invasive cervical cancers from 118 to 88 cases per 100 000; invasive carcinomas now account for less than one-third of the total incidence of cervical neoplasia.

The importance of sexual intercourse raises the question of a transmitted agent being responsible. Recent interest has centred around the herpes genitalis viruses Type 2 (HSV 2) which have been shown to produce morphological changes in human vaginal cells. A higher titre of antibodies to HSV 2 antigen is found in women with carcinoma of the cervix than in normal women; with a lower (but still elevated) level in patients with carcinoma *in situ*.

HSV specific RNA is found in the cells of most cases of carcinoma but in only 2% of samples of normal epithelial cells, and HSV-coded proteins have been found in the cytoplasm of cervical carcinoma cells. However, these studies do not prove that HSV 2 is a cause of cervical cancer. Infection with HSV 2 is common, and some women with cervical cancer have no evidence of HSV infection. It is possible that infection with HSV 2 renders women more susceptible to another (unidentified) carcinogenic stimulus which is itself associated with sexual activity. In recent years, interest has also centred on the carcinogenic importance of some types of human papilloma virus.

Pathology and spread

The widespread application of routine Papanicolaou screening cytology has taught us a great deal about pre-cancerous lesions in the cervix. These changes, collectively known as cervical intraepithelial neoplasia (CIN), can be graded according to the degree of cytological abnormality. Carcinoma *in situ* (now often referred to as CIN 3) represents the most severe of the intraepithelial changes. Though it may remain superficial for up to 20 years, a large proportion, possibly 30–40% of these lesions, will develop into true invasive carcinomas if left untreated (4). Invasive carcinoma of the cervix probably represents the extreme of a spectrum of cell changes from normality through to carcinoma *in situ*, which is clearly a pre-invasive malignancy.

The usual invasive lesion is a squamous carcinoma which accounts for over 90% of all cases. These are typical squamous cell carcinomas, arranged in nests and sheets of abnormal tissue and invading the cervical stroma. Adenocarcinoma accounts for a further 5%, and the remainder are much rarer lesions including mixed tumours, adeno-acanthomas and sarcomas. Although there is no firm evidence that adenocarcinomas should be treated differently from squamous cell carcinomas, they more frequently spread into the corpus uteri and myometrium, and surgery has in the past been preferred to radiation therapy. It is thought that the majority of adenocarcinomas of the cervix arise from the endocervical canal.

The major routes of spread are predictable, forming the basis of standard surgical and

Table 17.1. Clinical staging in carcinoma of the cervix.

Stage	Description
Pre-invasive carcinoma	
Stage 0	Carcinoma *in situ*
Invasive carcinoma	
Stage I	Disease confined to the cervix
Ia	Micro-invasive carcinoma
Ib	All other cases of stage I
Stage II	Disease beyond cervix but not to the pelvic wall. Upper 2/3 of vagina may be involved
IIa	No parametrial involvement evident
IIb	Parametrial involvement
Stage III	Extension to pelvic sidewall and/or lower third of vagina. Includes cases with hydronephrosis or non-functioning kidney (unless other known cause exists)
IIIa	No extension to pelvic side wall
IIIb	Extension to pelvic side wall and/or hydronephrosis or non-functioning kidney
Stage IV	Carcinoma beyond true pelvis or involving mucosa of bladder or rectum
IVa	Spread to local organs
IVb	Spread to distant organs

pathological staging (Table 17.1; Fig. 17.3). Direct and lymphatic spread occur much earlier than haematogenous dissemination. The most important direct routes of spread are downwards into the vaginal mucosa (often extending microscopically and submucosally beyond the limits of visible or palpable disease) and upwards into the myometrium of the lower part of the uterus. Direct extension also occurs laterally, beyond the paracervical tissues to the parametria, resulting in extension to the lateral wall of the true pelvis.

Lymphatic spread takes place via the paracervical lymphatics and from there to pelvic and para-aortic groups which largely follow the course of the major vessels. Surgical and lymphographic studies have confirmed a high incidence of nodal spread even in patients with localized disease with tumours apparently

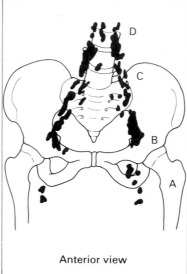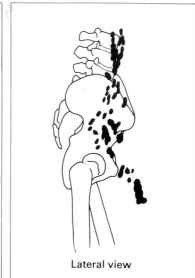

Anterior view   Lateral view

Fig. 17.3. *Lymphatic drainage of the cervix.* Lymphatic involvement in carcinoma of the cervix generally occurs in an orderly progression. The sequence is: (A) obturator, (B) internal, external and common iliac, (C) lateral sacral, (D) para-aortic.

confined to the cervix but with no obvious clinical extension into vagina, uterus or parametria. Nodal metastases can be identified in almost 20% of cases. Sites of blood-borne metastases include the lungs, liver and bone.

Clinical features

Women with dysplasia or CIN are generally free of symptoms. Such women have a clinically healthy looking cervix; the common condition of cervical erosion appears to bear no relationship to pre-malignancy. Women with CIN 3 also tend to be asymptomatic and this finding is almost invariably the result of a routine cervical smear examination.

Invasive cancers usually present with vaginal discharge, often offensive and discoloured. Many women consider it a normal feature of their lives and fail to seek advice until the discharge has been present for many months. Vaginal bleeding is an important symptom and often follows intercourse. Abdominal pain, dyspareunia or low back pain may also be present and suggest a bulky or advanced lesion. Urinary and rectal symptoms suggest locally extensive disease.

These tumours are usually visible with simple speculum techniques. *Exophytic* lesions are bulky in character, often forming large friable polypoid growths, making them easy to diagnose. *Infiltrative* tumours can show little in the way of visible ulceration due to a tendency for abnormal growth to be directed inwards towards the body of the uterus, often replacing the cervix and upper part of the vagina by a large confluent malignant ulcer. If the disease recurs following treatment a characteristic clinical syndrome may develop, with pelvic, back and buttock pain (often with an easily palpable pelvic mass), bowel disturbance, and leg oedema (usually unilateral) due to lymphatic and venous obstruction.

Staging procedures for invasive carcinoma

Careful staging is essential, yielding important prognostic information and facilitating attempts to compare results in centres using different approaches to treatment. The International Federation of Gynaecology and Obstetrics (FIGO) introduced a staging system in 1974 which is still in common use (Table 17.1), and the current TNM system is less widely used. Staging is based on colposcopy, inspection, palpation, and curettage, together with simple investigations such as chest X-ray and intravenous urography. Colposcopy has become an indispensible staging procedure, capable of disagnosing stage 0 and 1a cancers which might otherwise escape detection. Wherever possible, examination is performed under anaesthesia. Using these criteria, the reproducibility of assessment is excellent. Unsuspected involvement of the bladder is occasionally found in early cases. Oedema of the bladder mucosa is important since it may be caused by frank invasion of the bladder wall. Intravenous urography is particularly valuable since hydronephrosis and non-functioning kidneys are frequently asymptomatic, and can occur in patients with clinical stage I disease, placing the tumours into the stage III category. The value of lymphography is unclear, though it is a useful means of demonstrating pelvic node metastases. Several studies have shown close concordance between surgical and lymphographic findings, but the contribution to treatment is less certain since pelvic nodes are routinely treated either surgically or by external beam irradiation, even in the absence of firm evidence of involvement. Lymphographic studies have shown an increasing incidence of nodal metastases with advancing stage, with involvement in almost 20% of patients with stage I disease, and over 60% of patients with Stage III disease (5).

Other useful investigations include CT scanning and pelvic ultrasonography, but their value in staging is not yet entirely clear and they have not replaced the other staging procedures.

Management

For patients with CIN 3, therapeutic cone biopsy has been widely employed and usually results in complete excision and cure with preservation of reproductive function. However, newer approaches, particularly laser surgery or cryotherapy, can be expected to cure 70% of cases without cone biopsy. Occasionally, hysterectomy is performed in women beyond the childbearing age or in patients who have no wish for further children. Although hysterectomy is almost always successful, recurrences at the vaginal vault have been reported.

For patients with frankly invasive disease, the most important modalities of treatment are surgery and radiotherapy. Management details vary from one institution to another and it would be unrealistic to deny that local expertise and facilities play an important part in these decisions. Most centres rely on the FIGO staging system to provide guidelines for management.

Stages I and IIa cancers are particularly important, now accounting for over half of all carcinomas of the cervix. Surgery and radiotherapy are equally effective with high 5-year survival rates (over 85-90% in patients with stage I disease) following either method of treatment (6, 7). Although radiotherapy has become standard treatment in many institutions, few direct comparisons are available from the same source, and no randomized studies have been performed. In general, surgical series tend to be more highly selective—in some series, the operability rate of patients with Stage I disease is not much more than half of all patients referred for consideration of surgery. In patients who are suitable, a radical (Wertheim's) hysterectomy is usually recommended. This involves total abdominal hysterectomy with removal of a 2-3 cm cuff of vagina and all supporting tissues within the true pelvis. A complete pelvic lymphadenectomy is performed because 20% of patients have lymph node involvement. Bilateral oophorectomy is often performed but is not mandatory since the tumour rarely metastises to the ovary. Indeed, in young women, conservation of the ovaries is one of the advantages which surgery has over radical radiotherapy.

Care must be taken not to damage the ureters, and operations as extensive as this require great skill. It is probably better for a limited number of gynaecologists to maintain the technique and practice it frequently than for all gynaecologists to infrequently perform this sort of operation. An important advantage of surgery is the definition of the true state of spread which should allow more accurate overall planning of treatment; the radiotherapist never has such complete information. A further important advantage is that although early surgical morbidity is greater than that from radiotherapy, there are fewer late complications.

Surgery in skilled hands is a reasonable alternative to radiotherapy, particularly for young women in whom avoidance of late radiation reactions is particularly desirable. In some young women it may also be possible to conserve the ovaries in an otherwise radical operation. Surgery is often preferred for endocervical lesions and for tumours other than squamous carcinomas, including adeno-acanthomas and sarcomas.

Despite these advantages most centres now recommend that radiotherapy be employed as initial treatment for carcinoma of the cervix, even in early cases with clinical stage I disease.

For patients presenting with more *advanced stages of disease* (*IIb–IV*), radiotherapy is the treatment of choice. In some centres (mostly in North America), radical lymphadenectomy is performed in selected cases, but its therapeutic contribution is uncertain and it has no place in routine management. The claim that radiotherapy cannot deal with node-positive cases seems unfounded. Rutledge and colleagues studied 500 patients who underwent full pelvic irradiation followed by lymph node dissection (8). The number of histologically positive nodes was only one-third of that found in a series of patients treated by surgery alone, suggesting that the radiation therapy was successful in sterilizing pelvic nodes in the majority of cases.

Radiation technique and dosage

Radiotherapy is the most important single treatment for carcinoma of the cervix, and can cure substantial numbers of patients even including some with advanced disease and a small proportion of those who relapse following surgery. Both internal (intracavitary) and external treatments are used. Intracavitary radium treatment is of considerable historic importance in the evolution of modern radiotherapy techniques, but with improvement in equipment, external irradiation has assumed an increasing role. In general, intracavitary treatment is of greater importance in early disease and external beam treatment makes the greater contribution in advanced cases. Some patients with early disease are initially unsuitable for intracavitary treatment, particularly where there is distortion of local anatomy, where the vaginal vault is narrow or the cervical os is obliterated by tumour, making such treatment impossible in the first instance.

In most centres, intracavitary treatment consists of placement of an intra-uterine source (usually radioactive caesium rather than radium, because of its more suitable characteristics—see Chapter 5) together with radioactive sources placed adjacent to the cervix in the lateral vaginal fornices (Fig 17.4). Most centres perform these insertions under a general anaesthetic, except for those employing high dose-rate remote after-loading techniques (see below) where local anaesthetic may be sufficient. Radiotherapy departments now mostly employ after-loading techniques, whereby the plastic housing for both the intra-uterine and vaginal fornix containers are introduced first and the active source inserted only when the geometrical placement is perfect. These techniques produce a typical pear shaped isodose distribution (Fig 17.5). In this way the uterus, cervix and upper vagina all receive a high dose of radiation, with a decreasing but significant dosage to the paracervical and parametrial tissues including at least some of the regional lymphatics. Traditionally, two points, designated A and B, are used as a guide to dosimetry. Though variability in gynaecological anatomy necessarily makes dosimetry based on these arbitrary points difficult, they are widely used as a basis for dose calculation. Point A is located 2 cm from the midline of the cervical canal and 2 cm superior to the lateral vaginal fornix. Point B is

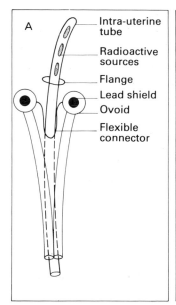

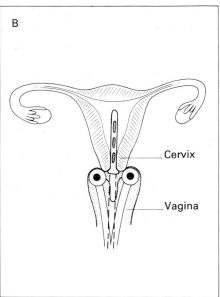

A
Intra-uterine tube
Radioactive sources
Flange
Lead shield
Ovoid
Flexible connector

B
Cervix
Vagina

Fig. 17.4. *Typical disposable after-loading system of intra-cavitary irradiation in carcinoma of the cervix. (A) Components. (B) In position. After placement, these sources act as a single irradiation source, and the components are packed into position to retain their location.*

3 cm lateral to Point A (i.e. 5 cm from the midline along the same lateral axis).

There is a great variety of applicators, some of which are now disposable. Most low dose-rate techniques employ a relatively short treatment time of the order of 2–3 days, though much longer applications, up to a week or

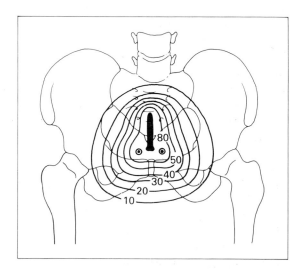

Fig. 17.5. *Typical isodose curves following intracavitary placement of caesium sources for carcinoma of the cervix. The numbers refer to the dose in Gray.*

more, are preferred by some. An alternative approach is the use of high dose-rate equipment such as the Cathetron, which allows remote control after-loading of ^{60}Co sources into manually placed applicators. This equipment certainly carries the advantage of a more rapid treatment and no risk of radiation exposure for staff. However, the patient has to accept the discomfort of repeated treatments, and the long-term complications of high dose-rate therapy have yet to be described in detail.

When external beam irradiation, is employed in conjunction with intracavitary irradiation, the pelvis is usually treated to a dose of 40–50 Gy (4000–5000 rad) over 4–5 weeks (or equivalent) and supplementary treatment to the parametrial region may also be indicated. Some centres employ higher dosage. Many departments employ a simple anterior and posterior parallel pair of fields with supervoltage equipment, though a multifield arrangement is usually better tolerated. A typical field size of 15×15 cm is usually adequate to cover the primary tumour and local nodes. Although some shielding may be possible, irradiation of significant volumes of small and large bowel (including rectum) is unavoidable. In general, it

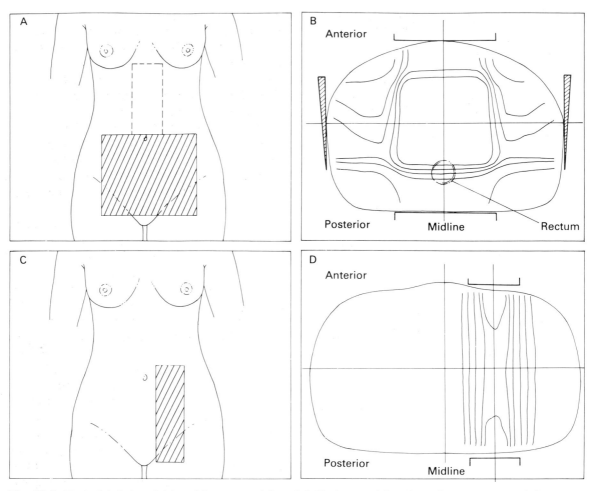

Fig. 17.6. *Typical 'whole pelvis' and 'parametrial boost' fields* (*external beam*) *used in carcinoma of the cervix.* Megavoltage equipment is employed but techniques vary widely. (A) and (B) Whole pelvis. Dotted lines show position of para-aortic field, if used. (C) and (D) Parametrial boost, often used if there is palpable residual disease (can be employed bilaterally).

is irradiation damage to these organs which limits whole pelvic dosage. Typical pelvic and parametrial fields are shown in Fig. 17.6. In advanced cases (stages III and IV), external irradiation is particularly valuable, often controlling pain, haemorrhage and discharge, within days. Additionally, intracavitary treatment may be rendered possible as a result of tumour shrinkage. Although some authorities recommend transvaginal or interstitial radiotherapy for haemorrhage, conventional external beam techniques are probably equally effective.

Combinations of intracavitary and external beam treatment are often employed, though the emphasis may vary in different departments. Fletcher's guidelines (Table 17.2) are based on considerable experience (9) and are widely followed, though they represent a more radical approach in terms of radiation dose, than most British departments would recommend. It is generally accepted that for patients with early stages of disease the intracavitary irradiation is of the greatest importance (additional external irradiation may be unnecessary) and that for

Table 17.2. Radiotherapeutic guidelines for management of carcinoma of the cervix. Values given are for maximum dose.

Stage	Intracavitary irradiation (mg–hr)*	External irradiation (Gy)	
		Whole pelvis	Parametrial boost
I (<1cm)	10 000	—	—
I (>1cm) ⎫	6 500–	0–40	0–40
IIa ⎭	10 000		
IIb	6 500	40–50	—
IIIa	6 500	50	0–15
IIIb	5 000	60	0–10
IV	4 000	70	—

Modified from Fletcher (9).

*Intracavitary irradiation using radium or (more commonly) caesium is traditionally given on two occasions 1–2 weeks apart though there are many variations both in sources and techniques since the advent of remote after-loading equipment.

Milligram-hour (mg–hr) is simply a convenient measure of radium dosage. It is derived from the product of the number of milligrams of radium multiplied by the number of hours of exposure. For example, a total of 4000 mg-hr could be achieved by an exposure of 40 mgm radium for a total of 100 hours. This would generally be attained in two procedures, each lasting 50 hours.

more advanced cases, particularly with lateral spread to the pelvic site wall, external radiation therapy to the whole pelvis contributes more to the final chance of cure. When both methods are employed—as in the majority of patients—some radiotherapists prefer the traditional approach of using the intracavitary irradiation first, whereas an increasing number always use external beam treatment initially. Certainly there will be a few cases in whom the attempt to insert radioactive tubes at the outset is unsuccessful, because of tumour bulk which can to some extent be reduced by treating with external irradiation first. However, the use of intracavitary treatment as primary therapy does allow for central shielding of this treated area when the external beam irradiation is added

later—a real advantage in terms of treatment-related side-effects without significantly reducing the overall radiation dosage to the cervix or upper vagina.

Although both early and late complications of irradiation have been reduced substantially by improved technique and understanding of radiation pathology, they cannot be avoided entirely, particularly if effective dosage schedules are rigidly adhered to. Early problems include diarrhoea, anorexia, nausea and vomiting, together with erythema, dry and (less frequently) moist desquamation of the skin. Most of these symptoms are easily controllable with symptomatic measures, and skin problems have been markedly reduced with the routine use of supervoltage equipment. Intracavitary treatment may produce proctitis and vaginal discharge though cystitis is less common. Late complications are much more important and include chronic proctosigmoiditis, small bowel damage and rectovaginal or vesicovaginal fistulae, which can require urinary or colonic diversion. Avascular necrosis of the femoral heads was a serious complication before the advent of supervoltage treatment, but is now rarely seen. Chronic skin changes, consisting of excessive fibrosis, depigmentation and telangiectasia, are common though rarely cause serious problems. After radiotherapy, the upper vagina usually becomes stenosed and dry. Sexual intercourse is possible but additional lubrication is often required. Radical surgery leads to a short but normally lubricated vagina. The frequency of radiation sequelae is dependent on dose and technique. When intracavitary irradiation is given before the external beam treatment, central shielding of the external beam can be introduced, (Fig 17.7), to avoid over-irradiation of the primary tumour and midline structures particularly the rectum. This seems reasonable since the dose to central structures is already considerable, because of the effectiveness of intracavitary treatment.

Radiation damage occurs even in the most experienced hands since malignant tumours are only marginally more sensitive to radiation

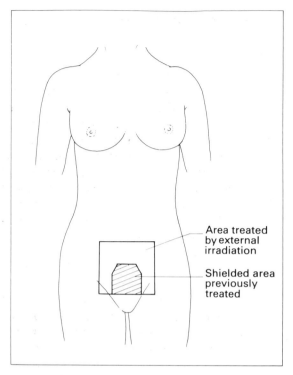

Fig. 17.7. *Central shielding of midline structures in external beam therapy of carcinoma of the cervix for use after intracavitary treatment.*

than normal tissues and radiation dosage is therefore limited by the tolerance of surrounding normal tissues such as bladder, bowel, kidneys and skin (see Chapter 5). Fortunately, with increasingly sophisticated planning and treatment techniques, severe complications such as fistulae and bowel necrosis are now seen less frequently.

Treatment of recurrent disease

In patients with recurrent post-irradiation local disease, but no evidence of distant metastases, pelvic exenteration represents the only chance of cure. This is a major operation with complete removal of the pelvic contents usually including the rectum and bladder, and with a permanent colostomy and ileostomy. Very few surgeons are prepared to undertake this formidable procedure, and careful selection of patients is essential.

Chemotherapy

Chemotherapy has been disappointing in carcinomas of the cervix and is not yet indicated in the initial management. In patients with advanced uncontrolled local disease, or those with widespread metastases, responses are frequently seen, particularly with methotrexate, bleomycin, cisplatin, cyclophosphamide, ifosphamide and doxorubicin. However, these responses tend to be temporary, so far making no real impact in survival. Up to two-thirds of patients show a subjective improvement (often including worthwhile relief of pain), though objective responses are less common. There is as yet no definate advantage for combination chemotherapy over treatment with single agents (10). The increased number of responses seen in recent years gives some hope that chemotherapy might find a role in initial management.

Prognosis

There was a fall in the overall death rate from carcinoma of the cervix between 1940 and 1960 (11), from 9.8 per 100 000 to 6 per 100 000 white US women, and 21.6 to 16 per 100 000 black US women. This was partly due to the 100% curability of CIN 3, which in recent years has been diagnosed more frequently as a result of routine cervical smear testing. For *invasive* carcinoma there have been no recent improvements in survival. Indeed in the increasing proportion of young patients in the 1970s and 1980s, the disease appears to be more aggressive and the prognosis worse. Five-year survival rates reflect the final outcome in the majority of patients, since most though not all, will recur before five years or not at all. The tumour stage is clearly the most important prognostic factor, and patients with stage I disease have a 5-year survival rate of 80–90%; the 10–20% who fail are probably those who have occult abdominal nodal disease. For patients with stages III or IV disease, the 5-year survival rates are of the order of 15–35%, and stage IV disease has a particularly bad prognosis.

Cancer of the cervix and pregnancy

Diagnosis of cancer of the cervix complicates one in 2500 pregnancies. Moreover, in about 1% of cases of cervical cancer, the diagnosis is made during pregnancy, and this proportion may rise as the mean age of diagnosis of cervical cancer falls. Management depends largely on the stage of disease at diagnosis, but also on the stage of the pregnancy and the mother's wishes regarding termination.

If carcinoma *in situ* is diagnosed in a young woman, it is usually safe to allow the pregnancy to continue, though regular cervical smears and colposcopy should be undertaken throughout the pregnancy. In older women, early surgical treatment (cone biopsy) has in the past been considered advisable though there is a 20% complication rate, particularly from haemorrhage. It is no longer considered necessary, providing regular colposcopy is undertaken.

For invasive carcinoma, treatment during the first and second trimester should generally be undertaken without regard for the foetus, providing the patient is prepared to accept termination. Pelvic irradiation usually causes foetal death and inevitable abortion within 6 weeks. Following evacuation of the uterus, intracavitary treatments can be undertaken in the usual way. If the diagnosis is made in the final trimester, most authorities agree that treatment can safely be delayed, with elective caesarian section before the 38th week. Treatment is by surgery (sometimes performed at the time of the caesarian section) or by irradiation following healing of the surgical wound. Unfortunately, delayed treatment cannot always be recommended in the third trimester, for example where severe haemorrhage may present a real threat to the mother's health. Provided that diagnosis and treatment are prompt, the results are as good as those obtained in non-pregnant patients.

CARCINOMA OF THE UTERUS

Aetiology

Endometrial carcinoma is commonest amongst women 50–70 years of age. Its incidence has risen slightly in the past 20 years, though the reasons are not clear (see below). There are wide variations in incidence, from a low of 0.6 per 100 000 Nigerian women, to 14 per 100 000 women living in the South of Great Britain. It is common in Jewish women. The death rate is low since this is a relatively slow growing and well-localized malignancy. Obesity, hypertension and diabetes have long been considered to be risk factors. Although there is uncertainty about the mechanisms, it seems likely that there is peripheral conversion of oestrogen precursors in fat, which may account at least for the rôle of obesity. A widely discussed possible aetiological factor is the presence of endometrial hyperplasia, particularly since the use of exogenous oestrogens for hormone replacement therapy at the menopause frequently produces such change. Of the two major types of endometrial hyperplasia, cystic glandular hyperplasia is generally thought to have a low rate of progression to malignancy, whilst in the other type, atypical adenomatous hyperplasia, at least 1 in 10 patients progress to develop endometrial carcinoma. Late menopause is also important as a risk factor, because of the excess and prolonged oestrogenic stimulus.

A number of studies have suggested an increased incidence of carcinoma of the endometrium in patients taking exogenous oestrogens. In several of these, the risk index for all women receiving oestrogens was over five times that of control subjects. However, there are a number of criticisms of these studies including the frequency with which control cases and patients taking exogenous oestrogen were examined, as well as the possibility that hyperplasia itself can be difficult to distinguish from frank malignancy, even by experienced pathologists. Although there is good evidence therefore that cyclical oestrogen therapy produces endometrial hyperplasia, its role in the development of invasive carcinoma has yet to be fully established. Unopposed continuous oestrogen replacement appears to be more dangerous in this respect than cyclical oestrogen used in conjunction with a progestogen. Low dose oestrogen probably carries little risk.

Pathology and staging

By far the commonest of tumours of the body of the uterus is the endometrial adenocarcinoma which constitutes at least 90% of all endometrial neoplasms. The next largest group of endometrial tumours is the adeno-acanthoma, which is an adenocarcinoma with areas of benign squamous metaplasia. Mixed mesodermal tumours occur. Other tumours include adeno-squamous carcinoma and a variety of soft tissue sarcomas, chiefly leiomyosarcoma which arises from the muscle wall.

The degree of differentiation of adenocarcinoma of the endometrium can be very variable. Conventionally, three grades or histological differentiations are recognized. The largest single group is the well-differentiated (grade I) adeno-carcinoma.

Lymphatic spread is chiefly to pelvic nodes, particularly the external and common iliac group (and thence to the para-aortic nodes), as well as the paracervical and obturator nodes. Lymph node 'skipping', i.e. with metastatic involvement of para-aortic nodes bypassing the pelvic node groups, is well described. Inguinal node metastases are also encountered. Morrow *et al.* (12) reviewed a large series of patients with localized carcinoma of the endometrium, noting an incidence of positive nodes of 11% with a particularly high likelihood in patients with grade III (the most anaplastic) lesions. It was also clear from this and other studies that deep myometrial invasion of tumour is associated with a high incidence of positive local nodes (Table 17.3). As these authors pointed out, this clearly implies that local nodal metastases are almost as common in endometrial carcinoma as in cancer of the cervix.

Table 17.3. Incidence of pelvic lymph node metastases in carcinoma of the endometrium: the relationship to tumour grade and depth of myometrial invasion. Figures refer to the number of patients in whom positive nodes were confirmed (n = 140).

Depth of myometrial invasion	Histological grade			Total number with +ve pelvic lymph nodes (%)
	I	II	III	
<1/3	1/60	4/42	4/14	9/116 (8)
>1/3	1/5	2/8	4/11	7/24 (29)
TOTAL	2/65	6/50	8/25	16/140 (11)

From Morrow (12).

As with other cancers, the histological grade, depth of invasion, frequency of nodal involvement and likelihood of local recurrence are interrelated variables. For this reason it is difficult to assess the separate contributions of histological grade and tumour stage to prognosis.

Myometrial invasion is important since its depth correlates closely with the incidence of recurrence. Patients whose tumour shows superficial invasion only, have a local recurrence rate of well below 10%, whereas with deep invasion the recurrence rate is approximately 25%. Although more common in patients with high grade tumours, myometrial involvement is sometimes seen in patients with well-differentiated lesions. Direct spread to the cervix and vagina also occurs though vaginal 'satellite' metastases (i.e. not as part of direct extension) are unusual at presentation. Vaginal deposits are commoner in patients with recurrent disease, and occur predominantly in patients who have not been treated with radiotherapy. Local spread to other pelvic structures such as the broad ligament, fallopian tubes and ovaries also occurs.

Blood-borne metastases are unusual, though more common than with carcinoma of the cervix. Peritoneal involvement, pulmonary deposits and even ascites are features of advanced disease. Late metastases to para-aortic nodes, lung, bone and supraclavicular nodes are in-

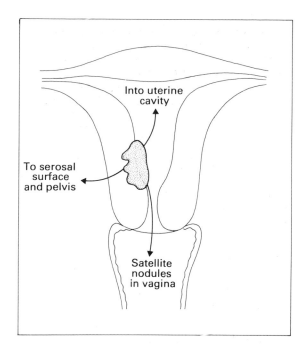

Fig. 17.8. *Local spread in carcinoma of the corpus uteri.*

creasingly encountered with greater survival time.

The routes of spread and current staging systems are summarized in Fig. 17.8 and Table 17.4. At present both the TNM and FIGO systems are used, though both suffer from the fact

Table 17.4. Clinical staging in carcinoma of the endometrium. T-stage (from TNM staging system) shown in brackets, but the staging definitions are essentially those of the FIGO.

Stage	Description
Stage 0	Carcinoma *in situ* (TIS)
Stage I	Carcinoma confined to the corpus uteri (T1)
Ia	Uterine cavity 8 cm or less in length (T1a)
Ib	Uterine cavity >8 cm (T1b)
Stage II	Extension to cervix only (T2)
Stage III	Extension beyond the uterus but disease confined to true pelvis (T3)
Stage IV	Extension beyond true pelvis, or invasion of bladder or rectum (T4)

that the limits of cancer spread cannot be determined by clinical means as easily as in carcinoma of the cervix. The large majority of patients with endometrial carcinoma have localized disease, and are potentially curable by surgery. For most carcinomas of the uterus, the clinical stage at presentation is Ia or Ib, and surgical staging at laparotomy is particularly important.

Clinical features and treatment

Postmenopausal bleeding is the cardinal symptom of endometrial carcinoma and is an indication for dilatation and curettage even if the bleeding is mild. Twenty per cent of cases occur in premenopausal patients so intermenstrual bleeding is also an important clinical feature. Other symptoms such as pain and vaginal discharge are uncommon and suggestive of more advanced disease. The uterus may be enlarged clinically and these patients should be investigated with particular urgency. The diagnosis is established by curettage, and the differential diagnosis includes postmenopausal bleeding from other causes, of which the most common is probably atrophic vaginitis.

Surgery is the most important treatment for endometrial carcinoma. Most gynaecologists agree that a total abdominal hysterectomy with bilateral salpingo-oophorectomy is the operation of choice. Because of the success of surgical treatment in localized cancers, the role of radiotherapy as routine additional treatment has been questioned. There seems little need for irradiation for localized well-differentiated tumours without evidence of myometrial invasion. On the other hand, where the histology is poorly differentiated or anaplastic, many gynaecologists refer such patients for postoperative irradiation because of the risk of local recurrence, particularly in patients with evidence of myometrial invasion beyond one-third of the thickness of the uterine wall. With myometrial penetration, or involvement of the cervix, the risk of node metastases is also high—at least 30% by a high-grade tumour.

Additional radiotherapy treatment can be either pre-operative, usually by means of intrauterine radioactive caesium insertion, or by external beam irradiation to the true pelvis. Pre-operative intracavitary irradiation reduces the volume of tumour and also reduces the probability of subsequent vaginal metastases. However, pre-operative treatment may be technically difficult because of enlargement of the uterus and/or widespread intrauterine involvement by the tumour. It may be necessary to pack the uterus with several irradiating sources rather than relying on the arrangement usually employed for carcinoma of the cervix. External beam irradiation may be an acceptable alternative and is probably equally effective for reducing the incidence of vaginal metastases. In one large series treated in this way (13), no vaginal recurrences were seen. Such treatment may result in up to 50% of patients being free of disease at the time of subsequent planned hysterectomy.

In Britain, many gynaecologists and radiotherapists advocate pre-operative intracavitary irradiation and a dose of 60 Gy (6000 rad) to Point A (see p. 292) is often recommended. The authors prefer the use of postoperative external irradiation in selected cases. After total abdominal hysterectomy with bilateral salpingo-oophorectomy, supplementary external radiation therapy is best reserved for patients with adverse risk factors such as deep myometrial invasion or poor histology, both of which can be better determined at operation. In most patients, a dose of 45–55 Gy (4500–5500 rad) in daily fractions over 4.5–5.5 weeks is well tolerated and effective.

In patients with recurrent disease, the use of further irradiation, endocrine therapy with progestogens, or chemotherapy can all be worthwhile. Vaginal recurrences, usually seen in previously unirradiated patients, respond to local therapy with intra-vaginal caesium loaded in a plastic (Dobbie) applicator, though some radiotherapists prefer to use interstitial radiotherapy (usually with 192-iridium).

Progestogen treatment may be beneficial for local recurrence but is particularly valuable for patients with distant metastatic disease. Several large series of patients have confirmed that about one-third show an objective response, and that responding patients have a much longer lifespan than patients who show no response. On the other hand, the use of progestogens as an adjuvant to surgery has not been shown to prolong survival. The most popular drug is medroxyprogesterone acetate, given by mouth at doses of the order of 100 mgm t.d.s. Pulmonary metastases seem particularly likely to respond.

In patients who fail to respond to progestogen therapy, chemotherapy has sometimes been of value. The most useful agents appear to be cyclophosphamide, 5-fluorouracil, vincristine and doxorubicin. Combination chemotherapy may produce more responses than treatment with single agents, but at the cost of increased toxicity. There is no place for chemotherapy in the routine treatment of early endometrial carcinoma.

For further discussion of uterine sarcomas and their management, see Chapter 23.

Prognosis

In white US women, the age-adjusted death rate is 1.4 per 100 000, with a total death rate of 3300 in 1975. About two-thirds of patients with endometrial carcinoma are cured by current treatments. As previously mentioned, the survival falls with extra-uterine spread, poorly differentiated tumours and those with deep myometrial invasion.

Unfortunately, no prospectively randomized study has been done to assess the value of pre- or postoperative radiotherapy as an adjunct to surgery. Taking together the large series of patients treated with pre-operative radiotherapy and surgery, the 5-year survival rate is over 75%. Indeed the results of radiotherapy alone have often surprised those who feel surgery to be essential. In Kottmeier's series of almost 1500 patients treated in Stockholm, the 5-year survival was 63% (14). The survival of 'operable lesions' (809 patients) was 79%, comparable to or better than many of the surgical series.

The relatively good prognosis of endometrial carcinoma is largely due to the preponderance of localized disease, which itself is probably a reflection of the slow growing nature of the tumour and the early concern aroused by its major symptom: postmenopausal bleeding.

The increasing incidence of adenosquamous carcinomas is of considerable concern since this particular group of tumours has a poor prognosis. The 5-year survival rate is less than 20%, compared to over 70% for well-differentiated adenocarcinomas and adeno-acanthomas. Patients with sarcomas of the uterus also do less well, with reported 5-year survival rates between 15% and 32%, but possibly with a slightly more favourable outlook in younger women. Once again, in this group the degree of myometrial invasion is important. If leiomyosarcoma is an incidental finding following removal of a uterine fibroid, the survival rate is over 80% whereas in patients with invasive leiomyosarcomas, survival is very poor indeed.

CARCINOMA OF THE OVARY

Little is known of the aetiology of this disease. It is commoner in nulliparous and subfertile women and there are wide demographic differences in mortality rates; for example, the mortality rate in Denmark is six times as great as in Japanese women. There is both a familial incidence and an increased frequency in women with breast cancer—possible also related to nulliparity. There is a 10% risk of ovarian tumours in patients with the Peutz-Jeghers syndrome.

Clinical features

These tumours usually present late and only one-third are localized at the time of diagnosis. Early ovarian cancer is often asymptomatic. When symptoms occur they are often vague and are overlooked by the patients even when the tumour is locally advanced and lower abdominal distension is obvious to the doctor. Lower abdominal pain, bloating and anorexia are common, but often insufficiently specific to raise suspicions which might then lead to further investigation. Signs such as ascites or palpable pelvic masses often indicate advanced disease. Even with more widespread use of cervical smear tests and annual examinations, the proportion of early diagnoses has not risen. At present there is no evidence that routine screening tests are able to uncover a significant number of women with early disease. Possibilities for the future include pelvic ultrasound, which is rapidly improving in its resolving power, as well as transvaginal aspiration with cytology of peritoneal washings. So far, rate of diagnosis in asymptomatic women is low but these and other methods may prove valuable in the future.

Pathology, staging and prognosis

There is great variety in the histological subtypes of ovarian cancer. The World Health Organization lists 27 subtypes for benign and malignant primary ovarian tumours (15). About 90% of ovarian carcinomas originate from the epithelial surface of the ovary, the remainder comprising the much less common group of germ cell tumours (both teratomas and dysgerminomas), ovarian sarcomas, granulosa cell tumours, thecomas, Leydig and Sertoli cell tumours. Of the epithelial carcinomas, the major types include serous cystadenocarcinoma, mucinous, endometrioid, clear cell (mesonephroid) and undifferentiated adenocarcinomas. For epithelial tumours there is little doubt that the tumour grade, or degree of differentiation, is of prognostic importance particularly in serous tumours. Within this group, the histological grade can vary from those which are barely malignant to highly undifferentiated invasive tumours. In general, tumours which are relatively well-differentiated are more likely to be operable.

Clinical staging is of considerable importance in ovarian cancer and is often considered the

Table 17.5. FIGO staging system in carcinoma of the ovary. From Tobias and Griffiths, 1976 (16).

Stage	Description
Stage I	Growth limited to ovary (26%)*
Ia	One ovary involved
Ib	Both ovaries involved
Ic	Ascites present, or positive peritoneal washings
Stage II	Growth limited to pelvis (21%)
IIa	Extension to gynaecological adnexae
IIb	Extension to other pelvic tissues
Stage III	Growth extending to abdominal cavity—including peritoneal surface seedlings, omentum etc. (37%).
Stage IV	Metastases to distant sites (including hepatic parenchymal disease) (16%)

*Figures in brackets refer to proportion of total cases presenting with each particular stage.

most important indicator of prognosis (16). The FIGO (International Federation of Gynaecology and Obstetrics) staging system is now widely accepted (Table 17.5), and Table 17.6 shows the relation between FIGO stage and prognosis. Patients with disease localized to the ovaries have an overall survival rate of 60%.

Table 17.6. Relationship between FIGO stage and prognosis in carcinoma of the ovary.

Stage	Number of patients	% 5-year survival
Stage I	751	61
Ia	528	65
Ib	130	52
Ic	80	52
Stage II	401	40
IIa*	40	60
IIb	205	38
Stage III	539	5
Stage IV	101	3

From Tobias and Griffiths (16).
* The distinction between stage IIa and IIb is a particularly important one prognostically, the 5-year survival of patients with stage IIa disease being similar to that of patients with stage I disease.

However, even within this group, further risk factors have been identified. For example, in a large series from the Mayo clinic, patients with intracystic tumours had a 5-year survival rate of 98%, whereas in those with intra-operative rupture or adherence of the tumour to surrounding structures, the 5-year survival was reduced by half. When the disease has spread outside the ovary but is still confined to the pelvis, there is an important distinction between tumours with minimal local spread to adjacent gynaecological organs (stage IIa) which carry a 5-year survival rate almost as good as stage I tumours, and those which have spread more widely (stage IIb) and which carry a very much poorer prognosis.

Once the tumour has disseminated beyond the pelvis into the peritoneal cavity, the outlook is very much worse, particularly in patients with bulky abdominal disease. Common sites of intra-abdominal tumour include the omentum, the peritoneal surface (often the site of multiple seedlings) and the undersurface of the diaphragm, a particularly important area for inspection at the initial operation (Fig. 17.9). Beyond the peritoneal cavity, important sites for metastasis include liver, lungs and occasionally the central nervous system. Lymph node spread is chiefly to pelvic and para-aortic nodes, and less commonly to supraclavicular, neck and inguinal nodes. Bone marrow dissemination is extremely unusual.

Surgical management

Operative treatment has always been the cornerstone of successful management in ovarian cancer. The initial operation has a greater bearing on outcome than any subsequent therapy, and the success of postoperative treatment largely depends on careful operative assessment and adequate removal of tumour.

Careful inspection of the whole of the abdominal cavity is an essential part of the initial procedure before removal of tumour. In particular, the infra-diaphragmatic surfaces and para-acolic gutters should be carefully inspected,

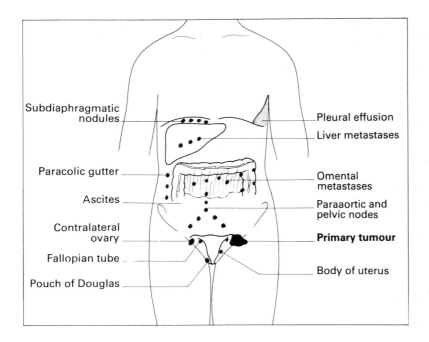

Subdiaphragmatic nodules

Paracolic gutter

Ascites

Contralateral ovary

Fallopian tube

Pouch of Douglas

Pleural effusion

Liver metastases

Omental metastases

Paraaortic and pelvic nodes

Primary tumour

Body of uterus

Fig. 17.9. *Common sites of metastasis in carcinoma of the ovary.*

since these are common but often overlooked sites of spread. Even when sub-diaphragmatic seedlings are not visible, peritoneal lavage may reveal malignant cells from this and other sites. The importance of such inspection cannot be overestimated; Rosenoff and others (17) have shown that using such procedures, a substantial proportion of patients initially thought to have localized disease have evidence of more widespread dissemination, making local treatment entirely inappropriate.

For stage I disease, surgery is often the only treatment recommended and usually consists of total abdominal hysterectomy and bilateral salpingo-oophorectomy. Even with unilateral tumours, the opposite ovary is normally removed as there is a 20% frequency of bilateral tumours or occult metastases. In young women, particularly anxious to retain fertility, conservative operations are occasionally performed, though the safety of this approach is uncertain. In one large series, the survival rate of 60% at 5-years following 'conservative' surgery was 10% below the survival rate following a more complete operation (18). In tumours of borderline malignancy, conservative operations can be

recommended with greater confidence though most gynaecologists understandably prefer to perform a full operation unless the patient is particularly anxious to become pregnant.

In patients with more advanced disease (stages II–IV) the consensus of opinion favours excision of as much tumour as possible at the time of initial operation. Good palliation may be achieved by the reduction of a heavy tumour burden but there is little evidence that surgical debulking procedures substantially improve survival unless all or nearly all of the tumour can be excised. Many of the technically operable tumours are of relatively low-grade which will itself imply a more favourable prognosis. Nonetheless, Griffiths and others have shown that the size of the largest postoperative residual tumour nodule is a good predictor not only of responsiveness to the subsequent postoperative treatment, but also of the ultimate outcome (19). Using a multiple linear regression equation with survival as the dependent variable, only histological tumour grade and size of the largest postoperative residual mass were factors of real importance; the operation itself contributed nothing to survival, unless it reduced the size of the largest tumour mass below an upper limit of 1.6 cm in diameter.

Most clinicians would agree that post-operative chemotherapy or radiotherapy in patients with residual palpable masses is extremely unlikely to be curative. For this reason many radiotherapists and oncologists recommend a second operative procedure in patients in whom the initial laparotomy did not include an attempt at removal of tumour. It therefore seems likely that expert surgeons will be needed to perform the definitive operation, wherever possible. Gynaecological oncologists have become increasingly radical in their surgical approach, and lengthy operations including removal of pelvic contents, omentectomy, bowel resection and excision of the entire parietal pelvic peritoneum, are now performed more frequently (20).

Quite apart from the critically important first operation, the gynaecologist has an increasingly accepted role in 'second-look' procedures. Despite the advent of abdomino-pelvic ultrasonography, lymphography, CT scanning and other imaging procedures, there is no reliable guide to the effectiveness of treatment in advanced ovarian cancer short of a further exploratory procedure. Such information is invaluable for several reasons. First, it indicates whether postoperative treatment has been successful in eradicating residual tumour. Secondly, it may be possible to perform further surgery at the second procedure. Finally, in patients who have achieved a complete remission confirmed by a second look procedure, it may be possible to discontinue chemotherapy. Laparotomy may not be required in all such cases, since laparoscopic re-evaluation sometimes shows residual disease even in patients who have achieved a complete clinical remission. Laparotomy is justifiable in cases where laparoscopic examination has failed to show residual disease and peritoneal washings have been negative. Nonetheless, it is difficult to demonstrate beyond doubt that 'second-look' laparotomy has contributed to improved survival in ovarian cancer, although treat-ment decisions have become more logical as a result.

In summary, the role of the gynaecological surgeon in the management of ovarian cancer has changed and continues to evolve. The initial assessment and operative procedure is a critically important part of management, both for localized and generalized disease. The surgeon also has an important role in the assessment of response. Although second-look laparotomy is the most reliable means of judging response, there remains doubt about its therapeutic value in patients with residual disease.

Radiotherapy

Radiotherapy has been used in several distinct ways: as definitive therapy, as an adjuvant to surgery, for recurrent disease and occasionally as pre-operative treatment. It has often been recommended as postoperative treatment for patients with disease confined to the pelvis, though evidence for its routine use is unconvincing (16). The two main techniques which have been used are first, pelvic irradiation (for patients with stage I or II disease) usually to a dose of 40–50 Gy (4000–5000 rad) over 4–5.5 weeks, using either anteroposterior or multifield techniques (Fig. 17.10); and secondly, whole

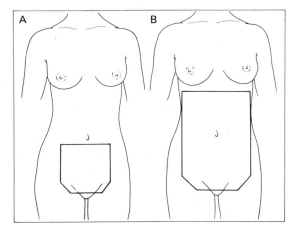

Fig. 17.10. *Commonly used radiotherapy treatments in carcinoma of the ovary.* (A) Pelvic field. (B) Whole abdominal irradiation.

abdominal irradiation. The latter is technically one of the most difficult techniques in clinical radiotherapy, and is always difficult to achieve, in view of the very large treatment volume (Fig. 17.10). Adequate irradiation including the sub-diaphragmatic areas results in a treatment volume extending from the pelvic floor to the domes of the diaphragm. The dose rate has to be low (usually 1 Gy/day) for patients to be able to tolerate this treatment without developing severe nausea and myelosuppression. It is especially difficult to deliver after chemotherapy because of the risk of radiation nephritis and hepatitis. The kidneys and liver are shielded after doses of 15–20 Gy and the total elsewhere has to be limited to doses of the order of 25 Gy (usually taking about 5 weeks daily treatment) together with boosting of the pelvis alone to a dose of 40–50 Gy (4000–5000 rad).

In FIGO stage I disease, retrospective studies of surgery alone *vs* surgery with postoperative irradiation have suffered from the usual difficulty that the two study groups may not have been similar enough for comparison to be valid. In most of these retrospective studies, the group receiving postoperative radiotherapy did less well than the group receiving surgery alone, which probably means that patients selected for postoperative irradiation were, in general, a higher risk group, because of cyst rupture at operation or other unspecified features. Five-year survival rates in patients with stage I disease vary from 50 to 65%, regardless of whether or not radiotherapy is given. Survival figures from prospective studies of surgery alone *vs* surgery plus local irradiation are beginning to emerge, though no clear differences have so far been demonstrated.

In stage II disease, there seems to be a genuine benefit from the use of postoperative pelvic irradiation (16). In almost all series, admittedly retrospective, the 5 year survival rate was improved (Table 17.7), particularly where adequate surgery had already been undertaken (see p. 302). Since these studies were performed before careful operative staging was a routine part of the initial assessment, many of these

Table 17.7. Adjuvant radiotherapy in FIGO stage II disease.

Number of patients		5-year survival (%)	
Operation alone	Operation + irradiation	Operation alone	Operation + irradiation
8	22	25.0	36.4
27	91	33.0	48.0
32	36	28.2	52.8
16	61	0	40.0
4	12	55.0	63.0
6	51	16.7	31.4
	18*		72†
	6‡		33†
	13		69
13	16	23.1	25

From Tobias and Griffiths (16)
* Palpable disease after operation
† 4-yr follow-up results only
‡ No palpable disease after operation

patients would in fact have had stage III disease. For this reason the results of postoperative radiotherapy in true stage II disease may be even better than these figures suggest. In patients with more advanced disease (stage III–IV) the value of postoperative irradiation is equivocal; although postoperative whole abdominal irradiation has been claimed to produce modest improvement in 5-year survival from about 5% to 10%, the evidence is unconvincing.

Recent work from Toronto has reawakened interest in radiation therapy for ovarian carcinoma (21). Patients undergoing surgery (total hysterectomy, bilateral salpingo-oophorectomy and omentectomy) were randomized to receive either chemotherapy with chlorambucil, pelvic irradiation alone, or radiotherapy to the whole abdomen with a boost to the pelvic region. There was a clear survival advantage for patients receiving abdomino-pelvic irradiation (Stages IIa–III) despite the difficulties in achieving more than a low dose of irradiation to such a large area (Fig. 17.11). There seems little doubt that the superior results from this study largely reflected the adequacy of initial surgical

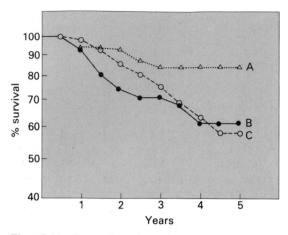

Fig. 17.11. *Survival in stage Ib and II carcinoma of the ovary treated with pelvic irradiation after surgery.* (A) Additional whole abdominal irradiation. (B) Pelvic irradiation alone. (C) Additional chlorambucil. (Modified from Dembo *et al.* (21). With permission.)

treatment. There was a highly significant survival difference in favour of patients without palpable postoperative tumour, regardless of whether chemotherapy or radiotherapy was used as the postoperative treatment. It is also possible that the 'moving strip' technique of radiotherapy employed by this group allowed a reasonable radiation dose to be delivered without undue toxicity though later data discounts this view. As expected the radiation dosage was limited by renal, hepatic and bowel tolerance. Most radiotherapists feel that the gastro-intestinal dysfunction and partial bowel obstruction so commonly associated with advanced ovarian cancer makes many patients poor candidates for whole-abdominal irradiation, with its high likelihood of additional gastro-intestinal side-effects. Unfortunately the incidence of recurrent subacute bowel obstruction appears to be increased by the use of abdominal radiation therapy (16).

An alternative form of radiotherapy is the use of intraperitoneal radioactive colloids such as gold (^{198}Au) or phosphorus (^{32}P). Originally used for treatment of malignant effusions, they have gradually been replaced by systemic treatment with chemotherapy. This approach is now more commonly used as adjuvant therapy in patients with small superficial intraperitoneal tumour inplants, particularly when recurrent ascites, not controlled by cytotoxic drugs, is a clinical problem. It has also been claimed that radioactive colloids are of value in patients with stage I disease either incompletely removed, or resected with intra-operative spillage from rupture of a malignant cyst (22).

Chemotherapy

For patients who present with disease outside the true pelvis (FIGO stages III and IV) the initial treatment after surgery is usually with chemotherapy. Ovarian cancer is moderately sensitive to cytotoxic agents but for most drugs information regarding response rates to single agents was gained, at a time when no attempt had been made to reduce tumour bulk before starting treatment. Since massive disease reduces responsiveness (see Chapter 6), the reported response rates to many agents may be lower than those which could be achieved under more favourable conditions. Stringent criteria of assessment were seldom used; complete response therefore usually meant no more than the clinical disappearance of disease, artificially raising the response rate. Nowadays response rate data should be based on careful pre- and post-treatment assessment of tumour size, including, where necessary, the use of imaging techniques and, if appropriate, second-look laparotomy.

SINGLE AGENTS

The response rates to the most useful single agents are shown in Table 17.8. Alkylating agents have been the most widely employed drugs. Chlorambucil, cyclophosphamide and melphalan have been used most frequently, with response rates for each in the range of 40%. Recent studies have not altered this figure. There is, however, some evidence that response rates are higher when the dose is given in high dose in a pulsed intermittent form (23). Of the antimetabolites, 5-fluorouracil and methotrexate

Table 17.8. Response to single agent chemotherapy in advanced ovarian carcinoma.

Agent	Response rate (%)
Alkylating agents	
Cyclophosphamide	50–60
Chlorambucil	50
Melphalan	45
Antimetabolites	
Methotrexate	25
5-fluorouracil	25
Others	
Cisplatin*	40–60
Doxorubicin*	30–40
Hexamethylmelamine	30–40

* Since much of the data regarding response rates of newer drugs has been obtained in patients already resistant to alkylating agents, the true single-agent response to cisplatin, doxorubicin and others may be higher.

have some activity but complete responses are rarely seen. The vinca alkaloids have not been tested extensively in ovarian cancer but reported response rates are low. Hexamethylmelamine is a drug with activity, though its side-effects are considerable (see Chapter 6). Of the newer drugs, cisplatin and its derivatives are the most promising. Response rates of 25–60% have been recorded, but the schedules of administration have varied widely. There is evidence that higher doses may be associated with increased response rates, though of course this incurs the penalty of increased toxicity. It is now clear that cisplatin is more effective than alkylating agents such as cyclophosphamide. Cisplatin is a toxic drug causing severe nausea and vomiting, renal and VIII nerve damage, and peripheral neuropathy. The newer analogues appear to have similar activity to the parent compound, but reduced toxicity (24). Doxorubicin has some activity (30% response rate) but is not useful in patients who have relapsed after failure with alkylating agents.

In ovarian cancer attempts have been made to predict tumour responsiveness *in vitro* using colony formation (see Chapter 6). It is too

soon to assess the potential of these techniques. At present it seems that they will only provide negative evidence—if a drug is inactive *in vitro*, it will be ineffective *in vivo* (25).

COMBINATION CHEMOTHERAPY

As in other malignancies, there has been an increasing tendency in recent years to use combinations of drugs for advanced ovarian cancer. In previously untreated patients, higher response rates have been achieved than with single agents (Table 17.9). However, where studies have been carried out in patients who have relapsed after treatment with a single agent, responses to the combinations have usually been poor.

Most of these studies have not made any formal comparison with a single agent so that an

Table 17.9. Combination chemotherapy in advanced ovarian cancer.

Drug	Dose	Response rate (%)
Doxorubicin	40 mg/m² day 1 ⎫ every	55
Cyclophosphamide [A–C]	500 mg/m² day 1 ⎭ 4 weeks	
Hexamethyl-melamine	150 mg/m² daily ×14 ⎫	
Cyclophosphamide	150 mg/m² daily ×14 ⎬ every 4 weeks	75
Methotrexate	40 mg/m² day 1, 8	
5-Fluorouracil [Hexa-CAF]	600 mg/m² day 1, 8 ⎭	
Cyclophosphamide	300 mg/m² daily 1 ⎫	
Doxorubicin	30–40 mg/m² day 1 ⎬ every 3 weeks	60–75
Cisplatin [CAP]	50 mg/m² day 1 ⎭	
Cyclophosphamide	300 mg/m² day 1 ⎫	
Hexamethyl-melamine	150 mg/m² daily ×14 ⎬ every 4 weeks	65–80
Doxorubicin	40 mg/m² day 1	
Cisplatin [CHAP]	50 mg/m² day 1 ⎭	

(Schedules and administration vary widely. Reported response rates also differ and figures are approximate.)

advantage in *survival* over simple alkylating agent therapy has not been shown. In the widely quoted study of Young *et al*, an early advantage was observed for combination chemotherapy over single agent treatment (26), but the toxicity was much greater and the final survival data have not yet been published. In a study from the Mayo Clinic, a similar advantage for a two drug regimen (cyclophosphamide and doxorubicin) was seen only in patients with minimal residual disease after surgery (27).

In future studies of combination chemotherapy, it will be essential to compare effective combinations with single agent therapy after 'debulking' surgery has been carried out. It is important to establish whether aggressive chemotherapy increases the chance of cure in patients who have had effective surgery. Studies which include a majority of patients with a poor prognosis (including those in whom the operation did not attempt any worthwhile removal of bulk disease) may obscure the potential benefits of intensive chemotherapy in the other patients. For patients with a poor prognosis, the substantial toxicity of combination chemotherapy may not be justified by the few extra months of life. The current position is that surgical removal of as much of the tumour mass as possible, followed by an effective single agent or combination chemotherapy regimen, will result in a minority of patients being free of tumour 1–2 years after the initial treatment, as judged by subsequent laparotomy or laparoscopy. The ultimate prognosis of these patients remains to be determined but there now seems little doubt that cure is possible though in a disappointingly small proportion.

A worrying sequel to long term treatment of ovarian cancer with alkylating agents (particularly melphalan) is the development of acute leukaemia, usually of the myeloid type. Frank leukaemia is often preceded by a period in which the blood count is abnormal, with mild neutropenia, thrombocytopenia and macrocytosis. The cumulative incidence in surviving patients after chemotherapy for 2 years is probably of the order of 5% (28).

Unresolved controversies in epithelial ovarian cancer

It will be apparent from the foregoing discussion that there are several important issues in management to be resolved over the next few years. These are:

1 The contribution of debulking surgery both to improving response rates to chemotherapy, and to overall survival.

2 The role of radiotherapy in stage II disease, in stage III disease after cytoreductive surgery, and in patients with minimal residual disease after second-look laparotomy.

3 The contribution of second-look laparotomy to treatment. Will further surgery at this stage, followed by additional treatment (either with further chemotherapy or whole-abdominal irradiation) result in long-term survival for some patients?

4 Definition of the place of combination chemotherapy compared with the best single agent therapy. Assessment of the role of new platinum analogues in combination.

5 Is second-line chemotherapy of any value in patients who fail to achieve complete remission or who relapse after treatment?

GERM CELL TUMOURS OF OVARY

A pathological classification of germ cell tumours of the ovary is shown in Table 17.10. Benign dermoid cysts are relatively common and are cured by surgical excision. Occasionally they consist largely of thyroid tissue, *struma ovarii*, which may even be functioning. Less than 5% of strumas are malignant—so-called *monomorphic* or *monodermal teratomas*. Rarely they may show secondary malignant change, most commonly squamous carcinoma.

Of the malignant tumours, *dysgerminoma* is much the commonest and histologically is a uniform clear cell tumour resembling seminoma in males. Lymphocytic infiltration is common. The endodermal sinus tumour (*yolk sac tumour*) is a highly malignant tumour which produces α-fetoprotein (AFP) which can be demonstrated

Table 17.10. Germ cell tumours of the ovary.

Tumour	% of all malignant germ cell tumours
Benign (20% of all ovarian tumours) Dermoid cyst—mature cystic teratoma	
Malignant (3% of all ovarian tumours)	
Dysgerminoma	50
Endodermal sinus tumour or yolk sac tumour	20
Embryonal carcinoma	3
Malignant (immature) tera-toma (includes malignant mono-dermal teratomas and carcinoids)	20
Mixed germ cell tumours	7
Choriocarcinoma	rare
Gonadoblastoma	

in the tumour and is detectable in the blood. Rupture of the tumour occurs early. *Embryonal carcinoma* consists of glandular and papillary masses, often with trophoblastic elements which secrete human chorionic gonadotrophin (HCG). It may occur in childhood and produce sexual precocity. AFP may also be produced by yolk sac elements in the tumour. *Immature teratoma* is a mainly solid tumour containing a multiplicity of different tissues. Primitive neuroectoderm often predominates but monomorphic forms consisting of thyroid tissue or malignant carcinoid also occur. Even when the tumour has not metastasized, carcinoid syndrome may occur because of the large size. The *mixed germ cell tumour* contains mixtures of the previous histological types. *Gonadoblastoma* is a small tumour arising in childhood, usually composed of several of the elements of the developing gonad. It may calcify, rarely metastasizes, but might cause virilization as it may contain functioning Leydig cells.

CLINICAL FEATURES

In dysgerminoma, as with other malignant ovarian tumours, the presentation is with an abdominal mass and pain, but the mean age is far lower; 75% of patients are between 10 and 30 years old (median 20 years). They do not usually produce marker hormones unless teratomatous elements are present, and they not infrequently present during or shortly after pregnancy. Other germ cell tumours (yolk sac, endodermal sinus tumours, teratoma, mixed germ cell tumour) are also tumours of adolescents and young women. Many of these patients have precocious puberty, menstrual disturbance and a positive pregnancy test (with pregnancy as a differential diagnosis of the pelvic mass!). These tumours grow rapidly causing abdominal pain.

MANAGEMENT

In dysgerminoma, management depends on stage. Ninety percent of patients with FIGO stage I are cured by unilateral oophorectomy but the recurrence rate is higher with large tumours, positive peritoneal washings at operation, or if the tumour contains mixed germ cell elements. If recurrence occurs, or if there are metastases, patients are usually treated with whole abdominal irradiation, often extending into the mediastinum and left supraclavicular region. The routine use of postoperative radiotherapy is questionable and more advanced stages of disease might well be better treated with chemotherapy as for teratoma (see below) but experience is very limited. Yolk sac, endodermal sinus and mixed germ cell tumours have a much worse prognosis with surgical treatment than dysgerminoma, even in stage I disease. The use of serum AFP and βHCG as markers has greatly improved the monitoring of chemotherapy, which is now an essential part of treatment for most patients (exceptions are discussed below).

The use of platinum-based regimens has followed the outstanding success achieved in testicular teratoma. Since the tumours are unilateral they can be managed by unilateral salpingo-oophorectomy followed by chemotherapy, with the possibility of preservation of fertility. Exceptions to the use of chemotherapy include teratomas which contain low mitotic activity, those with no embryonal or trophoblastic elements and where there are no detectable tumour markers after surgery. Such patients can be treated by surgery alone, but need careful follow-up. Ovarian choriocarcinoma is usually treated with chemotherapy as for other non-dysgerminomatous ovarian germ cell tumours.

At present, chemotherapy for these tumours consists of combination treatment with cisplatin, vinblastine and bleomycin, in a regimen identical to that used for testicular non-seminomatous germ cell tumours (see Chapter 19). Epipodophyllotoxin (VP-16213) is an active agent and is sometimes given as a substitute for vinblastine with the advantage of lesser toxicity.

Ovarian carcinoids and struma ovarii are treated by unilateral oophorectomy.

Granulosa cell tumours of the ovary

These tumours account for 3–5% of malignant ovarian tumours. The cell of origin is unclear. They are frequently hormone-producing. The granulosa-theca tumour is composed of cells which resemble the normal granulosa cell of the follicle. It may be difficult to decide whether the tumour is malignant or not because it often lacks the typical cellular features of malignancy. Capsular invasion and cellular atypia are the most reliable signs of malignancy, and probably influence prognosis. Granulosa-theca cell tumours produce oestrogen (mainly from theca cells), androgens and progesterone. Oestrogen-related symptoms include postmenopausal bleeding, menorrhagia and breast tenderness. Virilizing symptoms, which are rarer, include hirsutism and oligomenorrhoea.

The prognosis of these tumours is excellent as they are mostly cured by conservative surgery (unilateral salpingo-oophorectomy). Re-

sponses to chemotherapy have been recorded in patients with recurrence of tumour.

Sertoli-Leydig cell tumours of the ovary

These rare tumours representing 0.5% of ovarian cancers, are seen at the ages of 20–40 years and are sometimes termed *arrhenoblastomas*. Eighty percent of them are associated with virilization. The histological appearance varies and some are poorly differentiated though all contain Leydig cells identical to the male testicular cell. Occasionally, teratomatous elements are present.

Following surgical removal, the prognosis is excellent and over 90% of patients are alive at 10 years. The tumours are rarely bilateral so unilateral oophorectomy is usually adequate.

CARCINOMA OF THE FALLOPIAN TUBE

This uncommon gynaecological malignancy is sometimes considered as a 'variant' of ovarian carcinoma since the two diseases share the common aetiological feature of low fertility or nulliparity, with adenocarcinoma (solid, cystic or mixed) as the commonest histological type. Clinical symptoms include pelvic pain and vaginal discharge which is sometimes profuse and often blood-stained. Other symptoms, similar to those found in ovarian carcinoma, include abdominal distension, altered bowel habit or in occasional cases, dyspareunia.

Both staging and treatment are similar to the recommendations for ovarian cancer (see above). Where a carcinoma of the fallopian tube is encountered at the initial laparotomy, it is much more likely to be due to secondary involvement from a carcinoma of the ovary than a true primary fallopian tube cancer. As for ovarian cancer generally, stage is an important prognostic determinant.

CARCINOMA OF THE VULVA

This uncommon tumour accounts for about 4% of all gynaecological cancer (1% of all cancer) with about 1000 new cases annually in Britain, chiefly affecting the older age group. Invasive carcinoma is dinstinctly uncommon in patients under 50 years of age (Fig. 17.1) while carcinoma *in situ* occurs in younger women (average age 50 years).

AETIOLOGY AND PATHOGENESIS

Leucoplakia and other dystrophic changes in vulval skin can predispose to carcinoma. These skin changes can be *hypoplastic*, including lichen sclerosis and atrophic vulvitis, or *hyperplastic*, including leucoplakia as well as hypertrophic vulvitis. These are distinct from true intra-epithelial neoplasia, which is a group including carcinoma *in situ* (often multifocal), and Paget's disease. Most vulval cancers are squamous cell carcinomas, though other histological types are occasionally seen, including adenocarcinoma (usually arising in a Bartholin's gland), melanoma, basal cell carcinoma, fibrosarcoma and adenoid cystic carcinoma. Diabetes is not infrequently associated with carcinoma of the vulva.

DIAGNOSIS

Most patients present with pruitis vulvae, pain, ulcer or discharge though some patients are unaware of any vulval problem and seek advice about a lymph node in the groin. The most common sites of origin are the labia majora, though the labia minora and clitoris can be primary sites. All thickened, fissured, ulcerated or sloughing lesions should be viewed with great suspicion, particularly in elderly patients, and biopsied. The histological distinction between premalignant lesions (particularly leucoplakia and lichen sclerosus et atrophicus) and frank invasive carcinoma can be difficult, particularly since intra-epithelial cancer can occur in areas of hypertrophic leucoplakia. Vulval carcinomas are almost always visible so careful follow-up of suspicious lesions should not be difficult. Clinical photographs are useful to document slowly evolving changes.

Benign lesions can cause diagnostic confusion. These include chronic vulvitis, vulval condylomas of tuberculous, syphilitic, viral or unknown aetiology, lymphogranuloma inguinale, lymphogranuloma venereum (chiefly in younger patients) and vulval abscesses. The vulva is occasionally a site of secondary spread from carcinoma of the endometrium, cervix and large bowel.

PATTERNS OF SPREAD AND CLINICAL STAGING

The FIGO system is widely used (Table 17.11) and is based on the predictable behaviour of vulval carcinoma. Dissemination is chiefly via direct and lymphatic routes, and haematogenous spread is very unusual. Local spread occurs to contiguous areas of the vulva, vagina and urethra, or to the perineum and/or anus (Fig. 17.12). Local pubic tenderness results from infection and periostitis, though malignant bone erosion has been described. Nodal involvement may be bilateral or contralateral. Anteriorly placed lesions usually spread to the inguinal nodes whereas those of the deeper parts of the vulva tend to involve urethral and bladder lymphatics, thereby spreading to the internal iliac nodes. More posterior lesions may drain to the femoral nodes. Almost half of all patients with invasive vulval cancers have evidence of local lymphatic involvement (29), usually with superficial node involvement but occasionally with

Table 17.11. FIGO staging in carcinoma of the vulva

Stage	Description
Stage 0	Carcinoma *in situ*
Stage I	Tumour confined to vulva (<2 cm). No palpable nodes
Stage II	Tumour confined to vulva (>2 cm). No palpable nodes
Stage III	Tumour spread to urethra, vagina, or perineum. Palpable mobile nodes
Stage IV	Tumour infiltrates bladder or rectum. Fixed nodes

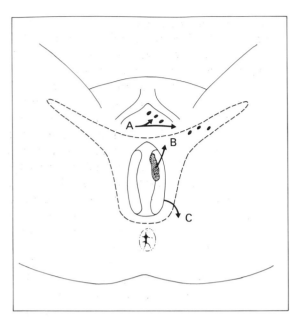

Fig. 17.12. *Local and nodal spread in carcinoma of the vulva.* (A) Nodal involvement: inguinal, femoral, deep pelvic and common iliac nodes. Bilateral spread is common. (B) Anteriorly to contiguous parts of the vulva, clitoris, vagina, urethra and bladder. (C) Posteriorly to posterior vulva and rectum.

Dashed line shows incision and resection in radical vulvectomy.

spread to the deep iliac nodes without evidence of superficial lymphadenopathy.

INVESTIGATION AND MANAGEMENT

Routine investigation should include full blood count, chest X-ray, blood urea and electrolyte estimation. Lymphography can be useful in delineating pelvic and para-aortic nodes, particularly in patients where there is doubtful clinical evidence of involvement and the gynaecologist is uncertain whether to proceed with surgery. Unfortunately the advanced age of many patients and the presence of gross infection with reactive lymphadenopathy limits the applicability and reliability of this technique, and a negative lymphogram cannot exclude microscopic nodal involvement. Needle aspiration of enlarged superficial nodes may occasionally help to decide whether surgery is appropriate though a positive result is more reliable than a negative one. CT scanning of the pelvis may also be useful in delineating suspicious areas of nodal or direct spread.

TREATMENT

Treatment is by surgical excision, preferably of the primary carcinoma and lymphatic drainage *en bloc*. Wide excision of vulval skin has been considered necessary since contiguous subdermal lymphatic spread is common; however, many gynaecologists are now less radical in their approach. Both superficial and deep node dissection are advocated by some surgeons although this need not be so extensive in stage I disease. Removal of the lower part of the urethra may also be necessary in more advanced stages. Because of the laxity of skin and subcutaneous tissue in this area, primary closure is usually possible despite the wide excision. Postoperative infection is common, and is the major cause of mortality. Some surgeons prefer to perform a simple vulvectomy if there is any doubt about the invasiveness of the carcinoma, though examination of the operative specimen may reveal obvious areas of invasion. A second surgical operation may then have to be performed in order to carry out lymph node dissection. Although surgical excision is the treatment of choice, many patients are unfit for these procedures, and palliative local irradiation can be valuable, particularly in patients with pain and ulceration. Local irradiation can also be considered as a substitute for surgery in unfit patients with obvious inguinal or pelvic node involvement, though radiation tolerance in these elderly patients is limited by bladder, bowel and other local structures. It is usually possible to achieve a total dose of 45–55 Gy (4500–5500 rad) in 4–5½ weeks, to the perineum and/or nodal sites. Where there is obvious local extension to the anus or rectum (stage IV), local irradiation is probably best preceded by a defunctioning colostomy which can sometimes be closed after completion of treatment.

PROGNOSIS

The survival rate largely depends on whether or not there is nodal involvement. About 75% of operable patients without lymphatic metastases are alive and free of disease at 5 years, whereas the 5-year survival of patients with inguinal or femoral node deposits is 30–40%, and less than 20% in patients with pelvic node involvement, even where pelvic lymph node dissection has been performed. Very occasionally further surgery (including pelvic exenteration) may be considered for patients with recurrent disease, though the end results are poor.

CARCINOMA OF THE VAGINA

This is a rare tumour, accounting for less than 1% of all gynaecological malignancy (i.e. about one-fiftieth as common as carcinoma of the cervix) and chiefly occurring in the 50–70 year old age group (Fig. 17.1). Little is known of the aetiology, but prolonged irritation from a vaginal ring pessary sometimes appears to predispose to malignant change. Vaginal carcinoma is almost invariably a squamous cell carcinoma, most frequently arising in the upper vagina, sometimes extensively involving the vaginal wall. Clear cell adenocarcinoma of the vagina has been reported in girls and young women whose mothers were taking exogenous stilboestrol in pregnancy—an example of a transplacental carcinogen with a latent period of 15–30 years. Secondary deposits are occasionally encountered in the vagina, usually as a result of lymphatic spread from endometrial carcinoma (often thought to occur at operation); vaginal deposits from malignant melanomas are also well-recognized and rarely, the vagina is the primary site of a melanoma. Direct extension may occur from carcinoma of the cervix or bladder.

SYMPTOMS AND MODE OF SPREAD

Blood-stained vaginal discharge is the commonest symptom, and is often unaccompanied by pain. In view of the typical age group, vaginal bleeding, when it occurs, is usually postmenopausal. Urinary complaints (chiefly frequency, nocturia and haematuria) or rectal discomfort occur with advanced disease.

As with carcinoma of the cervix, spread of the disease tends to take place chiefly by direct and lymphatic invasion (Fig. 17.13). Direct extension occurs to the parametria, pelvic side wall, and bladder. The lymphatic route varies with the site of the lesion. Lymphatic drainage of the upper part of the vagina is similar to that of the cervix, i.e. via the external, internal and common iliac nodes. Lesions placed lower in the vagina drain to pelvic inguinal and femoral nodes. Posteriorly placed lesions may spread towards the rectum because the lymphatic drainage of the posterior vaginal wall is to deep pelvic nodes (sacral, rectal and lower gluteal).

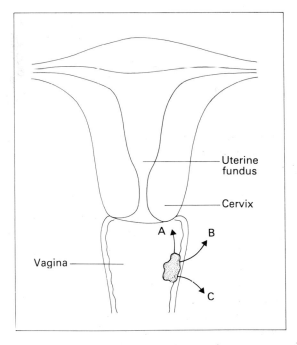

Fig. 17.13. *Local and lymph node spread in carcinoma of the vagina.* (A) Submucosal spread to adjacent parts of vagina and cervix. (B) Parametrial tissues, bladder, rectum and eventually to pelvic sidewall. (C) Lymphatic spread: upper vagina as for cervix (Fig. 17.3.). Posterior vagina as for rectal lymphatics. Anterior wall; towards lateral pelvic wall nodes. Lower vagina: to pelvic and inguino-femoral nodes.

As with carcinoma of the cervix, haematogenous spread is uncommon, and local control of disease tends to be the major clinical problem.

DIAGNOSIS AND STAGING

Careful vaginal examination should always be performed in patients presenting with vaginal bleeding and discharge, with direct inspection using a vaginal speculum. Colposcopy and biopsy can be extremely valuable, particularly where the speculum examination is inconclusive. Cytology of vaginal smears can be diagnostic. Where there is no obvious visible lesion, but definite cytological abnormalities, carcinoma *in situ* (now often termed vaginal intra-epithelial neoplasia, VAIN) of the vagina must be suspected. This condition should also be considered where cervical cytology has yielded malignant cells but colposcopy-directed biopsy of the cervix has proved negative—particularly where subsequent high vaginal smears are still abnormal.

Important investigations include examination under anaesthetic with cystoscopy, cervical dilatation and uterine curettage and biopsy of the cervix to exclude a primary carcinoma of the cervix. CT scanning, lymphography, sigmoidoscopy and peritoneal cytology may help to confirm the extent of spread in doubtful cases.

A FIGO staging system is generally used. This clinical staging system (Table 17.12) has been in use for over 10 years.

Table 17.12. FIGO staging of carcinoma of the vagina.

Stage 0	Carcinoma *in situ**
Stage I	Vaginal wall only
Stage II	Subvaginal tissue involved
Stage III	Extension to pelvic side wall
Stage IV	Spread beyond true pelvis—
IVa	to adjacent organs
IVb	to distant organs

* Vaginal intra-epithelial neoplasia, VAIN.

TREATMENT

Both radiotherapy and surgical removal can be effective though the surgical operation has to be very radical to stand a real chance of success and it is not often employed as a primary procedure. Total vaginectomy, pelvic lymphadenectomy and abdominal hysterectomy would be necessary, with reconstruction of the perineum and vagina where possible. This operation is only suitable for early lesions (stage I) or in a few highly selected cases following radiation failure. For most patients, radiotherapy is considered to be the treatment of choice.

Carcinoma in situ. The whole of the vaginal mucosa is usually irradiated using a vaginal applicator containing radioactive sources (often termed Dobbie applicators after their originator). The intravaginal mould can be differentially loaded to treat the area at greatest risk to a higher dose, but irradiation of the whole mucosa is usually advised as there may be more than one neoplastic site. Complications of treatment include vaginal stenosis, lack of lubrication and proctitis. A radical dosage of at least 60 Gy (6000 rad) mucosal dose is usually recommended.

Invasive carcinoma of the vagina. For stage I tumours, surgery, as described above, is occasionally recommended, particularly in younger patients with more distal lesions (lower-third of vagina). For the large majority of patients, treatment by intracavitary caesium insertion is combined with external beam irradiation as for carcinoma of the cervix (see above). This applies particularly to tumours of the upper part of the vagina. In tumours of the lower-third, it may be more difficult to deliver adequate local irradiation by intracavitary applications. Irradiation of the whole pelvis, using external beam multifield techniques, may be the best means of achieving adequate and homogeneous treatment to the primary site and local node groups. In patients with more advanced disease (FIGO stages II–IV), a pelvic nodal dose of 45–50 Gy (4500–5000 rad) given in daily fractions over 4.5–5 weeks is usually well tolerated and generally considered adequate for sterilizing *microscopic* direct or local lymphatic extension, though it is essential to give additional irradiation to the primary site and any area which is obviously clinically involved. This is achieved either by intracavitary treatment or by additional external beam radiotherapy to encompass the whole of the vagina, treating the primary site if possible to a total of 60 Gy (6000 rad) in daily fractions over 6 weeks.

Despite the use of lead shielding techniques to minimize the rectal dose, acute proctitis must be expected in a substantial proportion of patients, and late radiation-induced rectal stricture may result. Other complications include increased urinary frequency with cystitis (often sterile and poorly responsive to antibiotics) and as later complications, local fistula formation, proctitis or sigmoid colitis, any of which may require bowel diversion though local intrarectal steroid preparations may relieve symptoms. In view of the poor results and high complication rate when treating patients with very advanced (stage IV) disease, the treatment of these patients is usually palliative and lower doses, consistent with symptom relief, are generally felt to be more appropriate. Overall, the results of treatment are disappointing. Even with a radical approach, the 5-year survival rate falls from 75% for patients with stage I disease, to 25% with stage II disease and less than 5% for patients with stage IV tumours.

CHORIOCARCINOMA

This rare tumour has received considerable attention because of its extreme chemosensitivity, placing it in the small group of solid tumours which can be cured even when metastatic. In addition, the secretion of a tumour marker (human chorionic gonadotrophin, HCG, see Chapter 4) in 100% of cases of choriocarcinoma, permits a logical treatment approach based on a reliable index of tumour bulk.

The tumour most frequently follows pregnancies which have resulted in a hydatidiform mole (occurring in approximately 1 in 1400 normal pregnancies in Britain), though it may rarely accompany a normal or ectopic pregnancy, or even a termination. It is more common in Asia than Europe or the USA, and following pregnancy in 'elderly' subjects (i.e. over 40 years).

PATHOLOGY

Histopathologically, the tumour consists of malignant syncitio- or cytotrophoblast cells, which can be shown immunocytochemically to contain HCG. Following successful evacuation of a hydatidiform mole, sequential determination of plasma HCG provides reliable information as to the completeness of the evacuation. In some cases, the HCG level falls more slowly to normal than would be predicted by the half-life of HCG (24–36 hours), suggesting that spontaneous regression of a tumour may have occurred. In other cases, local or distant invasion of tumour supervenes and the HCG level remains elevated.

The traditional classification of trophoblastic tumours was based on morphology: *hydatidiform mole*, *invasive mole* or *true choriocarcinoma*. However, the availability of the quantitative HCG assay has largely supplanted these terms, since the diagnosis is made as a result of persistently raised HCG and tissue is now rarely available. It is probably better to use the term 'gestational trophoblastic tumour' instead. Abnormalities such as mitotic activity, degree of cellular atypia and local invasiveness appear to correlate fairly closely with prognosis.

Although the tumour may remain localized within the uterus, local extension into myometrium or even the serosal surface or vagina may take place, sometimes causing severe intra-uterine or intraperitoneal bleeding. More distant blood-borne secondary deposits occur, chiefly to lung, liver and brain, with a frequency which depends on the antecedent history; possibly as many as 1 in 20 molar pregnancies, but excessively rarely following normal or ectopic pregnancy.

DIAGNOSIS AND STAGING

Vaginal bleeding during or after pregnancy, particularly if associated with a 'large-for-date' uterus, should be regarded with suspicion. Some patients appear to suffer from particularly marked symptoms of pregnancy, or pre-eclampsia. Ultrasound examination may lead to an almost certain diagnosis of a molar pregnancy before delivery. Evacuation of a hydatidiform mole and/or persistent elevation of post-partum HCG levels should lead in Britain to registration of the patient with the Royal College of Obstetrics and Gynaecology. The patient will then be followed closely, sending regular samples of blood and/or urine to one of three designated centres. Staging investigations include repeat estimations of β HCG, with chest and abdominopelvic CT scanning. Isotope bone scanning is not routinely performed as less than 1 in 1000 cases involve bone. Pelvic ultrasound may be valuable since it is easier and safer for repeated estimations than CT scanning.

Risk classification is important since optimal treatment is different for patients at varying risk of drug resistance. Clinical staging systems are no longer used. Important prognostic factors include age (older patients do worse), interval between antecedent pregnancy and start of chemotherapy, height of initial HCG level, number and sites of metastases (the brain is a particularly adverse site) and previous administration of chemotherapy (30).

TREATMENT

Patients with *low-risk* disease are treated either by chemotherapy (generally single agent chemotherapy with methotrexate) or hysterectomy in older patients who have no wish for further children. Where surgery is performed, it is often recommended that the hysterectomy be 'covered' by administration of methotrexate. If methotrexate is the definitive method of treatment it is usually given daily or every other day

for one week, the response assessed by serial HCG measurement, and treatment repeated until the marker has been undetectable in the serum for 6-8 weeks. Patients should be advised to avoid further pregnancy for at least 1 year.

Patients with more advanced *moderate-risk* disease are treated with combination chemotherapy, once again using serial HCG assays as a means of monitoring response. Surgery (hysterectomy) may be necessary if vaginal bleeding is troublesome.

Most drug regimens include methotrexate, actinomycin-D and an alkylating agent (cyclophosphamide or chlorambucil). Higher doses of methotrexate (with folinic acid rescue) are generally given for patients with early disease. Newer regimens include vinca alkaloids cisplatin and etoposide (VP-16213). One hundred per cent of patients in this category respond to combination chemotherapy usually resulting in cure, and a small number of patients who develop drug resistance to 'conventional' combination regimens respond to newer drugs (31).

In patients with pulmonary metastases but no other adverse features, single agent chemotherapy with methotrexate and folinic acid remains the treatment of choice. For patients with involvement at other distant sites (or other features placing them in the *high-risk* category), intensive multidrug combination chemotherapy should be given, together with local irradiation, e.g. to brain, if indicated.

PROGNOSIS

Prior to treatment with chemotherapy, patients with localized disease were treated by surgery and/or pelvic irradiation and the cure rate was 40%. Patients with more advanced disease were virtually never cured. With current treatment, 100% of patients with localized disease should be cured, as are over 70% of all patients with more advanced stages. Even with Stage 4 disease, the majority of patients survive, and the number of tumour deaths in England and Wales is now under 10 per annum. For the most part, fertility of choriocarcinoma survivors is well maintained, and these patients do not appear to be at increased risk of second tumours (32).

REFERENCES

1 Chamberlain G. (1981) Aetiology of gynaecological cancer, *Journal of the Royal Society of Medicine* **74**, 246–61.
2 DiSaia P.J. (1981) The Cervix. In Romney S.L., Gray M.J., Little A.B., Merrill J.A., Quilligan E.G. & Stander R.W. (eds) *Gynaecology and Obstetrics—The Health Care of Women.* p. 1017. McGraw-Hill, New York.
3 Terris M., Wilson F., Smith H., Sprung E. & Nelson J.H. (1967) The relationship of coitus to carcinoma of the cervix. *American Journal of Public Health* **57**, 840.
4 Peterson O. (1956) Spontaneous course of cervical precancerous conditions. *American Journal of Obstetrics and Gynecology* **72**, 1063.
5 Piver M.S., Wallace S. & Castro J.R. (1971) The accuracy of lymphangiography in carcinoma of the uterine cervix. *American Journal of Roentgenology* **111**, 278.
6 Brunschwig A. (1968) The surgical treatment of cancer of the cervix stage I and II. *American Journal of Roentgenology* **102**, 147–51.
7 Brady L.W. (1975) Advances in the management of gynaecological cancer-radiation therapy. *Cancer* **36**, 661–8.
8 Rutledge F.N., Fletcher G.H. & MacDonald E.J. (1965) Pelvic lymphadenectomy as an adjunct to radiation therapy in treatment for cancer of the cervix. *American Journal of Roentgenology* **93**, 607–614.
9 Fletcher G.H. (1971) Cancer of the uterine cervix. *American Journal of Roentgenology* **111**, 225–42.
10 Wasserman T.H. & Carter S.K. (1977) The integration of chemotherapy into combined modality treatment of solid tumours. VIII, Cervical cancer. *Cancer Treatment Reviews*, **4**, 25.
11 Cutler S.J., Myers M.H. & Green S.B. (1975) Trends in survival rates of patients with cancer. *New England Journal of Medicine* **293**, 122.
12 Morrow C.P. (1980) Endometrial carcinoma stages I and II: is surgery adequate? *International Journal of Radiation Oncology Biology Physics* **6**, 365.
13 Del Regato J.A. & Chahbazian C.M. (1972) External pelvic iradiation as a preoperative surgical adjuvant in treatment of carcinoma of the endometrium. *American Journal of Roentgenology* **114**, 106.
14 Kottmeier H.L. (1959) Carcinoma of the corpus uteri—diagnosis and therapy. *American Journal of Obstetrics Gynaecology* **78**, 1128.
15 Serov S.F., Scully R.E. & Solvin L.H. (1973) *Histological Typing of Ovarian Tumors.* International histological classification of tumours, No. 9. World Health Organisation, Geneva.
16 Tobias J.S. & Griffiths C.T. (1976) Management of ovarian carcinoma: current concepts and future prospects. *New England Journal of Medicine* **294**, 818–23; 877–82.
17 Rosenoff S.H., Young R.C., Anderson T., Bagley C., Chabner B., Schein P.S., Hulibaud S. & DeVita V.T. (1975) Peritoneoscopy: a valuable staging tool in ovarian carcinoma. *Annals of Internal Medicine* **83**, 37.
18 Munnel E.W. (1969) Is conservative therapy ever justified in stage I (IA) cancer of the ovary? *American Journal of Obstetrics and Gynecology* **103**, 641.
19 Griffiths C.T. (1975) Surgical resection of bulk tumor in the primary treatment of ovarian carcinoma. *National Cancer Institute Monograph* **42**, 101.
20 Hudson C.N. (1973) Surgical treatment of ovarian cancer. *Gynaecologic Oncology* **1**, 370.
21 Dembo A.J., Bush R.A., Beale F.A., Bean H.A., Pringle J.F., Sturgeon J. & Reid J.G. (1979) Ovarian carcinoma: improved survival followed abdominopelvic irradiation in patients with a completed pelvic operation. *American Journal of Obstetrics and Gynaecology* **134**, 793.
22 Keettel W.L., Fox M.R., Longnecker D.S. & Latourette H.B. (1966) Prophylactic use of radioactive gold in the treatment of primary ovarian cancer. *American Journal of Obstetrics and Gynaecology* **94**, 766–79.
23 Buckner C.D., Briggs R., Clift R.A., Fefer A., Funk D.D., Glucksberg H., Neiman P.E., Storb R. & Thomas E.D. Intermittent high-dose cyclophosphamide (NSC-26271) treatment of stage III ovarian carcinoma. *Cancer Chemotherapy Reports* **58**, 697–703.
24 Wiltshaw E., Evans B.D., Jones A., Baker J.W. & Calvert A.H. (1983) JM8, successor to cisplatin in advanced ovarian carcinoma? *Lancet* **i**, 587.
25 Alberts D.S., Chen H.S.G., Salmon S.E., Surivit E.A., Young L., Moon T.E. & Meyskens F.L. (1981) Chemotherapy of ovarian cancer directed by the human tumor stem cell assay. *Cancer Chemotherapy and Pharmacology* **6**, 279.
26 Young R.C., Chabner B.A. & Hubbard S.P. (1978) Prospective trial of melphalan (L-PAM) versus combination chemotherapy (Hexa-CAF) in ovarian adenocarcinoma. *New England Journal of Medicine* **299**, 1261–66.

27 Edmonson H.J., Fleming T.R., Decker D.G., Malkasian G.D., Jorgensen E.O., Jeffries J.A., Webb M.J. & Kvol L.K. (1979) Different chemotherapeutic sensitivities and host factors affecting prognosis in advanced ovarian carcinoma versus minimal residual disease. *Cancer Treatment Reports* **63**, 241–7.

28 Reiumer R.R., Hoover R. & Fraumeni J.F. (1977) Acute leukaemia after alkylating agent therapy in ovarian cancer. *New England Journal of Medicine* **297**, 117.

29 Parry-Jones E. (1960) Lymphatics of vulva. *Journal of Obstetrics and Gynaecology, British Commonwealth* **67**, 919.

30 Rustin G.J.S. & Bagshawe K.D. (1986) Gestational trophoblastic tumours. *Critical Reviews in Oncology and Haematology (in press)*.

31 Newlands E.S. & Bagshawe K.D. (1979) Activity of high-dose cis-platinum (NC1 119875) in combination with vincristine and methotrexate in drug resistant gestational choriocarcinoma. *British Journal of Cancer* **40**, 943–5.

32 Rustin G.J.S., Rustin F., Dent J., Booth M., Salt S. & Bagshawe K.D. (1983) No increase in second tumours after cytotoxic chemotherapy for gestational trophoblastic tumours. *New England Journal of Medicine* **308**, 473–6.

Chapter 18

Genito-urinary Cancer

Cancers of the kidney, bladder, prostate and testis represent an important group of tumours which together constitute over a quarter of all cancers in males. Due to important advances in the management of testicular tumours this topic is dealt with separately in Chapter 19. Other rare sites of cancer include the urethra, penis and epididymis. Genito-urinary cancer presents a considerable challenge in management, and although surgery has traditionally been the corner-stone of treatment, both radiotherapy and cytotoxic chemotherapy are assuming an increasing importance. These tumours are currently the object of a good deal of study since surgical and radiotherapeutic techniques have changed markedly during the past 20 years.

TUMOURS OF THE KIDNEY

Incidence and aetiology of renal tumours

Tumours of the kidney account for about 2% of all cancers (Fig. 18.1) and represent particular problems of management both to surgeons and others since their developments. Clinical evolution and pattern of dissemination is sometimes measured over many years, with apparent success followed by late recurrence, often several years later. In adults, the commonest type of renal tumour is the *renal cell carcinoma (hypernephroma)* which accounts for 75% of adult renal concer. Tumours of the renal pelvis are uncommon (10%) and are discussed later. In children, *nephroblastoma (Wilms' tumour)* is amongst the commonest of

malignant paediatric tumours, and is discussed in Chapter 24.

Renal cell carcinoma is about three times as common in men as in women, and there is increasing evidence that it is aetiologically related to cigatette smoking (1). Little else is known about its pathogenesis, though it is common in patients with von Hippel-Lindau syndrome (characterized by haemangioblastomas in the cerebellum and retina, associated with phaeochromocytoma). Stone formation in the renal pelvis, carcinogenic derivatives of aromatic amines or tryptophan, and phenacetin abuse, are all thought to be important in the aetiology of renal pelvic tumours.

Renal cell adenocarcinoma (hypernephroma, grawitz' tumour)

PATHOLOGY AND STAGING

Although Grawitz considered that the tumour arose from cell rests of adrenal tissue, this view is no longer held, particularly since electron microscope studies have revealed the presence of brush border characteristics, making it almost certain that these tumours arise from the epithelium of the renal tubules themselves. For this reason, the term *renal cell adenocarcinoma* is now increasingly preferred to hypernephroma.

Local, lymphatic and haematogenous spread are all important, making surgery unwise or technically impossible in about one-third of all cases (2). In a series of over 100 patients, direct invasion into peri-renal tissues was seen in 21%,

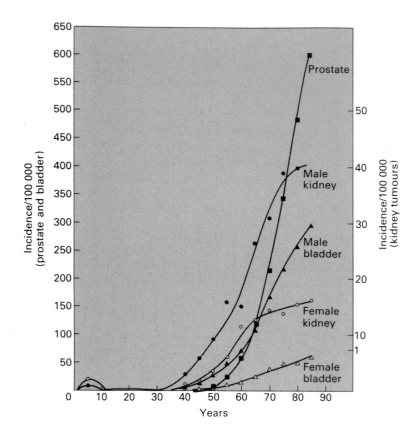

Fig. 18.1. *Age-specific incidence of renal, bladder and prostatic cancer.*

and local lymph node metastases in 8%. Renal vein invasion is also common and cords of tumour cells are sometimes seen growing directly into the inferior vena cava, though this is not usually detectable pre-operatively. The likelihood of local or lymphatic spread correlates with—and may be determined by—the histological differentiation, and in patients with low-grade carcinomas the incidence of metastatic disease at presentation is very low.

A number of staging systems have been proposed, chiefly relying on the information obtained at operation. A straightforward TNM staging system has been suggested which is simple enough to be reproducible but also yields important prognostic information (Table 18.1). Prognosis is closely related to stage (see p. 325).

Table 18.1. Renal carcinoma—TNM staging system.

T0	No evidence of primary tumour
T1	Small tumour surrounded by normal kidney
T2	Large tumour with deformity and kidney enlargement
T3	Perinephric or renal vein involvement
T4	Invasion of neighbouring structures (diaphragm and abdominal wall)
N0	No involvement
N1	Ipsilateral node involvement
N2	Contralateral or bilateral nodes
N3	Fixed node involvement
M0	No distant metastases
M1	Distant metastases

TNM Stage Grouping

	T	*N*	*M*
Stage I	0 or 1	0	0
II	2	0	0
III	3	0 or 1	0
IV	4	0–3	0 or 1

CLINICAL FEATURES OF RENAL CELL
ADENOCARCINOMA (HYPERNEPHROMA)

These tumours present with a wide variety of symptoms. Approximately 50% of all patients have haematuria, which may be very slight but occasionally is sufficiently severe to produce anaemia. Loin pain and a palpable mass are classical features, and a large mass may be palpable even when the tumour is confined to the kidney, without extracapsular spread. Apart from these local symptoms, many patients initially present with complaints resulting from metastases, such as a pathological fracture through a bone deposit, dyspnoea and cough from mediastinal, hilar or lung metastases, or epilepsy from an intracerebral deposit. Renal cell tumours are a well known cause of pyrexia, and fever without other symptoms is not uncommon. Hypertension, polycythaemia and hypercalcaemia may also occur in about 5% of patients. Liver

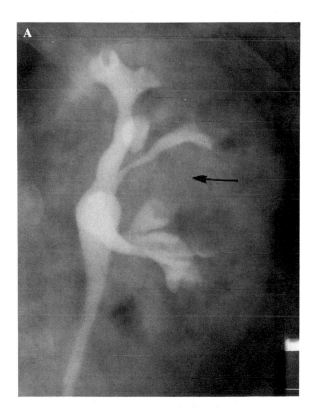

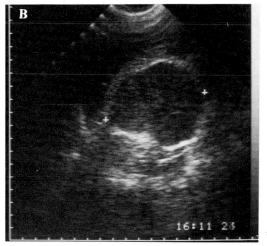

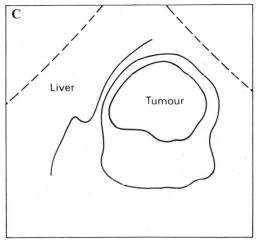

Fig. 18.2(A). *Intravenous urogram in renal carcinoma.* The left kidney contains a tumour (arrowed) which displaces the calyces. (B) Transverse ultrasound scan showing a large renal carcinoma below the liver. (C) Line Drawing of (B).

function tests may be abnormal even in patients without metastatic disease, though they are unreliable as tumour markers.

Even when a renal cell carcinoma is suspected, the diagnosis can be difficult. Intravenous urography (IVU) usually demonstrates a space-occupying mass in the renal cortex, often with distortion of the calyceal system (Fig. 18.2), though a negative IVU is unreliable since these tumours can be small. IVU with tomography may help in these cases, and can usually distinguish a solid tumour from a renal cyst. This distinction is particularly well made by ultrasound examination of the kidney (Fig. 18.2), which is a useful examination in iodine-sensitive patients in whom IVU would be hazardous. Renal calcification particularly if 'rim-like' is a common finding. In difficult cases, further radiological investigations using CT scanning (or very occasionally, ascending ureterography) may give additional information (Fig. 18.3). These techniques, coupled with cyst puncture and aspiration cytology, have reduced

the need for renal angiography as a routine investigation, though some urological surgeons still request a pre-operative angiogram in order to obtain the maximum anatomical detail. Before surgery, a chest X-ray must always be obtained in case pulmonary metastases are already present. There may be a place for routine whole-lung tomography or CT scanning, since pulmonary metastases have to be at least 2 cm in diameter to be visible on a standard chest X-ray. Isotope bone scanning may reveal unsuspected bony metastases particularly in patients whose primary lesions is palpable. Biochemical tests of renal and liver function are important, and it is also wise to perform isotope renography pre-operatively, to assess the function of the contralateral kidney.

MANAGEMENT OF RENAL CELL CARCINOMA

Surgical resection is unquestionably the most effective method of treatment, though over 25%

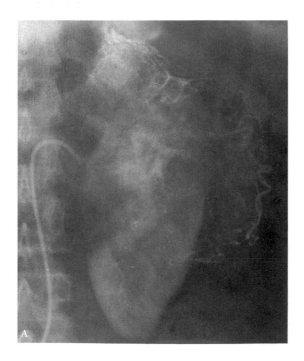

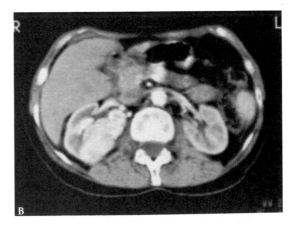

Fig. 18.3. *Renal arteriogram* (late arterial phase). (A) A tumour circulation is seen due to a large carcinoma occupying the upper two-thirds of the kidney. (B) *CT scan of the abdomen* (with contrast) in a patient with a carcinoma of the right kidney.

of renal carcinomas are technically unresectable. Many surgeons still follow the guidelines set out by Robson (3), who advocated *en bloc* resection of the kidney with as little disturbance as possible, coupled with wide lymphatic dissection of local nodes from the aortic bifurcation to the diaphragm, and with prevention of tumour dissemination by early ligation of the renal artery and vein. Although still controversial, lymph node dissection seems advisable since it has been noted that the incidence of regional lymph node involvement can be as high as 15%. In general, an aggressive surgical approach is usually justifiable since other methods of treatment are at best palliative. In cases where the tumour is large, or difficult to remove, it may be necessary to perform nephro-ureterectomy, with removal of part of the bladder if indicated. Where evidence of involvement of the renal vein or inferior vena cava is apparent (about 10% of patients), attempts at radical surgical removal are often justified, since renal vein involvement without other evidence of extrarenal extension appears to have little effect on the prognosis at 5 and even 10 years (4). Difficulties arise where a renal carcinoma occurs in a solitary or horseshoe kidney, and the commonest approach is to perform a partial nephrectomy. Occasionally, if the tumour is too large for a conservative resection, total nephrectomy is unavoidable, with transplantation of an allogeneic kidney (if available) at a later procedure.

In patients with obvious clinical or radiological evidence of metastases elsewhere, the choice of initial treatment is more difficult. The primary lesion may be technically operable, and providing the patient's condition is reasonably good, nephrectomy is by far the most effective and simplest means of securing control of the primary, particularly when there are troublesome symptoms such as renal pain or haematuria. Although there are sporadic case reports of regression of secondary lung deposits following resection of the primary tumour, this phenomenon is in fact very rare and the possibility of its occurrence should never be used as the sole rationale for surgery. Since this capricious tumour can remain quiescent for many years (even decades) before metastases become apparent, it is sometimes recommended that solitary metastases should be surgically removed. In patients with obvious widespread metastatic disease in whom nephrectomy seems unwise, the recently developed technique of renal artery embolism or occlusion is worth considering since it leads to partial or complete infarction of the kidney and offers a reasonable chance of temporary control of the tumour. Some urologists prefer to use this technique routinely as a pre-operative adjunct to nephrectomy. Several other methods of occlusion are currently in use, including intra-arterial balloon catheter occlusion, induction of an autologous local thrombus, or insertion of foreign material such as gelatine sponge or polyacrylamide gel.

Radiotherapy has a limited role in renal cell cancer, though it can be useful, particularly with stage II tumours where there is evidence of extrarenal local invasion, and in cases where complete surgical removal is technically impossible. However, renal cell adenocarcinomas are only marginally sensitive to radiotherapy, and radical irradiation of the kidney in totally inoperable cases does no more than delay the onset of local progression of disease. In operable tumours, the routine use of postoperative irradiation remains controversial. In a prospective trial of postoperative irradiation following apparently successful nephrectomy, Finney was unable to demonstrate any useful benefit, even in the incidence of local recurrence (5). In another trial using pre-operative irradiation (which may be expected to lead to a lower rate of dissemination of viable tumour cells at operation), no survival advantage was seen, although the proportion of technically complete operations was higher in patients undergoing radiation therapy (6). On the other hand, Rafla (7) demonstrated an improvement in survival following radiotherapy for patients where capsular invasion was noted at surgery with no other evidence of distant disease—the one group in whom postoperative radiotherapy might be expected to be beneficial. When radiotherapy is employed postoperatively, either because of incomplete removal or as an 'adjunct' to surgery, the typical radiation field should cover the renal bed, taking care to avoid treatment of the contralateral kidney (Fig. 18.4). Doses are generally in the range 35–50 Gy (3500–5000 rad) over 3–5 weeks depending on the volume treated as well as patient tolerance.

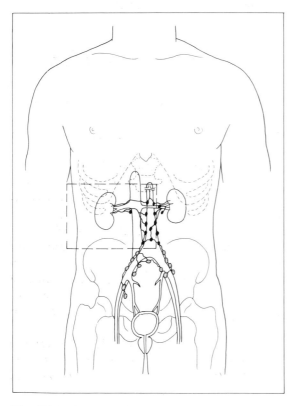

Fig. 18.4. *Anatomical relations of the kidney with lymphatic drainage pathways and typical volume treated when irradiating the renal bed. In most cases the kidney will have been surgically removed. Particular care must be taken with right-sided tumours because of the risk of radiation hepatitis. Commonly affected lymph nodes are shown in black.*

SYSTEMIC TREATMENTS AND PALLIATIVE THERAPY

In spite of early reports of response to hormone preparations, the overall response rate to pro-gestogens and androgens is very low, of the order of 5%. Despite this disappointing figure, these agents are non-toxic and therefore worth considering in patients with widespread metastases. Medroxyprogesterone acetate is widely used (100 mg t.d.s. by mouth).

CHEMOTHERAPY

Chemotherapy has had little success. The most widely used agents are doxorubicin, nitro-sureas, cyclophosphamide and hydroxyurea. None of these agents has significant activity on its own and in combination the response rate is still very low (20%). Alpha interferon is the most effective agent, with responses in 20–30% of patients.

Although cytotoxic drugs have no established role in palliation, treatment with radiotherapy may be very successful, particularly in the relief of bone pain. Bone metastases are very common and internal orthopaedic fixation of long bones is invaluable in prevention or treatment of pathological fractures, thereby allowing early mobility.

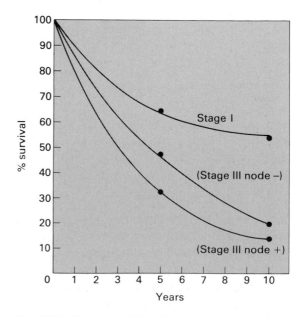

Fig. 18.5. *Prognosis of renal adenocarcinoma related to stage and lymph node involvement.*

PROGNOSIS

The prognosis in renal cell cancer depends on the stage and grade of the tumour, and the completeness of surgery (Fig. 18.5). For stage I tumours, the 5-year survival is >60%, whereas if the regional nodes are involved this falls to 30%. For stage IV tumours, there are very few 5-year survivors. With high-grade tumours, only 30% of patients are alive at 5-years whilst with low-grade tumours, 80% of patients survive.

Carcinoma of the renal pelvis

These tumours are uncommon (about 7% of all renal carcinomas) and are usually transitional cell carcinomas (80%) or squamous cell carcinomas, which may be more common in women. Clinical symptoms include haematuria (90%) and loin pain due to obstruction of the renal pelvis. On examination, in advanced cases, there may be a palpable loin mass.

Investigation includes an IVU, which usually shows a filling defect in the collecting system and occasionally non-functioning kidneys where there has been long-standing post-renal obstruction by tumour. Fifty per cent of all patients have malignant cells in the urine and cytological examination of the urine is therefore a mandatory investigation.

For tumours of the renal pelvis, surgery is again the most important method of treatment. Nephro-ureterectomy is usually required; for transitional tumours a part of the bladder wall is also usually removed since, as with all such cell tumours, a wide area of epithelium is at risk. As the histology of the renal pelvic tumour is not usually known pre-operatively, the operation is the same for both transitional cells and squamous carcinomas. However, local ureteric stump recurrence is reportedly less frequent with squamous carcinomas.

Radiotherapy may be worth considering for inoperable or recurrent cases but there is little evidence that it is ever curative in these situations. It may, however, temporarily retard the local progression of disease. In the follow-up care of patients with renal pelvic tumours, the possibility of a contralateral lesion must always be borne in mind. Repeated cystoscopy and cytological examination of the urine are both important, since 50% of patients will later develop a carcinoma of the bladder at some stage. About 10% of patients with transitional cell carcinoma of the renal pelvis have a synchronous bladder carcinoma as well.

CARCINOMA OF THE URETER

This rare tumour is usually a transitional cell carcinoma though sarcomas are occasionally encountered. Typically, the disease presents with frequency and dysuria. Ureteric colic is unusual.

The diagnosis is usually made by IVU which shows ureteric dilatation or distortion, or a non-functioning kidney. Retrograde pyelography demonstrates the site of the block. Urinary cytology may also be helpful in diagnosis.

Treatment is by nephro-ureterectomy, but occasionally the kidney may be preserved. In removing the ureter a cuff of bladder should be taken. Radiotherapy has occasionally been employed in patients with inoperable tumour, but with little success.

The prognosis depends largely on the cellular differentiation of the tumours, The 5-year survival is 80% with well-differentiated tumours but only 10% with the most anaplastic forms.

CANCER OF THE URINARY BLADDER

Aetiology and incidence

At the end of the 19th century it was recognized that workers in the aniline dye industry had a higher incidence of bladder cancer than expected, and the active carcinogen to which they were exposed was later identified as β-naphthylamine (8). Workers in the rubber industry form another important occupational group (see also p. 9 and p. 24). Chronic bladder infection or infestation also predisposes to malignant change; world-wide, the most important of these causes is schistosomiasis. There is no doubt that bladder cancer is more frequent amongst cigarette smokers, and this may partially explain its much higher incidence in males. In the United States, the disease is reportedly four times as common in white men than in blacks, and is commoner in urban than in rural areas.

Pathology and staging

Over 90% of bladder tumours are derived from transitional cell epithelium. In Western countries, transitional cell carcinoma (TCC) of the bladder is at least five times as common as squamous cell carcinoma, though in Egypt where schistosomal infestation is common, the squamous carcinoma is more frequent. Other histological types such as adenocarcinoma, leiomyosarcoma and rhabdomyosarcoma are rare. TCCs may be single or multiple, and are sometimes pedunculated, whereas squamous carcinomas are usually sessile and often necrotic in appearance. Multiple papillomatous tumours are often of low-grade, though there is general agreement that they should be regarded as pre-malignant lesions.

In TCC, pathological grading is of considerable importance, though pathologists may differ in their methods of classification. Well-differentiated tumours clearly carry a better prognosis than anaplastic ones, quite independent of the stage of the tumour. Further important prognostic information can be obtained from a knowledge of the depth of infiltration of the bladder wall, with a direct correlation between pathologically-verified depth of penetration (P-stage) and survival.

The TNM staging notation (Table 18.2) allows a convenient shorthand description of bladder tumours, based largely on the degree of local spread at presentation (Fig. 18.6). The most important distinction lies between T2 and

Table 18.2. TNM and P-staging for Bladder Cancer.

Tis	Pre-invasive carcinoma (carcinoma *in situ*)
Ta	Papillary non-invasive carcinoma
T0	No evidence of primary tumour
T1	Tumour limited to the lamina propria (P1) Bimanual examination may reveal a mobile mass which cannot be felt after TUR
T2	Tumour limited to superficial muscle (P2) Mobile induration of the bladder wall may be present, but should be impalpable following TUR.
T3	Invasion of deep muscle layer of the bladder wall (P3). On bimanual palpation a mobile mass is felt which persists after TUR.
T3a	Deep muscle invasion
T3b	Invasion through the muscle wall
T4	Invasion of prostate or other local structures (P4); tumour fixed or locally extensive
T4a	Tumour infiltrates prostate, uterus or vagina
T4b	Tumour fixed to pelvic and/or abdominal wall
N0	No regional lymph node involvement
N1	Involvement of a single ipsilateral regional node group
N2	Contralateral, bilateral or multiple regional node involvement
N3	Fixed regional lymphadenopathy (i.e. a fixed space between this and the tumour)
N4	Involvement of juxta-regional nodes
M0	No distant metastases
M1	Distant metastases

T3 tumours, since over 50% of all patients with T2 tumours will be alive at 3 years from diagnosis, whereas <25% of patients with T3 tumours (i.e. with invasion of the deep muscle of the bladder) will survive. In addition to TNM stage, pathological grade and histological type, the size, location and number of bladder tumours will influence the management. Multiple bladder tumours are so frequently encountered that the whole of the transitional cell epithelial surface may be considered to be at risk, and in some instances where tumours are widespread throughout the bladder, total cystectomy may be required even though the local invasiveness of each one may be unimpressive.

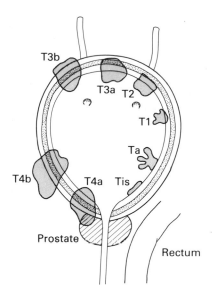

Fig. 18.6. *T staging of bladder cancer.* Tis: *in situ* carcinoma; Ta: non-invasive papillary carcinoma; T1: limited to lamina propria; T2: superficial muscle involvement; T3a: deep muscle involvement; T3b: full thickness of bladder wall; T4a: invading neighbouring structures (prostate, vagina); T4b: involvement of rectum, fixed to pelvic wall.

The major sites of distant metastasis are lymph nodes, lung, liver and bone.

Clinical features

The majority of patients with bladder cancer complain of haematuria, usually painless, though other symptoms such as urgency of micturition, nocturia, and frequency or reduction of the urinary stream may also be present. Loin or back pain may be a feature, particularly if tumour obstruction has led to hydronephrosis or if large intra-abdominal lymph node metastases are present. Even single episodes of haematuria should be fully investigated by cystoscopy.

Definitive diagnosis usually requires cystoscopy with biopsy, which gives a clear indication of the site, size, general appearance and multiplicity of bladder tumours. This procedure is normally performed under general anaesthesia, permitting a full examination including thorough rectal and bimanual palpation which are essential for accurate staging. Urinary exfoliative cytology is a valuable addition to diagnosis and is currently being evaluated as a means not only of diagnosis but also of monitoring response to treatment.

An intravenous urogram should routinely be performed, giving essential information regarding the anatomy and functioning of the kidneys and ureters, and often some degree of information as to the site and extent of the primary tumour. Renal function should also be assessed by measurement of blood urea and creatinine clearance (or other form of assessment such as DTPA clearance). Very few centres now perform pelvic arteriography, but lymphography and CT scanning are increasingly used, and the latter is particularly useful for accurate visualization of extravesical spread (Fig. 18.7). The technique is less satisfactory in visualizing enlarged lymph nodes, since the nodes of the external and internal iliac, and paravesical/obturator groups are less well surrounded by adipose tissue than the regional lymph nodes higher up in the abdomen. Nonetheless, CT scanning has rapidly become established as an important investigation in patients with deeply invasive bladder cancer, and is particularly valuable if radical irradiation is being contemplated.

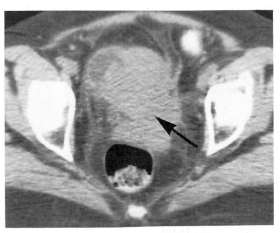

Fig. 18.7. *CT scan in advanced bladder cancer.* The tumour (arrowed) is shown extending posteriorly to the rectum and laterally to the side walls of the pelvis. We are grateful to Dr Janet Husband for this figure.

Management of carcinoma of the bladder

Management of superficial bladder tumours is almost entirely the province of the surgeon. Small papillary tumours can be repeatedly treated by cystodiathermy, often for many years, though other methods such as cryo-surgery or laser treatment are becoming more widely used. Intravesical chemotherapy using thiotepa, ethoglucid, doxorubicin and other cytotoxics is receiving increasing attention, since these agents are sometimes able to prevent or treat small recurrences of superficial bladder tumours. Although such tumours are rarely fatal, up to 10% of patients will develop widespread intravesical recurrence after repeated cystodiathermy, necessitating further treatment either with radiotherapy or even by total cystectomy. In these patients, intravesical chemotherapy may prove helpful in avoiding or delaying such treatment, thereby improving the quality of survival.

In patients with invasive carcinoma of the bladder (T2–3), the choice usually lies between a surgical procedure, radiation therapy, or a combination of both. In some patients with small lesions located in a mobile portion of the bladder, partial cystectomy is possible. An adequate cuff of normal bladder must be removed, and the procedure is usually only recommended where the initial capacity of the remaining bladder is >300–400 ml. Surgical technique is important in order to avoid implantation tumour nodules developing at the anastomosis, and the operation is less widely used now than formerly. Interstitial irradiation is an alternative to partial cystectomy in patients with T2 and early T3 lesions. A large study from van der Werf-Messing has provided a 5-year survival rate of 40% (T2) and 25% (T3), using interstitial (intravesical) irradiation with radium implants (sometimes with low-dose external irradiation) (9).

The introduction in the 1950s of a satisfactory method of total cystectomy led to rapid acceptance of this operation as the treatment of choice for patients with deeply invasive (T3)

tumours without extravesical or distant spread. This major procedure involves complete removal of the bladder, prostate and seminal vesicles (or bladder and urethra in the female), though some surgeons prefer a still more radical approach which combines total cystectomy with a pelvic lymph node dissection. Urinary diversion is usually achieved by fashioning a conduit from a section of resected ileum into which the ureters are implanted and which opens onto the abdominal wall (ileostomy), or by implanting the ureters directly into the sigmoid colon or rectum (Fig. 18.8).

One of the largest series of patients treated

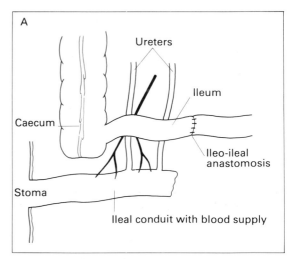

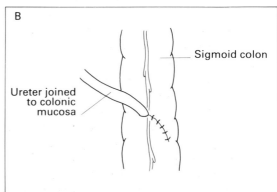

Fig. 18.8. Common procedures for ureteric diversion following total cystectomy. (A) Formation of an ileal conduit; (B) implantation into sigmoid colon.

Table 18.3. Survival of patients with deeply invasive carcinoma of the bladder treated (*a*) by surgery (total cystectomy with or without pre-operative irradiation); or (*b*) by radical irradiation alone, using external beam treatment.

(*a*) *Present status of all patients* (%)

	Group I (137 cases)	Group 2 (109 cases)	Group 3 (119 cases)	Group 4 (86 cases)
Alive and no evidence of disease after 5 or more years	10	28	27	38
Dead with no evidence of disease in <5 years	18	25	18	18
Dead with no evidence of disease in >5 years	22	7	11	2
Dead of disease in <5 years	48	32	39	2
Dead of disease in >5 years	1	3	5	41
Lost to follow-up in <5 years	1	5	0	1

Treatment details:
Group 1   radical cystectomy alone
Group 2   radical radiotherapy (60 Gy) with 'salvage' surgery for local failure
Group 3   planned pre-operative irradiation (40 Gy) followed by radical cystectomy
Group 4   planned intensive one-week pre-operative irradiation (20 Gy) followed by radical cystectomy

(*b*) *Urinary bladder cancer* (*radiotherapy 1957–1970*) *corrected survival rates* (*Karolinksa Hospital*)

Category (T-stage)	Interval (yrs)	Number of patients	Survival (%)
T1/2	5	188	31
	10	151	22
T3	5	283	20
	10	220	14
T4	5	129	10
	10	103	4

Data for (a), Whitmore *et al.* (10) and for (b), Edsmyr (11).

by surgery alone was reported by Whitmore (10). Of 137 patients treated by surgery alone, the operative mortality was 14% with an overall 5-year survival of 10% (Table 18.3). In three further groups of patients, pre-operative irradiation was used in an attempt to improve these results; three different techniques and dose schedules were employed, and in each group the 5-year survival rate was at least doubled. Although this study was not randomized, these data have persuaded most urologists that combinations of surgery and radiotherapy offer superior results to the use of total or radical cystectomy alone. More recently, several large radiotherapy centres have reported the results of treatment with radical radiotherapy alone, which seem comparable to those achieved by surgery. A large series of over 500 patients were reported by Edsmyr (11) with similar results to those obtained by Whitmore (Table 18.3). In several of these patients who later suffered local recurrence it was possible to perform a total cystectomy with successful 'salvage' (i.e. a significant additional recurrence-free period, or even a cure) in a substantial proportion.

In view of the effectiveness of radical radiotherapy for carcinoma of the bladder, it seems reasonable to ask whether cystectomy as primary management can be avoided altogether. A large cooperative study based at the Royal Marsden Hospital has attempted to answer this question. Nearly 200 patients were allocated either to receive radical radiotherapy alone— 60 Gy (6000 rad) over 6 weeks—or pre-operative irradiation—40 Gy (4000 rad) over 4 weeks—followed by a radical cystectomy a month later (12). At 5 years, there was a trend in favour of the group of patients receiving both radiotherapy and surgery, with a survival rate of 38% compared with 29% for the group undergoing radical radiotherapy. Although the overall result did not reach statistical significance, the combination of pre-operative irradiation and surgery seemed more effective in younger patients and in males. The difference between the two groups may also have been exaggerated because 20% of patients randomized to radiotherapy and surgery could not complete the treatment as planned. After local recurrence with radiotherapy alone, it was possible to perform salvage cystectomy with the impressive result of a 52% 5-year survival post-cystectomy.

The biological effectiveness of radiotherapy for bladder cancer is also shown by the phen-omenon of post-irradiation tumour 'down-staging'. Several groups have shown that after radiotherapy, the pathological (P) stage of the excised surgical specimen is frequently lower than the initial tumour (T) staging would suggest. For example, in one study (12), 47% of the bladder specimens excised after radiotherapy demonstrated this effect. Sterilization of locally involved lymph nodes can also be achieved by radiotherapy, the same study showing an incidence of node metastasis of 23% (the expected proportion would be 40–50% with unirradiated T3 tumours). Only 8% of patients who had been judged to be good responders to radiotherapy had histologically positive local nodes at cystectomy, suggesting that pre-operative irradiation may be particularly useful for patients with limited or microscopic regional or local lymph node deposits. Perhaps the most important result of all was that where down-staging could be demonstrated, the 5-year sur-

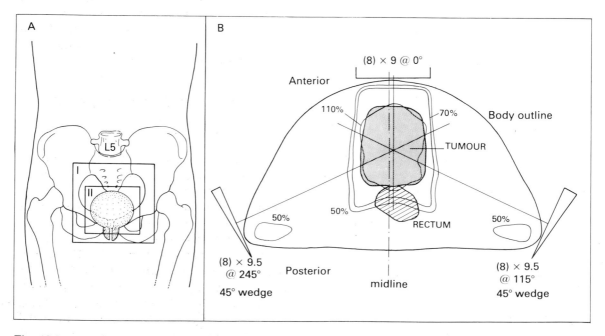

Fig. 18.9. *Typical external irradiation treatment technique for invasive (T3) carcinoma of bladder.* (A) Vertical representation of treatment volume. I: for first phase of treatment bladder and pelvic nodes are treated; II:for second phase of treatment the bladder is boosted to radical dose. Phase I is treated with the bladder full to minimize radiation damage to small bowel. (B) Typical treatment plan in phase II of radical treatment (field sizes in cm).

vival rate was 51%, whereas in patients who showed no such change, the survival at 5 years was only 22%.

Although cystectomy remains a widely practised treatment for T3 tumours, these and other data suggest that radiotherapy may be its equal, with considerable advantages in terms of morbidity. The quality of life with an ileal conduit is of course less satisfactory than for patients who micturate by the usual route. Common additional difficulties include odour, leakage, psychological adjustment to the stoma, and feelings of loss of sexual attractiveness. Many of these problems can be reduced by careful surgical technique but these patients naturally require a great deal of explanation and support pre- and postoperatively.

Radical external beam irradiation of bladder cancer should always be carried out using supervoltage equipment and requires a multifield technique employing 3 or 4 fields (Fig. 18.9). There is considerable debate as to whether it is essential to treat the local pelvic nodes as well as the bladder itself. Although it is difficult to show any evidence of improved survival when the pelvic nodes are treated, the demonstration of down-staging as described above certainly strengthens the case. Treatment-related morbidity is of course greater when the pelvis is treated, even to the relatively modest dose of 40 Gy (4000 rad). Apart from the importance of radiation treatment with curative intent, symptoms such as pain, haematuria and frequency usually respond well, and radiotherapy is the most valuable palliative treatment even in advanced (stage IV) tumours where there is virtually no prospect of cure.

CHEMOTHERAPY IN CARCINOMA OF THE BLADDER

The usefulness of systemic chemotherapy for advanced bladder cancer remains controversial. Cyclophosphamide, doxorubicin, mitomycin C, 5-fluorouracil, methotrexate and cisplatin all produce responses of the order of 20–30%. Many groups have attempted to improve the

results still further with combination regimes (13), but no clearcut survival advantage has yet been demonstrated although there are recent encouraging early reports. The results of combination regimes including cisplatin seem to be almost identical with those of cisplatin therapy alone (14). Further studies will be required to determine whether any groups of patients really benefit from such intensive treatment. At present, chemotherapy for advanced bladder tumours cannot be considered as conventional or established therapy, particularly since these patients tend to be in poor health and often with impaired renal function.

Prognosis

Important prognostic determinants include histological grade, tumour stage and presence of nodal spread. T1 tumours have a 5-year survival of about 75% with surgery alone. In T2 and early T3 lesions the 5-year survival is 35% while with more advanced disease, particularly where there is nodal involvement at diagnosis, only 10–15% will survive. There are virtually no long-term survivors when distant metastases are present at diagnosis.

CARCINOMA OF THE PROSTATE

Incidence and aetiology

Carcinoma of the prostate is among the commonest of all cancers in men (Fig. 18.1), and is the third largest cause of death from cancer in males, exceeded only by deaths from cancer of the lung and large bowel. In the United States, the mortality rate is almost twice as high in blacks as in whites and in 1977, 57 000 new cases were registered, with over 20 000 deaths (American Cancer Society figures). In both England and Australia there is strong evidence to suggest an increasing mortality during the past 50 years (15), though the death rate appears to have stabilized since 1960. The current death rate is 15–20 per 100 000 men.

Little is known of the aetiology of prostatic carcinoma. It does not occur in castrated men and is also thought to be less common in hepatic cirrhosis which is accompanied by impaired oestrogen degradation.

Pathology and staging

Adenocarcinoma is overwhelmingly the most common cell type, though transitional cell carcinoma may arise in the large prostatic ducts. Seventy-five percent of all prostatic cancers arise in the posterior or peripheral part of the prostate, and about 10% of these tumours are discovered during prostatectomy for an apparently benign prostatic hypertrophy. Such cases tend to be more localized than when the diagnosis of carcinoma is suspected clinically.

Histological grading is of considerable im-portance, though the majority of prostatic cancers are moderately well-differentiated. In a series of specimens reviewed at the Mayo Clinic, well-differentiated tumours accounted for 20%, and anaplastic cancers accounted for less than 5% of the total, with the remainder showing a moderate degree of differentiation (16). The incidence of lymph node metastases increases with the degree of anaplasia and there is no doubt that patients with low-grade lesions survive substantially longer (60% 5-year survival in the Mayo Clinic study, compared with 5% 5-year survival for patients with high-grade lesions).

No clinical or surgical staging system has yet found universal acceptance. The pattern of local invasion is shown schematically in Fig. 18.10.

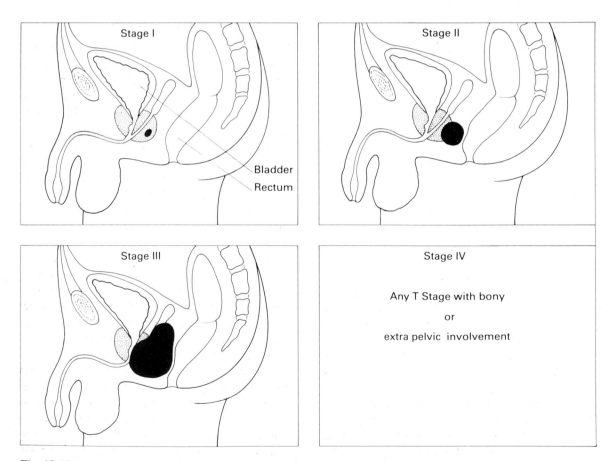

Fig. 18.10. *Local extension and clinical staging in carcinoma of the prostate.*

Table 18.4. TNM staging system for cancer of the prostate

T0	No palpable tumour
T1	Intracapsular tumour surrounded by normal prostatic tissue
T2	Tumour confined to the gland but with deformity and with minimal capsular invasion.
T3	Tumour extends locally beyond the capsule (including invasion of seminal vesicles)
T4	Tumour fixed or involving local structure
N0	No lymph node involvement
N1	Regional lymph node involvement (single)
N2	Regional lymph node involvement (multiple)
N3	More widespread nodal involvement
M0	No known metastases
M1	Distant metastases (usually bone)

The TNM system is increasingly employed (Table 18.4), but can be difficult in practise, particularly in determination of the T-stage of the tumour. The American system (17) is simpler and correlates fairly closely with the TNM staging. In this classification, the stages are defined thus:

Stage I carcinoma: microscopic cancer arising in a prostate gland which is not indurated on rectal examination. There are no metastases present.

Stage II carcinoma: a well-defined nodule or area of induration is present, confined to the prostate on rectal examination and without evidence of metastatic disease.

Stage III carcinoma: there is local extension beyond the confines of the prostate gland, usually with involvement of the bladder neck or seminal vesicle, but without clinical evidence of distant metastases.

Stage IV carcinoma: metastatic disease is present, usually in the bones or in other extra-pelvic sites.

There is some evidence that clinical staging is an accurate reflection of the true degree of spread. Where radical prostatectomy has been performed and the specimen carefully analysed, close agreement between surgical and clinical findings is discovered in about three-quarters of all cases, though sometimes with unsuspected local invasion—usually of the seminal vesicles. Invasion of pelvic lymph nodes may be clinically silent but is increasingly likely with advanced stages of disease as the prostate has an unusually rich lymph node network. Drainage is most commonly to the obturator-hypogastric group and then to the external and common iliac nodes. Distant metastases are predominantly osseous, particularly to the pelvic and lower lumbar vertebrae though ribs, dorsal spine and skull are not uncommonly involved. The bone metastases are typically osteosclerotic, as a result of the relatively slow clinical evolution of disease, though the pattern may be chiefly lytic or mixed.

Clinical features and investigation

Prostatic carcinoma is often asymptomatic, and is increasingly diagnosed at routine rectal examination. The typical finding is of a firm, indurated or craggy gland which is usually enlarged. There may be obliteration of the median sulcus or spread to the lateral pelvic walls. Many patients present with bone pain from secondary deposits particularly in the back and pelvis. In patients with local prostatic symptoms, the commonest complaints are urinary infection or obstruction, with changes in the urinary stream including hesitancy or urgency of micturition.

Histological diagnosis is always required and biopsy by the transrectal route is widely favoured. If fragments from a transurethral resection of a hypertrophic gland show evidence of malignancy, further confirmation is not usually necessary. Other methods of biopsy include the perineal or retropubic routes.

Although some clinicians do not carry out routine staging investigations in carcinoma of the prostate, it is important to assess the local extent of disease as well as the presence of distant metastases in order to decide on the correct treatment, and to identify cases in which a local approach to treatment could be curative. Serum acid phosphatase is valuable since if raised, it can be useful in monitoring the effectiveness of treatment. An isotope bone scan should always be done since bone metastases are often asymptomatic, particularly in the skull, ribs and upper part of the vertebral column. Skeletal X-rays give further details of these deposits but are not usually essential to management decisions unless local therapy for the metastasis is being considered. Routine tests of renal function are often revealing, and an IVU may show prostatic irregularity and back-pressure on the kidneys.

For patients who are candidates for surgery or radiotherapy of the primary tumour (with curative intent), it is essential to determine the full extent of the local disease. Routine lymphography has not become an established part of pre-treatment investigation. Its chief value probably lies in the demonstration of unequivocal lymph node metastases in a proportion of patients with clinically early disease, in whom radical treatment by prostatic surgery or intensive radiation therapy might otherwise have been carried out but with little chance of success. Unfortunately, false-positive and false-negative lymphograms are not uncommon in this disease. CT scanning may also be useful in detecting unsuspected nodal metastases, but also gives more detailed information regarding local extent of disease, particularly with respect to the degree of periprostatic invasion. It is not however generally considered to be as valuable an investigation as it is with bladder cancer.

Management of prostatic cancer

There are few areas in clinical cancer management today where such diversity of opinion exists, even amongst experts. Most would agree that in patients with clinically localized prostatic cancer, and without evidence of bone or extrapelvic metastases, some attempt at curative therapy should be made. However, some urologists believe (rightly or wrongly) that the true incidence of early (T1) disease is so low that a localized approach is never really justifi-

able, preferring palliative methods of treatment in every case. More aggressive surgeons will consider radical surgical techniques even in patients with local periprostatic extension (T2–T3, i.e. up to stage III disease), sometimes using hormonal treatment in an attempt to produce tumour shrinkage pre-operatively.

There are only two possible approaches for patients in whom radical treatment with curative intent is considered justifiable; radical prostatectomy or radical radiotherapy. The radical surgical approach has evolved since the turn of the century, and consists of *en bloc* resection of the prostate, prostatic urethra and seminal vesicles with part of the surrounding connective tissue (Denonvillier's fascia). Only patients with disease confined within the prostatic capsule and without lymph node metastasis can be considered suitable, and the operation has always been more popular in the United States than in Britain. The surgical approach can be either retropubic or perineal. The suprapubic approach also allows for pelvic lymphadenectomy, if this is considered appropriate. Complications are discussed below.

Radical radiation therapy, though more recently introduced, is certainly more widely applicable than surgery since minimal extracapsular extension or periprostatic invasion do not represent contraindications to treatment. Although any form of radical treatment should be considered with care since the majority of these patients are over 65 years of age, there seems no doubt that radical surgery demands a greater general level of medical fitness than the radiotherapeutic approach. It is known that the normal prostate tolerates high dosage of radition without prostatic symptoms developing, though excessive irradiation of surrounding tissues (bladder, prostatic urethra or large bowel) can cause serious problems (see Chapter 5).

In patients suitable for radical radiotherapy, a high dosage has to be given to the whole of the gland and periprostatic area. Although interstitial approaches using radium implants into the gland were initially employed by early

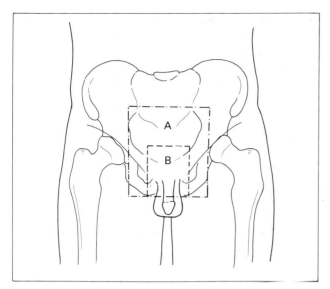

Fig. 18.11. *Typical treatment volume for radical irradiation of carcinoma of the prostate using external beam therapy.* (A) First phase of treatment (to 40 Gy/ 4 weeks) treats prostatic lymph node drainage as well as prostate and prostatic urethra. (B) Prostate and peri-prostatic area boosted to total of 60 Gy/6 weeks. Field arrangement similar to Fig. 18.9.

workers, external beam irradiation is now usually preferred (but see below).

There is general agreement that a total dose of at least 60 Gy (6000 rad) over 6 weeks (or equivalent over a shorter period) is required for eradication of prostatic cancer and even higher doses have been recommended. In addition, the pelvic contents are often irradiated (Fig. 18.11), to a dose of 40 Gy (4000 rad) over 4 weeks, because of the possibility of unsuspected peri-prostatic or lymphatic spread; some radio-therapists recommend a minimum of 50 Gy (5000 rad) to the whole pelvic contents, with a final boost to the periprostatic and prostatic region when the pelvic irradiation has been completed. A variety of techniques have been used to achieve these high dosages. Multifield arrangements are invariably required, often employing three or four fields of treatment as for treatment of bladder cancer, always using supervoltage equipment.

An alternative approach receiving increasing attention, is the use of permanent interstitial implants, usually employing ^{125}I seeds, to the prostate (and periprostatic area if necessary), (Fig. 18.12). This treatment delivers a very high local dose (>100 Gy, 10 000 rad) with remarkably low morbidity, and clearly warrants

further trial, possibly in conjunction with external irradiation of the pelvic lymph nodes.

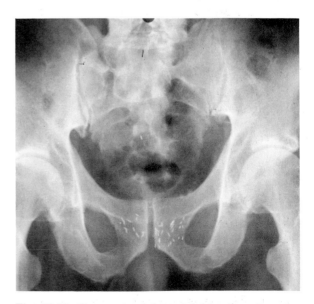

Fig. 18.12. *Transperineal interstitial implantation of the prostate.* ^{125}I seeds are used to obtain a high local dose (in excess of 100 Gy (10 000 rad). Intra rectal ultrasound is used for localization of the gland avoiding the need for open operation.

RESULTS OF RADICAL TREATMENT

It is difficult to assess the results of treatment in carcinoma of the prostate, because of its uncertain and often indolent natural history and the high death rate in any group of elderly men. Among the best results of radical surgery are those of Jewett (18), who noted 28 long survivors (15 years or more) amongst a group of 86 patients. Despite very careful selection, the operation failed to control the local disease in approximately 25% of cases. Several centres have reported large series of patients treated by radiotherapy, in whom a proportion appear to have been cured (19) though 'cure' is difficult to define in this elderly population. In following up these patients, it is important to realise that in the irradiated prostate, subsequent biopsy may show evidence of persistent malignant cells for up to a year, without any supportive clinical suggestion that the treatment has failed. In one series, 60% of patients with locally advanced disease had positive biopsies up to 9 months after treatment, falling to only 24% at 12–30 months, without further treatment (20). Selection of patients for definitive radiation therapy is less stringent than selection for surgery, and patients with T1, T2 and T3 lesions may be suitable. One of the largest radiation series, by Bagshawe and colleagues (21), described the results in over 400 patients (Fig. 18.13) showing a difference in survival between patients whose disease was limited to the prostate and those who had extra-capsular extension. Survival at 5 years approached 60%, with 40% of patients alive at 10 years.

Complications of radical surgical treatment include an operative mortality rate of up to 5%, permanent impotence in at least 90% of patients, and urinary incontinence in at least 5%. Rectovesical fistula and ureteric damage may also occur. Important complications of radical radiotherapy include side-effects of diarrhoea, dysuria and perineal skin reaction (sometimes severe), commonly occurring during the latter part of treatment. Long-term sequelae also occur, and a degree of subcutaneous fibrosis, urethral stricture and fibrotic reduction of bladder capacity may have to be accepted. Treatment with a full bladder will help to keep the small bowel out of the irradiated volume. The avoidance of impotence as a side-effect is a valuable advantage since with either radical surgery or hormonal treatment for prostatic cancer, impotence is almost certain.

HORMONAL THERAPY IN PROSTATIC CANCER

In 1941, Huggins discovered that prostatic cancers were almost always hormonally dependent (22). Both oestrogen therapy and orchidectomy were found to be useful for palliation, particularly in patients with bone metastases. Since the majority of patients are unsuitable for radical surgery, the use of oestrogen derivatives or orchidectomy (sometimes both) became increasingly widespread as part of standard therapy both for early and advanced cases.

Hormonal manipulation has been increas-

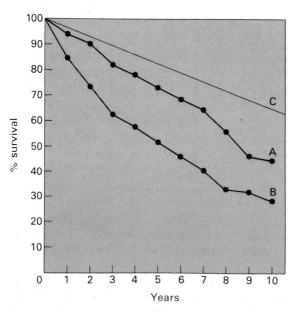

Fig. 18.13. *Results of radical radiation therapy for carcinoma of the prostate.* (A) Disease limited to prostate; (B) extra-capsular extension; (C) expected survival, adjusted for age. (From Bagshawe *et al.* (21), with permission.)

ingly widely used as definitive treatment for advanced disease (stages III and IV), though many radiotherapists prefer to offer local irradiation to patients with stage III disease who have no evidence of metastases elsewhere, and whose clinical condition warrants an attempt at radical treatment. There has been an increasing trend towards bilateral orchidectomy instead of oestrogen treatment, in order to avoid the cardiovascular complications of oestrogens as well as the troublesome gynaecomastia which usually occurs (though admittedly preventable by low dose irradiation to the breasts, providing this is done before oestrogen therapy is started). It came as something of a surprise when the Veterans' Administration Urological Research Group demonstrated in the 1960s that the prophylactic use of hormone treatment did not improve the overall survival (23). Although the hormone therapy had a slight beneficial effect on survival from the prostate cancer, this was counterbalanced by the increased death rate from cardiovascular disease. There was some evidence that the use of orchidectomy and oestrogen therapy together was preferable to either modality alone. In a later study it was shown that a lower dose of diethylstilboestrol (1 mg rather than 5 mg daily) was still effective but without the attendant cardiovascular mortality. Nonetheless, many urologists prefer to delay treatment in locally advanced cases either until symptoms appear or the disease progresses.

In palliative treatment of metastatic prostatic cancer, radiotherapy has an important role since the majority of the metastases are bony, and likely to be painful. These deposits generally respond well to moderate doses of radiotherapy. In recent years, single fraction hemi-body irradiation has been shown to be valuable, particularly since widespread metastases in the lower spine are so common. Treatment of the lower half of the body to a single fraction dose of 7.5–10 Gy (750–100 rad) is well tolerated and often dramatically effective for pain relief.

In patients with widespread metastatic problems unresponsive to oestrogens or palliative irradiation, there is every reason to consider bilateral orchidectomy since worthwhile responses are often seen.

Occasionally, the use of phosphorylated oestrogens such as 'Honvan' may produce a response where ethinyl oestradiol or stilboestrol has failed, and may delay the need for orchidectomy. A more recent addition to therapy is the conjugated nitrogen mustine derivative of oestradiol (estramustine) which has given promising results and needs further evaluation. In one study, 50% of 65 patients with refractory tumours responded subjectively, with significant palliation of pain and in some cases, objective responses such as a reduction in serum acid phosphatase (24).

Other agents of probable value include cyproterone acetate and flutamide (anti-androgens which interfere with testosterone binding to the androgen receptor), and aminoglutethimide which inhibits adrenal steroid synthesis as well as acting as a peripheral aromatase inhibitor. Considerable interest has followed the demonstration that analogues of gonadotrophin-releasing hormone (so-called LHRH agonists) may interfere with gonadotrophin release, leading to a fall in circulating testosterone (25). These agents appear to be as effective as the commonly used hormonal approaches, but with fewer side-effects than either stilboestrol or orchidectomy. They are now available by slow-release preparation given by monthly implant. They are often given with an anti-androgen to prevent a flare of the disease.

Chemotherapy for prostatic carcinoma has been disappointing although a number of agents show modest levels of activity, including cyclophosphamide, methotrexate, 5-fluorouracil, nitrogen mustard and cisplatin.

In patients with unresponsive widespread bone pain, treatment with radioactive phosphorus may be of value, and up to 75% of all patients have been reported to benefit (26), though remissions tend to be short. Hypophysectomy is also effective and can be done without craniotomy using a transphenoidal approach. In a review of nine separate series comprising well over 200 patients, a total response rate of 63% was observed (27), a remarkable figure since the majority of these patients had undergone previous hormone treatment.

CANCER OF THE URETHRA

Male urethra

This very rare tumour may arise in the prostatic, bulbar or penile urethra, and is thought to be commoner in patients with a history of chronic inflammation or stricture. In the prostatic urethra, the tumour is a transitional cell carcinoma but in the penile urethra, squamous carcinomas are more common. The tumour spreads by direct invasion into the perineum and penile tissues.

The penile urethra drains to inguinal lymph nodes, and the prostatic urethra to pelvic nodes.

Urethral carcinomas present with a urethral mass, obstruction, fistula, pain and haematuria. The age range is 50–80 years. Prostatic urethral tumours are treated either by radical prostatectomy or cystoprostatectomy, or by radical radiotherapy. This latter method is increasingly employed, using doses of the order of 60–70 Gy (6000–7000 rad) to the prostate. Radiation technique is similar to that employed for carcinoma of the prostate (Fig. 18.11).

Distal penile urethral carcinomas are usually treated by amputation of the distal part of the penis. Lesions of the bulbomembranous urethra are generally treated by radical excision.

Female urethra

The tumour is twice as common in females, and the histological pattern is more varied. Squamous carcinoma is the predominant form in the distal two-thirds, and transitional cell carcinoma in the proximal third. Adenocarcinoma may arise from the periurethral glands, and melanoma and sarcoma occasionally occur. Leukoplakia of the urethra is regarded as a pre-malignant change, as are urethral papillomas and polyps.

The tumour typically presents with a mass or with bleeding and offensive discharge. Lymphatic involvement occurs late, tumours of the distal urethra draining to the inguinal nodes and those of the proximal urethra to the iliac nodes.

Tumours of the anterior urethra are sometimes treated by partial urethrectomy but there is a high risk of local recurrence and nodal spread frequently occurs. There is increasing interest in the use of radical radiation therapy since surgical control of the more extensive tumours is hard to achieve and the results are very poor. Interstitial radioactive implants are sometimes used for small tumours, and external beam radiation therapy for larger lesions. The usual tumour dose is of the order of 60 Gy (6000 rad), carefully fractionated to avoid stricture formation.

CANCER OF THE PENIS

Incidence and aetiology

Carcinoma of the penis is uncommon in Britain and United States. It accounts for less than 0.2% of all male cancer deaths in Britain. It is, however, much more frequent in South East Asia, and in parts of India and Africa. It is thought that general hygiene has a bearing on its incidence, and early circumcision is known to be associated with a very low risk. There is slight concordance between the incidence of penile and cervical carcinomas in sexual partners. In addition, there are several premalignant conditions which predispose to the development of the tumour. These include Bowen's disease (intra-epithelial carcinoma), erythroplasia of Queyrat, leukoplakia and Paget's disease. Leukoplakia may coexist with an invasive carcinoma. These premalignant lesions should be treated by local excision.

Clinical features

Presentation is usually with an exophytic, or occasionally an excavating, ulcerated lesion, most commonly arising in the glans or the inner surface of the prepuce. There is often wide surface extension before deeper invasion to the urethra and corpora cavernosa. Some carcinomas of the penis are clinically obvious with a circumferential exophytic necrotic tumour, whereas in other cases only careful inspection with retraction of the prepuce will allow the tumour to be visualized. Local invasion to the inguinal nodes is common, but lymph node enlargement may be due to local infection rather than metastasis. The superficial inguinal nodes drain the prepuce and most of the penile skin, whereas the glans and corpora cavernosa drain chiefly to the deep inguinal nodes. A biopsy should always be performed since non-malignant conditions, such as lymphogranuloma venereum, trauma, penile warts (condylomata) or leucoplakia can cause diagnostic confusion.

A TNM staging classification has been proposed (Table 18.5), but can be difficult to apply in practise, particularly since palpable inguinal lymph nodes are often due to local infection. Though relatively unlikely to disseminate widely, the commonest sites of blood-borne metastases (M1) are the lungs and bone,

Table 18.5. TNM staging cancer of the penis

T0	No evidence of primary tumour
T1S	Carcinoma *in situ* (include Bowen's disease and erythroplasia of Queyrat)
T1	Superficial tumour < 1 cm diameter
T2	Larger tumour but remains superficial
T3	Tumour invades underlying tissues
T4	Tumour invades local tissues including corpora cavernosa, urethra or perineum
N0	No regional lymphadenopathy
N1	Unilateral regional node involvement
N2	Multiple unilateral node groups involved, or bilateral nodes
M0	No distant metastases
M1	Distant metastases present

and a chest X-ray should always be performed as part of the investigation. The value of lymphography is limited by the frequent concurrent infection.

Treatment

In the past, surgery has been considered the treatment of choice, though amputation of the penis has never been a popular method of treatment and radical local irradiation has increasingly been used as an alternative. As the tumour is uncommon, few surgeons or radiotherapists have a large experience. Treatment is often individualized: a small non-infiltrating tumour, which can be surgically excised without amputation, is probably best treated by surgery, with local irradiation given wherever there is doubt about the adequacy of the resection edge of the specimen. Many radiotherapists are disinclined to offer radical irradiation in bulky lesions because of the probability of hypoxia within the necrotic part of the tumour which limits the prospect of radiocurability; such tumours are probably best dealt with surgically, particularly if partial amputation will suffice. More proximal lesions would require total amputation, but many surgeons are prepared to agree to radical irradiation in the first instance, with surgery if there is local recurrence.

A variety of radiotherapy techniques has been described, including superficial X-rays (with single or opposed direct fields), treatment by radium mould, or by orthovoltage or supervoltage irradiation using photons or electrons. A wax block can be used to improve dose homogeneity. Interstitial implants with radioactive iridium or other sources can also be used. The total dose of external irradiation is usually 60 Gy (6000 rad) in daily fractions over 6 weeks, or the equivalent over a shorter treatment period. With mould treatments using iridium wire or radium, the treatment can usually be completed within 10 days (the patient wearing the mould for 8–10 hours per day), to a total dose of the order of 60 Gy. The major complications of radiation therapy for carcinoma of the penis include urethral stricture (10–12% of patients), fibrosis, ulceration and local recurrence (10–40% depending on the size of the tumour). For larger and more infiltrating tumours, surgery is probably the treatment of choice, particularly where the inguinal nodes are obviously involved by tumour. Where the inguinal nodes are mobile, block dissection is generally preferable to local irradiation though it is probably wise to perform aspiration cytology to confirm that the nodes are indeed metastatic. Before the advent of aspiration cytology, delay in inguinal block dissection was often advocated to allow infected palpable nodes to settle. Where the inguinal nodes are clearly fixed and surgery is not possible, local irradiation of the inguinal node groups can be useful as a palliative procedure. Although remissions have been documented in such cases, survival is poor. The majority of patients with stage I (T1 or T2, N0) tumours are free of inguinal metastases but the incidence in stage II (T3, N0 or N1a) is well over 50%, and it is these patients who probably benefit most from block dissection.

Prognosis

Early carcinoma of the penis has an excellent cure rate with surgery and/or radiotherapy. Although few large series of patients have been reported, it seems probable that T1 and T2 N0 cases are equally well treated by surgery or radiotherapy. In one series, 18 out of 20 patients treated by radical irradiation were free of disease at 3 years (27), which compares closely with surgical figures. Patients with deep involvement of penile structures or inguinal node involvement do far less well, and the survival rate is approximately 50%. Where there are inoperable inguinal metastases or distant involvement, the 5-year survival rate is well under 10%.

REFERENCES

1 Doll R. & Peto R. (1981) *The Causes of Cancer: Quantitative Estimates of Avoidable Risks of Cancer in the United States Today.* Oxford University Press.

2 Selli C., Hinshaw M.W., Woodard B.H. & Paulson D.F. (1983) Stratification of risk factors in renal cell carcinoma. *Cancer* **52**, 899.

3 Robson C.J., Churchill B.M. & Anderson W. (1968) The results of radical nephrectomy for renal cell carcinoma. *Transactions of the American Association of Genito-urinary Surgeons* **60**, 122.

4 Skinner D.G., Colvin R.B., Vermillion C.D., Pfister R.C. & Leadbetter W.F. (1971) Diagnosis and management of renal cell carcinoma. *Cancer* **28**, 1165.

5 Finney R. (1973) An evaluation of postoperative radiotherapy in hypernephroma treatment—a clinical trial. *Cancer* **32**, 1332–40.

6 Van der Werf-Messing B. (1973) Carcinoma of the Kidney. *Cancer*, **32**, 1056.

7 Rafla S. (1970) Renal cell carcinoma: natural history and results of treatment. *Cancer* **25**, 26–40.

8 Hueper W.C., Wiley P.H. & Wolfe H.D. (1938) Experimental production of bladder tumors in dogs by administration of beta-naphthylamine. *Journal of Industrial Hygiene and Toxicology*. **20**, 46.

9 Van der Werf-Messing B. (1978) Cancer of the urinary bladder treated by interstitial radium implant. *International Journal of Radiation Oncology Biology Physics* **4**, 373.

10 Whitmore W.F., Batata M.A., Ghoneim M.A., Grabstald H. & Unal A. (1977) Radical cystectomy with or without prior irradiation in the treatment of bladder cancer. *Journal of Urology* **118**, 184–7.

11 Edsmyr F. (1981) Radiotherapy in the management of bladder carcinoma. In Oliver R.T.D., Hendry W.F. & Bloom H.J.G. (eds) *Bladder Cancer*, pp. 139–49. Butterworths, London.

12 Bloom H.J.G., Hendry W.F., Wallace D.M. & Skeet R.G. (1982) Treatment of T3 bladder cancer: controlled trial of pre-operative radiotherapy and radical cystectomy versus radical radiotherapy. Second report and review (for the Clinical Trials Group, Institute of Urology). *British Journal of Urology* **54**, 136–51.

13 Merrin C. (1981) Adjuvant post-surgical chemotherapy with cyclophosphamide, doxorubicin hydrochloride, and cisdiamminedichloroplatinum in patients with bladder cancer. In Oliver R.T.D., Hendry W.F. & Bloom H.J.G. (eds) *Bladder Cancer* pp. 255–60. Butterworths, London.

14 Yagoda A. (1980) Chemotherapy of metastatic bladder cancer. *Cancer*, **45**, 1879.

15 Holman C.D.J., James I.R., Segal M.R. & Armstrong B.K. (1981) Recent trends in mortality from prostate cancer in male populations of Australia, England & Wales. *British Journal of Cancer* **44**, 340.

16 Pool T.L. & Thompson G.J. (1956) Conservative treatment of carcinoma of the prostate. *Journal of the American Medical Association* **160,** 833.

17 Rubin P. (1969) Cancer of the urogenital tract: prostatic cancer. *Journal of the American Medical Association* **209**, 1695.

18 Jewett H.J., Bridge R.W., Gray G.F. & Shelley W.M. (1968) The palpable nodule of prostatic cancer. Results fifteen years after radical excision. *Journal of the American Association* **203**, 403.

19 Taylor W.J., Richardson R.G. & Hafermann M.D. (1979) Radiation therapy for localised prostate cancer. *Cancer* **43**, 1123–7.

20 Cox J.D. & Stoffel T.J. (1977) The significance of needle biopsy after irradiation for stage C adenocarcinoma of the prostate. *Cancer* **40**, 156–60.

21 Bagshaw M.A., Ray G.R., Salzman J.R. & Meares E.M. (1975) Extended-field radiation therapy for carcinoma of the prostate: a progress report. *Cancer Chemotherapy Reports*. **59,** (Part I), 165–73.

22 Huggins C. & Hodges C.F. (1941) Studies on prostatic cancer. I: The effect of castration, of estrogen and of androgen injection on serum acid phosphatase in metastatic carcinoma of the prostate. *Cancer Research* **1**, 293.

23 The Veterans Administration Co-operative Urological Research Group (1967) Treatment and survival of patients with cancer of the prostate. *Surgery, Gynecology and Obstetrics*, **124**, 1011.

24 Mittelman A., Shukla S.K., Welvaart K. & Murphy G.P. (1975) Oral estramustine phosphate (NCS-89199) in the treatment of advanced (stage D) carcinoma of the prostate. *Cancer Chemotherapy Reports* **59**, 219.

25 Editorial (1985) Dilemmas in the management of prostatic carcinoma. *Lancet* **ii,** 1219.

26 Blackard C.E. (1974) Management of cancer of the prostate. *British Journal of Hospital Medicine* **11,** 357.

27 Brendler H. (1973) Adrenalectomy and hypophysectomy for prostatic cancer. *Urology* **2**, 99–102.

28 Duncan W. & Jackson S.M. (1972) The treatment of early cancer of the penis with megavoltage x-rays. *Clinical Radiology* **23**, 246–8.

Chapter 19

Testicular Cancer

Although testicular tumours are uncommon, with a frequency of just over 2 per 100 000 males per year, they have an importance beyond their low incidence. First, they represent the most common malignant disease of young men between the ages of 25 and 35 years; second, they are exceptionally chemosensitive tumours with a high cure rate even with disseminated disease; and thirdly, because they often manufacture tumour markers which can be used to monitor treatment and to predict recurrence before it is clinically evident.

GERM CELL TUMOURS

Aetiology and incidence

The vast majority of testicular tumours are *germ cell tumours* which are believed to arise in the pluripotent germ cell. This cell, when malignant, can give rise to tumours which have somatic or trophoblastic features or both. Somatic differentiation gives rise to the mixture of tissues seen in teratomas, and choriocarcinoma comes from trophoblastic differentiation. *Non-germ cell tumours* are discussed on p. 354. While most male germ-cell tumours arise in the testis they may occasionally be *extragonadal* in origin, and these are described on p. 353.

The presence of an undescended testis (cryptorchidism) is associated with a ten-fold increase in the incidence of testicular tumours. Orchidopexy reduces, but does not abolish, this risk. Data from North America suggests that testicular tumours are rarer in blacks than in

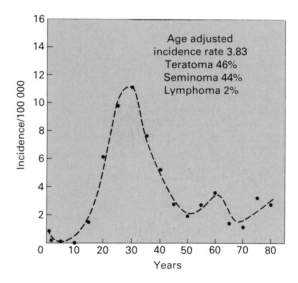

Fig. 19.1. *Age-specific incidence of testicular tumours.*

US whites. Teratomas of the testis present at an earlier age (peak age 20–30 years) than seminomas (peak age 30–50 years). The age-adjusted incidence in Britain is 3.8 per 100 000; incidence at different ages is shown in Fig. 19.1. Teratoma and seminoma are the usual tumours at 10–40 years of age, but in older age groups lymphoma is the commonest tumour.

Pathology

A variety of different systems of classification are in current use (Table 19.1). In Britain, the commonest classification is that of the British Testicular Tumour Panel, whilst in the United States, the Dixon and Moore classification is widely used (1). Each is the result of

Table 19.1. Pathological Classification of Testicular Tumours.

British Testicular Tumour Panel
  Seminoma
  Malignant Teratoma Undifferentiated (MTU)
  Malignant Teratoma Intermediate (MTI)
  Maligant Teratoma Trophoblastic (MTT)
  Teratoma Differentiated (TD)

Dixon and Moore (1)
  Pure seminoma
  Embryonal carcinoma (pure or with seminoma)
  Teratoma (pure or with seminoma)
  Teratoma with embryonal carcinoma, choriocarcinoma or seminoma
  Choriocarcinoma pure or with seminoma embryonal carcinoma (or both)

World Health Organization
  1 Tumours of single cell type
    Seminoma
    Embryonal carcinoma
    Teratoma
    Choriocarcinoma
  2 Mixed histological appearances
    Embryonal carcinoma with teratoma
    Embryonal carcinoma with teratoma and seminoma
    Embryonal carcinoma with choriocarcinoma
    Teratoma with seminoma
    Choriocarcinoma with any other cell type

a review of a large number of patients, and both are based on light microscopic criteria, and attempt to identify the predominant cell type. A major problem with these classifications is that the tumours are often heterogeneous, the teratomas displaying pleomorphism and a tendency to multiple cell types. Future classifications may depend increasingly on histochemical criteria, particularly in those tumours which produce tumour markers.

Most testicular tumours are of germ-cell origin (Fig. 19.2). These can usually be classified into seminomas (40%), teratomas (32%), or combined tumours with elements of both (14%). The non-germ cell tumours include lymphomas (predominantly large cell lymphomas), Sertoli cell tumours, Leydig cell tumours and paratesticular rhabdomyosarcomas.

Although it has always been thought that the histological type of germ cell tumour carries prognostic significance, particularly in the distinction between seminomas and the teratomas, the recent dramatic improvements in treatment (particularly of teratomas) have reduced these disparities. Apart from the cell type, the most important prognostic feature, from the operative specimen at orchidectomy, is the presence of tumour cells either at the cut end of the cord or within its vessels (intravascular invasion). Such tumours have an adverse prognosis.

SEMINOMA

Seminomas tend to be encapsulated and firm, with the cut surface pale grey and often featureless, and with little or no necrosis or haemorrhage. The microscopic appearance shows large round cells with distinct cell borders, clear cytoplasm, and large nuclei often with conspicuous nucleoli (Fig. 19.2). Lymphocytic infiltration is frequently seen. When spread beyond the testis occurs, it is almost invariably to pelvic and para-aortic lymph nodes followed by involvement of mediastinal and supraclavicular nodes. Although chiefly testicular in origin, primary extra-gonadal seminomas are occasionally encountered in the retroperitoneal region, mediastinum, and suprasellar region or pineal area of the brain.

TERATOMA (NON-SEMINOMATOUS GERM-CELL TUMOURS)

Malignant Teratoma Undifferentiated (MTU, embryonal carcinoma) is the commonest non-seminomatous germ-cell tumour. These are often firm and nodular, showing areas of haemorrhage and necrosis. Microscopically, large anaplastic cells are usually seen, with less distinct cell borders and an eosinophilic cytoplasm containing nuclei of widely varying shapes. Some form of differentiation may occur, often with a glandular pattern (Fig. 19.2).

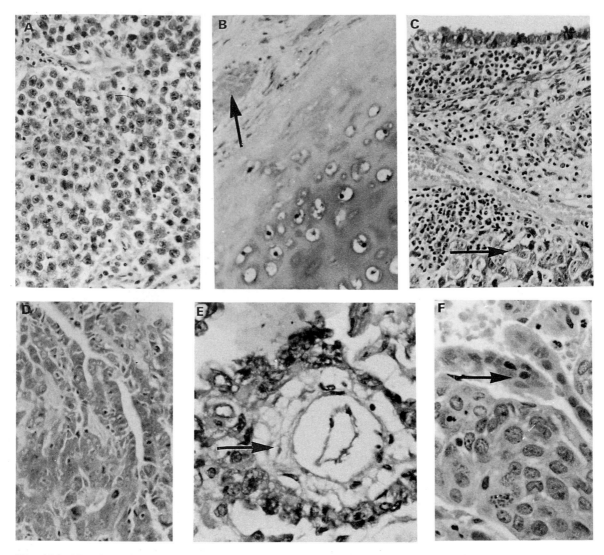

Fig. 19.2. *Histological appearances of testicular germ cell tumours.* (Original magnification ×200.) (A) pure seminoma; (B) malignant teratoma differentiated, showing cartilage and smooth muscle (arrowed); (C) malignant teratoma intermediate, showing differentiated epithelium and embryonal carcinoma (arrowed); (D) malignant teratoma undifferentiated, showing embryonal carcinoma; (E) Yolk sac tumour, showing a Schiller-Duval body (arrowed); (F) choriocarcinoma, showing syncytiotrophoblast (arrowed) and cytotrophoblast.

Malignant Teratoma Intermediate (MTI or teratocarcinoma) usually shows characteristic differences from MTU, with a nodular appearance which, on sectioning, frequently feels gritty because of the presence of cartilage and/ or bone. There is often a wide variety of germ cell types, including cells derived from all three of the primitive germ cell layers, including bone, cartilage, connective tissue and smooth muscle as well as cells suggestive of respiratory or gastro-intestinal epithelium.

Malignant Teratoma Trophoblastic (MTT, choriocarcinoma) is very much less common, and is histologically distinct because of the typical elements of cytotrophoblast and/or syncytiotrophoblast cells. These tumours are highly malignant, metastasising early and widely. It is extremely unusual to encounter a true trophoblastic testicular tumour which is confined to the testis. They tend to be bulky tumours at presentation and are more often associated with brain metastases than other types of teratoma. They may develop drug resistance early, and should probably be treated with regimens containing methotrexate. A prognostic distinction can be drawn between MTT and the commoner teratoma types (MTI and MTU). MTU probably has a more rapid doubling time than MTI, more commonly presents with lung deposits, seems more responsive to chemotherapy, and carries a somewhat better prognosis.

Occasionally, a fully mature or differentiated testicular teratoma is encountered, in which mature bone, bone marrow and cartilage, and other tissues may all be present. Even these tumours should be regarded as 'potentionally malignant'.

Patterns of metastases

Clinical staging is based on a relatively predictable pattern of progression (Fig. 19.3). Typically, the mode of spread is lymphatic, along the lymphatics of the spermatic cord to the para-aortic lymph nodes, and thence to the retroperitoneal and retrocrural nodes, thoracic duct, posterior mediastinum and supraclavicular nodes (usually left-sided, though bifid or right-sided thoracic ducts occur in a small percentage of the population). Blood-borne spread frequently occurs, especially in MTT and MTU. In over 90% of cases this is associated with demonstrable nodal spread; in the remainder, metastases develop in the lungs, in the absence of abdominal lymphatic disease. Although liver involvement is not frequent, it is exceptional in patients without lung deposits. Intracerebral and bone metastases are occasionally encountered. MTU is more commonly associated with locally invasive primary

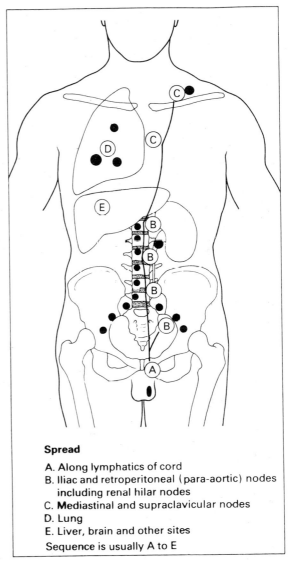

Spread

A. Along lymphatics of cord
B. Iliac and retroperitoneal (para-aortic) nodes including renal hilar nodes
C. Mediastinal and supraclavicular nodes
D. Lung
E. Liver, brain and other sites
Sequence is usually A to E

Fig. 19.3. *Pathways of spread of testicular germ cell tumours.*

tumours and with haematogenous spread than MTI.

Clinical features

Patients typically present with a painless swelling of the testis, although pain may be a feature particularly in rapidly growing tumours. There seems to be a great difference in level of concern, some young men presenting with a tumour of only 2–3 cm whilst others are unaware of the change until the testis is well over twice its normal size. Although small hydroceles are frequently present, invasion of the scrotal skin is extremely unusual and the tunica albuginea is rarely breached. Occasionally a spermatocele or varicocele may cause diagnostic difficulties.

The lymphatic drainage of the testis can be traced to the original embryonic site of origin in the abdomen (pelvic, common iliac and para-aortic nodes), rather than to adjacent nodes. Dissemination of tumour into these lymph node groups is common and may cause low back pain. Patients may also notice lymphadenopathy in other sites, particularly the left supraclavicular nodes. In patients with a previous history of inguinal or testicular surgery (usually herniorrhaphy or orchidopexy), inguinal lymph node involvement may occur due to interference with the normal lymphatic pathways. Occasionally, abdominal swelling may occur as a result of massive nodal deposits from an unsuspected primary testicular tumour. The presenting symptoms will then be different and may include ureteric obstruction, acute abdominal pain or retrograde ejaculation as a result of pressure on the presacral plexus.

When patients present with obvious abdominal lymph node disease, it is sometimes the case that the only sign of the primary tumour is testicular atrophy rather than a mass. An unusual presentation is with gynaecomastia, presumably due to ectopic hormone production by the tumour. Rarely, patients present with symptoms due to secondary spread in lung or brain or other sites. Infertility, due to azoospermia, may be the presenting complaint and clinical examination of the testes should be a routine procedure in the infertility clinic.

Tumour markers

An important advance in the management of these tumours has been the recognition that they manufacture tumour markers of which alpha-fetoprotein (AFP) and beta human chorionic gonadotrophin (beta-HCG) are the best known (2). AFP is synthesized by the foetal yolk sac, and plasma levels are elevated in about 70% of patients with MTU or MTI. It is never raised in patients with pure seminoma, and detection of AFP in such cases must be assumed to be due to foci of occult teratoma. β-HCG, which is produced by trophoblastic elements in the tumour, is detectable in the plasma of about 50% of patients with testicular teratomas and can also be modestly raised in patients with pure seminomas. With modern radioimmunoassay techniques it is possible to measure these hormones at nanogram levels. The levels of these markers may vary independently, reflecting their differing cell of origin. This may be confusing since treatment may lead to a fall in one marker without affecting the other.

In those patients whose tumours manufacture a marker, repeated measurements give a quantitative indication of tumour responsiveness and activity, and have become an established part of the management of these tumours. At presentation it is very important to obtain a *pre-operative* plasma sample for measurements of tumour markers.

In patients with marker-producing tumours, these levels will fall after orchidectomy to within the normal range provided the patient has no metastases (Fig. 19.4). If the pre-operative levels of AFP and/or HCG are very high, the return of these values to normal may not be complete for several weeks since the half-life of AFP is 6–7 days, and that of HCG is 16 hours. For this reason a single, elevated postoperative marker level does not always imply that there is residual disease. It is now clear that the level of both AFP and HCG at diagnosis is an indication of prognosis. Patients with levels of AFP above 500 units/ml and/or HCG above 10000 units/ml have a worse prognosis.

Tumour markers are also of great importance in the early diagnosis of relapse (Fig. 19.4). Almost all patients with marker-producing tumours will develop elevated plasma

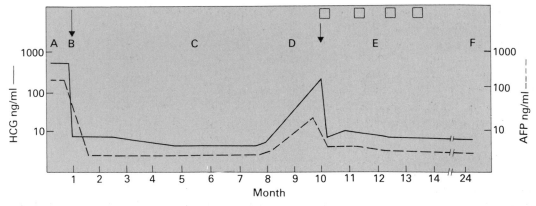

Fig. 19.4. *Serum markers in testicular teratoma.* (A) Presentation with left testicular swelling HCG = 623 ng/ml, AFP = 246 ng/ml. (B) Orchidectomy: HCG falls in 6 days to 10 ng/ml; AFP falls more slowly (t/2 = 6 days) to 4 ng/ml. (C) No rise in markers, clinical remission. (D) HCG and AFP rise, CT scan confirms enlargement of para-aortic nodes. (E) Cyclical intermittent combination chemotherapy produces rapid fall in HCG and slower fall in AFP, both to normal values. (F) Two years after presentation: normal markers, clinical remission, probable cure.

levels as the first, and most sensitive, indication of relapse. Occasionally patients with recurrent disease will develop raised levels of only one marker even though both may previously have been elevated. This can be due either to the differing sensitivity of components of the teratoma to chemotherapy or to a differential metastatic potential of the various elements of the primary tumour. Tumour markers are particularly valuable in the diagnosis of extragonadal primaries since the differential diagnosis from other causes of a retroperitoneal, mediastinal or suprasellar mass is so wide.

Staging

Clinical staging systems vary widely, but all depend on the anatomical extent of spread at diagnosis (Table 19.2). In Britain a simple system analogous to that used for Hodgkin's disease and other lymphomas (see Chapter 25) is often used. Greater detail can be incorporated into this system, to take account of the importance of tumour volume both in the abdomen and lungs, since these characteristics are increasingly understood as being crucial to the outcome.

Increasingly sophisticated non-surgical stag-

ing methods such as lymphography and CT scanning have helped our understanding of the natural history of these tumours. For example, the frequency of spread to the mediastinum was not appreciated until the advent of CT scanning and it is now recognized that nearly 30% of patients with testicular teratomas have evidence of involvement. This technique has also led to more accurate diagnosis of pulmonary deposits. Other important investigations include lymphography and intravenous urography. These are particularly important in seminomas where irradiation of the para-aortic nodes is an important part of treatment and care must be taken to avoid irradiation of the kidneys as far as possible. Isotope and/or ultrasonic scanning of the liver can also be helpful. The staging notation in Table 19.2 is based on investigations including lymphography and CT scanning.

In the USA retroperitoneal lymph node dissection is usually performed, partly for its value in staging and partly for its possible therapeutic effect. The TNM system is therefore partly surgically based (Table 19.2). In Britain a greater emphasis is placed on non-surgical approaches and the operation is rarely performed. The accuracy of lymphography and CT

Table 19.2. Staging of Testicular Tumours.

UK Notation

Stage I	Tumour confined to testis. (Tumour markers not elevated after orchidectomy, all investigations negative.)
Stage II	Tumour in pelvic and abdominal (retroperitoneal) nodes. (Tumour markers may be persistently elevated. Positive lymphogram or CT scan of abdomen.)
IIa	Nodes <2 cm diameter
IIb	Nodes 2–5 cm diameter
IIc	Nodes >5 cm diameter
Stage III	Mediastinal and/or supraclavicular nodes
Stage IV	Distant metastases*
	L1 <3 metastases, maximum diameter <2 cm
	L2 >3 metastases, maximum diameter <2 cm
	L3 maximum diameter >2 cm

TNM Staging Notation

T1	Confined to testis and adjacent spermatic cord
T2	Tumour detected in spermatic cord at level of inguinal ring
T3	Testicular capsule breached (or scrotal orchidectomy)
N0	No pathological involvement
N1	Normal size nodes, microscopic involvement
N2	Enlarged nodes but no extranodal extension (A: less than 2 cm and less than 5 nodes) (B: more than 2 cm and more than 5 nodes)
N3	Extranodal extension
N4	Retroperitoneal nodes with residual disease after surgery
M0	No distant metastases
M1	Distant metastases

*The number and size of lung metastases should be noted, in view of the prognostic importance of this observation.

scanning is demonstrated by comparison with American data which indicates that about 25% of lymph node dissection specimens in patients clinically thought to be free of extra-testicular spread are indeed positive; a figure remarkably similar to British data from non-surgical series.

Management of testicular tumours

The last ten years have seen major changes in the management of testicular tumours. Increased understanding of the importance of scrupulous staging, coupled with the advent of highly effective but hazardous chemotherapy and the routine use of tumour marker studies has led to widespread acceptance that this is a tumour best treated by a multimodal approach, in which expert surgeons, radiotherapists and medical oncologists play an important and complementary role. Since these tumours are uncommon and expert attention is so crucial, many feel that they are best treated in special units, or at least by study groups which will ensure some uniformity of approach.

SURGERY

For patients with a suspected testicular tumour, the proper operation is a radical inguinal orchidectomy. Scrotal procedures, though still sometimes performed, should never be considered since trans-scrotal orchidectomy carries a real risk of scrotal recurrence or later development of inguinal node involvement. The spermatic cord should be excised as high as possible to provide information regarding the possibility of direct or intravascular spread of tumour, which will have important implications for both management and prognosis. Before orchidectomy it is desirable that the surgeon request AFP and HCG levels, for the reasons described above.

Surgery in seminoma. If the tumour proves to be a pure seminoma, it is generally accepted that the surgeon has no further part to play, except perhaps for biopsy procedures if, for example, a supraclavicular node is discovered. Although American authorities sometimes recommend surgery in seminomas with bulky abdominal lymph node metastases or seminomas in which the HCG level is modestly raised, this is not usual practice in Britain. Radiotherapy alone will usually cure even bulky disease, and the addition of chemotherapy will increase this cure rate still further (see below).

Surgery in teratoma. For malignant teratomas there has been an important difference of opinion between British and American authorities. For patients with no evidence of abdominal node involvement, or evidence of only minimal node deposits (usually detected at lymphography or CT scanning), standard British practice has been to recommend treatment by irradiation (see below). In the US most of these patients would be treated by extended retroperitoneal lymphadenectomy, removing all lymphatic and connective tissues along the great vessels from the diaphragm to the level of the iliac vessels, a formidable surgical procedure. Many American urologists claim that a lymph node metastatic rate of 25% fully justifies radical lymphadenectomy in all cases. In Britain it is generally felt that combinations of radiotherapy and chemotherapy can effectively sterilize small volume metastases in abdominal lymph nodes, and that the postoperative problems of aspermia (dry ejaculation) render such surgery unjustifiable.

Although it has been claimed that results of treatment by lymphadenectomy are superior to those in patients treated primarily by para-aortic irradiation, careful study of the literature does not bear this out. Comparisons are difficult since British patients are staged by clinical investigation while American urologists rely greatly on lymphadenectomy as a staging operation as well as a potentially therapeutic procedure. In malignant teratomas the lymphogram is positive in about one-third of cases and it seems inescapable that many patients undergoing radical lymphadenectomy will have done so unnecessarily, in addition to having to face the unpleasant sexual difficulties that the operation may bring. Reasonable comparison is possible between patients where lymphadenectomy confirms histologically positive para-aortic nodes and those from British series who have obviously positive lymphographic appearances (stage II). Comparison of such cases confirms

similar overall survival rates, regardless of treatment.

Surgery is being used increasingly after initial chemotherapy has been completed in order to reassess the state of residual intra-abdominal disease. This approach is discussed further on p. 352.

RADIOTHERAPY

Radiotherapy in seminoma. For patients with testicular seminoma there is little argument that radiotherapy can be curative, even in patients with advanced disease. For patients with stage I seminoma, modest dosage of irradiation to bilateral para-aortic nodes and the ipsilateral common iliac chain is routinely performed (Fig.

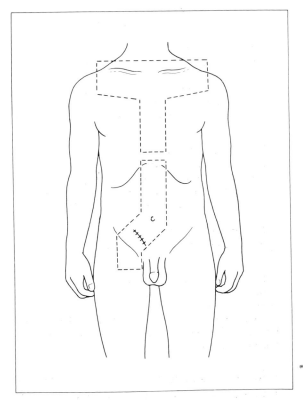

Fig. 19.5. Widely used radiation fields in seminoma. The fields are designed to cover the lymph node groups illustrated in Fig. 19.3. Seminoma is highly radiosensitive and a dose of 30 Gy over 3–4 weeks is generally sufficient.

19.5) since there can be no guarantee that orchidectomy alone will have cured these patients. Seminoma is among the most radiosensitive of all tumours; a dose of 30 Gy (3000 rad) delivered by anterior and posterior fields over a 3-week period (daily fractions of treatment) is normally considered adequate and leads to few, if any, acute or chronic side-effects. Some centres recommend treatment to even lower doses. Infertility is not normally a problem provided that the contralateral testis is protected from scattered irradiation by means of lead shielding. For this and other reasons, supervoltage radiotherapy is essential, though one or two specialized centres are beginning to adopt a 'watch-and-wait' policy (i.e. without any radiotherapy at all) for patients with stage I seminoma since a substantial proportion of patients are presumably cured by orchidectomy alone.

Where a scrotal operation such as orchiopexy, transcrotal biopsy or scrotal orchidectomy has been performed, the scrotal sac and ipsilateral inguinal nodes must also be treated. Some authorities also irradiate the inguinal nodes if there has been a herniorrhaphy. Although preservation of fertility cannot be guaranteed, an attempt at shielding the contralateral testis should once again be made.

Many radiotherapists adopt a policy of 'keeping one step ahead' of known nodal involvement from a seminoma. In patients with stage II disease, orthodox practice includes para-aortic and pelvic node irradiation, followed by radiotherapy to the mediastinum and supraclavicular nodes. Although this approach can be curative such wide field irradiation can be a real drawback if chemotherapy is subsequently required for recurrent disease, since a large volume of bone marrow will have been treated thus compromising haematological tolerance. For this reason, in many centres (including the authors'), patients with bulky abdominal disease are now routinely treated with chemotherapy prior to irradiation. Indeed, some centres omit irradiation entirely, relying on chemotherapy for patients with bulky abdominal disease. It is not yet clear whether this approach will prove superior.

The same alternative approaches also apply in patients with stage III though one would now recommend chemotherapy as unequivocally the better treatment. In stage IV disease, chemotherapy has been increasingly accepted as representing the best opportunity of cure, though some centres have reported encouraging results with total body irradiation.

Occasionally patients with 'pure' seminoma have an elevated serum βHCG, and HCG can be demonstrated immunocytochemically (3). This does not appear to be associated with a worse prognosis. An elevated serum AFP is usually regarded as an indication for treatment as for non-seminomatous germ cell tumours (see below).

Radiotherapy in teratoma. The place of radiotherapy in the management of teratomas is much less clear. In stage I disease the traditional British approach has been to offer postoperative radiotherapy as for seminomas although often to a higher dose (40–45 Gy in 4–5 weeks). With the increasing use of tumour markers to detect recurrence coupled with the highly effective chemotherapy now available for patients who do relapse, many large centres are increasingly adopting a policy of careful follow up after orchidectomy, without postoperative radiotherapy. In patients with stage II disease of small volume (<2 cm maximum diameter, radiologically demonstrable but without palpable lymphadenopathy) radiotherapy will be curative in about 80% of patients. However, chemotherapy is curative in over 90% of these patients, though there has been no formal comparison of these two treatments. Radiotherapy in stage II disease is compatible with normal fertility (4) which is an important advantage over radical lymph node dissection. With bulky stage II disease, control by radiation is much less certain and the case for chemotherapy is established. A further disadvantage of irradiation is the large volume of marrow included in the treatment field, making later chemotherapy, should it be necessary, much more hazardous. Patients with stage III and IV disease are treated, and often cured, with chemotherapy although radiotherapy may still have a role in the control of bulky abdominal disease (see below).

CHEMOTHERAPY

The emergence of chemotherapy for testicular teratoma has been one of the most exciting advances in cancer medicine over the past 20 years. In the early 1960s one or two agents were available with known but limited activity. Li and his colleagues (5) described a combination regimen comprising actinomycin D, chlorambucil and methotrexate, which was the first major advance in the treatment of widespread testicular teratoma. Mithramycin was introduced at about this time and, although no longer widely used, is capable of producing regression of metastases particularly in patients with MTU (embryonal carcinoma) with long-term survival (probably complete cure) in a small number of patients.

The next important step was the recognition of further agents of quite different classes, each of which had major activity (Table 19.3). Vinblastine, bleomycin, and later cisplatin have all been indentified as independently effective. Samuels and colleagues investigated combinations of vinblastine and bleomycin, demonstrating very high response rates even in patients with advanced disease, particularly when the bleomycin was given as an infusion (6).

This effective but highly toxic regimen was a major advance. It was replaced by a regimen which added cisplatin to the two-drug combination. Cisplatin is not only a highly effective agent but also relatively free from toxicity to the bone marrow, making it particularly suitable as part of a combination regimen. In 1974 Einhorn and colleagues at Indiana began evaluation of a combination of cisplatin, vinblastine and bleomycin in patients with advanced disease (7); this regimen is now widely used. Analysis of a group of 50 patients showed an

Table 19.3. Cytotoxic drugs in germ cell testicular tumours.

	Response rates (complete and partial)
*Single agents**	
Actinomycin D	40%
Vinblastine	20%
Cisplatin	>60%
Methotrexate	20%
Bleomycin	40%
Etoposide	40%
Alkylating agents	30%
Combination therapy	
Platinum, bleomycin, vinblastine (PVB)	98% (70% CR)
PVB and etoposide (see text)	100% (70% CR)
Vinblastine, bleomycin	75% (50% CR)

PVB regimen
Cisplatin 20 mg/m² i.v. daily for 5 days every 3 weeks
Vinblastine 0.3 mg/kg i.v. every 3 weeks
Bleomycin 30 mg i.v. weekly × 3 (four complete courses are usually given)

BEP regimen
As for PVB, but substituting etoposide (VP-16-213) at a dose of 120 mg/m² i.v. × 3 days for vinblastine, which is omitted

* Of historical interest. No longer employed singly for non-seminomatous tumours.

overall response rate of 98%, with complete responses in 68% of patients, of whom all but three remained free of disease with a minimum follow-up of a year. Despite these remarkable results, the toxicity of all these regimens is a serious problem, with gastro-intestinal disturbance, granulocytopenia and infection, nephrotoxicity and pulmonary fibrosis as the major hazards. In Einhorn's earlier series four patients died in complete remission and two of these deaths were clearly drug related. Reduction of vinblastine dosage led to a significant improvement in tolerance without jeopardizing responsiveness. Bleomycin is used in large doses in these regimens and as haematological toxicity has diminished pulmonary toxicity from bleomycin has become the main toxicity (see Chapter 6).

Patients with bulky widespread disease, and particularly those with MTT (choriocarcinoma), have a poor prognosis despite treatment with combination chemotherapy. In these patients newer agents have been investigated and the epipodophyllotoxin VP-16 213 (etoposide) is of particular interest since it clearly produces responses and appears to act in a different way from the other major agents (8). It has been successfully combined with them, producing a four-drug regimen for adverse cases which has shown early promise. Still more complicated regimens are currently in use for these resist ant cases. Examples of common drug regimens are given in Table 19.3.

The use of chemotherapy for patients with less advanced disease needs further exploration, particularly where there is modest para-aortic involvement (stage IIa and IIb). We still know little of the proper role of chemotherapy in advanced *seminomas* though it is now clear that seminoma is highly chemosensitive. Most cases of seminoma present early with radiocurable disease but for the few that present with advanced disease or later develop recurrence, there was little effective chemotherapy until the advent of cisplatin-based regimens. The current practice is to use combinations of drugs similar to those used for teratoma, and to employ radiotherapy subsequently, to sites of bulk disease. However, the use of single-agent cisplatin may be as effective for metastatic seminoma as the more complex combination regimens.

SURGERY AFTER CHEMOTHERAPY AND RADIOTHERAPY

As survival times lengthen, surgery has become increasingly aggressive in young patients, particularly where there is evidence of residual disease after orchidectomy. Abdominal 'debulking' surgery, and even excision of pulmonary metastases by repeated thoracotomy, are frequently performed. Combinations of chemotherapy and surgery are increasingly used, and

it is now clear that chemotherapy should precede surgery (9). Postponing surgery to the end of treatment, after administration of repeated courses of combination chemotherapy, gives both an accurate histological picture of the effect of preceding treatment, as well as removing tumour in patients with residual disease. Ideally, such surgery should be performed only after tumour markers have fallen to undetectable levels and at least one additional course of chemotherapy given beyond this point.

In a large proportion of these cases there is evidence of treatment-induced differentiation into mature teratoma, and though this obser-

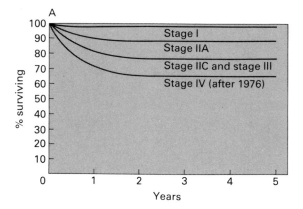

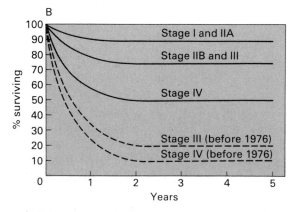

Fig. 19.6. Prognosis of testicular germ cell tumours related to stage. (A) Seminoma; (B) teratoma (all types). These survival curves illustrate the dramatic improvement with advanced stages since the introduction of combination chemotherapy.

vation is encouraging, its significance and implications for long-term survival are not yet clear. Many such patients appear to be cured, showing no evidence of relapse after several years' follow-up.

Prognosis of testicular tumours

Stages I and II seminoma are nearly always curable by radiotherapy. The prognosis of bulky stage II (stage IIC) and stages III and IV is improving with chemotherapy (Fig. 19.6A). The majority of patients are now cured even in these more advanced stages.

In non-seminomatous germ cell tumours the prognosis is excellent for stage I and early stage II disease. Approximately 70% of all patients with stage III disease will be cured, but bulky disease and stage IV patients are still at risk or incomplete drug response and relapse. Nevertheless the last decade has seen a great improvement even in this poor prognosis group (Fig. 19.6B). Results from large centres in Britain are amongst the best reported, with overall survival of 80 to 90% following treatment with combination regimens containing cisplatin, bleomycin, vinblastine, etoposide and/or other drugs.

EXTRA-GONADAL GERM CELL TUMOURS

Primary extra-gonadal germ cell tumours are extremely uncommon, but have been described in a variety of sites including the retroperitoneum, anterior mediastinum, suprasellar or pineal area and the pre-sacral region. Although the pathogenesis is not entirely clear, it is possible that these tumours result from malignant change in primordial germ cells which have migrated incompletely (cell 'rests') or in cells displaced during embryogenesis.

The commonest site is probably the anterior mediastinum, followed by the retroperitoneum. In occasional cases, an associated congenital or developmental abnormality is present. The tumours comprise only 1% of all mediastinal

tumours. The largest single group are mixed tumours, but pure seminomas are more common than pure teratomas or choriocarcinomas. Since primary testicular tumours can be small and impalpable, one should always be wary when diagnosing a germ cell tumour apparently arising from an extra-testicular site, since metastasis from an occult primary is an alternative diagnosis.

Both teratomas and seminomas are encountered and in general show the same radiosensitivity and chemosensitivity as primary testicular tumours. For mediastinal seminomas, surgery followed by radiotherapy appears effective, with long-term survival rates of about 50%. However, in bulky disease chemotherapy can be extremely effective at reducing tumour volume thus eliminating the need for wide field irradiation of the lungs. Although the long-term effectiveness and morbidity of chemotherapy has yet to be determined, this approach will probably prove to be extremely valuable. At present, treatment with cisplatin, bleomycin and either vinblastine or etoposide seems most effective, though more complicated regimens have been used.

For primary mediastinal non-seminomatous germ cell tumours, radiotherapy is relatively ineffective. Several reports have appeared showing a dismal prognosis with no cures and an average survival of only 5 months from diagnosis. However, recent reports show good response to modern chemotherapy, usually including cisplatin, vinblastine, etoposide, bleomycin, and actinomycin D. Primary germ cell tumours of the brain are treated quite differently. Most of these are pineal or suprasellar tumours, and both teratomas and seminomas occur. These can sometimes be cured by wide field irradiation, including full irradiation of the whole central nervous system. The 5-year survival rate in children with radiosensitive pineal tumours (usually not biopsied but assumed to be seminoma or the less common pinealoblastoma) is 50%. With proven pineal teratomas (i.e. biospy-proven or where the AFP or βHCG are clearly raised) the outlook is less good, though response to chemotherapy can be dramatic. It is certainly possible that for these rare tumours which are only partly or doubtfully radiosensitive, combination chemotherapy could become standard initial management over the next few years.

The apparent rarity of extra-gonadal germ cell tumours may have to be revised in the light of recent reports describing patients originally thought to have undifferentiated carcinomas but with a clinical course and response to chemotherapy much more suggestive of extragonadal germ cell tumours. This has been described as the 'atypical teratoma syndrome' and none of these patients have clinically apparent testicular tumours. In the majority of cases serum markers (AFP and βHCG) are raised, and subsequent staining of tissue sections by immunoperoxidase techniques shows intracellular AFP and βHCG. Treatment with cisplatin, vinblastine and bleomycin is effective, with a high proportion of complete responders. In young men with mediastinal tumours which on biopsy prove to be 'poorly differentiated carcinoma' it is therefore essential to consider this diagnosis and to measure plasma βHCG and AFP. Even if these are negative, it is so important not to overlook this potentially curable tumour that response to platinum-based regimens should be fully assessed.

MANAGEMENT OF NON-GERM CELL TUMOURS OF THE TESTIS

Orchidectomy alone is usually sufficient for Leydig and Sertoli cell tumours since these rarely metastasise. Lymphomas of the testis are usually large cell centroblastic B cell neoplasms. As they are frequently bilateral, irradiation of the contralateral testis is usually recommended if the disease appears localized. These patients need careful staging as for other lymphomas (see Chapter 26). With paratesticular rhabdomyosarcomas occult metastasis is so frequent that adjuvant combination chemotherapy is an essential part of management (see Chapter 24).

REFERENCES

1 Dixon F.J. & Moore R.A. (1953) Testicular Tumours: a Clinicopathological Study. *Cancer* **6**, 427.

2 Lange P.H., McIntire K.R., Waldmann T.A., Hakala T.R. & Fraley E.E. (1976) Serum alpha-fetoprotein and human chorionic gonadotrophin in the diagnosis and management of non-seminomatous germ-cell testicular cancer. *New England Journal of Medicine* **295**, 1237–40.

3 Javadpour N., McIntire, K.R. & Waldmann T.A. (1978) Human chorionic gonadotrophin (HCG) and alpha-fetoprotein (AFP) in sera and tumour cells of patients with testicular seminoma: a prospective study. *Cancer* **42**, 2768.

4 Smithers D.W., Wallace E.N.K. & Wallace D.M. (1971) Radiotherapy for patients with tumours of the testicle. *British Journal of Urology* **43**, 83.

5 Li M.C., Whitmore W.F., Golbey R. & Grabstald H. (1960) Effects of combined drug therapy on metastatic cancer of the testis. *Journal of the American Medical Association* **174**, 1291–9.

6 Samuels M.L., Johnson D.E. & Holoye P.Y. (1975) Continuous intravenous bleomycin therapy with vinblastine in stage III testicular neoplasia. *Cancer Chemotherapy Reports* **59**, 563.

7 Einhorn L. & Donohue J.P. (1977) Cisdiamminechloroplatinum, vinblastine and bleomycin combination chemotherapy in disseminated testicular cancer. *Annals of Internal Medicine* **87**, 293–8.

8 Newlands E.S. & Bagshawe K.D. (1977) Epipodophyllin derivative (VP-16–213) in malignant teratomas and choriocarcinomas. *Lancet* **ii**, 87.

9 Javadpour N., Ozols R.F., Anderson T., Barcock A., Wesley R. & Young R.C. (1982) A randomised trial of cytoreductive surgery followed by chemotherapy versus chemotherapy alone in bulky stage III (poor prognosis) testicular cancer. *Cancer* **50**, 2004–2010.

Chapter 20

Thyroid and Adrenal Cancer

This group of diseases is exceptional in many ways. First of all, some thyroid cancers are very indolent, with a long natural history, often over many decades, even where complete control of the tumour has not been achieved. Secondly, because most thyroid cancers take up iodine, the administration of oral radioactive iodine—a highly specific therapy—results in sterilization of both normal and neoplastic thyroid cells and may be used for total ablation of the tumour, usually resulting in excellent 20-year survival rates. Thirdly, in the majority of patients with metastases from well-differentiated thyroid carcinomas, the metastatic lesions retain the important characteristic of radio-iodine uptake, so that even patients with metastatic disease at

Table 20.1. Clinical characteristics and survival in thyroid tumours.

Histological type	Response to radio-iodine	Clinical behaviour	10-year survival
Papillary	+ + +	Young patients. Often slow to evolve. Metastases usually lymphatic	95%
Follicular	+ + +	Young, middle-aged patients. Metastases often haematogenous (bone, lung).	90%
Medullary	—	Young patients. Familial. Produces calcitonin as marker. C-cell tumour. Often a rapid clinical evolution. Surgery very important as radioresponsiveness variable.	40%
Anaplastic	—	Elderly patients. Predominantly local invasion with pressure symptoms.	5%
Small cell	—	Rapid but very radiosensitive. Usually localized	5%
Lymphoma	—	Middle-aged group (Highly radiosensitive)	

presentation can still be treated successfully. If necessary, these treatments can be repeated several times, using whole-body isotope scanning as an accurate method of assessment of progress and to determine whether further therapy is required.

There are important histological and behavioural differences between the major types of thyroid cancer and these differences help to determine treatment strategy (Table 20.1). Although these tumour subgroups are well defined, several types of thyroid carcinoma have been recognized only recently, and further histopathological refinements seem likely. The clinician needs a complete histopathological description of the tumour which should include not only the tumour type but also the degree of differentiation. If a thyroidectomy specimen is available, the degree of local invasion into blood vessels, local structures and adjacent lymph nodes should also be described.

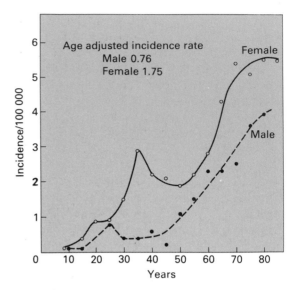

Fig. 20.1. *Age-specific incidence of thyroid cancer.*

AETIOLOGY AND INCIDENCE

A number of aetiological factors have now been described. Like other thyroid diseases it is commoner in women than in men (Fig. 20.1), with a bimodal age distribution. The lower age peak of incidence is due to papillary and follicular tumours, and the rise in incidence in older patients is chiefly due to anaplastic cancers. Both thyrotoxicosis and Hashimoto's thyroiditis share a similar age distribution with well-differentiated thyroid carcinomas. It has been described as being more frequent in survivors of the atomic bomb, and has also been reported following irradiation of the neck, usually with a latent period of 10–30 years. Therapeutic neck irradiation, usually to the thymus or tonsils, was generally taken to only a low dose. The risk of carcinogenesis is higher in females, or where the radiation exposure occurred in very young children, and also increases with increasing length of follow-up. Medullary thyroid carcinoma has both a familial and a sporadic incid-

ence and may form part of the syndromes of multiple endocrine neoplasia (see Chapter 15).

PATHOLOGY

Papillary carcinoma

The commonest type of cancer is papillary carcinoma (Fig. 20.2), which comprises about 60% of all thyroid cancers, and a slightly greater proportion of those occurring in childhood. In at least 20% of cases the tumour appears to be multifocal in origin, and in older patients tends to have a more aggressive clinical course, with correspondingly poorer survival than in children and young adults. Papillary carcinomas are almost three times as common in women as in men, with a peak incidence in the 3rd and 4th decades. Any differentiated thyroid tumour that contains neoplastic papillae is by definition a papillary carcinoma, regardless of the presence of neoplastic follicles. The tumour is made up of cuboid cells and often contains psammoma bodies. A characteristic feature of papillary tumours is large empty nuclei—so-called 'orphan Annie' nuclei. Over 90% of these tumours appear to be encapsulated, but lymph node invasion is common though this finding is thought to be prognostically unimportant. Occasionally, papillary microcarcinomas (even up to 1 cm in size) are discovered in thyroidectomy specimens where a neoplasm was not suspected pre-operatively. It is generally accepted that these small clinically undetected tumours can be ignored (from the point of view of further treatment) unless a tumour is found adjacent to one of the resection margins of the specimen. Larger tumours, with evidence of extrathyroid invasion and/or invasion of the thyroid capsule, are associated with a worse prognosis, particularly in older patients. However, in general this is a slowly growing tumour, usually completely resectable and with a low overall mortality.

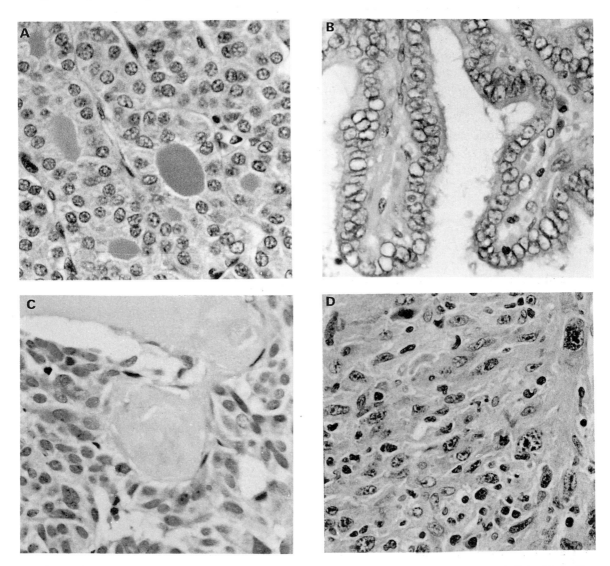

Fig. 20.2. *Histological appearances in thyroid cancer.* (A) Follicular carcinoma showing follicle formation ($\times 200$); (B) papillary carcinoma showing characteristic 'empty' nuclei ($\times 200$); (C) medullary carcinoma showing small cells with masses of amyloid ($\times 200$); (D) anaplastic carcinoma ($\times 200$).

Follicular tumours

Follicular tumours (Fig. 20.2) are much less common, accounting for about 15% of all cases and often found in patients with a long history of goitre. These tumours are unusual in children and are seen in a rather older age group than the papillary carcinomas, again with a slight female predominance. Overall prognosis is good (Table 20.1). Lymph node involvement is uncommon, as the main route of dissemination is via the bloodstream with lung and bone as the commonest sites of metastasis. This is often reflected in the histological appearance of the tumour, since microangio invasion can frequently be demonstrated even though, as with papillary carcinomas, over 90% of these tumours appear macroscopically to be encapsulated. The presence of plugs of tumour within the lumen of the capsular venous sinusoids is associated with a higher risk of dissemination, as is permeation of extra-thyroidal veins. These are important adverse prognostic features. The tumour can be difficult to distinguish histologically from atypical adenomas, since the presence of nuclear pleomorphism and even bizarre nuclear forms is not necessarily tantamount to true malignancy, in the absence of evidence of microangio invasion.

Medullary thyroid tumours

Medullary thyroid tumours (Fig. 20.2) have a quite different derivation and are thought to arise from the parafollicular or C-cells. The disease is often familial (see below). Typically, the stroma of the tumour has an amyloid appearance and the tumour itself may be bilateral. Medullary thyroid tumours tend to have a high metastatic potential both to lymph nodes and also the bloodstream. The large majority secrete calcitonin, a particularly important tumour marker in view of the familial incidence of the disease and the obvious importance of identifying affected family members as early as possible (1). Equally important is the use of the calcitonin assay for monitoring results of therapy.

In the past most patients reached the age of 30 years by the time of diagnosis. The mean age at diagnosis is expected to drop in the future, since the familial nature of the tumour is well understood and the use of the calcitonin assay has now become widespread.

In some familial forms of the disease other abnormalities have also been noted, particularly phaeochromocytoma and hyperparathyroidism—the so-called multiple endocrine neoplasia (MEN) syndromes. These can be associated either with the sporadic or the familial form of medullary thyroid cancer. The disorders are inherited as an autosomal dominant with a high degree of penetrance but variable expression. The commonest variant of MEN, *Wermer's syndrome*, can involve the thyroid and parathyroid glands as well as the pancreatic islets, pituitary and adrenal cortex (see Chapter 15). Two-thirds of these patients have tumours of at least two of the endocrine glands. The second type of MEN, *Sipple's syndrome*, includes more patients with medullary thyroid carcinoma; approximately 50% of these patients have parathyroid hyperplasia and/or phaeochromocytoma. Medullary thyroid cancer may be associated with ectopic hormone production from the thyroid tumour itself, and may produce ACTH, VIP and also prostaglandins and serotonin.

Anaplastic carcinoma

Anaplastic carcinoma of the thyroid (Fig. 20.2) is the predominant form of thyroid cancer in elderly people, and approximately 75% of patients with this disorder are over 60 years old at the time of diagnosis. These tumours form about 15% of all thyroid cancers, and are seen more frequently in women, in the ratio of 3:2. Unlike well-differentiated thyroid cancer, they are generally rapidly growing tumours, often painful and with pressure symptoms as an early feature. In some cases the tumour appears to arise in a longstanding goitre. The course of these tumours is quite different from that of the more slowly-growing varieties commoner in younger patients, and several histological sub-types of anaplastic carcinoma have been recognized, including spindle and giant cell carcinomas in which there may be areas of well-differentiated carcinoma, supporting the suggestion that these tumours may sometimes arise from transformation of pre-existing well-differentiated thyroid cancer.

A very small number of 'anaplastic' carcinomas are characterized by infiltration with small lymphocyte-like cells, and are generally known as *small cell* carcinomas of the thyroid. These are typically found in elderly patients and are rapidly growing and locally invasive. *Thyroid lymphomas* are discussed in Chapter 26.

DIAGNOSIS AND INVESTIGATION

Patients may present with a firm mass in the neck, due either to the primary thyroid mass or to an involved cervical lymph node. It is some-times possible to classify the thyroid mass on clinical grounds as obviously benign, suspicious of cancer, or 'probable' (2), though rather few thyroid cancers present with symptoms or signs which are of real prognostic value. The most one can say clinically is that most cases prove not to be malignant. In making these distinc-tions, useful clinical criteria include the size and position of the mass, its mobility, and the pres-ence of signs of compression of vital structures in the neck.

Non-malignant conditions can simulate thy-roid cancer; these include benign adenomas and multinodular goitres, as well as less common causes such as thyroglossal or colloid retention cysts. These may cause particular difficulty since they also produce the 'cold' nodule on thyroid isotope scanning so characteristic of malignant neoplasms (Fig. 20.3). Ultrasound scanning will reliably distinguish between cystic and solid lesions. The circulating thyroglobulin level may be elevated, but the test is unreliable as a marker of malignancy. Evidence of micro-calcification in a soft tissue X-ray, though rarely seen, is strongly suggestive of papillary

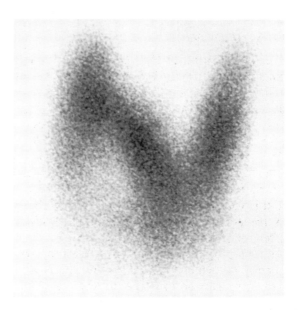

Fig. 20.3. ^{123}I *scan of thyroid, showing a cold nodule in the enlarged right lobe.*

carcinoma, and is due to the psammoma bod-ies. Apart from the mass itself, and the pressure-effects such as stridor or recurrent laryngeal nerve involvement, patients with med-ullary carcinoma may occasionally present with systemic endocrine symptoms from an associ-ated MEN syndrome. The great majority of patients with thyroid cancer are clinically eu-thyroid. Autoimmune thyroiditis can usually be identified by the presence of a high level of anti-thyroglobulin antibodies as well as a low ^{131}I uptake and diffuse, tender or painful glandular enlargement.

In general, patients with thyroid scans suggestive of a 'cold' nodule, i.e. one which fails to take up radio-iodine, should be referred for a surgical opinion in order to exclude a cancer. At most, only 20% of these patients will prove to have a malignant neoplasm. Aspiration cy-tology and needle biopsy are very useful though not entirely reliable, and in order to make the diagnosis, hemithyroidectomy may be neces-sary, or, in the case of larger lesions, partial or subtotal removal of the gland. For papillary can-cers (the largest single subtype), medullary and anaplastic cancer, needle aspiration may be sufficient, whereas in follicular carcinoma, important histological features may not be recognizable in such small specimens.

SURGICAL MANAGEMENT OF THYROID CANCER

In making the diagnosis of thyroid cancer a substantial thyroid resection has usually been undertaken, often consisting of unilateral thyroid lobectomy (hemithyroidectomy) with resection of the isthmus. However, there is no clear agreement, once the diagnosis has been established, as to whether the surgeon should then consider a further operation to complete a total or near total thyroidectomy. The risk of surgically-induced hypoparathyroidism is low— probably about 3% in experienced hands. Repeated operations by inexperienced surgeons undoubtedly increase this hazard.

In small cancers, completely enclosed by normal tissues, it may seem unjustifiable to advocate further surgery in view of the risk of a second operation in a difficult site. Nonetheless, routine total thyroidectomy has sometimes been recommended, even for *well-differentiated papillary tumours*, because of the high incidence of microscopic foci in the contralateral lobe (3). A common recommendation in British centres is that a near total or subtotal thyroidectomy be performed (4).

For *follicular carcinomas* total thyroidectomy is usually best even in cases where metastases are present at the time of diagnosis, though this carries a risk of permanent hypoparathyroidism. In cases of papillary and follicular carcinomas, any obviously enlarged lymph nodes should be removed at the initial operation. *En bloc* resection of the thyroid gland and pathological nodes should be attempted even if bilateral lymph nodes are present. Despite the high incidence of histologically confirmed malignancies in clinically impalpable lymph nodes (probably of the order of 50%), prophylactic lymph node dissection is not usually recommended since recurrence after subsequent postoperative treatment with radio-iodine will occur in less than 30% of patients.

In *papillary carcinoma* it is important to remember that the presence of palpable lymph nodes at diagnosis does not affect the prognosis. There is no difference in outcome between patients treated by prophylactic neck dissection in whom lymph node involvement is confirmed histologically, and those with a later nodal recurrence who may then be treated by therapeutic lymph node dissection (and possibly other methods as well). This is particularly true of the largest group of good risk patients, i.e. women under 40 years of age with well-differentiated tumours.

With *medullary carcinomas* routine neck node dissection is sometimes recommended, in addition to total thyroidectomy (5), a view substantiated by the high local recurrence rate in the order of 25%. For *anaplastic carcinomas* surgical removal of the tumour should be attempted wherever possible, though this is often technically difficult since early direct extension is the rule and tissue planes may be hopelessly destroyed. These tumours are only partly responsive to external beam irradiation so surgical removal of as much tumour as possible is increasingly performed even where this involves cutting directly across tumour. Because of the frequency of compression of the oesophagus, pharynx and trachea, maintenance of the airway by tracheostomy is often required.

For true *small cell carcinomas* and *lymphomas* of the thyroid, thyroidectomy is unnecessary though occasionally performed for biopsy purposes. Where these tumours are suspected, 'tru-cut' or other needle biopsy procedures are now more often employed in order to avoid thyroidectomy wherever possible. They are highly radiosensitive and surgery plays a correspondingly small part in the management.

THE ROLE OF RADIOTHERAPY IN THYROID CANCER

Radio-iodine therapy[131]I

Postoperative management depends on the histological findings, the extent of disease and the completeness of surgery. In most cases of well-differentiated thyroid cancer (both papillary and follicular), ablation of residual thyroid tissue, together with neck and whole body scanning should be carried out postoperatively, using oral radioactive iodine. This is particularly important if there is any doubt as to the completeness of surgery. About half of all follicular carcinomas fall into this category, and rather fewer of the papillary group. Treatment with ^{131}I is not necessary for all of the well-differentiated tumours, since occult and intra-thyroid carcinomas have an excellent prognosis following surgery alone, and high doses of radioactive iodine can generally be avoided with safety in these predominantly young patients for whom radiation dose is a particularly important consideration.

For patients in whom ^{131}I treatment is required, a moderately large dose (a common recommendation is of the order of 80 mCi) is given. This is to ablate the residual thyroid tissue which always takes up iodine more avidly than the tumour, making therapeutic use of ^{131}I impossible in the presence of a significant volume of active residual thyroid tissue (Fig. 20.4). If thyroxine (T4) has been administered postoperatively, this must be discontinued well before (usually 4 weeks) any attempt at thyroid ablation with radio-iodine, in order to ensure that the TSH rises. It is the rise in TSH rather than the hormone withdrawal that is important. After the ^{131}I radio-ablation has been performed, a short 6-week course of tri-iodothyronine (T3) is then given (in preference to T4 which has a much longer duration of action and is therefore less flexible). After withdrawal of T3 for 10 days, neck and whole body scanning is once again performed, and residual uptake in the neck or elsewhere provides evidence of metastatic or unresected primary cancer. If this is demonstrated a therapeutic dose of [131]I (150-200 mCi) is indicated. This can be repeated at approximately 3-monthly intervals (discontinuing exogenous T3 10 days beforehand) for as long as the repeat scans confirm residual active disease, i.e. until the metastases are totally eradicated or treatment fails.

Despite the dangers of significant radiation doses to the neck, marrow, gonads and other

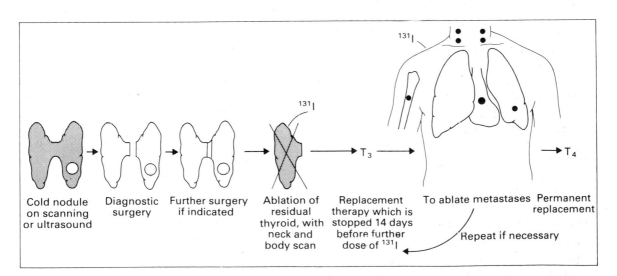

Fig. 20.4. *The use of* [131]*I in management of thyroid cancer.*

sites, it is important to realize that this specific and cytotoxic form of irradiation has produced many cures even in patients with widely metastatic disease. These patients (indeed most patients with thyroid cancer) need life-long T4 replacement since all thyroid tissue will have been ablated long before the final therapeutic dose. In a proportion of patients no longer responsive to radio-iodine but with residual or metastatic disease, hormone replacement with T4 may produce further regression of disease (particularly in those under 40 years old) since many of these tumours retain at least a partial dependency on TSH, which is suppressed by exogenous T4. Occasionally it is necessary to give treatment with therapeutic doses of ^{131}I when the patient has only just discontinued taking T3 or T4. In these cases TSH should be given for 2–3 days (by injection) before the ^{131}I is administered.

The contribution of radio-iodine was well demonstrated by Mazzaferri and his colleagues in a study of 576 patients with papillary carcinoma (6), all with several years of follow-up. The excellent prognosis was confirmed by the fact that only five of the patients died as a result of the cancer although, like most studies, there was patient selection. Most patients, for example, were less than 40 years old at diagnosis. Adverse features included age 40 years or over, a large primary tumour, and extracapsular extension. Local recurrence was more than twice as common after subtotal as after total thyroidectomy and, more important, resulted in an increased mortality. In addition, the use of radio-iodine ablation was strongly recommended where adequate uptake could be demonstrated in patients with multiple, locally invasive, or large primary tumours, as well as those with distant metastases. Finally, the routine use of T4 was of value even in patients who had not undergone total thyroidectomy and did not require it for physiological replacement.

External irradiation

In patients with thyroid cancers which do not take up radio-iodine, and particularly those which are locally unresectable (including almost all cases of anaplastic carcinoma and a high proportion of medullary carcinomas), external irradiation has an important role. A radical dose is required, typically of the order of 50–65 Gy (5000–6500 rad) in 5–7 weeks (7). Such treatment is valuable both to delay local recurrence and also to treat or prevent troublesome symptoms from local obstruction. It can be curative, though rarely in patients with anaplastic carcinoma. In patients with thyroid lymphomas and small cell tumours, both of which are highly radiosensitive, external beam irradiation is the definitive treatment (8). For these tumours a lower dose is adequate, of the order of 40 Gy (4000 rad) in 4 weeks. Since the total volume treated can be very substantial and at a site where spinal cord damage is a real threat, radical irradiation of the thyroid is technically difficult, especially if homogeneity of dosage is considered important. For this reason several groups have developed sophisticated techniques using wedged field arrangements or arc rotation planning. Others prefer a more straightforward approach with a single anterior direct field, shaped by lead blocks in order to protect the larynx and, if necessary, the lungs. The radiation fields should cover the whole thyroid gland, and it is conventional to include the first-stage supraclavicular or cervical lymph nodes. The field may have to be extended inferiorly to include the upper mediastinal area if there is evidence of disease at this level. Intratracheal deposits, for example, are well described and can lead to haemoptysis.

RESULTS OF TREATMENT FOR THYROID CANCER

For well-differentiated tumours the results of treatment are remarkably good. One substantial subgroup of patients, i.e. those below the age of 40 years with well-differentiated papillary carcinoma, have a normal survival pattern equal to that of a comparable population. The prognosis is affected by the age at diagnosis (the lower the better) and by the sex of the patient. In one large European co-operative study, 5-year survival rates were 60% for men and 75% for women (9). Histological type also correlates with survival and, in general, the more well-differentiated the tumour the better the prognosis. Both papillary and non-invasive follicular carcinomas have a 10-year survival rate of the order of 75%. For papillary carcinoma, evidence of extrathyroid disease reduces the 10-year survival to about 50%. For medullary carcinomas the survival is only about 40%, a reflection of its early metastatic potential and the ineffectiveness of ^{131}I therapy, itself a reflection of its different histogenesis. Worst of all, anaplastic carcinoma has a very poor prognosis with about 5% of patients surviving 5 years and essentially no 10-year survivors. It is important to distinguish small cell carcinomas and thyroid lymphomas from the truly anaplastic group, since their prognosis is undoubtedly better, and thyroid lymphoma, though uncommon, has an extremely good prognosis. For anaplastic carcinoma even highly aggressive treatment including surgery, external irradiation (and sometimes chemotherapy) has failed to improve the outlook.

It is difficult to assess the separate contributions of surgery and radiation therapy since they tend to be used in a complementary fashion, and radiotherapy is usually offered only to patients in whom surgery has not been complete, i.e. those with a higher than usual risk of local recurrence and poorer ultimate survival. Nonetheless, Tubiana's group (10) achieved a 10-year survival rate of over 70% in patients with papillary carcinoma who had undergone incomplete surgery. In follicular and medullary carcinoma the 10-year survival was 51% and 60% respectively. For patients presenting with metastases, treatment with radio-iodine (sometimes in combination with external irradiation to the primary tumour) may be very

successful and gives an overall survival rate of about 22% at 12 years. This reflects not only the effectiveness of ^{131}I therapy but also the indolent nature of this tumour, even when metastatic.

Chemotherapy for recurrent or metastatic thyroid cancer has so far been disappointing. The most active single agent is doxorubicin, with a response rate of about 30%, and with proven activity in all cell types. In addition, bleomycin has produced well documented responses, and combinations of these and other agents have now been employed by several groups, reportedly with better response rates than with single agents alone. The difficulty with this approach is that the durations of response are on the whole very short, quite apart from the fact that many of these patients are elderly and with rapidly advancing disease. Chemotherapy has only a limited role in the management of metastatic carcinoma of the thyroid and treatment with external irradiation, radio-iodine and exogenous thyroxine should all be considered first.

CANCER OF THE ADRENAL GLAND

These rare tumours arise either from the adrenal cortex or the medulla, and in adults the ratio of adrenocortical carcinoma to malignant medullary tumours (malignant phaeochromocytoma) is approximately 2:1. Neuroblastoma, a common childhood tumour chiefly arising from the medulla, is discussed in Chapter 24.

Adrenocortical carcinoma

About a quarter of patients with adult Cushing's syndrome who have no obvious source of ectopic hormone production have an adrenal tumour, of which less than half are malignant. Fewer than thirty cases are diagnosed in Britain per annum, and most of these are hormonally active, presenting with the features of Cushing's syndrome. In some patients virilization, feminization or hyperaldosteronism (Conn's syndrome) are more obvious clinical features, though 10% of cases are non-functional. Benign adrenocortical tumours are typically yellowish in appearance and are adenomas often with large cell or giant cell patterns. Malignant tumours are usually more obviously necrotic or haemorrhagic, sometimes with pleomorphic morphology and frequent mitoses. Vascular invasion and distant dissemination (chiefly to bone, lung and liver) can occur. The diagnosis is usually made by biochemical measurement (persistent hypercortisolaemia with no suppression in response to dexamethasone, and a low plasma ACTH), CT scan confirmation of an adrenal tumour (Fig. 20.5) and, ultimately, tissue diagnosis following laparotomy or CT-guided needle biopsy. Adrenal hyperplasia is usually bilateral, so unilateral adrenal enlargement is strongly suspicious of a benign or malignant tumour. Other imaging techniques include ultrasound and selective angiography with venous sampling. Non-functional tumours are more difficult to diagnose pre-operatively; clinical features are of a palpable abdominal mass (often a substantial size because of the 'silent' nature of the tumour), weight loss or

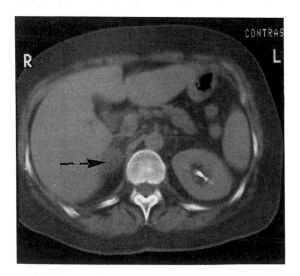

Fig. 20.5. *CT scan of abdomen showing adrenal tumour (arrowed).* Normal anatomy of other structures is also clearly shown.

fever. These patients are generally below the age of 20 years.

Treatment is primarily surgical, with wide resection which may necessitate a substantial thoracoabdominal incision. A short course of pre-operative steroid therapy is often advocated. If there is evidence of metastatic disease, systemic treatment with o,p-DDD (a derivative of the insecticide DDT) can be beneficial (11). In the majority of patients both a reduction in corticosteroid production and a documented tumour regression can be demonstrated. However, the normal dosage of 8–10 g/day frequently produces toxic side-effects of anorexia, nausea, diarrhoea, confusion and lethargy, limiting the acceptability of the treatment. Steroid replacement is usually necessary. Where there is failure of response to o,p-DDD, or if treatment has to be discontinued because of side-effects, palliation may be achieved by agents which interfere with steroid synthesis such as metyrapone or aminoglutethimide. Surgical resection or embolization of bulk disease should also be considered, as well as palliative radiotherapy for patients with painful bone metastases.

Adrenal medulla

The cells of the adrenal medulla have a different derivation from those of the cortex, developing from neuroectodermal tissue and giving rise to both benign and malignant tumours. In adult life these include *phaeochromocytoma* (benign in 90% of cases), *ganglioneuroma* or *neuroblastoma*. In childhood, neuroblastoma is much the commonest of the adrenal medullary tumours and is discussed in Chapter 24.

Phaeochromocytomas can arise from the adrenal medulla (90%), organ of Zuckerkandl or adrenal medullary cell rests in the pelvis. They can occur sporadically or as part of a familial syndrome of multiple endocrine neoplasia (see Chapter 15). Other associated diseases are neurofibromatosis, von Hippel-Lindau and Sturge-Weber syndromes, cerebellar ataxia, and tuberose sclerosis/astrocytoma.

About 10% are histologically malignant though the light-microscopical appearances are an unreliable guide to their clinical behaviour.

Phaeochromocytoma can occur at any age but patients are usually aged 40–60 years. Most patients are diagnosed as a result of investigation for hypertension, but the secretion of catecholamines by the tumour also causes symptoms (Table 20.2). These symptoms are

Table 20.2. Symptoms caused by phaeochromocytoma.

Skin
  Attacks of sweating, flushing, blanching

Cardiovascular
  Hypertension, tachycardia, paroxysmal rhythm change, slow forceful beating chest pain, postural hypotension.

Central Nervous System
  Headache, tremor, irritability, mood change, psychosis, anorexia

Metabolic
  Weight loss, increased metabolic rate, glycosuria

the same for benign and malignant tumours and include intermittent or paroxysmal headache, severe sweating attacks, postural hypotension, dysrhythmias and chest pain. Some patients present primarily with an abdominal or pelvic mass.

Confirmation of the diagnosis is made by demonstration of excess catecholamines (adrenaline, noradrenaline and metabolites in both urine and blood. The paroxysmal nature of the disorder may lead to false-negative plasma catecholamine measurement, and 24-hour urine collections are essential. The measurement of urine vanilyl mandelic acid (VMA) will give a diagnosis in 85% of patients. In the others it may be necessary to resort to provocative tests using pharmacological agents. Phentolamine in *very small doses* (0.5–1.0 mg) will produce a fall in blood pressure of 25 mmHg lasting 5 minutes to 4 hours. Histamine and tyramine provoke hypertension in these patients by liberating the excess catecholamines stored in nerve

endings (but not in the tumour). The use of these drugs requires extremely careful monitoring.

Selective angiography and venous sampling may be necessary to localize the tumour though CT scanning generally gives excellent visualization of the adrenal. In most cases the diagnosis of malignancy can be made only when the resected specimen is examined histologically, but occasionally a patient may have clinically obvious metastases.

Treatment of malignant phaeochromocytoma is by surgical resection with careful dissection and microscopical inspection of excision margins to ensure adequate surgical clearance. Surgical excision of single metastatic deposits has also been recommended. Pre-operatively the blood pressure is controlled by gradually increasing doses of phenoxybenzamine (to produce alpha receptor blockade). In patients with arrhythmia, a beta blocking agent is added after the blood pressure is brought under control. (Fig. 20.6) Used alone they can precipitate severe hypertension. After good blood pressure control has been achieved for 10 days the resection is performed. During operation it is advisable to have continuous intra-arterial blood pressure monitoring with treatment of hypertension with phentoalamine and arrhythmias with a beta blocking agent. A fall in blood pressure following removal can usually be controlled by blood transfusions.

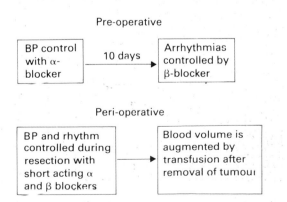

Fig. 20.6. *Pre- and peri-operative management of phaeochromocytoma.*

The use of chemotherapy for metastatic disease is purely anecdotal but alkylating agents and doxorubicin have been reported to be effective. In patients with symptomatic inoperable phaeochromocytoma both α and β blockers are valuable in controlling symptoms and may have to be maintained for several years in patients with slow-growing tumours. Although long-term survival has been recorded, the majority of patients with malignant phaeochromocytoma die of the disease; extra-adrenal primary sites are said to have a particularly poor prognosis.

CANCER OF THE PARATHYROID GLANDS

This tumour is very rare with less than 100 cases in the world literature. Fewer than 5% of all parathyroid tumours are malignant. The disease has been reported following irradiation of the neck. Most parathyroid carcinomas secrete PTH, causing hyperparathyroidism sometimes with a florid form of osteitis fibrosa cystica. The tumour tends to be slow growing, and long-term survival frequently occurs if complete surgical removal is performed. Local recurrence can lead to severe pressure symptoms in the neck, but can be surgically resectable. Distant metastases occasionally occur, chiefly to lung and liver.

REFERENCES

1 Melvin K.E.W., Miller H.H. & Tahjian A.H. (1971) Early diagnosis of medullary carcinoma of the thyroid gland by means of calcitonin assay. *New England Journal of Medicine* **285**, 1115–20.
2 Staunton M.D. & Greening W.P. (1973) Clinical diagnosis of thyroid cancer. *British Medical Journal* **4**, 532–5.
3 Clark L., Ibanez M.L. & White E.C. (1966) What operation for carcinoma of the thyroid? *Archives of Surgery* **92**, 23–6.
4 Leading article (1976) Thyroid cancer. *British Medical Journal* **1**, 113–14.
5 Chong G.C., Beahrs O.H., Sizemore G.W. & Woolner L.H. (1975) Medullary carcinoma of the thyroid gland. *Cancer* **35**, 695–704.
6 Mazzaferri E.L., Young R.L., Oertel J.E., Kemmerer W.T. & Page C.P. (1977) Papillary thyroid carcinoma: the impact of therapy on 576 patients. *Medicine (Baltimore)* **56**, 171–96.
7 Moss W.T., Brand W.N. & Battifora H. (1979) The Thyroid. In *Radiation Oncology—Rationale, Technique, Results* (5th Edn) Mosby, St. Louis, pp 233–242.
8 Souhami L., Simpson W.J. & Carruthers J.S. (1980) Malignant lymphoma of the thyroid gland. *International Journal of Radiation Oncology Biology Physics* **6**, 1143–8.
9 Byar D.P., Green S.B., Dor P.R., Williams D., Colon J. *et al* (1979) A prognostic index for thyroid carcinoma—an EORTC study. *European Journal of Cancer* **15**, 1033–42.
10 Tubiana M., Lacour J., Monnier J.P., Bergiron C., Gerard-Marchant R., Roujeau J., Bok B. & Parmentier C. (1975) External radiotherapy and radio-iodine in the treatment of 359 thyroid cancers. *British Journal of Radiology* **48**, 894–907.
11 Modlin I.M., Farndon J.R., Shepherd A., Johnston I.D.A., Kennedy T.L., Montgomery D.A.D. & Welbourne R.B. (1979) Phaeochromocytomas in 72 patients: Clinical and diagnostic features, treatment and long-term results. *British Journal of Surgery* **66**, 456.

Chapter 21

Metastases from an Unknown Primary Site

In the majority of patients who present with symptoms from metastases, routine examination and investigation quickly disclose the underlying primary. However, 1–5% of all patients with cancer present with symptoms and signs due to metastases and, after initial investigation, the primary site remains undetected. In these cases the primary tumour is too small to be clinically apparent and simple investigations such as chest X-ray, full blood count and liver function tests fail to give the diagnosis. Usually the histological diagnosis, obtained from the metastasis, is of an adenocarcinoma or poorly differentiated carcinoma.

There are few situations in medicine which are a greater test of clinical judgement. Faced with this situation, many physicians resort to a battery of investigations designed to disclose the primary site, but at the same time are aware that if and when they find the primary tumour, it will make little or no difference to the management of the patient. Investigation is undertaken, almost as a ritual, to reassure both the physician and the patient that something is being done.

SITE OF PRESENTATION

For the purposes of this chapter cases will be considered in which, despite full and appropriate examination, no primary site has been disclosed. The extent and nature of this preliminary investigation will depend on the site of the metastasis. The common metastatic sites include lymph nodes, bone, brain, liver and skin. Table 21.1 shows the most frequent primary

tumours presenting at these sites. With each metastatic site, investigation will have a different

Table 21.1. Sites of metastases from unknown primary.

Site of metastasis	Likely primary site
High cervical nodes	Head and neck cancer Thyroid Lung
Lower cervical nodes	Head and neck Lung, Breast Gut (especially L. supra- clavicular node)
Axillary nodes	Lung Breast
Skin	Breast Lung Melanoma
Bone	Myeloma Breast Kidney Prostate Lung
Brain	Lung Breast Prostate Melanoma
Inguinal nodes	Vulva Anorectal Prostate Ovary
Disseminated intra- abdominal adenocarcinoma (including liver metastasis)	Ovary Stomach Pancreas Gut

emphasis. For example, a squamous carcinoma in a cervical node will lead to a strong suspicion that the nasopharynx or lung is the likely primary site and full examination including the larynx, pharynx and post-nasal space will often give the diagnosis. Similarly an inguinal node or malignant ascites will lead to careful gynaecological examination. Management will then be as for the underlying malignancy. When initial investigation has failed to give any clue as to the primary cancer, the physician must ask himself the question 'If I find the primary, will there be any treatment which offers a reasonable chance of palliation or cure?'

THE SITES OF ORIGIN OF METASTASIS FROM AN UNKNOWN PRIMARY

Curiously, the distribution of cancers which present as metastases from an occult primary is not the same as the overall distribution of cancer. In Table 21.2 the frequency of presentation of metastasis from an unknown primary is shown compared with the frequency of cancers in general. It is clear that the commonest tumours to present in this way are pancreas,

lung, liver, stomach and colo-rectal cancer. Common cancers such as breast and prostate are much less frequent causes of metastasis from an unknown primary. This is probably because primary tumours in the breast are relatively easily detected clinically, while prostatic cancer is associated not infrequently with an elevation of the acid phosphatase which is a straightforward investigation often giving the diagnosis.

PROGNOSIS OF METASTASIS FROM AN UNKNOWN PRIMARY

Several studies have shown that the survival of patients who present in this way is extremely poor. The median survival is usually only 3–5 months and only 10% of patients are alive at 2 years. This poor prognosis is probably related to the malignant potential of these tumours since at autopsy the primary is sometimes only very small. The tumour is presumably rapidly growing, with a tendency to early metastasis. The tumours which are associated with a less catastrophic prognosis are shown in Table 21.3 and it is these tumours in particular which one must not miss. Investigation must therefore be directed towards the confident exclusion of these tum-

Table 21.2. Sites of origin of carcinomas presenting as metastases from unknown site.

	% of all unknown primary cases	% of all cancers
Pancreas	20	2
Lung	20	10
Unknown	15	
Liver	10	2
Stomach	10	5
Colo-rectal	8	15
Breast	3	26
Thyroid	3	1
Renal	3	2
Prostate	3	18
Ovary	2	5
Other	3	14

Table 21.3. Treatable cancers which may present as metastases from an unknown primary

---

Curable tumours which must not be missed
  Germ cell and trophoblastic tumours
  Lymphomas
  Well-differentiated thyroid cancer

Tumours which can be palliated by chemotherapy
  Breast
  Ovary
  Small cell carcinoma of the bronchus

Tumours which can be palliated by hormone therapy
  Breast
  Prostate

---

ours and, this having been done, there is probably no point in pursuing investigation further.

Several studies have shown that the yield of investigation is low when applied routinely to all patients in this situation. In one report the primary site was identified in only 10% of cases and in only 14 out of 266 cases was a treatable cancer detected (1). In none of these was cure possible but palliation might have been considered. In most cases, therefore, a primary will not be found at presentation and even if it is, it is extremely unusual for a treatable disease to be discovered. A further problem in adopting an attitude of intensive investigation for all these patients is that the clinical studies frequently sometimes give false-positive and false-negative results, and the patient is then subjected to a number of further investigations, often invasive and invariably expensive, the end result usually being failure.

INVESTIGATION AND MANAGEMENT

The following is a guide to management of this difficult problem. It must be emphasized that the degree to which investigation will be pursued will vary greatly with individual patients. The patient's age, fitness and degree of anxiety will all influence the decision as well as the possibility of finding a treatable tumour.

Review of histology

The most important first step is to discuss the biopsy with an experienced pathologist. Sometimes the pathologist may have a shrewd idea where the primary site might be, but because of lack of clinical information, has left the diagnosis open. Special stains may be useful in providing further information, for example, immunocytochemical staining for large cell lymphomas. These tumours are often difficult to distinguish from anaplastic carcinoma, but are very responsive to chemotherapy. Mucin stains may demonstrate intracellular mucin and point to an origin from the gut, pancreas or stomach. Immunohistochemical techniques using monoclonal antibodies are likely to prove increasingly valuable in the future. Already there are reagents which react with most haemopoietic tumours such as lymphomas, and enable them to be distinguished from anaplastic carcinoma (see Chapter 3). Some of these reagents will work on paraffin sections, but many require frozen tissue. This is another reason why biopsy material should not be placed entirely in formalin when cancer is a possible diagnosis. Antisera to epithelial membrane antigens are available which help to define epithelial tumours such as breast cancer or other poorly differentiated adenocarcinomas. Antibodies to prekeratin may be helpful in determining whether the tumour is of squamous origin or not; others react with melanoma associated antigens. If the node is taken from an axillary or a supraclavicular site, examination for oestrogen receptor positivity may be helpful in proving a breast origin of the tumour. Occasionally electron microscopy may help, for example in showing premelanosomes in malignant melanoma, or intercellular bridges in poorly differentiated squamous carcinoma. Undifferentiated germ cell tumours are curable cancers of young people which are easily overlooked. They may contain human chorionic gonadotrophin (HCG) and alphafetoprotein (AFP) and can be stained for the intracellular presence of these peptides by immunocytochemical techniques.

Biochemical and haematological investigation

Certain tests should be carried out as a routine. These include an acid phosphatase measurement in men over 40 years old to detect carcinoma of the prostate; HCG and AFP determinations in young patients in case the tumour is of germ cell type, and immunoelectrophoresis and examination of the urine for Bence Jones protein if myeloma is a possibility. The blood film may show evidence of leucoerythroblastic anaemia and this is most commonly seen with breast cancer, occasionally in carcinoma of the lung and much less commonly in any other tumour. Polycythaemia and thrombocytosis may occur with renal carcinoma and hepatoma. Hepatomas also produce AFP (see Chapter 15).

Other Investigations

The urine should always be examined. A fresh sample should be taken to look for red cells, which may indicate an underlying renal carcinoma. A chest X-ray is of course an essential examination and may disclose a carcinoma of the bronchus or enlarged mediastinal lymph nodes suggestive of a lymphoma.

Other more invasive investigations are of much more doubtful benefit. Although there is a temptation to go further and perform contrast radiology of the gut and kidneys, and CT scans of the chest and abdomen, these are seldom valuable or useful contributions to management since, by definition, the disease is disseminated at the time of presentation. There is a place for mammography if carcinoma of the breast is a serious differential diagnosis since the presence of a supraclavicular or axillary node does not rule out effective treatment of the tumour. In the final analysis the decision is one which requires judgement and skill. In the main, the less experienced the physician, the greater the number of investigations performed. It requires considerable clinical authority and careful explanation to help the patient understand that further investigation is not needed after the metastasis has been discovered and treatable causes excluded.

TREATMENT

The diagnosis of cancer presenting as metastasis poses a considerable burden on the patient and the doctor. The element of uncertainty in the situation and the serious nature and poor prognosis of the complaint make management difficult. Symptomatic treatments are always available and include local radiotherapy, analgesics and steroids, as used in metastatic cancer of known origin when it recurs. If the diagnosis has been established as a germ cell tumour or other treatable condition as outlined in Table 21.3, then of course treatment is along the appropriate lines. In young males with poorly differentiated carcinoma, a trial of germ-cell tumour chemotherapy (see Chapter 19) is justified even when tumour markers are negative since an early response would be highly suggestive of a germ cell tumour.

In many cases, however, no diagnosis will will be reached, and the issue will then be to decide if chemotherapy should be used in an attempt to delay the progress of the disease. This depends very much on the clinical state of the patient and on the intensity of the patient's anxiety for treatment. Undoubtedly regressions can be induced with the use of drugs such as doxorubicin and mitomycin in combination, or combinations such as cyclophosphamide, methotrexate and 5-fluorouracil. Such regressions are usually short-lived and it is by no means clear whether the overall prognosis of patients will be improved even though it is likely that responders will live longer than non-responders. The single most useful agent is doxorubicin, but this of course has the unwanted effects of nausea and alopecia. Our practise is to use a combination including doxorubicin in those patients who are young, relatively fit, and who have a strong desire for treatment (2). All too often, however, there is a failure of response or only a short-lived response, and palliative treatment is all that can be offered.

In women in whom the histological diagnosis is adenocarcinoma, a trial of endocrine therapy with tamoxifen or aminoglutethimide is worthwhile even if there is no clinical or radiological evidence that the breast is the primary site.

REFERENCES

1 Nystrom J.S., Weiner J.M. & Wolf R.M. (1979) Identifying the primary site in metastatic cancer of unknown origin. Inadequacy of roentgenographic procedures. *Journal of the American Medical Association* **241,** 381.
2 Woods R.L., Fox R.M., Tattersall M.H.N., Levi J.A. & Brodie E.N. (1980) Metastatic adenocarcinomas of unknown primary site. A randomised study of two combination chemotherapy regimens. *New England Journal of Medicine* **303,** 87.

AETIOLOGY AND PATHOGENESIS

It is perhaps not surprising that skin cancers are the commonest of all malignancies, since the skin is the largest and most accessible organ of the body, directly exposed to whatever carcinogens are in our environment. It has been recognized for over 200 years that skin cancers can develop as a result of directly applied carcinogens, and the earliest described and perhaps best known example, noted by Percivall Pott in 1775, is the carcinoma of scrotal skin which affected chimney sweeps who came into direct contact with soot in the chimney flue. In the 19th century, an increase in the incidence of skin cancers was reported in patients who had been treated with medicines containing arsenic, and arsenical fumes had already been implicated as a contributing factor in the scrotal cancers of copper miners and smelters. Towards the end of the century, it was suggested that strong sunlight might be a promoter of skin cancer, and shortly after the discovery of radium, Becquerel proposed that ionizing radiation might be the component of sunlight responsible for malignant change. More recently, the carcinogenic roles of ultraviolet radiation, X-rays and chemicals has been confirmed; most important of all was the work of Yamagiwa and Ichikawa who were the first to demonstrate the carcinogenic properties of coal tar when applied directly to the skin of experimental animals (1), though it was Kennaway who isolated and identified the carcinogen as 3:4 benzpyrene.

Sunlight

Epidemiological studies have provided important clues to the aetiology of skin cancer. In general, its incidence varies directly in proportion to the intensity of sunlight, with the result that skin cancers are much more common in Australia and South Africa than in more temperate areas. The importance of sunlight is further suggested by the high proportion of skin cancers (particularly basal cell carcinomas) which occur in exposed areas of the body. In addition, certain races such as the fair-skinned Celts are particularly prone to developing skin cancer, probably due to a relative lack of protection by melanin pigment; in contrast, skin cancers are relatively uncommon in black races, (both Negroes and Indian), presumably as a result of effective shielding by pigment in the superficial skin layers. In Negroes, the distribution of skin cancers is much less determined by sunlight exposure than in caucasians, and is almost as common in unexposed areas such as the trunk and lower limbs. The use of psoralens and ultraviolet light (PUVA) in psoriasis is associated with a risk of cutaneous malignancy, and not only in cases where other carcinogens (such as X-rays) have been given in the past.

Occupational factors

Occupational carcinogens have in the past been an important cause of skin cancers, though increasing awareness of the hazards has substantially reduced these risks. However, industrial carcinogens such as petroleum derivatives, arsenicals, and coal tar are still in common use, and protective clothing is still important in prevention. Even more critical is the need to keep radiation exposure to an absolute minimum, particularly for those working with X-rays; including medical, nursing and radiographic personnel who require regular monitoring of radiation exposure throughout their working lives.

Immune suppression and viral causes

Recipients of renal allografts have an increased risk of cancer—possibly as great as 100 times that of the general population. The most common malignancies are those of the skin including squamous carcinoma, melanoma, basal cell carcinoma and Bowen's disease. The squamous carcinomas are more frequent than basal cell (a reverse of the usual pattern) and occur twenty times more often than in normal people. Sometimes the disease is severe and multifocal running an aggressive course.

Recently considerable interest has been aroused in the role of the wart viruses, *Human Papilloma Virus* (HPV), in the aetiology of cancers of the skin and genital tract. A pattern is now emerging in which HPV appears to be associated with the appearance of cancer in particular clinical settings. The genome of HPV type 5 has been found in squamous carcinoma of the skin in a renal allograft recipient and also in the squamous cancers which occur in the rare inherited skin disorder *epidermodysplasia verruciformis* in which patients develop multiple warts.

Pre-malignant lesions

A group of pre-malignant skin lesions has been recognized in which malignant change, though not inevitable, is sufficiently common to justify very close surveillance. These lesions include:

INHERITED DISORDERS

Xeroderma pigmentosum. This autosomal recessive disease is characterized by greatly in-creased sensitivity to ultraviolet light leading to multiple solar keratoses, pre-malignant and ultimately frankly malignant skin lesions on exposed surfaces. The cancer can be squamous or basal cell carcinoma, or malignant melanoma. The defect appears to be due to UV-induced DNA damage causing a deficiency in the excision-repair mechanism for DNA.

Naevoid basal cell carcinoma syndrome (Gorlin's syndrome). This syndrome is characterized by multiple basal cell carcinomas particularly on the face and trunk, associated with cleft lip and skeletal abnormalities which include frontal bossing, mandibular cysts and bifid ribs. It is inherited as an autosomal dominant characteristic. The skin tumours often develop in young adult life.

Albinism. This group of congenital diseases is associated with defective skin pigmentation and an increased tendency to solar keratosis and squamous carcinoma *in situ*.

Epidermodysplasia verruciformis. This is an autosomal recessive disease characterized by multiple flat warts. These and even non-affected skin may evolve into squamous carcinoma (see above).

CARCINOGEN-INDUCED DISORDERS

Arsenical keratoses. After exposure to inorganic arsenicals, keratotic lesions may develop 10 years or more later on the palms and soles. These lesions are pre-malignant although overt cancer is uncommon. The patients often have Bowen's disease and superficial basal cell carcinomas at other sites.

Solar keratoses. Although histologically similar to arsenical keratoses, the incidence of frank malignant change is much greater. The distribution is also different, since these lesions chiefly occur on the face and dorsal surfaces of the hands. Other changes of prolonged exposure to sunlight are present: furrowed elastic leathery skin, with wrinkling, atrophy and hyper- or depigmented patches.

Radiation Dermatitis. Following exposure to modest doses of superficial radiation (often given many years before, for benign conditions, e.g. ringworm, acne or hirsutism), the skin may assume a characteristic appearance, with depigmentation, atrophy of the skin, hair and sweat glands, and telangiectasia. These areas are more susceptible to malignant change. Basal cell carcinomas on the scalp are usually related to previous irradiation and may arise in skin which shows no evidence of radiation change.

MISCELLANEOUS DISORDERS

Bowen's Disease. Often considered with the pre-malignant skin disorders, this disease is more properly considered as a squamous cell carcinoma *in situ*, and is a superficial intraepidermal carcinoma usually found on the trunk or limbs. Characteristically, this lesion spreads laterally within the cutis, commonly arising at several sites, and evolving slowly from a small erythematous papule to a crusting lesion. Histologically, the basal layer is intact but the epidermis shows premature keratinization and is disrupted with homogeneous cells with basophilic cytoplasm, small nuclei and frequent mitoses. There is an important association with internal malignancies, and as many as a quarter of all patients with Bowen's disease may develop a deep-seated carcinoma during the 10 years following diagnosis.

Leukoplakia. These are indurated whitish plaques, often fissured and with sharply defined borders, found on mucus membranes of the mouth. They may result from local irritation—ill-fitting dentures and smoking are frequently associated. The histology shows hyperplasia, hyperkeratosis and dyskeratosis; carcinoma *in situ* may arise, sometimes progressing to squamous cell carcinoma.

Genital carcinoma in-situ. This presents as a persistent red papule or plaque on the penis. Pathologically there is an abnormal epidermis with an absent granular layer and small densely packed cells similar to those found in Bowen's disease. The lesion used to be called erythroplasia of Queyrat. Intra-epithelial neoplasia may also be found on the vulva.

BASAL CELL CARCINOMA

Basal cell carcinoma (rodent ulcer) accounts for over 75% of all cases of skin malignancy in the Western world. The age specific incidence is shown in Fig. 22.1. They are epithelial tumours without any histological evidence of maturation or tendency to keratinization, and almost cer-

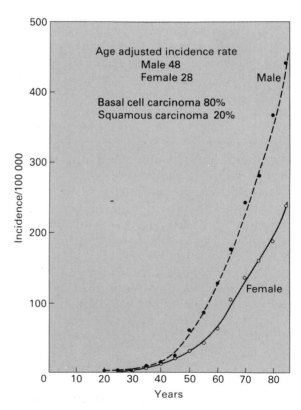

Fig. 22.1. *Age-specific incidence of basal cell carcinoma and squamous carcinoma of the skin.*

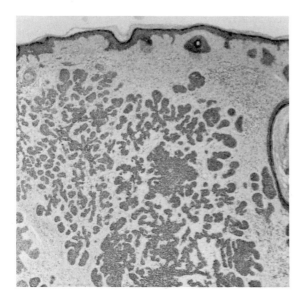

Fig. 22.2. *Basal cell carcinoma of skin.* Showing small nests of invading basal cells (× 20).

tainly arise from the undifferentiated basal cells of the skin, which normally differentiate into mature structures such as hair or sweat glands. Microscopically, these tumours are characterized by uniform cells with darkly stained nuclei and little cytoplasm. The cells form a characteristic palisade (Fig. 22.2). The tumour generally arises on exposed areas, particularly the skin of the face and most characteristically around the nose, forehead, cheeks and lower eyelid although they may sometimes occur on the limbs. Macroscopically, these lesions are often described as being either nodular, pigmented, sclerosing (morphoeic), cicatrizing, infiltrating or ulcerative. The most typical appearance is that of a firm pink papule with a distinct raised edge, often serpiginous, with a pearly and telangiectatic appearance and with a slightly depressed or frankly ulcerated centre with or without a central crust. Although non-inflammatory and typically painless, they may irritate and will often bleed repeatedly if scratched.

Untreated, these tumours invade laterally with local destruction of cartilage or even bone; less commonly, such destruction may also result from deep extension. In the sclerosing variety, the typical features may be absent and the margin indistinct—making diagnosis more difficult. Superficial basal cell carcinomas, often multiple, also have an unusual appearance and are more commonly encountered on the trunk with characteristically, a more plaque-like configuration, often with reddish scaling patches and a typical fine pearly edge. Very occasionally, cystic degeneration occurs in a basal cell carcinoma.

Despite the characteristically highly malignant microscopic appearance of basal cell carcinomas, metastasis to local lymph nodes or distant sites is exceptionally rare, a remarkable fact in view of the large size that many of these cancers can achieve, and an important contrast from the behaviour of squamous cell carcinomas.

SQUAMOUS CELL CARCINOMA

Squamous cell carcinomas of the skin are less common than basal cell carcinomas (Fig. 22.1) though they share many characteristics of aetiology and site. Sunlight exposure, arsenic ingestion, and occupational carcinogens are all known to be important, as well as direct exposure to X-rays. Multiple squamous cell carcinomas of the hand were common among radiation scientists in the early years of this century until these hazards were recognized and methods of dosimetry improved. Histologically, these are typical keratinizing squamous lesions (Fig. 22.3) quite unlike the basal cell carcinoma, though diagnostic difficulties can occasionally occur with basal cell carcinoma and other lesions such as melanoma since more invasive and aggressive tumours may lack this characteristic feature. To some extent, the likelihood of local lymph node metastases can be predicted from the histological appearance, being more common with less well-differentiated tumours.

As with basal cell carcinomas, the commonest sites include the exposed areas of the head and neck, particularly the nose, temples,

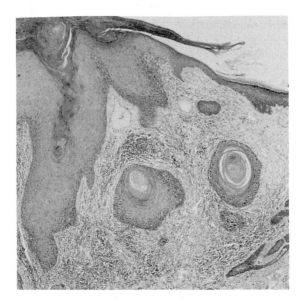

Fig. 22.3. *Squamous cell carcinoma of skin.* Showing invading masses of squamous epithelium forming keratin pearls (× 20).

rim of the ear and lip, as well as the side and back of the neck, and the dorsal surfaces of the hand and forearm. The appearance of these lesions tends to resemble either a crusted scaly ulcer or a more nodular exophytic type of lesion, which can fungate if untreated. Small lesions may be impossible to distinguish macroscopically from basal cell carcinomas but the site of the tumour may be diagnostically helpful since squamous cell carcinomas, though commonest on the face, have a much more widespread distribution than basal cell carcinomas and a shorter history. A skin tumour of the hand or forearm is much more likely to be of squamous cell origin. Squamous cell carcinoma may also be difficult to distinguish macroscopically from the usually benign condition of kerato-acanthoma, characterized by a locally rapidly advancing, discrete and often bulky papule, usually occurring on the face or neck, and typically with a central plug of keratin filling the ulcerated central part of the lesion.

Squamous cell carcinomas arising in an area of radiation dermatitis are both clinically and histologically more aggressive than other varieties, though the mean latent interval is about 20 years. In one large series of nearly 400 patients, the mortality was 10% (2). These tumours are now less frequent because of higher energy radiotherapy equipment, and the infrequent use of radiotherapy for benign skin disorders and arthritic conditions. This is also true of squamous carcinomas arising from chronic burn ulcers, *Marjolin's ulcer*, though this used to be a common problem, typically with a lengthy period of quiescence terminated by a highly aggressive phase with metastases to the lungs and other sites. A similar type of squamous cell carcinoma occasionally develops in chronic sinus tracts of osteomyelitis or other chronic infections (3). Squamous carcinomas can also develop in dysplastic or scar areas resulting from chronic skin diseases such as lupus vulgaris, and are also reportedly more common in areas of vitiligo, particularly in blacks.

Squamous carcinomas arising at muco-cutaneous junctions such as anus and vulva tend to be aggressive, as do those developing in areas of radiation-damaged skin, patches of Bowen's disease, or against a background of carcinoma *in situ*. In many cases, deep invasion and early metastasis takes place even though the primary lesion may appear unchanged. Sweat gland carcinoma, an uncommon condition, may also behave unpredictably. These tumours most commonly arise in the axilla and anogenital regions, and should be distinguished from the rare sebaceous gland cancers.

Treatment of basal cell and squamous cell carcinoma

Because of the frequency and characteristic appearance of these tumours, treatment without firm histological diagnosis is sometimes advocated. In general this is an unwise policy although elderly patients are sometimes too unwell to withstand even the mild trauma of a surgical or drill biopsy under local anaesthetic. In all other cases, a biopsy should first be obtained. Benign conditions such as papillomas, sclerosing haemangiomas and kerato-acanthomas can all be macroscopically confused with a basal or squamous cell carcinoma, and occasionally these two major types of skin cancer can themselves be difficult to distinguish from each other.

There are several effective methods of treatment, including electrocautery and curettage, cryosurgery, excisional surgery, chemosurgery, radiotherapy and topical chemotherapy. Since all of these methods have their strong adherents and each method yields a very high success rate, formal comparisons are difficult. In addition, approaches such as electrocautery and cryosurgery are in general confined to such small lesions (usually under 5 mm diameter) that the very high success rate of over 95% (4) is not representative of an unselected group of patients.

Electrocautery is not usually used for tumours at difficult sites such as the margin of the eyelid or nasolabial fold, or for deeply infiltrating tumours. Cryosurgery, usually using liquid nitrogen, is also effective for small lesions, particularly for superficial tumours such as Bowen's disease and the most superficial of basal cell carcinomas. Chemosurgery, an interesting technique first described by Mohs (5), employs a zinc chloride paste fixative which is applied to the tumour, partly destroying it and allowing easy removal from the underlying skin whilst preserving its histological pattern. Further zinc chloride paste is then applied to any area of the residual tumour, and the whole process can be repeated. Currently the zinc fixative is often omitted. This method can be useful even for fairly large tumours and at sites where radiotherapy may be hazardous (see below), though the technique is time-consuming and laborious, and demands great expertise and care particularly in the histological assessment.

For basal cell and squamous cell carcinomas too large to be treated by electrocautery, most dermatologists would agree that the real choice in therapy lies between excisional surgery and radiotherapy. Each has its advantages. Excisional surgery is quick, and is the only method producing a complete specimen for the pathologist to ensure that total microscopic excision has been achieved. On the other hand, for tumours of large size a general anaesthetic is usually required, and for still larger lesions, skin grafting or flap rotation may well be necessary, contributing to a less acceptable final cosmetic result as well as the risk of a higher postoperative complication rate than with simple excision alone. With tumours at difficult sites such as the inner canthus of the eye, surgery is probably best avoided since there is a risk of damage to the nasolachrymal duct, and surgical reconstruction can be very difficult. In general, however, the results of surgery are very good and an excellent cosmetic result can be achieved. This is true for both basal cell and squamous cell carcinomas, though a wider excision of squamous cell carcinomas is usually recommended because of the possibility of local lymphatic spread. Despite the known tendency of squamous cell carcinomas to metastasise to local lymph nodes, there is no place for routine lymph node dissection, though surgical excision is undoubtedly the treatment of choice for clinically involved regional lymph nodes.

Radiotherapy treatment is also highly effective, with a cure rate of over 90% (6). It is especially useful for tumours on the face, particulay around the eye, nose and nasolabial fold where tumours may infiltrate deeply. Both the columella of the nose and the ala nasae are difficult surgical sites, and radiotherapy is highly effective and gives excellent cosmetic results. One advantage enjoyed by radiotherapists is the versatility of modern radiotherapy equipment, offering an energy and effective depth dose of the irradiation beam which can be chosen to suit the individual tumour. Simple lead cut-outs can be tailor-made so that irregularly shaped tumours may be adequately treated without unnecessary treatment of large volumes of normal skin (Fig. 22.4). For tumours of the lower eyelid and other sites where shielding of deeper structures

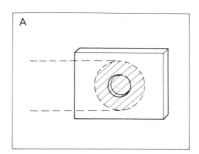
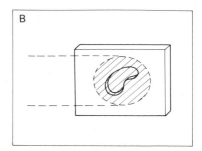

Fig. 22.4. *Typical lead cut-outs for treatment of basal or squamous carcinoma.* (A) Regularly shaped; (B) irregularly shaped.

is desirable (e.g. gums, teeth and tongue in treatment of cancer of the lip), simple shielding can be repeatedly introduced, for each treatment session. Fig. 22.5 shows a lead shield inserted under local anaesthetic into the lower conjunctival sac, to protect the eye whilst a tumour of the lower lid is treated. For tumours overlying bone or cartilage where low to moderate energy X-ray beams carry a risk of radionecrosis (see Chapter 5), direct electron beams can be employed with equally good results and far less risk of damage. The major disadvantage of radiotherapy is that in order to produce the

best cosmetic result, most radiotherapists feel that it is necessary to employ fractionated regimes of treatment over 2 weeks or more. Most patients are able to attend the radiotherapy department for several treatment sessions during this period, but for the elderly or infirm, the travelling may be tiring and a quick operation or treatment by a single large fraction of radiotherapy may be preferable.

Treatment with less highly fractionated course of radiotherapy (such as the Sambrook split course, in which two fractions of radiation are given some 6 weeks apart), have a very

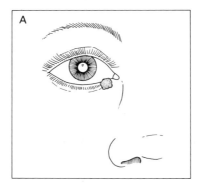
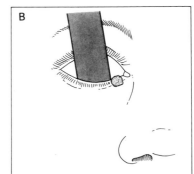
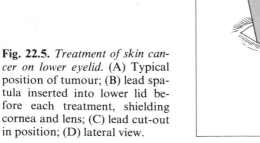
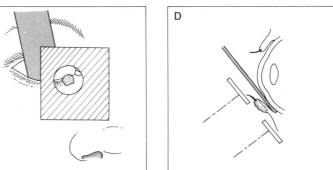

Fig. 22.5. *Treatment of skin cancer on lower eyelid.* (A) Typical position of tumour; (B) lead spatula inserted into lower lid before each treatment, shielding cornea and lens; (C) lead cut-out in position; (D) lateral view.

good cure rate but an undoubtedly higher incidence of late skin changes such as telangiectasia, atrophy and depigmentation. The aim of longer courses of radiotherapy is to decrease these late effects to a minimum, particularly important for facial skin cancers where a very high cure rate, coupled with a perfect cosmetic result, should be the aim of every radiotherapist. Acute skin changes are much less important (though sometimes irritating and occasionally painful to the patient), and usually consist of intense local erythema and inflammation, leading to early crusting, and finally, resolution with healing which may take several months to complete, particularly with larger lesions. Common fractionation regimens are shown in Table 22.1; they often reflect the capacity of the radiotherapy department to treat these common tumours, as much as the individual preference of the radiotherapist. Expressed in terms of the nominal standard dose (see Chapter 5), these treatments aim for a total of 1500–1900 ret. It is generally accepted that squamous cell carcinomas require a wider treatment field than basal cell carcinomas, though most radiotherapists treat both lesions to the same doses and their radiocurability is probably identical (7). Radiotherapy is not indicated in the naevoid-basal cell carcinoma syndrome in which it gives poor results with marked skin damage.

Topical chemotherapy, usually using 5-fluorouracil, has been increasingly employed in recent years (8), particularly for recurrent lesions where surgery and/or radiation therapy have already been used. Although its precise role has not yet been determined, the advantages of topical cytotoxic therapy include the possibility of repeated use where necessary, as well as its value in pre-malignant lesions and large areas of carcinoma *in situ* where other methods of treatment might be difficult. It is also valuable in treatment of multiple lesions, particularly of the superficial basal cell carcinoma type, but is not usually recommended for thick or infiltrating lesions. Topical cytotoxic therapy produces inflammation which is a disadvantage, although steroids are helpful in alleviating this.

Overall results of treatment of both basal cell and squamous cell carcinoma are excellent. Cure rates of 90–95% are regularly achieved by surgery or radiotherapy; for smaller tumours treated by curettage, cryosurgery or electrocautery the figures are claimed to be higher still. Sadly, the occasional tumour is encountered (particularly with basal cell carcinoma) which proves resistant to all methods of treatment, usually with multiple recurrences of tumour, often at the margins of the treated area and sometimes over a period of 10 years or more. These cases are characterized by relentless local invasion and destruction both laterally and deeply. Distant metastases to bone, lung or elsewhere, are occasionally seen.

MALIGNANT MELANOMA

Epidemiology and pathogenesis

Malignant melanoma is a far less common skin tumour than the true carcinomas discussed above, but has a much worse prognosis. At present, it accounts for less than 2% of all skin cancers, with an annual incidence in Britain of about 3 per 100 000 population (Fig. 22.6). Its incidence appears to have risen sharply during the last decade (9). There is a wide international variation and the disease is almost ten times as common in Australia and New Zealand as it is in Europe. It occurs most frequently in patients between 40 and 70 years old, and is slightly

Table 22.1. Fractionation regimens in basal and squamous cell carcinoma. Single fraction or 2-fraction policies are generally adopted in elderly patients for whom repeated visits may be difficult. In general, however, better cosmetic results are achieved with more prolonged fractionation.

20–22 Gy × 1
14 Gy × 2 (6 week gap)
7.5 Gy × 5 (7–10 days)
6.75 Gy × 6 (alternate days)
6 Gy × 9 (over 3 weeks)
4.5 Gy × 10 (over 3 weeks)

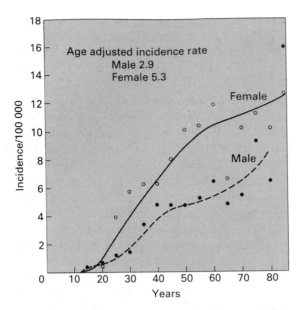

Fig. 22.6. *Age-specific incidence of melanoma in Britain.*

more common in females than males. This is in contrast to basal cell and squamous carcinoma (Fig. 22.1) and implies that there is a difference in the relative importance of external factors, such as sunlight, in aetiology in these types of skin cancer. Like other skin cancers, melanoma is more common in Whites than Blacks, possibly as a result of the effectiveness of pigmented skin in screening out solar UV which has long been thought to be the most important factor in its aetiology (10). About 75% of all malignant melanomas occur on an exposed site, chiefly affecting pale complexioned Whites especially with red hair and freckles. Families have been described in which the disease occurs with unusual frequency (11). In Australia, epidemiological studies have shown that the amount of received sunlight, as measured by distance from the Equator, correlates well with the incidence of the disease. Although trauma to superficial skin naevi has frequently been implicated as a cause of malignant change, there is little evidence to support this view. The most common skin sites of melanoma in Whites are the head and neck, trunk and limbs. In blacks the bodily distribution is different, with a greater likelihood of a primary site on the palms of the hands, soles of the feet and mucous membranes.

Clinical and pathological features

Although more than half of all melanotic lesions arise from a pre-existing benign naevus, some undoubtedly develop at sites of previously normal skin; in many cases the primary site is never discovered, the patient presenting either with lymphadenopathy or with more widespread involvement. Post mortem studies have shown that most of the organs of the body are capable of harbouring a primary melanotic focus: larynx, oesophagus, trachea, bronchus, gastro-intestinal tract, and leptomeninges have all been implicated. Certainly all these organs (and many more) contain clusters of melanocytes, but why these should undergo malignant change remains completely unknown.

Diagnosis of malignant melanoma is not always straightforward. Almost all of us have pigmented melanocytic naevi (approximately twelve in the average Caucasian), and many innocent pigmented naevi appear to enlarge slowly over the years. They are maximal in number in the third decade of life and then slowly disappear. Those undergoing any form of rapid change, particularly with ulceration or bleeding, must be regarded with great suspicion, and most dermatologists will advise excision biopsy. Other important skin conditions may be difficult to distinguish from malignant melanoma unless a biopsy is obtained; these include the pigmented basal cell carcinomas, solar keratoses, blue naevi, juvenile melanomas, pyogenic granulomas, sclerosing angiomas and benign pigmented melanocytic naevi.

The benign melanocytic naevi are derived from the intra-epidermal melanocyte whose origin is from the neural crest. There are important differences between the various types of naevus, which may have a bearing on the pathogenesis of malignant melanoma. *Junctional naevi* are well circumscribed small, flat, pigmented lesions arising from clumps of pigmented cells at the junction of dermis and epidermis. The normal skin lines are not distorted. Their proliferation and penetration into the true dermis results in a *compound naevus*. These lesions are larger than junctional naevi and may be raised. Coarse hair may arise from these naevi and although the junctional activity may then abate, the pigmented cells deep in the dermis may then continue to multiply, resulting an *intradermal naevus*. Here the melanocytes are no longer in contact with the epidermis. Clinically the lesion has very little pigmentation. It is usually a raised papule and is commoner in the older age groups. Although junctional naevi are certainly capable of malignant change, this happens only rarely. It is not clear how frequently melanoma arises in a common melanocytic naevus. A history of enlargement of a pre-existing naevus can be obtained in 10–40% of patients with melanoma but this is not a reliable guide. A more definite precursor, though numerically far less frequently encountered, is the *lentigo maligna*, or Hutchinson's melanotic freckle. This is an epidermal lesion resulting from the maturation of atypical melanocytes, thought embryologically to result from neural crest tissue. It is one of three well recognized macroscopic varieties of malignant melanoma, accounting for up to 10% of all cases and, if suspected, demanding immediate surgical excision. The lesion is found in sun-exposed areas in elderly patients. At first there is a flat pigmented area on the skin which appears to represent a radial growth phase of the tumour. This expands slowly over many years. Later an invasive vertical growth develops, visible as nodules within lesion. Surgical excision in the radial growth phase is often curative. *Superficial spreading melanomas* are usually larger lesions, often 2–3 cm in diameter, and chiefly occurring in middle aged people. They have an irregular edge often with a pale central area. After 1–2 years the lesion may itch or ulcerate and may become nodular. The superficial growth phase has then given way to a deeper vertical penetration of the lesion. In general these melanomas evolve

gradually in the first instance, though more rapidly than Lentigo maligna. *Nodular melanomas* develop more rapidly still, and are almost always characterized by deep dermal invasion by the time of diagnosis. There is no histologically recognizable radial growth phase. The patients are usually middle aged (Fig. 22.6) and areas of skin not exposed to light are often affected. Typically there is a raised nodule on the skin surface and the normal skin markings are disturbed. Ulceration occurs after 2–3 months and deep penetration occurs early. The association with a pre-existing naevus is less strong than in superficial spreading melanoma.

These three major types of melanoma account for almost 90% of all cases, the remainder arising from other types of naevus (congenital, blue, compound or intradermal), or from mucus membranes, meninges or other internal sites.

Stage of melanoma

The most important prognostic characteristics in malignant melanoma are the level of invasion (or microstage) and the clinical stage of the tumour.

MICROSTAGE

Clark and colleagues (12) described five separate levels of invasiveness (Fig. 4.1), and demonstrated that prognosis correlated well with the depth of invasion, though subsequent work by Breslow suggests that vertical tumour thickness in millimetres may be an even better guide (13). Tumours less than 0.75 mm in thickness very rarely metastasise. In addition, the *type* of primary melanotic lesion may also influence the prognosis, and nodular primary lesions in general have a worse prognosis stage for stage than the more common superficial spreading variety, which may well reflect the increased probability of nodal involvement with nodular lesions (14).

CLINICAL STAGE

No single clinical staging system has been universally accepted, though patients with obvious lymphadenopathy undoubtedly do less well than patients with cutaneous disease only. A simple scheme is shown in Table 22.2. Involve-

Table 22.2. Clinical Stage of Malignant Melanoma.

Stage I   Disease confined to local site
Stage II Involvement of regional lymph nodes
Stage III Distant metastases

ment of regional nodes is usually judged clinically, but patients with palpable and histologically positive regional lymph nodes have a 5-year survival of less than 20%, whereas those with non-palpable local lymph nodes but microscopically confirmed lymph node invasion have a 5-year survival of over 50% (14).

In reality the problem of classification and case-comparison is far more complex, since a surprising number of features are thought to have prognostic significance even in clinical stage I disease (Table 22.3). The clinical diagnosis of regional lymphadenopathy or disseminated disease is undoubtedly of over-riding prognostic significance. Important metastatic sites include liver, lung, spleen, heart and cen-

Table 22.3. Prognostic factors in clinical stage I malignant melanoma.

Low risk
    Radial (lateral) growth phase
    Thickness less than 0.76 mm
    or Clark level 2

Intermediate risk
    Level 3 invasion
    Up to 1.5 mm thickness

High risk
    Level 4 or 5
    1.5–4.0 mm invasion
    High mitotic rate
    Satellite lesions
    Ulceration
    Axial location or hands or feet

tral nervous system (particularly brain but also meningeal involvement). Malignant melanoma can also metastasise to bone and solitary bony metastases, in the absence of any other sign of dissemination, are well described.

STAGING INVESTIGATIONS

Once the diagnosis of melanoma has been established, clinical staging should naturally take account of these routes of spread, and simple investigations such as full blood count, chest X-ray and liver function tests should be undertaken in all patients. A fuller assessment, including liver and brain scanning, will undoubtedly reveal an occasional case of unsuspected occult disease. Lymphography, abdominal CT scanning and/or abdominal ultrasonography may demonstrate unsuspected local or para-aortic lymphadenopathy. Although these investigations are difficult to justify as a routine, their increasing availability should allow for better prognostic detail. In particular ultrasonography in skilled hands is a very valuable, simple and non-invasive technique in melanoma since it provides reliable information regarding both the liver and abdominopelvic lymph nodes.

Treatment of malignant melanoma

SURGERY

Local excision. For localized (stage I) malignant melanoma, confined to the primary site, surgical excision is unquestionably the cornerstone of management. Because of the propensity of local lymphatic invasion, most surgeons recommend *wide* excision of the primary lesion, with a particularly generous clearance proximally. Although it can be difficult to confirm the need for this in every case, at least one study has demonstrated an increase of melanocytes in clinically and histologically normal epidermis surrounding a significant proportion of primary malignant melanomas, supporting the view that wide excision is essential (15). Wide excision usually requires split-skin graft coverage, and some authorities feel that for relatively good prognoses (i.e. Clark's level 1 or 2 (Fig. 4.1) and lentigo maligna lesions), a less generous surgical excision, with primary closure, is adequate.

Depth of excision is also contentious, and will depend not only on the type of primary lesion but also the site. Nodular lesions almost always invade deeply and demand deeper excision than primary lentigo maligna melanomas. Lesions of the hands and feet, for example subungual melanomas, are generally best dealt with by partial amputation of the digit. Nodular melanomas present a particular problem in view of their early deep invasiveness, and have usually invaded as far as the papillary-reticular junction (Clark level 3) or more by the time of diagnosis. These lesions should therefore always be excised with wide clearance, and deeply down to at least as far as deep fascia. Skin grafting will almost always be required.

Regional lymph node dissection. Apart from primary surgical excision of the cutaneous lesion, the question of elective regional lymph node dissection frequently arises. Is it wise to undertake local lymphadenectomy in all cases of malignant melanoma? In patients with stage I disease where no clinical lymphadenopathy is present, lymphadenectomy undoubtedly gives useful *prognostic* information. The presence of microscopic disease worsens the prognosis; 70% of cases with true stage I (node negative) lesions are alive at 5 years while only 50% of patients with occult regional lymph node involvement (proven only by surgery) survive this long.

Whether or not regional lymphadenectomy makes any therapeutic contribution to prognosis also remains uncertain. In general, there is agreement that for patients with good risk melanoma, i.e. a small lesion of a limb, not nodular in character and of Clark's level I, there is nothing to be gained by lymphadenectomy. For deeper lesions, for example, nodular and spreading melanomas of Clark's levels III, IV or V, lymphadenectomy is often recommended.

Certainly most surgeons would favour dissec-

tion if there are clinically involved lymph nodes in the primary nodal drainage area, though it is doubtful whether such dissection genuinely adds to survival. Only 10% of patients with clinically detectable lymphadenopathy, confirmed at lymphadenectomy, are alive 5 years later (16). This unhappy situation is closely analogous to what we know from breast cancer studies, in that local lymph node involvement undoubtedly implies disseminated (though often clinically undetectable) disease. In both of these illnesses, this prognostic information is gained by a procedure which is itself of doubtful benefit. Despite this dispiriting state of affairs, radical lymph node dissection for clinical stage II melanoma is the only practical means of therapy with any serious chance of success at present. For the highly selected group of patients with bad risk clinical stage II lesions of the distal portion of a limb, amputation may give the best chance of cure.

In Britain, few surgeons favour prophylactic lymph node dissection even in patients with high risk lesions even though it provides useful prognostic information. This view is borne out by careful analysis of a large group of Australian patients (17). The extremely high incidence of this disease in Australia and New Zealand has led to a special experience in the larger Australian centres, and the 5-year survival rates from Queensland appear better than for anywhere else in the world (Queensland 81%; England 61%; United States 37%). Although this might suggest particular expertise, it is also true that a higher proportion of Australian patients have primary melanotic lesions confined to the epidermis, and therefore likely to have a relatively good prognosis.

RADIOTHERAPY

There are few reports of the use of radiotherapy as an alternative to surgery for primary melanomas, though it is known that melanoma cells *in vitro* are not radioresistant (18), contrary to a long-held clinical belief that radiation therapy is of no value. Several reports have demonstrated the clinical usefulness of radiotherapy, which has in general been employed for patients in whom surgery is unsuitable often because the lesion is too advanced. Radiotherapy may be especially valuable in lentigo maligna melanoma.

Since many lesions are on the extremities, a high dose can usually be reached without danger to internal structures. Further evidence for the potential value of radiotherapy for surgically unsuitable lesions comes from assessments of radiation treatment for recurrent or disseminated melanomas (see below). In treating melanoma large infrequent fractions of treatment (greater than 5 Gy) are used in an attempt to overcome the shoulder effect which is thought to be largely responsible for resistance (see Chapter 5).

CHEMOTHERAPY

Management of disseminated disease represents at present an almost insoluble problem. The median survival for all patients with disease beyond the regional lymph nodes is of the order of 5 months, though patients with predominantly skin involvement have a median survival of almost a year. Although malignant melanoma is frequently cited as a tumour in which spontaneous regression has been documented, the actual incidence of the phenomenon is no more than 1%, and lengthy survival is exceptionally rare. Nonetheless, with the demonstration in the early 1970s of some degree of sensitivity to cytotoxic chemotherapy, the use of anticancer drugs for disseminated malignant melanoma became widely adopted though objective responses were low (Table 22.4), and the overwhelming majority of these responses were less than complete. Furthermore responses are usually seen in skin, but are very uncommon in liver, brain, bone and lung—the sites which are the main cause of death.

At present, the more active agents are thought to be DTIC and vindesine, with response rates of 25–35%. It is not clear whether the use of drugs in combination offers genuinely superior

Table 22.4. Chemotherapy in melanoma.

Drug	Response Rate*
Single agents	
DTIC	22%
Alkylating agents	10%
Methotrexate	7%
Cytosine Arabinoside	10%
Actinomycin D	13%
Vindesine	15%
Vincristine	10%
Mitomycin C	14%
Hydroxyurea	10%
Nitrosoureas	14%
*Combination chemotherapy**	
DTIC + vinca	17%
DTIC + nitrosourea	17%
DTIC + vinca + nitrosourea	24%
Vinca + nitrosourea	24%
Vinca + nitrosourea + procarbazine	30%

* Complete and partial response together. Most response rates refer to cutaneous lesions. Responses are uncommon in visceral lesions.
** Typical regimens.

results to treatment with single agents alone, though improved results have been claimed in some series.

REGIONAL LIMB PERFUSION

An alternative approach, for patients with primary melanoma of an extremity and with loco-regional or recurrent disease, is to consider the use of regional perfusion with cytotoxic drugs. This was first described by Creech in 1959, and proved an effective method of palliation (19). Although this led to enthusiastic work in the 1960s and 1970s, employing this technique as an adjuvant to primary surgical treatment, there is no convincing evidence that it reduces the likelihood of metastatic disease. The drug most frequently used is melphalan and regressions are frequently seen. Its use is reserved for unresectable limb lesions with recurrent disease or widespread satellite tumours.

IMMUNOTHERAPY

Reports of occasional spontaneous regression of disease in melanoma, coupled with the demonstration of antigen and antimelanoma antibodies in the sera of a few patients with the disease (20), have led a number of groups to consider the use of 'active immunotherapy' in this disease. Non-randomized clinical trials using immunization with allogeneic melanoma cells or transfusions of allogeneic or autologous 'sensitized' leucocytes were inconclusive and generally suggestive of, at best, transient benefit. More recently, non-specific intralesional treatment with BCG has undoubtedly produced local responses in patients with recurrent cutaneous or nodal disease where direct injection of BCG is feasible. Unfortunately, most of these responses are short-lived, and of little or no value for patients with recurrent visceral or bone metastases.

Other forms of 'immunotherapy' including the use of levamisole and *Corynebacterium parvum*, are also currently under study. In addition, combined treatment of disseminated disease, using simultaneous administration of both chemotherapy and immunotherapy, are in progress at several centres, though the results have so far been discouraging. It seems that immunotherapy has at present little to offer patients. Claims for effectiveness have been from uncontrolled studies and randomized studies have failed to confirm any value.

PALLIATIVE RADIOTHERAPY

Palliative irradiation is undoubtedly useful in some patients with troublesome deposits, particularly for those with brain or osseous metastases. Although melanoma is not amongst the more radiosensitive of malignant diseases, it has been claimed that resistance can partly be overcome by the use of large infrequent fractions of treatment (21). Where surgical treatment of the primary site is considered unsuitable, radiation therapy is the only possible alternative, and long-term control, both of primary and meta-static lesions, is achieved in about 25% of these cases. Newer approaches, including neutron and charged particle therapy, radiosensitizers and hyperthermia, are all being investigated. Finally, use of hormone therapy has become an intriguing possibility for patients with disseminated melanoma. Women with melanoma have a better prognosis than men, and the use of non-toxic hormonal manipulation such as tamoxifen and other hormones is at present under study. Although the results have in general been discouraging, some reports have suggested that this approach may be worth pursuing and response rates in the region of 10–15% have been reported.

Prognosis

Prognosis in melanoma is always difficult to determine, a reflection of the multitude of potentially important features (Table 22.2). For patients with stage I, about 50% will survive 5 years free of recurrence (Fig. 22.7). About a quarter of patients with clinical stage I disease have lymph node involvement at diagnosis (pathological stage II), as shown by surgical series in which elective lymphadenectomy has been undertaken. Seventy-five percent of these lymph node positive patients will later develop evidence of dissemination, and a further 20% of patients with true stage I disease will develop distant metastases without ever having had local lymph node enlargement. About 20% of all patients destined to develop recurrent disease will remain disease free during the first 5 years from diagnosis. For this reason a 5-year survival rate of 60% for stage I melanoma signifies an overall cure rate of about 50% i.e. only 50% of all patients presenting with the earliest stage of melanoma.

For patients with regional lymphadenopathy (stage II) at diagnosis, the true cure rate is probably no more than 15% whilst those with disseminated disease at presentation have a median survival of less than 6 months. These dreadful figures will only improve with increased public and professional awareness re-

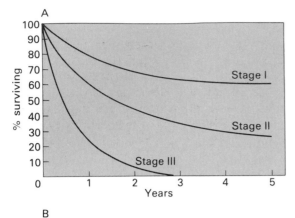

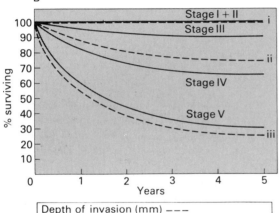

Depth of invasion (mm) ---		
i 0-0.76	ii 0.76-1.5	iii 2.25-3.0

C	5 year survival
Trunk	40%
Arm	60%
Leg	60%
Head and neck	50%
Male	40%
Female	50%

Fig. 22.7. *Prognosis in melanoma.* (A) Prognosis related to stage grouping; (B) prognosis related to microstage; (I–V) and depth of invasion (dashed lines); (C) prognosis related to site and sex.

sulting in earlier diagnosis and treatment. Although both chemotherapy and 'immunotherapy' are at present relatively ineffective, it is at least now widely accepted that disseminated melanoma is not totally resistant to treatment.

One possible approach for the future is the use of intensive chemotherapy supported by autologous marrow grafting. Very high doses of melphalan can safely be used in this way. However, even though drug responses are seen in some patients, durability of remission has so far been disappointingly short.

SKIN LYMPHOMAS

These are discussed in Chapter 26.

MISCELLANEOUS RARE TUMOURS

Dermatofibrosarcoma protuberans

This is a soft tissue sarcoma arising in the skin. It develops as firm nodules which grow slowly and may become large and be locally invasive. In general it does not metastasise but may recur after simple excision. Wide excision is the treatment of choice. Radiotherapy may be useful if major surgery (e.g. amputation) would otherwise be required.

Kaposi's sarcoma

Originally described by Kaposi in 1872, this sarcoma was a rarity in Europe until recently. Kaposi described the tumour in elderly Ashkenazi Jewish men. Its incidence in Europe was about 0.3 per million until the AIDS (acquired immune deficiency syndrome) epidemic. In Africa however it is common and may account for 10% of all cancers in Kenya and Uganda. There is a much higher frequency in renal allograft recipients and in patients with AIDS. In both these situations the tumour appears to be sustained by the immune suppression which if discontinued may allow regression of the neoplasm.

Pathologically the tumour is a proliferation of endothelial vascular channels with numerous spindle cells which are thought to be proliferating endothelial cells. There is often an infiltrate of lymphocytes and macrophages and if the spindle cell predominates, differentiation from a fibrosarcoma may be difficult. In the classic form of the disease a pigmented nodule appears on the leg or foot and grows very slowly. It may ulcerate but lymph node spread is unusual until multiple new lesions have appeared and the disease is more advanced. A form of the disease results in a brawny infiltration with diffuse swelling of the thigh or lower leg. This is a very indolent, unresponsive type of tumour.

The nodular form may become locally aggressive with invasion of deep tissues and formation of large masses. Another form occurs in children which affects lymph nodes early with a clinical picture similar to lymphoma. In AIDS the disease is a mixture of the nodular and lymphadenopathic forms and lesions may also appear on the mucous membranes. Some cases progress very rapidly indeed, others have a slow tempo.

Nodular localized disease is treated with radiotherapy. It is a sensitive tumour and single fractions of 8 Gy (800 rad) using electrons is effective with a complete response rate of 60–90%. The tumour is also sensitive to chemotherapy. The most effective agents (with response rates) are actinomycin D (90%), DTIC (60%), bleomycin (60%). Combination chemotherapy gives a high proportion of complete responders. The usual combinations are actinomycin D and vinblastine, or actinomycin, vincristine and DTIC. Alpha interferon produces tumour responses in about 40% of patients who have AIDS.

In the classic form of the disease patients live for many years. In AIDS related cases the prognosis is worse, patients dying of opportunistic infection in addition to the sarcoma.

Extra-mammary Paget's disease

These lesions are located near apocrine sweat glands, in the ano-genital region, breast areola and axillae. They are probably a form of carcinoma *in-situ*, and present as red, scaly plaques, slowly increasing in size. They are usually removed surgically.

Metastatic carcinoma

Nodules of secondary carcinoma are not infrequently found in the skin especially with cancer of the breast and melanoma. If the diagnosis is in doubt excision biopsy is essential. If any treatment is necessary this will be of the underlying disease if possible. Radiotherapy is useful for ulcerating or painful deposits.

REFERENCES

1 Yamagiwa K. & Ichikawa K. (1918) Experimental study of the pathogenesis of carcinoma. *Cancer Research* **3**, 1.
2 Martin H., Strong E. & Spiro R.H. (1970) Radiation-induced skin cancer of the head and neck. *Cancer* **25**, 61–71.
3 Sedlin E.D. & Fleming J.L. (1963) Epidermoid carcinoma arising in chronic osteomyelitic foci. *Journal of Bone and Joint Surgery* **45**(A), 827–38.
4 Crissey J.T. (1971) Curettage and electrodessication as a method of treatment for epitheliomas of the skin. *Journal of Surgical Oncology* **3**, 287.
5 Mohs F.E. (1956) *Chemosurgery in cancer, gangrene and infections.* C. Thomas, Illinois.
6 Spittle M.F. & Russell R.C.G. (1982) Skin. In Halnan K. (ed) *Treatment of Cancer*, pp. 587–606. Chapman and Hall, London.
7 Von Essen C.V. (1960) Roentgen therapy of skin and lip carcinoma: factors influencing success and failure. *American Journal of Roentgenology, Radium Therapy and Nuclear Medicine* **83**, 556–70.
8 Klein E., Stall H.L., Milgrom M., Melin F. & Walker M.J. (1971) Tumours of the skin XII. Topical 5-fluorouracil for epidermal neoplasms. *Journal of Surgical Oncology* **3**, 33.
9 Elwood J.M. & Lee J.A.H. (1975) Recent data on the epidemiology of malignant melanoma. *Seminars in Oncology* **2**, 149–54.
10 Lancaster H.O. & Nelson J. (1957) Sunlight as a cause of melanoma: A clinical survey. *Medical Journal of Australia* **1**, 452–6.
11 Anderson D.E., Smith J. & McBride C.M. (1967) Hereditary aspects of malignant melanoma. *Journal of American Medical Association*, **200**, 741.
12 Clark W.H., From L., Bernadino E.A. & Mihn N.C. (1969) The histogenesis and biologic behaviour of primary human malignant melanomas of the skin. *Cancer Research* **29**, 705.
13 Breslow A. (1975) Tumor thickness level of invasion and node dissection in stage I cutaneous melanoma. *Annals of Surgery* **182**, 572.

14 DeVita V.T. & Fisher R.I. (1976) Natural history of malignant melanoma as related to therapy. *Cancer Treatment Reports* **60,** 153–7.

15 Wong C.K. (1970) A study of melanocytes in the normal skin surrounding malignant melanomata. *Dermatologica* **141,** 215–25.

16 Everall J.D. & Dowd P.M. (1977) Diagnosis, Prognosis & Treatment of Melanoma. *Lancet* **ii,** 286–9.

17 Davis N.C., McLeod R., Beardmore G., Little J., Quinn R. & Holt J. (1976) Melanoma is a word, not a sentence. *Australia and New Zealand Journal of Surgery* **46,** 188.

18 Barranco S.C., Romsdahl M.M. & Humphrey R.M. (1971) Radiation response of human melanoma cells grown in vitro. *Cancer Research* **31,** 830.

19 Creech D., Ryan R.F. & Krementz E.T. (1959) Treatment of melanoma by isolated perfusion technique. *Journal of the American Medical Association* **169,** 339.

20 Morton D.L., Eilber F.R., Joseph W.L., Wood W.C., Trahan E. & Ketchan A.S. (1970) Immunological factors in human sarcomas and melanomas: A rational basis for immunotherapy. *Annals of Surgery* **72,** 740–9.

21 Overgaard J. (1980) Radiation treatment of malignant melanoma. *International Journal of Radiation Oncology Biology Physics* **6,** 641.

Chapter 23

Bone and Soft Tissue Sarcoma

INCIDENCE AND AETIOLOGY

Sarcomas are cancers of mesenchymal tissues. Although they are uncommon there is a great variety and a working classification is given in Tables 23.1 (below) and 23.2 (on p. 390). They occur in both children and adults and some types, particularly malignant bone tumours, occur most frequently in adolescents. There is a slight male preponderance. The age specific incidence is shown in Fig 23.1.

Table 23.1. Primary malignant bone tumours.

Osteosarcoma
   Variable malignancy, most benign form is parosteal osteosarcoma. Usually metaphyseal. Can be in flat bones. Age 10–20.

Ewing's Sarcoma
   High grade malignancy. Diaphyseal in long bones, often in flat bones. Age 10–20.

Chondrosarcoma
   Variable malignancy. Usually metaphyseal. Age 40–60.

Other Spindle Cell Tumours
   Malignant fibrous ⎫ Age 30–50. Long
      histiocytoma ⎪ bones. Metaphyseal
   Fibrosarcoma ⎬ usually, similar
   Haemangiopericytoma ⎪ distribution to
   Haemangioendothelioma ⎭ osteosarcoma

Other Round Cell Tumours
   Primary lymphoma of bone
   Mesenchymal chondrosarcoma
   Angiosarcoma

Giant Cell Tumour
   Occasionally malignant. Epiphyseal. Age 30–40.

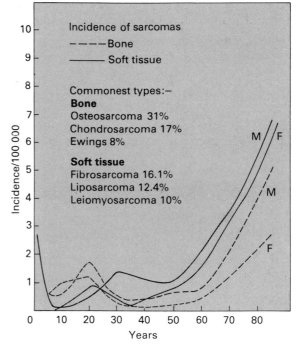

Incidence of sarcomas
- - - - Bone
——— Soft tissue

Commonest types:-
Bone
Osteosarcoma 31%
Chondrosarcoma 17%
Ewings 8%

Soft tissue
Fibrosarcoma 16.1%
Liposarcoma 12.4%
Leiomyosarcoma 10%

Fig. 23.1. *Age-specific incidence of soft tissue and bone sarcomas.*

Very little is known of their aetiology. Most cases are sporadic though a few families have been reported where two siblings have developed a soft tissue sarcoma. Patients with von Recklinghausen's disease have a tendency towards malignant change in fibromatous or neurofibromatous lesions (neurofibrosarcoma is the typical tumour type). Osteosarcoma may develop in long standing Paget's disease, usually in the elderly. Occasionally, a soft tissue or bone sarcoma develops in a previously irra-

Table 23.2. Soft tissue sarcoma.

Tissue of origin	Benign neoplasm	Sarcoma(s)
Fibrous tissue	Fibroma (single or multiple, as in fibromatosis)	Fibrosarcoma (including dermatofibrosarcoma protruberans)
Muscle *Striated*	Rhabdomyoma	Rhabdomyosarcoma Embryonal Alveolar Pleomorphic Botryoidal
Smooth	Leiomyoma (including uterine 'fibroids')	Leiomyosarcoma
'Histiocytic' tissue		Malignant fibrous histiocytoma of soft tissue or bone
Fat	Lipoma	Liposarcoma
Blood vessels	Angioma, haemangioma	Haemangiosarcoma, Kaposi sarcoma, lymphangiosarcoma, haemagiopericytoma
Peripheral nerves	Neuroma, neurofibroma neurilemmoma (incl Schwannoma)	Neurofibrosarcoma, malignant neurilemmoma (including malignant Schwannoma and neuroepithelioma)
Pleura and peritoneum		Mesothelioma
Synovium		Synovial cell sarcoma
Others		Alveolar soft parts sarcoma (malignant non-chromaffin paraganglioma)

diated area, e.g. chondrosarcoma of scapula following post-mastectomy irradiation of the chest wall. Osteosarcoma of the jaw was reportedly more common in patients in the luminous watch dial trade who regularly ingested radioactive material and angiosarcoma of the liver occurs more frequently in workers who are chronically exposed to polyvinylchloride (PVC). Patients with gross lymphoedema may rarely develop a lymphangiosarcoma of the oedematous limb (Stewart-Treves syndrome). Kaposi's sarcoma is one of the malignant tumours most characteristically seen in the acquired immune deficiency syndrome (AIDS). Kaposi's sarcoma is a hundred times more frequent in Africans than in Caucasians and is also more frequent in Jewish and Italian males. It is more common in patients with Hodgkin's disease.

PRIMARY MALIGNANT BONE TUMOURS

Although rare, primary malignant bone tumours are very important and their management is changing. Until the late 1960s the treatment was usually by amputation or radiotherapy alone, and the results were poor, osteosarcoma and Ewing's tumour being cured in only 10–20% of patients.

In recent years the management of malignant bone tumours has changed considerably. Local control of disease can now sometimes be achieved without amputation by the use of internal prosthetic replacement. The use of intensive chemotherapy pre- and postoperatively has prolonged survival in both Ewing's tumour and osteosarcoma.

These changes have meant that the management of these uncommon tumours has become highly specialized. There is, therefore, a great deal to be said for treating these cases in centres with special experience in the complex surgery and chemotherapy which is increasingly employed.

Osteosarcoma

This is the commonest malignant tumour of bone (31%) and accounts for 3–4% of all childhood malignancies. In Britain there are approximately 150 new cases each year. The term *osteosarcoma* is now preferred to osteogenic sarcoma which is confusing because many different bone tumours make bone within their substance.

PATHOLOGY

The tumour consists of malignant osteoblasts which make osteoid. Within the tumour there may be areas of chrondroblastic or fibroblastic differentiation so that small biopsies may not be representative. The histological differential diagnosis includes other forms of primary malignant bone tumour or soft tissue sarcoma, especially malignant fibrous histiocytoma if the biopsy obtains only soft tissue. Histological grading of the degree of malignancy gives a rough guide to prognosis and is a prognostic variable which is taken into account in assessing comparisons between treatments. The tumours characteristically spread to the soft tissue around the bone and also along the medulla. Metastases to the lung are extremely common and usually occur within the first 18 months. Bone metastases also occur but less frequently.

Juxtacortical (parosteal) osteosarcoma is an unusual variant in which new bone formation is especially dense and which presents as a large exostosis. The pathology and clinical behaviour is less malignant (1). A further variant, *periosteal osteosarcoma*, has an intermediate degree of malignancy. Osteosarcoma arising in Paget's disease occurs in an older age group and often

occurs in flat bones. The tumours are usually agressive and metastases occur early.

CLINICAL FEATURES

The disease mostly affects adolescents, the peak incidence being in the age range 10–20 years during the adolescent growth spurt. Boys are affected more often (1.5:1). Most of the tumours occur round the knee and the lower femur and upper tibia account for 60% of all cases. The presentation is with pain and swelling, often brought to attention by a minor trauma. On examination there is usually a firm swelling which may be warm and tender with limitation of movement of the joint (2).

RADIOLOGICAL APPEARANCES

Generally there is a destructive lesion in the metaphyseal region, usually but not always

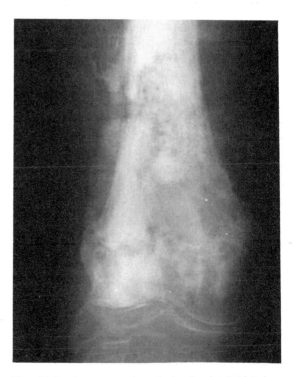

Fig. 23.2. *Osteosarcoma of the lower left femur.* There is extensive bone destruction with elevation of the periosteum and new bone formation.

with new bone formation in spicules. There may be a Codman's triangle caused by elevation of the periosteum (Fig. 23.2). The parosteal variety is associated with slow growth, exostosis and dense new bone, and the telangiectatic type with rapidly progressive destruction. The way in which the radiological appearances are produced by the tumour extension is clearly shown in X-rays of thin sections taken though the whole specimen (Fig. 23.3).

INVESTIGATION

Routine investigation should include chest X-ray which will show pulmonary metastases in approximately 20% of cases, isotope bone scan which may show skeletal metastases and a CT scan of the thorax. This should be performed before surgery since CT scanning is a more sensitive method of detecting pulmonary metastases than conventional whole lung tomogra-

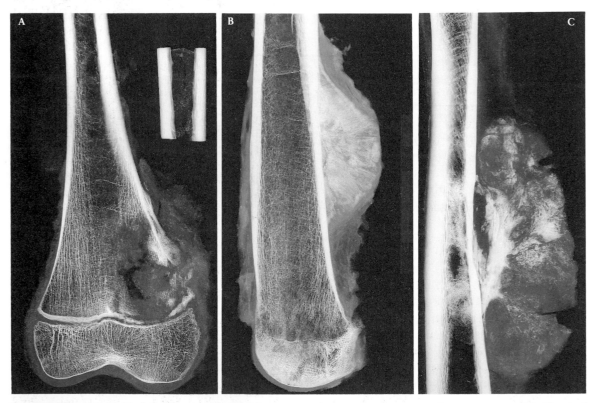

Fig. 23.3. *Fine detail X-rays of sagittal longitudinal slabs of resection specimens of osteosarcoma.* (A) Classical osteosarcoma of distal femur in a boy aged 14 years. The lesion stops at the unfused epiphysis. It is destroying the cortex and extends subperiosteally, lifting the periosteum and forming a Codman's triangle. There are spicules of new bone formation. This is the commonest site for osteosarcoma. (B) Parosteal osteosarcoma in an 18 year old male, arising from the posterior aspect of the distal femur (the typical site of this tumour). The tumour is confined to the outer aspect of the cortex and contains trabecular bone which is covered with fibrous tissue on the outer surface. The bone cortex is intact and the medulla is not involved. The fused epiphysis is visible. (C) Periosteal osteosarcoma of the mid femur in a woman aged 50 years. The tumour is made up of radiolucent tumour cartilage and shows patchy calcification. In a few places there is a trabecular pattern with mineralized tumour osteoid. There is involvement of the subadjacent medulla.
(We are greatly indebted to Dr Jean Pringle and Mr Hugh Kemp of the Royal National Orthopaedic Hospital, for these preparations.)

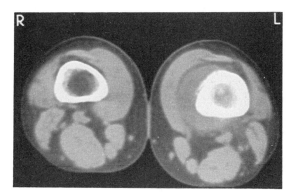

Fig. 23.4. *CT scan of osteosarcoma of the left femur.* At this level the bone X-ray was only slightly abnormal. The scan shows erosion of the cortex, periosteal reaction and considerable soft tissue swelling.

phy. If local resection is contemplated (see below) a CT scan of the affected limb may help to delineate tumour extent (Fig. 23.4). The serum alkaline phosphatase is frequently elevated and can be used as an approximate guide to disease activity.

TREATMENT

Surgery. Until recently, amputation was the main surgical treatment. For tumours around the knee the amputation is at mid-thigh level. To be of value the stump must extend at least 10 cm from the ischial tuberosity. Higher tumours, or those which extend high up the femoral shaft, are treated by disarticulation.

There is increasing use of conservative surgery in which a massive internal prosthesis is inserted after removal of the tumour (Fig. 23.5.). The functional results are excellent for the lower femur and upper tibia, but less satisfactory in the upper humerus. Local recurrence of the tumour is unusual in skilled hands and with the use of pre-operative chemotherapy, and local recurrences can still be successfully treated by amputation. Pathological fractures and/or extensive infiltration along the bone shaft or into soft tissue make prosthetic replacement less feasible.

Radiotherapy. In the days before chemotherapy, high dose radiotherapy to the primary

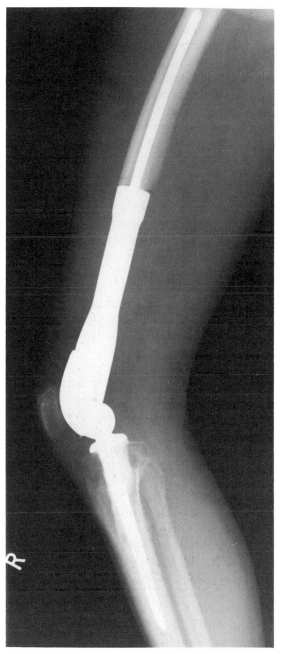

Fig. 23.5. *Endoprosthetic replacement of osteosarcoma of the distal femur.* Following chemotherapy the tumour was resected and the lower femur and knee replaced by the prosthesis. Chemotherapy was then continued for 3 months. This patient walks normally, can run, and climb stairs. (We are indebted to Mr Hugh Kemp and Professor John Scales for permission to show this X-ray.)

tumour was employed in order to avoid amputation in those destined to die of metastases (3). If these did not occur within 6–12 months a delayed amputation was performed. Unfortunately, local radiotherapy seldom provides long lasting control of the primary and local recurrence and fractures often occur. Radiotherapy is still of great value in palliation of an advanced tumour and in treatment of painful bone metastases.

There has been considerable interest in the use of low dose whole lung irradiation in the 'prevention' of pulmonary metastases. In reality the radiotherapy is to treat established but invisible metastases. Doses around 17.5 Gy in 20 fractions are usually used—which does not result in radiation pneumonitis. Some studies have shown prevention, or delay in onset, of pulmonary metastases, others have not and the value of this treatment is undecided. Its use has been superceded by chemotherapy.

Chemotherapy. Early experience with alkylating agents indicated that metastatic osteosarcoma was seldom responsive to chemotherapy (4). In the early 1970s very high dose methotrexate with folinic acid rescue was shown to produce regression in 40% of patients with pulmonary metastases from osteosarcoma (5), though these responses were usually short-lived. Methotrexate was then used as adjuvant therapy after amputation. Although the results looked encouraging at first (Fig 23.6), it later became apparent that metastasis with this regimen was delayed but not prevented (6).

Other drugs have also been shown to have activity in established disease. Cisplatin is associated with a response rate of about 25% and doxorubicin about 30%. Full dosage seems to be essential to produce regression and this may be a problem when the drugs are combined and the dose of effective agents reduced to prevent cumulative toxicities. Numerous other adjuvant studies have been undertaken using various combinations of methotrexate, doxorubicin and cisplatin, as well as other agents. In general most studies have shown over 50% freedom

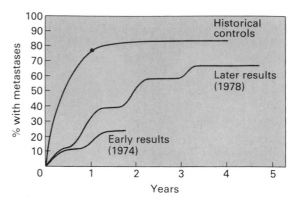

Fig. 23.6. *Probability of lung metastases in osteosarcoma treated by surgery alone (historical controls), or by surgery with adjuvant chemotherapy. The initial results (1974) seem to have been over-optimistic.*

from relapse at 1–3 years. It is now clear that this represents a significant advance over surgery alone since the natural history of osteosarcoma does not seem to have changed for the better in the last 10–15 years (see below).

Recently there have been attempts to produce tumour reduction by intensive pre-operative chemotherapy (Fig. 23.7). These intensive regimens usually employ very high dose methotrexate given weekly, combined with doxorubicin and other agents such as cisplatin. The aim is to use chemotherapy early to attack micro-metastases, to assess the clinical and pathological response of the primary tumour to drugs, to facilitate surgery because of reduction in tumour mass and soft tissue infiltration, and to allow time for prostheses to be made. The very intensive drug regimens have given 50–75% disease free survivals at a median follow-up of 3 years (7). It is perhaps too soon to know if metastases are delayed rather than prevented and if the use of chemotherapy pre-operatively, rather than after surgery, really offers an advantage. The early results are undoubtedly impressive but other factors than the chemotherapy have almost certainly contributed. These include earlier diagnosis, better staging and careful selection for surgery. However, a recent study has now been performed in which there was an untreated control arm. This study

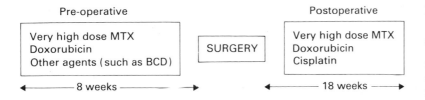

Pre-operative		Postoperative
Very high dose MTX Doxorubicin Other agents (such as BCD)	SURGERY	Very high dose MTX Doxorubicin Cisplatin
←——— 8 weeks ———→		←——— 18 weeks ———→

Fig. 23.7. *Schematic representation of a typical chemotherapy programme for osteosarcoma.* BCD is a combination of bleomycin, cisplatin and actinomycin D. Limb preservation surgery is increasingly employed.

has demonstrated unequivocally that chemotherapy delays recurrence and increases survival.

Intra-arterial infusions have also been used to produce regressions of the primary before prosthetic replacement but the technique is still in the developmental stage. In summary, the role of adjuvant chemotherapy in osteosarcoma is still being evaluated. It is now clear that metastases are delayed or prevented by cytotoxic drugs, and probable that very intensive regimens are necessary to achieve good results.

Treatment of pulmonary metastases. Patients who develop pulmonary metastases may still be curable by surgery (8). If a patients develops a pulmonary metastasis, CT scanning should be used to see if it is solitary and operable. Adjuvant chemotherapy after amputation may not only delay or prevent pulmonary metastases but may also benefit patients by reducing the number of pulmonary metastases when they do occur. This may allow a potentially curative resection. When a metastasis is detected chemotherapy is started using agents which have not previously been given, and if no new metastases have appeared within 2–3 months, thoracotomy should be undertaken. This approach helps to prevent needless thoracotomies in patients destined to develop further pulmonary metastases soon and to die quickly of their disease.

Chondrosarcoma

This is the second commonest bone tumour but occurs later in life than osteosarcoma, with a peak incidence at 40–60 years. It may arise *de novo* as a sarcomatous transformation of benign enchondromata, in multiple enchondro-matosis (Ollier's disease) and, rarely, in Paget's disease.

PRESENTATION

These tumours are usually slow growing. The commonest site is the pelvis, followed by the femur, humerus, scapula and ribs. The most usual symptom is of a painful swelling, but in

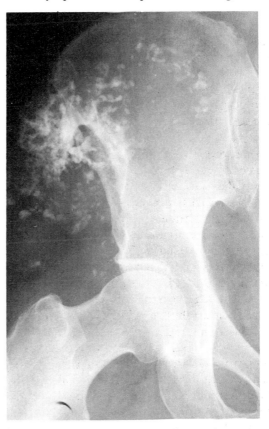

Fig. 23.8. *Chondrosarcoma of the ilium.* The ilium is eroded by the tumour which shows patchy calcification. The tumour extends into the soft tissues laterally.

slow growing lesions pain may not be a symptom at first. The disease tends to grow more rapidly in younger patients.

The X-ray typically shows a destructive bone lesion with areas of calcification normally as flecks (rather than spicules as in osteosarcoma) (Fig. 23.8).

PATHOLOGY

This is a spindle cell sarcoma containing cartilage but without tumour osteoid being formed. Low-grade tumours tend to be locally invasive and not to metastasise but pulmonary metastases are frequent in high-grade tumours. Sometimes low-grade tumours change to a more malignant variety after repeated local recurrence. Some types of chondrosarcoma have areas of small cell differentiation similar to Ewing's sarcoma. In young adults the histology is usually higher grade and the tumours tend to be in flat bones and unresectable.

TREATMENT

The mainstay of treatment is surgery with complete removal of the tumour with associated soft tissues. In a long bone this can sometimes be accomplished, without amputation, by *en bloc* resection and insertion of an endoprosthesis. In the pelvis a surgical approach is often impossible. Radiotherapy is used as a palliative treatment but the tumour is radioresistant and local control is usually short-lived. From the little evidence available the tumour also appears to be resistant to cytotoxic drugs.

Ewing's sarcoma

This is a malignant round cell tumour of bone whose aetiology is unknown. The peak incidence is 10–20 years of age and like osteosarcoma it is slightly more common in males (1.5:1).

PRESENTATION

Pain and swelling are the usual symptoms and may be present for many months before diagnosis. Pulmonary symptoms, due to metastases,

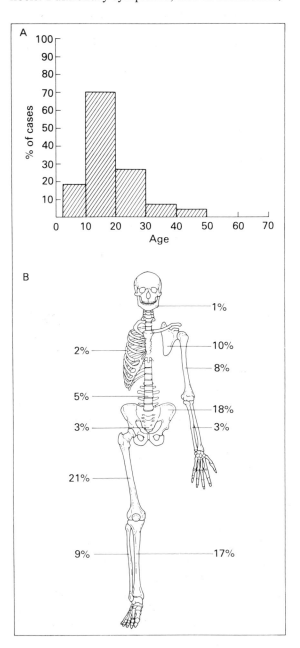

Fig. 23.9. *Ewing's sarcoma* (A) Age at onset; (B) site of primary tumour.

may first bring the patient to the doctor. The flat bones of the pelvis are the commonest site of involvement though the femur is the commonest single bone to be involved, and the tibia and humerus less frequently. The diaphyseal region is usually affected. The tumour can also arise in the vertebrae, skull and ribs (Fig. 23.9). Fever and weight loss are not infrequent and nodal spread may occur.

PATHOLOGY

The tumour usually arises in the diaphysis and occasionally the metaphysis. Epiphyseal involvement is exceptional. Histologically it consists of small round cells. It resembles, and has to be distinguished from, non-Hodgkin's lymphoma, metastatic neuroblastoma and some types of rhabdomyosarcoma. Glycogen can often be demonstrated in the cytoplasm by the PAS stain and the distinction from these other tumours can usually be made on clinical, radiological and biochemical grounds. Occasionally the diagnosis can be very difficult and newer techniques of diagnosis of lymphomas (by demonstrating surface immunoglobulin for example) and neuroblastoma (by monoclonal antibodies against cell surface antigens) may prove valuable in the future.

From the point of view of treatment, the whole bone should be regarded as involved due to spread through the medullary cavity. Metastases to lung and to other bones occur frequently.

INVESTIGATION

Diagnosis is by biopsy and expert opinion on the histology. The X-ray usually shows a diffuse erosion in a flat bone (Fig. 23.10) or in the diaphyseal region of a long bone (Fig. 23.11). There is a marked periosteal reaction sometimes with an 'onion skin' appearance, usually with evidence of a soft tissue mass which is often extensive.

Further investigation should include a full blood count which may show anaemia and leu-

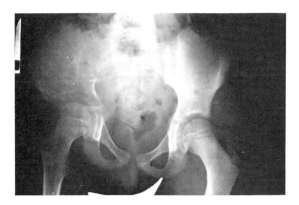

Fig. 23.10. *Ewing's sarcoma of the right ilium.* The bone is diffusely expanded by a large radiolucent tumour

cocytosis in advanced or rapidly progressive cases; chest X-ray, CT scan of the primary site and of the thorax which may show single or multiple metastases; isotope bone scan to detect bone metastases which are common; plasma LDH and liver function tests; and urine VMA if there is a possibility that the diagnosis is neuroblastoma.

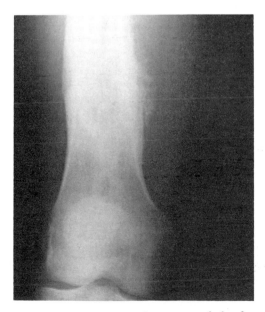

Fig. 23.11. *X-ray of Ewing's tumour of the femur.* Note the diaphyseal position, the periosteal elevation, and the new bone formation.

TREATMENT

This must be both local and systemic. Local treatment alone is associated with cure in only 10–20% of cases (9) and the prognosis has been improved considerably by the addition of adjuvant combination chemotherapy.

Local treatment. Unlike most primary bone sarcomas Ewing's sarcoma is highly radiosensitive. For this reason the mainstay of treatment is radical megavoltage radiotherapy. Doses of 60–70 Gy are given to the primary site in 2 Gy fractions, over 6–8 weeks. Care must be taken not to irradiate all the soft tissues of a limb to this dose, or troublesome oedema will occur below the irradiated site. In practice this involves careful avoidance of a strip of soft tissue the whole length of the treatment field (Fig. 23.12). Additionally the last 15–20 Gy are given to a smaller field around the residual tumour,

i.e. using a 'shrinking field' technique. Surgical excision of the lesion is often impractical but small, accessible tumours in, for example, the clavicle or rib, can sometimes be excised. In recent years troublesome late local recurrences have been seen in some patients after treatment with radiotherapy and chemotherapy. For this reason there is some interest in surgical excision and endoprosthetic replacement of bone as an adjuvant to chemotherapy and radiotherapy.

Chemotherapy. Adjuvant chemotherapy is an essential part of management and has been responsible for the improved prognosis in recent years (10). The four most useful agents are doxorubicin, cyclophosphamide, vincristine and actinomycin D. Responses are also seen with methotrexate and nitrosoureas. A variety of different combinations are in use, with none showing a clear superiority. It is probable that all four first line agents should be used, that the dose of drugs should be kept as high as possible. In recent years the tendency has been to use chemotherapy very intensively over a period of 6 months rather than to use lower doses for 1–2 years. The patient must be kept under regular review during this time with regular

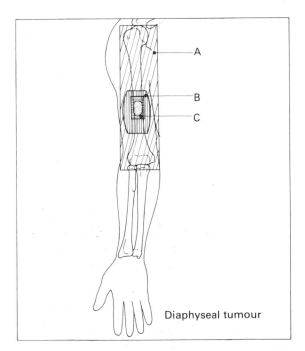

Fig. 23.12. *Radiation fields in Ewing's sarcoma.* (A) The whole bone is irradiated to a modest dose (30 Gy). (B) The field is shrunk down to the tumour and adjacent bone to 45 Gy. (C) The tumour itself is boosted to 60–70 Gy.

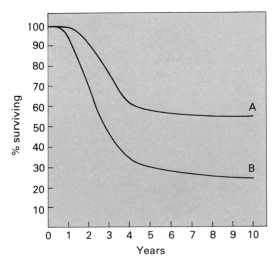

Fig. 23.13. *Prognosis in Ewing's sarcoma.* All cases treated with radiotherapy and combination chemotherapy. (A) Limb tumours. (B) Axial skeleton tumours. (Data from several sources.)

blood counts and chest X-rays, with bone scans when clinically indicated.

PROGNOSIS

In localized disease, the use of radical local treatment with the most intensive chemotherapy regimens (11) has led to 30–60% 5-year survival (Fig. 23.13). Most of these children have probably been cured. Although many factors have contributed to this improved survival there is little doubt that chemotherapy has been the major influence. Pelvic lesions have a worse prognosis than limb tumours.

Giant cell tumour of bone (osteoclastoma)

This tumour occurs at the age of 20–40 years and typically involves the epiphysis of a long bone (12). It causes a well defined lytic lesion which eventually erodes the cortex of the bone, giving rise to soft tissue extension. The presentation is with pain and swelling typically around the knee, the tumour occurring with equal frequency on the lower femur and upper tibia. X-ray shows a lytic lesion. Similar cystic changes can be caused by aneurysmal bone cysts or the cystic lesion of osteitis fibrosa cystica (primary hyperparathyroidism).

Pathologically the tumour consists of giant cells and spindle cells. Occasionally the appearances are frankly malignant and the tumour is then more locally invasive and metastases may occur. The tumours can be graded (I–III) according to the appearance of the stromal cells. There is some dispute about whether radiation treatment encourages malignant transformation. This is an uncommon development in the tumour and usually it is the more aggressive (grade III) tumours which are irradiated, so the issue is not clear.

The treatment is usually by thorough curettage of the entire cavity of a localized lesion. The cavity can be obliterated by bone chips. More extensive lesions can be treated by excision and endoprosthetic replacement of bone. Some tumours are not amenable to surgery, for example those in vertebrae. In these cases, ra-

diothapy at modest dose (40–50 Gy) over 4–5 weeks is the mainstay of treatment. There is no known effective chemotherapy although methotrexate has been used.

Other malignant spindle cell tumours of bone
(Malignant fibrous histiocytoma, fibrosarcoma, haemangiopericytoma, haemangioendothelioma)

These tumours have a similar anatomical distribution to osteosarcoma but occur in the age range 30–50 years, and in the diaphysis a little more commonly. The fibrosarcomas are often of very low grade. Many of the tumours are associated with a long history of pain before the diagnosis is established by X-ray followed by biopsy. Haemangioendothelioma has a propensity to occur in many bones at presentation, or with patchy involvement at several sites in the same bone. Treatment is by excision. High-grade tumours and malignant fibrous histiocytoma are often treated with chemotherapy as well, but the rarity of the tumours makes it difficult to be sure whether any benefit is conferred by systemic treatment. Like osteosarcoma they tend to be resistent to radiotherapy, though radiotherapy may be helpful as an adjuvant to surgery, or for local recurrence.

Other round cell tumours of bone (Primary lymphoma of bone, mesenchymal chondrosarcoma, angiosarcoma)

This heterogenous group of tumours are usually of high-grade malignancy with a propensity for metastasis, so systemic treatment with chemotherapy is usually employed.

NON-HODGKIN'S LYMPHOMA OF BONE

Non-Hodgkin's lymphoma may occur in bone and may be completely localized with no evidence of disease elsewhere, even with extensive investigation. Nevertheless, the risk of spread is great. The tumours are lytic and destructive typically having ill defined margins. A soft tissue mass is often present. Radiotherapy in a modest dose (30–40 Gy) controls the local disease but in young adults or children systemic chemotherapy is given if there is any doubt about whether the tumour is localized (see Chapter 26). In the older patients with clinically localized disease it is permissible to follow an expectant policy and treat with cytotoxic agents only when signs of spread appear.

MESENCHYMAL CHONDROSARCOMA

Pathologically this is a small round cell tumour of bone within which are areas of rudimentary cartilaginous differentiation. The tumours occur in the skull, ribs and pelvis, but are uncommon in long bones. They may also occur in soft tissues and in the meninges. Treatment is normally with resection, if possible, or by radiation therapy. Chemotherapy may be given subsequently, with agents effective against soft tissue sarcoma.

ANGIOSARCOMA

This is an exceedingly rare undifferentiated tumour. Treatment is normally with radiation and chemotherapy using similar agents to those effective against Ewing's tumour.

SOFT TISSUE SARCOMAS

Progress in the management of adult sarcomas has been hampered by the relative rarity and heterogeneity of these tumours, which makes it difficult for any single clinic or cooperative group to develop a large experience. In addition, they are unresponsive to radiotherapy and chemotherapy and many of these tumours have a high incidence of local recurrence after surgery. Although few advances have been made in adults the clinical behaviour of these tumours is at least becoming clearer, and one or two important points in management have begun to emerge over the past few years. In childhood sarcomas the picture is different,

with some degree of responsiveness to chemotherapy proving the rule, leading in many instances to an improvement in survival rate (see Chapter 24). This difference is largely due to a recognition of important differences in histological subtypes between typical childhood and adult sarcomas, of which the childhood preponderance of embryonal rhabdomyosarcoma is perhaps the best example.

Pathology and clinical features (13)

Soft tissue sarcomas can arise wherever mesenchymal tissue is present (Table 23.2). The commonest varieties in adults result from malignant transformation of fibrous tissue (fibrosarcomas); striated muscle (rhabdomyosarcoma); smooth muscle (leiomyosarcoma); 'histiocytic tissue' (malignant fibrous histiocytoma); fat (liposarcoma) and blood vessels (haemangiopericyoma, angiosarcoma and Kaposi's sarcoma). Tumours of peripheral nerves (Schwannoma, neurofibrosarcoma, etc.) are discussed in Chapter 11 and mesothelioma in Chapter 12. Other rarer tumours occur and are discussed below.

FIBROSARCOMA

These tumours are composed of fusiform fibroblasts which form collagen strands and reticulin. The histological definition of malignancy may be difficult and well-differentiated tumours such as dermatofibrosarcoma protruberans seldom metastasize but may be locally invasive. Anaplastic tumours invade locally and also spread rapidly to the lungs.

These tumours usually arise on the limbs or trunk but may occur in any soft tissue. Typically, the patient notices a painless firm lump. In dermatofibrosarcoma protruberans, the history is of a slowly enlarging skin nodule becoming violaceous and later ulcerating.

MALIGNANT FIBROUS HISTIOCYTOMA

In the last 10 years this has become more widely recognized as a pathological entity. It is not a new disease and cases previously diagnosed as poorly differentiated fibrosarcoma or pleomorphic rhabdomyosarcomas are now often included in this category. The cell of origin is not known. The typical histological pattern is one of malignant spindle cells often arranged in a 'storiform' or herringbone fashion. As with fibrosarcomas the presentation is usually with a painless lump or nodule though this tumour can also occur as a primary bone tumour (see p. 399).

LIPOSARCOMA

These tumours arise in fat. The well-differentiated neoplasm has areas of mature fat and myxoid cells and may remain localized for several years. Poorly differentiated tumours are pleomorphic, contain numerous giant cells and metastasize to the lungs. Clinically, these tumours present in middle age and occur in subcutaneous fat and in retroperitoneal tissues. They do not arise from pre-existing lipomas.

RHABDOMYOSARCOMA

This is a complex group of tumours with several distinct subtypes:

Embryonal rhabdomyosarcoma. These tumours occur in early childhood and young adult life. They consist of malignant spindle and round cells, and usually occur in the head and neck and orbit (see Chapter 24).

Alveolar rhabdomyosarcoma. This tumour is composed of large, round and polygonal cells. It occurs in adolescents and young adults and has a wider distribution, often presenting in the trunk. They are highly malignant and metastasize early.

Pleomorphic rhabdomyosarcoma. In these tumours the cells vary greatly in size and shape and giant cells are often present. Many are now classified as malignant fibrous histiocytoma.

They occur in adult life (over the age of 30 years), usually on the limbs, arising from deep muscle groups.

Botryoidal rhabdomyosarcoma ('sarcoma botryoides'). These tumours consist of polypoid growths in the urinary and genital tracts, usually in young children. Histologically the tumour consists of an area of cells with high mitotic activity surrounded by acellular oedematous tissue.

LEIOMYOSARCOMA

The uterus is much the commonest site of origin, and it is thought that the tumours usually occur as a result of malignant change in a uterine fibroid (leiomyoma). The histological diagnosis is usually made after hysterectomy for fibroids. Other leiomyosarcomas arise from smooth muscle at other sites such as subcutaneous tissue and retroperitoneum.

SYNOVIAL SARCOMA

These tumours arise in synovial tissue of joints, bursae and tendon sheaths. They occur in young adults, especially in the hands, feet and knees but do not involve the joint lining. They present as hard lumps near a joint. Local spread and metastasis occur and local recurrence after excision is frequent.

ANGIOSARCOMA AND HAEMANGIOPERICYTOMA

Angiosarcomas are rare, highly malignant neoplasms arising from the vascular endothelium itself. Rarely, they arise in the liver (see Chapter 15). Haemangiopericytoma (glomus tumour) is thought to arise from the contractile cells (pericytes) in small blood vessels. They usually occur in the extremities and retroperitoneal space but are also found in the head and neck.

KAPOSI'S SARCOMA

This important tumour is dealt with in Chapter 22. It arises from endothelial cells and presents as pigmented skin lesions which grow slowly. Formerly, the tumour was commonest in Jewish and Italian men, and was much more frequent in West Africa than in Europe or the United States. This has changed with the recognition of the acquired immune deficiency syndrome (AIDS), in which Kaposi's sarcoma frequently occurs with a much more aggressive course.

ALVEOLAR SOFT PARTS SARCOMA

This rare neoplasm occurs in young adults, usually women. It is usually a slowly growing tumour, occurring typically in the extremities. Although lung metastases usually occur, they grow slowly and may be compatible with long survival.

EPITHELIOID SARCOMA

This is a rare tumour, recently described, occurring on the extremities and with a tendency to spread to skin, bone and draining nodes. The cell of origin is unknown, but the histological appearances can be similar to a carcinoma or chronic inflammatory lesion.

Investigation and staging

Clinical staging in soft tissue sarcoma is important for management and also offers a guide to prognosis. Chest X-ray is the most important investigation since many of these tumours metastasize to the lungs. Lymph node metastases are frequent, particularly in alveolar rhabdomyosarcoma, and Ewing's sarcoma. Other important distant sites include the liver, bone marrow and brain.

Staging investigation should therefore include chest X-ray and CT scan of the thorax if

possible, since the latter is the most sensitive means of detecting pulmonary metastases. Lymphangiography is occasionally indicated. Xeroradiography and CT scanning of the limb or other primary site may be useful to demonstrate the extent of the tumour and may be invaluable in planning the surgical approach.

Although there is no generally accepted staging system the classification proposed by Russell *et al* (14) is useful prognostically (Table 23.3).

Table 23.3. Staging of soft tissue sarcoma.

Stage 1	Low-grade tumour, no nodal or distant spread
Stage 2	Moderate grade tumour, no nodal or distant spread
Stage 3	High-grade tumour, no nodal or metastatic spread or tumour of any grade or size with nodal spread
Stage 4	Tumour of any grade with local invasion or tumour with distant metastases

Management of the primary tumour

Surgical biopsy is always required for an accurate diagnosis. Where a sarcoma is suspected pre-operatively and confirmed by frozen section, it is unwise to attempt an excision biopsy at the same procedure since such surgery is inadequate and definitive surgery must be undertaken at a second operation. This is also true when excision biopsy of a 'benign' mass has been attempted, and the diagnosis of malignancy was not suspected even at operation. Examples are leiomyosarcoma of the uterus which is usually diagnosed after hysterectomy for fibroids, and soft tissue sarcomas of the head and neck region, which frequently present with cervical lymphadenopathy rather than with the primary tumour itself.

Traditionally, radical surgery has usually been recommended for soft tissue sarcomas arising in the extremities, and amputation has been widely used. For high lesions of the thigh, this may require disarticulation or even hemipelvectomy in an attempt to control the tumour. These radical operations were introduced because of the risk of local recurrence. The common problem of distant metastases, coupled with the realization that radiotherapy can play a useful part in local control, has led over the past 10 years, to an important modification of this view. Wide surgical excision, coupled with high dose irradiation, is now increasingly accepted as a satisfactory alternative with of course a far happier outcome than can be achieved by amputation. The radiation dose must be high (at least 60 Gy in 6 weeks) to minimize the risk of local recurrence. For tumours of the limbs the dose can often be taken to 70 Gy. The affected compartment should be considered at risk and uniformly irradiated to this high dose. A strip of skin and subcutaneous tissue should be left unirradiated to allow adequate lymphatic drainage from the distal limb. A proportion of these patients develop local recurrence which may well require amputation, but wide local excision plus radical radiotherapy offers a satisfactory method of local control in the large majority (80–90%) of all patients with soft tissue sarcomas of the extremities. Surgical removal of the whole of the affected compartment ('compartmentectomy') is usually recommended. These are often technically more difficult operations than amputation, in view of the important structures which have to be preserved, as well as the need to resect a large volume of tissue with primary closure wherever possible (Fig. 23.14).

Radiotherapy treatment is also particularly valuable in soft tissue sarcomas with multiple or extensive primary sites, such as soft tissue angiosarcomas or Kaposi sarcoma. Recent reports in both of these tumours confirm a high degree of local control using wide field irradiation, sometimes in combination with surgery, with durable remissions (possibly cures) lasting 10 years and more, even in patients with multifocal sites of primary disease, for example on the scalp.

The management of soft tissue sarcomas of childhood is further discussed in Chapter 24.

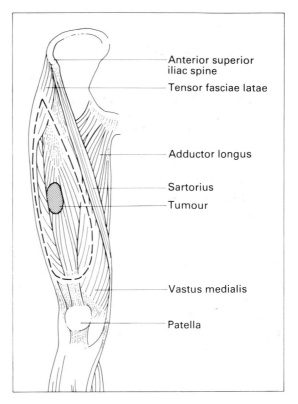

Fig. 23.14. *Compartmentectomy.* The diagram illustrates the wide surgical excision of soft tissue situated, in this case, in the rectus femoris.

CHEMOTHERAPY FOR SOFT TISSUE SARCOMAS

The past 10 years have seen a renewed interest in the chemotherapy of soft tissue sarcomas. A number of agents are effective in producing partial (or occasionally complete) remissions in patients with local recurrence and/or metastatic disease. A wide variety of agents has been shown to have activity, though in general the response rates to single agents are low and of brief duration. In the occasional patient a complete and durable response to chemotherapy is obtained. Responses of metastatic tumour lasting several years have been observed. Many classes of drug have activity (Table 23.4) including vinca alkaloids (vincristine), alkylating agents (cyclophosphamide and particularly ifosfamide), antimetabolites (particularly meth-

Table 23.4. Chemotherapy in soft tissue sarcoma.

	Response rate
Single agents	
Doxorubicin	30%
DTIC	15-20%
Cyclophosphamide	10%
Vincristine	5%
Methotrexate	15%
Cis-platinum	10%
Ifosfamide	35%
Combination Chemotherapy	
AD: doxorubicin-DTIC	30%
VAC: vincristine, actinomycin, cyclophosphamide	5%
VAC: vincristine, doxorubicin, cyclophosphamide	20%
VADIC: vincristine, doxorubicin, DTIC	40%
ACM: doxorubicin, cyclophosphamide, methotrexate	30%
CYVADIC: cyclophosphamide, vincristine, doxorubicin, DTIC	45%
CYVADACT: cyclophosphamide, vincristine, doxorubicin, actinomycin	35%

otrexate) and antitumour antibiotics (including actinomycin D and doxorubicin).

Undoubtedly, the most responsive of these tumours are the embryonal rhabdomyosarcomas, in which the success of combination regimens (particularly employing vincristine, actinomycin D, doxorubicin and cyclophosphamide) for metastatic disease has led to their routine use as adjuvant treatment immediately following local radiotherapy and/or surgery. At least 60% of patients with embryonal rhabdomyosarcomas can be cured with modern adjuvant chemotherapy and cure is even possible in patients with evidence of residual disease postoperatively and some patients with metastatic disease. The majority of these patients will be children or young adults, and these encouraging results have not so far been seen with other forms of soft tissue sarcoma.

A wide variety of single agents and combination regimens have been used (Table 23.4).

Although some groups have claimed a 42% response rate with doxorubicin and dacarbazine, a careful review of over 350 patients has indicated that the response rate is approximately 25% of patients. A much smaller proportion of patients will achieve complete response and the addition of cyclophosphamide and vincristine to these two drugs has increased the complete response rate only to about 14%, at the cost of considerable toxicity. Nonetheless it is worth reiterating that complete responses may last for years. Remissions are seen more frequently in young women with pelvic tumours (often leiomyosarcomas) than with other varieties of tumours.

New agents under active study include ifosfamide, with a reported response rate of 40%, making it perhaps the most active of all single agents yet encountered. In other centres, attempts at improving these figures have centred on the substitution of drugs in combination, for example to remove the unpleasant drug dacarbazine (DTIC) and replace it with actinomycin D. The Houston Group have studied over 400 patients treated with combinations of cyclophosphamide, vincristine, doxorubicin and either DTIC or actinomycin D (CYVADIC, CYVADACT). They concluded that the original CYVADIC regime, with a complete response rate of 14% and overall response rate of 52% was superior (15). Clearly, other large studies will be necessary to elucidate small but possibly important differences in chemotherapy effectiveness and also to monitor toxicity. If the initial promising results with ifosfamide can be confirmed, it may be possible to increase the response rate further by incorporating it into a combination programme with other active agents. These possibilities, together with a more humane approach to the management of the primary lesion, may allow us to view the next 10 years with guarded optimism.

Survival

The survival correlates with stage and site, 5-year survival for stage 1 is 80%; stage 2, 60%;

stage 3, 30%; stage 4, 10%. The more distal the tumour the better the prognosis, lymph node spread is important prognostically and is commoner in rhabdomyosarcoma and synovial sarcoma.

REFERENCES

1 Ahuja S. C., Villacin A. B., Smith A. L., Bullough P. E., Huvos A. E. & Marcove R. C. (1977) Juxtacortical (parosteal) oeteogenic sarcoma. Histological grading and prognosis. *Journal of Bone and Joint Surgery* **59**(A), 632

2 Marcove R. C., Mike V., Hajek J. V., Levin A. G. & Hutter R. V. P. (1970) Osteogenic sarcoma under the age of 21. A review of 145 operative cases. *Journal of Bone and Joint Surgery* **52**(A), 411.

3 Sweetnam R., Knowelden J & Seddon H. (1971) Bone sarcoma: treatment by irradiation, amputation or a combination of the two. *British Medical Journal* **2**, 363.

4 Friedman M. A. & Carter S. K. (1972) The therapy of osteogenic sarcoma: current status and thoughts for the future. *Journal of Surgical Oncology* **4**, 482.

5 Jaffe N. (1972) Recent advances in the chemotherapy of metastatic osteogenic sarcoma. *Cancer* **30**, 1627.

6 Jaffe N., Frei E., Watts H. & Traggis D. (1978) High dose methotrexate in osteogenic sarcoma. A 5 year experience. *Cancer Treatment Reports* **62**, 259.

7 Rosen G., Marlowe R. C. & Caparros B. (1982) Primary osteogenic sarcoma. The rationale for pre-operative chemotherapy and delayed surgery. *Cancer* **43**, 2163.

8 Goorin A. M., Delorey M. J., Lack E. E., Gelher R. D., Price K., Cassady J. R., Levey R., Tapper D., Jaffe N., Link M. & Abelson H. T. (1984) Prognostic significance of complete surgical resection of pulmonary metastases in patients with osteogenic sarcoma: analysis of 32 patients. *Journal of Clinical Oncology* **2**, 425.

9 Falk S. & Alpert M. (1967) Five-year survival of patients with Ewing's sarcoma. *Surgery, Gynaecology and Obstetrics* **124**, 319.

10 Rosen G., Caparnos B., Nirenberg A., Marlore R. C., Muvos A. G., Kosloff C., Lane J. & Murphy M. L. (1981) Ewing's sarcoma. Ten year experience with adjuvant chemotherapy. *Cancer* **47**, 2204.

11 Jaffe N., Traggis D., Sallan S. & Cassady J. R. (1976) Improved outlook for Ewing's sarcoma with combination chemotherapy (vinblastine, actinomycin D and cyclophosphamide) and radiation therapy. *Cancer* **25**, 1061.

12 Dahlin D. C., Cupps R. E., Joynson E. W. (1970) Giant cell tumours: a study of 195 cases. *Cancer* **38**, 1925.

13 Marsden H. B. (1985) The pathology of soft-tissue sarcomas with emphasis in childhood tumours. In D'Angio G. J & Evans A. E. (eds) *Bone and Soft-tissue Sarcomas*, p. 14–46, Edward Arnold, London.

14 Russell W. O., Cohen J., Enzinger F., Hajdu S. I., Heise H., Martin R. G., Meissner W., Miller W. T., Schmitz R. L. & Suit H. D. (1977) A clinical and pathological staging system for soft-tissue sarcomas. *Cancer* **40**, 1562.

15 Benjamin R. S., Gottlieb J. A., Baker L. O. & Sinkovics J. G (1976) CYVADIC *vs* CYVADACT–a randomized trial in metastatic sarcomas. *Proceedings American Association of Cancer Research and ASCO* **17**, 256.

FURTHER READING

Huvos A. G. (1979) *Bone tumours; Diagnosis, treatment and prognosis*. Saunders, Philadelphia.

D'Angio G. J & Evans A. E. (1985) *Bone and Soft-tissue sarcomas*. Edward Arnold, London.

Chapter 24
Paediatric Malignancies

INTRODUCTION: AN APPROACH TO CANCER IN CHILDREN

The diagnosis of cancer in a child is an exceptional and painful test of the strength of family life. Happy families usually cope better with the shock, grief and disruption. When the diagnosis has been made, the physician must take time to be alone with the parents explaining the diagnosis, prognosis and approach to investigation and treatment. About half of all children with cancer are cured; with many diseases a cautiously optimistic account can be given. The parents will sometimes feel angry about the diagnosis and may direct this towards the doctor. Often they feel that they have been responsible in some way, in that there is a genetic factor to which they have contributed, or that the cancer has arisen as a result of avoidable physical or mental trauma or faulty diet. They need to express these feelings and must be reassured that they are not to blame.

Talking to children and their parents requires tact, humanity, patience and a clear head. Every new case will prove an additional test of these qualities, and the doctor will have to deal with the guilt, anguish and anger of the parents as well as the physical and emotional suffering of the child. All children, except for the very youngest, need some account of why they are in hospital and what is likely to happen, and with older children and adolescents these explanations will need to be accurate and complete. It is impossible to make any generalization about how much to tell. Children of 6–8 years will understand that they are ill, and grasp the elements of treatment. At 10–11 years they will know more, and teenagers will know about cancer and leukaemia. The physician must talk to the child and try to gauge his or her feelings and understanding. For children of about 11 years or more, a personal and private relationship with the doctor is important. They often want to ask questions directly, and are anxious to avoid upsetting their parents. At other times they may feel that the truth is being filtered by their parents. The doctor should try to encourage the family to be open with each other with respect to the illness. Honesty and frankness are important in gaining the parents trust and in helping them to participate, whereas glossing over of the facts will leave them with insufficient detail to help them understand the implications of the diagnosis and treatment.

The complexity of treatment makes it difficult for any doctor to provide detailed answers to all the questions which a parent or the child might ask, but it is essential that a single experienced clinician should be seen to be in charge, so that both the patient and the parents can identify with an individual rather than a committee—always a danger whenever a large number of doctors are involved in a single patient's care.

With most childhood cancers, the disease is brought under control and the child feels and looks well, except for the side-effects of treatment. These side-effects come to dominate the illness, since the acute anxiety about the diagnosis fades with time and with the induction of a remission or disappearance of the tumour.

The nausea, vomiting and hair loss, and the disruption of school and family life because of frequent hospital trips all place a great strain on the child and family who will need support and reassurance from the medical team.

After successful treatment the long term sequelae of treatment may bring problems—intellectual and neurological impairment following brain tumours such as medulloblastoma (see Chapter 11), growth defects after extensive radiation (see Chapter 5) and infertility after chemotherapy.

If the disease recurs the implications for prognosis are usually grave. If there is still a chance of cure, intensive treatment may be needed again and the depression of morale in the child and family will make extra support necessary. If the chance of cure is slim, or non-existent, the parents must of course be told and the aims of palliative treatment explained. Many parents still hope that a cure will be found, yet they must at the same time begin to accept the likelihood of the child's death. The conflict may be great and there must be an opportunity for the family to express their feelings.

Parents may be angry that relapse has occurred and feel that they had been wrong to allow aggressive treatment with its attendant side-effects and all to no avail. This anger may be directed to the medical and nursing staff. Even at this difficult stage, gentle explanations remain important and the clinician in charge of the child will also need to remember that less experienced staff may themselves need to be reassured and supported. It is important for parents to know that freedom from pain or discomfort is usually possible, and that the child's survival will not be uselessly prolonged.

Very young children do not have an idea of death but may express their fears of separation in play or in conversation. Adolescents will usually have an adult perception of death. In dealing with a dying child the doctors should allow the patient and family to indicate how far and fast they wish to go in discussion and should not force unpalatable facts upon them.

Many families need to retain some hope of recovery in dealing with the situation. At the same time 'anticipatory mourning' may begin and the doctor must be prepared to listen to expressions of anger and grief as part of the process of acceptance that the child will die.

TUMOURS OF CHILDHOOD

Although all childhood tumours are uncommon, cancer is the commonest natural cause of death in childhood, and, of all causes, second only to accidents. Despite this chilling statistic, extraordinary advances have been made in the management of almost all of the common childhood tumours. Whereas 30 years ago it was unusual even to see the slightest response to treatment, nowadays with a better understanding of the diseases and far more effective treatments, some degree of responsiveness is the rule, and cure is frequently achieved (Table 24.1). As treatment policies become more sophisticated, paediatric oncology has become a specialized branch of cancer treatment. The purpose of this chapter will therefore be to outline general treatment principles and to emphasise the multimodal or team approach.

Table 24.1. Relative frequency and survival in childhood cancer.

Tumour	% of total cases	% 5-year survival
Leukaemia	31	
acute lymphoblastic		50
acute myeloblastic		15
Brain tumours	19	40
Lymphoma	13	
Hodgkin's disease		85
non-Hodgkin's		68
Neuroblastoma	7	25
Soft tissue sarcoma	7	60
Wilms' tumour	6	80
Bone sarcoma	4	45
Retinoblastoma	3	95
Germ cell tumour	2	77

There is little doubt that childhood cancer is best treated in a specialized paediatric oncology centre. With some tumours, the chances of survival are possibly improved by 10–15%. Conversely in cancers such as Wilms' tumour, while results are equal in non-specialist and specialist centres, this is at the expense of overtreatment in the non-specialist hospitals.

Aetiology and incidence

Little is known of the aetiology of childhood tumours. Ionizing radiation may be a predisposing cause, either when given during pregnancy or as a result of deliberate irradiation, for example to the thymus for thymic hyperplasia which has been responsible for an increased risk of thyroid carcinoma. Transplacental carcinogens have long been thought to be a possible cause of childhood cancer, but have been difficult to identify until the recent demonstration of the association of adenocarcinoma of the vagina with treatment of the mother 20 years previously with diethylstilboestrol for early threatened abortion (1).

Genetic factors are occasionally involved. These are discussed in more detail in Chapter 3 and are listed in Table 3.2. One of the best known examples is retinoblastoma, which has a marked familial incidence particularly in the bilateral form of the disease, where half the offspring of affected children will themselves develop the disease. Some congenital malformations appear to be associated with paediatric tumours. There is a greatly increased risk of tumours (usually neurogenic sarcomas) developing in children with Von Recklinghausen's disease. The rare syndrome of hemihypertrophy may be associated both with Wilms' tumour and hepatoblastoma. Wilms' tumour can be associated with aniridia and a wide variety of congenital abnormalities.

Apart from inherited chromosomal abnormalities (Table 3.2), there is some evidence of a familial risk in childhood cancer. One study (2) identified 38 families (from more than 5000 patients) where there was cancer in 2 or more

children. Siblings of children with brain tumours have an excess mortality from sarcomas and gliomas. If a child with an identical twin develops acute leukaemia, then the risk of the twin also developing this disease is high. The overall risk of cancer in childhood is 1:600, but in siblings 1:300.

Geographic and racial variations also exist, which may eventually throw further light on aetiology. Liver cancer is commoner in the Far East, retinoblastoma in India, intestinal lymphoma in Israel and Burkitt's lymphoma in Uganda. In Britain and United States the proportion of various groups of tumours is reasonably constant; 20–25% consist of tumours of the CNS and eye, 33% are leukaemias, and 35% are solid tumours (chiefly Wilms' tumour and neuroblastoma). Most of these tumours have their maximal incidence at ages 0–4 years, though some, such as bone tumours and lymphomas have a later peak, between 6 and 14 years. In general, younger children appear to have a better survival than older groups particularly with neuroblastoma and retinoblastoma. With the relative improvement in treatments of other paediatric illnesses, cancer has assumed an increased importance as a cause of death despite the many advances in management.

Childhood tumours of the CNS are common, and are discussed with adult brain tumours in Chapter 11; leukaemia in Chapter 28, and paediatric lymphomas in Chapter 26.

Neuroblastoma

After brain tumours, leukaemia and lymphoma, neuroblastoma is the commonest of paediatric tumours, accounting for some 7% of the total. Over 80% of cases occur below 4 years of age. Most cases are sporadic but there are reports of twins with both affected, as well as families with 2 or more affected siblings.

PATHOLOGY

Neuroblastomas arise from neural crest tissue, which normally develops into the adrenal med-

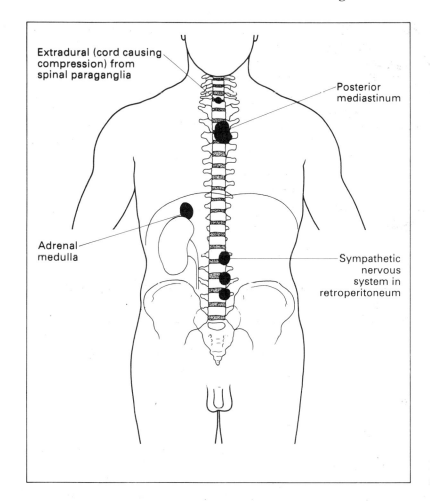

Extradural (cord causing compression) from spinal paraganglia

Posterior mediastinum

Adrenal medulla

Sympathetic nervous system in retroperitoneum

Fig. 24.1. *Common primary sites of neuroblastoma.*

ulla and sympathetic ganglia. The common primary sites are therefore the adrenal medulla and in sympathetic nervous tissue in the retroperitoneum. However, tumours may also arise in the posterior mediastinum and spine, predominantly extradurally from paravertebral ganglia (Fig. 24.1). Because of the common cell of origin, neuroblastomas are closely related to both ganglioneuromas, which are seldom malignant, and phaechromocytomas. Because of their derivation from the adrenal medulla, elaboration and secretion of adrenal medullary hormones or metabolites are characteristic of this tumour (see below).

The tumour is composed of small cells with scanty cytoplasm, often in lobules with inter-vening fibrous or fibrovascular septa and with evidence of neurofibrillary tissue, often arranged as rosettes. Wide variations in degree of differentiation are seen, sometimes in a single specimen. Neuroblastomas are almost always PAS negative, unlike Ewing's sarcoma, rhabdomyosarcoma or ganglion cell tumours. Immunocytochemical techniques, using monoclonal antibodies to neuroblastoma-associated antigens, have proved helpful in diagnosis of difficult cases. Electron microscopically, the tumour cells contain electron-dense granules and in this respect are similar to tumours of the APUD system (see Chapter 15). Whilst adrenal primaries tend to be encapsulated, those arising retroperitoneally and in the mediastinum tend to infiltrate and become fixed so that surgery is usually more difficult.

Neuroblastomas tend to spread very widely (Fig. 24.2), by local, lymphatic and haemotogenous routes, and important sites of blood borne dissemination include the bone marrow (often forming clusters of large, poorly differentiated cells), the liver (sometimes resulting in enormous hepatomegaly) and bone (often with a single destructive lesion as the typical neuroblastoma deposit). Unlike other paediatric soft tissue tumours, the lungs are seldom the site of metastases. Skin and periorbital metastases are common. An unusual characteristic is the abil-

ity of this tumour to undergo spontaneous remission and cure, even when disseminated. Although frequently described, this phenomenon is in fact a rarity with an incidence of about 3% and almost exlusively confined to infants under the age of 12 months.

CLINICAL FEATURES

Clinical presentation is unusually varied, due to the variety of primary sites, the early wide dissemination and the secretion of pharmacologically active metabolites (Table 24.2). The commonest presentation is of an abdominal mass sometimes painless but often accompanied by mild or recurrent abdominal pain. Other common syndromes include irritability, fever, lethargy, anaemia or bone pain from a metastasis. Occasionally, lymph node or skin metastases, hepatomegaly or proptosis are the first clinical signs. Subcutaneous metastases often have a blue/black colour. Liver metastases may be painful. Other primary sites of

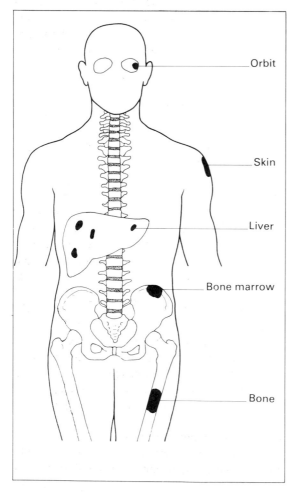

Fig. 24.2. *Common sites of distant metastasis in neuroblastoma.*

Table 24.2. Presenting symptoms of neuroblastoma.

Constitutional
    Fever, malaise, weight loss, anaemia

Primary site
    Adrenal: pain and abdominal mass
    Presacral: loss of bladder control, frequency of micturition
    Paravertebral: spinal cord compression
    Cervical sympathetic: Horner's syndrome
    Olfactory bulb: unilateral nasal block and epistaxis

Metastases
    Liver: Pain, weight loss, fever
    Bone: Pain (preceding x-ray change), anaemia, pathological fractures
    Orbit: Proptosis
    CNS: Malignant meningitis

Remote effects
    Diarrhoea: ? due to secretion of vasoactive intestinal polypeptide
    Myoclonus or opsoclonus
    Hypertension

presentation include presacral neuroblastomas causing urinary frequency or obstruction, posterior mediastinal tumours causing dyspnoea; intraspinal tumours causing spinal cord compression; cervical sympathetic tumours causing Horner's syndrome and olfactory bulb tumours (esthesioneuroblastoma) causing nasal obstruction and epistaxis. There is an association between neuroblastoma and myoclonic or opsoclonic movements, though the mechanism is unclear.

DIAGNOSIS AND INVESTIGATION

The definitive diagnosis is by biopsy of the affected site but a confident diagnosis may already have been made biochemically. Catecholamine metabolites are produced in about 90% of all children with neuroblastomas and screening for urinary metabolites should be undertaken if the diagnosis is suspected. Homovanillic acid (HVA) or vanillyl mandelic acid (VMA) are the most reliable and widely used measurements. Although the diagnosis can often be made on a random urine sample, 24-hour estimation is far more useful, and is often estimated repeatedly during treatment as a semi-quantitive test for monitoring progress. Both HVA and VMA should be measured since either metabolite may be raised; total catecholamine secretion should also be estimated. This will summate the output of metabolites of adrenaline, noradrenaline, metanephrine and normetanephrine, DOPA and dopamine as well as HVA and VMA. Carcino-embryonic antigen may also be elevated in serum but is of limited value in diagnosis.

Radiological investigations are often extremely valuable. Plain X-ray of the abdomen will frequently demonstrate calcification in the primary tumour, typically with a diffuse pattern. Liver metastases may also calcify. Chest X-ray is often normal, though abnormal mediastinal shadowing often occurs with primary intrathoracic tumours (typically in the posterior mediastinum). Parenchymal lung metastases are very unusual. Skeletal survey and isotope bone scanning are useful in detecting osseous metastases. Bone marrow aspiration is mandatory in all cases of neuroblastoma. Over 40% of children have marrow involvement even when bone X-rays are normal. Marrow examination often yields the only evidence of secondary spread. Intravenous urography may show renal displacement often without intrinsic distortion of the renal calyces, though hydronephrosis or non-functioning kidneys may also occur with large obstructing tumours. Before the advent of CT scanning, aortography was abnormal in more than 80% of cases with an obvious mass, and abnormal tumour circulation could often be demonstrated. CT scanning and abdominal ultrasonography are now more frequently performed, giving excellent delineation of tumour as well as providing accurate imaging of the liver.

DIFFERENTIAL DIAGNOSIS

The clinical diagnosis of neuroblastoma is not always straightforward, particularly if the child presents with failure to thrive and without other obvious abnormalities to suggest a diagnosis of malignancy. The most important distinction in children presenting with an obvious abdominal mass lies between neuroblastoma and Wilms' tumour. Although the urinary and radiological investigations usually give a firm answer, it can be difficult to distinguish between the two, especially where urinary catecholamines are normal and where CT scanning fails to confirm that the mass is unequivocally renal or adrenal. Other abdominal tumours which may cause diagnostic difficulty include hepatoblastoma and intestinal lymphoma. If the child presents with bone metastases, these may be difficult to distinguish radiologically from a primary Ewing's tumour, bone lymphoma or even a non-malignant cause such as osteomyelitis or tuberculosis.

Difficulty may also occur when the child presents with spinal cord compression when a variety of malignant and non-malignant causes must be considered. These include intraspinal cysts, neurofibroma, spinal tuberculosis, primary intraspinal tumours, medulloblastoma and other CNS tumours which seed within the CNS (see Chapter 11), or other rare causes of extradural compression, such as Hodgkin's disease.

CLINICAL STAGING

Clinical staging of neuroblastoma is important both prognostically and also as a means of selecting the most appropriate treatment. Although several classification schemes have been suggested, all are based on an accurate assessment of the detailed extent of spread. Although it is known that the degree of histological differentiation (i.e. tumour grade) may influence prognosis (3), this information, though potentially useful is difficult to fit into a simple staging classification. The same can be said for catecholamine excretion and age, though age at diagnosis is probably the single most important prognostic factor (4). The most widely used classification (5) is based entirely on extent of disease so as to produce a system that is practical for clinical use (Table 24.3).

Up to 70% of children have disseminated tumour at diagnosis, often in the bone marrow. The prognosis worsens with increasing stage. However, the IV-S category has been defined because these children have a surprisingly good prognosis with a survival rate similar to patients with stage 1 tumours. This might suggest a difference in sensitivity to treatment, dependent on the site of dissemination. However, it is also important to realize that most IV-S patients are under the age of 1 year, and patients of this age have a much better prognosis and a higher incidence of spontaneous regression.

In addition to age and disease extent, the primary site is also prognostically important. Tumours arising in the mediastinum and the neck have a better prognosis than those in the abdomen, probably since more are localized at the time of diagnosis. This is particularly true with thoracospinal lesions which produce early spinal cord compression (so-called dumb-bell

Table 24.3. Staging system for neuroblastoma (Evans' staging).

Stage I	Tumour confined to the organ or tissue of origin.
Stage II	Tumour extending beyond the primary site but not crossing the midline. Ipsilateral lymph nodes may be involved and tumours arising in midline structures such as the organs of Zuckerkandl but without extension, are included in this stage.
Stage III	Tumour extending across the midline or with metastases in regional lymph nodes bilaterally.
Stage IV	Distant metastases, for example bone, distant lymph nodes, liver or bone marrow.
Stage IV-S	This includes patients where the tumour is localized to one side of the midline but with evidence of remote involvement including liver, skin and/or bone marrow but without evidence of bony metastases.

tumours). Oddly enough, pelvic tumours also appear to have a better prognosis, and more frequently undergo differentiation to ganglioneuroma or even a spontaneous remission (6); again, this may relate to the fact that most of these children are under the age of 15 months.

CLINICAL MANAGEMENT

Current clinical management of neuroblastoma is unsatisfactory and refinements in treatment are continuously being suggested. Unlike many of the paediatric malignancies, chemotherapy has not yet made a significant improvement in the survival of these children, though the chemosensitivity of this tumour is not in doubt.

Local treatments with surgery and/or radiation therapy are therefore critically important, and may be curative in children with localized disease. In one surgical series, a 2-year survival rate of 84% was achieved by the use of surgery alone in apparently localized cases (7). Radiotherapy is usually recommended after incomplete excision, but probably best avoided where surgery appears complete. Long-term survivors have certainly been documented where surgery was incomplete, but supplemented by postoperative radiotherapy, though the contribution of radiotherapy is difficult to quantify since almost all patients will have had at least a partial or subtotal surgical excision. Most children with clinical stage II and III disease will be in this category. Even in children with stage IV disease, in whom chemotherapy may be the most important part of treatment, attention must be paid to controlling the primary disease.

In stage IV cases chemotherapy is usually the first treatment but radiotherapy and surgery will often be required at a later stage in order to achieve control of the bulky primary tumour. Many surgeons feel in this situation, that preoperative irradiation makes surgery technically easier. In these more advanced cases, the local treatment is usually withheld until at least 2 cycles of chemotherapy have been given, though low-dose hepatic irradiation may be useful if there is gross hepatomegaly.

Guidelines for treatment of neuroblastoma are given in Table 24.4. Combinations of vincristine, cyclophosphamide, actinomycin D and doxorubicin are usually used. Newer agents such as cisplatin, etoposide and ifosfamide are increasingly used in combination therapy. All of these drugs have been shown to be active as single agents in neuroblastoma. Most drug combinations contain vincristine, actinomycin D and cyclophosphamide (Table 24.5) often with other agents. These are generally well tolerated and yield higher response rates than treatment either with single agents or pairs of

Table 24.4. Guidelines for treatment of neuroblastoma.

Stage I	Surgery alone.
Stage II	Surgery with postoperative irradiation if surgery incomplete. Chemotherapy sometimes used.
Stage III	Chemotherapy followed by 'debulking' surgery with local irradiation and further chemotherapy.
Stage IV	As for Stage III, but intensive chemotherapy is the mainstay of treatment.
Stage IV-S	Uncertain. Early chemotherapy advisable but intensive hazardous treatment should be avoided because of the relatively good prognosis. Vincristine is often used alone. Surgery may be helpful in selected cases.

Table 24.5. Chemotherapy for neuroblastoma.

Single Agents Vincristine Actinomycin D Doxorubicin Cyclophosphamide High dose melphalan Cisplatin Etoposide	Response rates are not well characterized for any of these agents but are in the range of 30% with few maintained complete responses.
Combination Chemotherapy VAC I Vincristine, actinomycin and cyclophosphamide. VAC II Vincristine, doxorubicin and cyclophosphamide.	With both these regimens response rates appear to be approximately 60% with 10–20% maintained complete responses.

drugs, though the overall cure rate of only 10–20% is disappointing. Recent attempts to intensify treatment, either by the use of more agents (such as cisplatin and etoposide) or by increasing the drug dosage (sometimes using autologous marrow support) are of interest, though the effect on long-term survival is not known.

Although overall results remain disappointing, survival has improved in recent years, as a result of better diagnosis, treatment strategy, biochemical monitoring and possibly chemotherapy. Survival is clearly related to age and stage (Fig. 24.3), and children living beyond 3 years from diagnosis are usually considered cured.

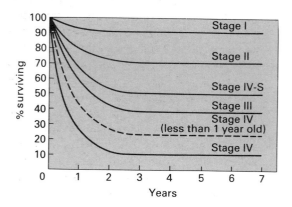

Fig. 24.3. *Survival related to stage in neuroblastoma.*

Wilms' tumour

INCIDENCE AND AETIOLOGY

Wilms' tumour (nephroblastoma) accounts for about 6% of all paediatric tumours, and has been recognized as a distinct clinical entity since the end of the last century. With neuroblastoma it forms much the largest group of intra-abdominal malignancies of childhood. Nonetheless there are pronounced differences between the behaviour of these two tumours, particularly in their response to treatment.

Although most cases are sporadic, a familial predisposition has been noted. Aniridia, hemihypertrophy, hamartoma, genitourinary and musculo-skeletal malformations are other well

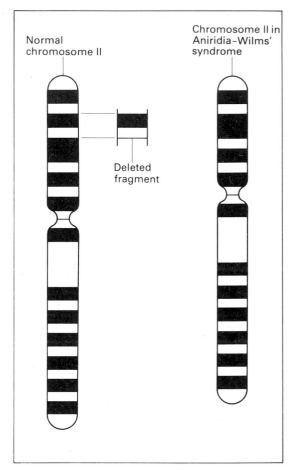

Fig. 24.4. *Deletion of part of the short-arm of chromosome 11 in aniridia-Wilms' syndrome.*

known associations. Chromosomal abnormalities may be present in children with Wilms' tumour including trisomy 8 or 18, XX/XY mosaicism, or deletion of the short arm of chromosome 11 in the aniridia-Wilms' syndrome (Fig. 24.4). The peak age of incidence is 3–5 years, though rarely, it has been discovered at birth. There is a slight male preponderance.

PATHOLOGY

Almost the whole kidney can be replaced either by a centrally or peripherally placed tumour, often exhibiting areas of patchy haemorrhage or degeneration, and sometimes with a lobulated appearance. Necrosis and cystic change are both common and although a very large size may be attained without obvious extrarenal involvement, extension of solid cores of tumour cells along the renal vein and inferior vena cava are common. Other direct sites of spread may include the perinephric fat, colon, adrenal gland or liver as well as the renal pelvis itself, and the local draining lymph nodes. Occasionally the tumour may be extrarenal in origin, presumably arising in ectopic cell rests from mesonephric crest migration. Bilateral presentation occurs in 5-10% of cases which are usually regarded as being bilateral synchronous primary tumours rather than secondary spread. Children with bilateral tumours are younger and have ten times the incidence of associated congenital anomalies.

Histologically, the tumours contain both mesenchymal and epithelial elements, often admixed and with differing stages of maturity. Within the epithelial element, there is usually evidence of a renal origin with embryonic tubular or glomerular structures sometimes lined by recognizable epithelium and occasionally arranged in rosettes. Undifferentiated stroma may form a large proportion of the tumour though this too may show areas of differentiation to form smooth muscle, bone or cartilage. A variety of histological types has been described, which probably represent differing degrees of differentiation. Some tumours (about 25%) are so undifferentiated as to defy unequivocal histological diagnosis. Typically, such tumours have a great propensity to metastasis. More highly differentiated forms also occur, and a specific group of 'mesoblastic nephromas' has been described, with only minimal nuclear pleomorphism and mitotic activity, a very low metastatic potential, and often surgically curable (8).

CLINICAL FEATURES

As with neuroblastoma, the common presentation is with a symptomless, painless abdominal mass more commonly on the left and often discovered by the parent or during a routine examination. There may be recurrent abdominal pain of moderate severity. Abdominal distension is common, though unlike neuroblastoma, these tumours tend not to cross the midline. Haematuria occurs in 30% of cases. Hypertension is unusual but is occasionally severe and sometimes accompanied by complications such as retinopathy or encephalopathy. It is thought to be due to excess renin production by the tumour or to renal ischaemia from renal artery stenosis. Fever, anorexia and lethargy are also common presenting symptoms.

About one-fifth of children with Wilms' tumour have evidence of distant metastases at presentation, though figures from central referral hospitals suggest a much higher incidence (up to 60-70%), representing a preponderance of advanced and complicated cases. Direct spread to extrarenal fat and other local organs is common, and local nodal spread occurs predominantly to the para-aortic and other intra-abdominal lymph node groups. Haematogenous spread occurs typically to the lung parenchyma, brain and bone, though liver, mediastinum, vagina and testis are well known secondary sites (Fig. 24.5). Bilateral renal involvement in the absence of another evidence of metastatic spread is well recognized.

INVESTIGATION AND STAGING

Plain chest and abdominal X-rays will help to define the extent of the primary tumour and demonstrate obvious pulmonary metastases. CT scanning of the chest is advisable since it is more sensitive in detecting pulmonary spread. Intravenous urography, abdomino-pelvic ultrasonography and in selected cases renal angiography, will give accurate pre-operative information as to the size and extent of disease.

Routine urine examination often reveals microscopic haematuria, and measurement of catecholamine excretion may be necessary in cases which are difficult to distinguish clinically from neuroblastoma. Isotope bone scanning is usually recommended since symptomless bone secondaries may be present. These investiga-

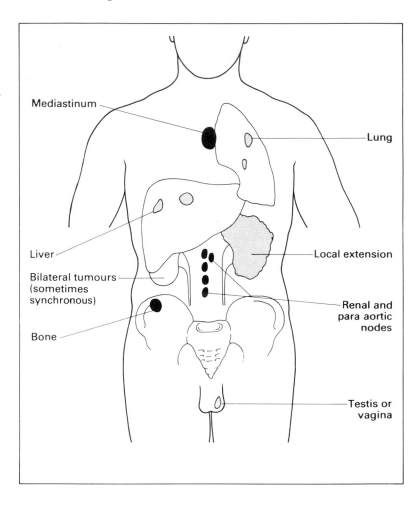

Fig. 24.5. *Common sites of metastasis in Wilms' tumour.*

tions should help distinguish the true Wilms' tumour from a variety of malignant and non-malignant conditions which it may clinically resemble.

Although neuroblastoma is the most important differential diagnosis, other intra-abdominal childhood tumours may cause difficulty, such as retroperitoneal sarcoma, hepatoblastoma and phaeochromocytoma. Important non-malignant causes of childhood abdominal masses include renal haematomas, hydronephrosis, multilocular cystic kidney, horseshoe kidney, perirenal haematoma and splenomegaly, almost all of which are uncommon though frequent enough as a group of disorders to cause diagnostic problems.

Staging systems have become more logical with increased understanding of the natural history of these tumours and of the importance of complete surgical removal. At present, the National Wilms' Tumour Study Staging System (Table 24.6) is most widely used (9).

This staging system has now been successfully used for 10 years, and data are accumulating to suggest that extent of disease at operation and the presence of lymph node involvement are the most influential prognostic factors. Large referral centres which treat a substantial number of children undoubtedly have better results than smaller hospitals where the occasional case is treated, a finding with the unavoidable implication that non-specialist cli-

Table 24.6. Staging of Wilms' tumour.

Stage I	Tumour limited to the kidney, and completely resected. Renal capsule intact, tumour removed without rupture, no residual disease.
Stage II	Tumour extends beyond kidney but is completely resected. Penetration is into the perirenal soft tissue or fat; infiltration of renal vessels outside the kidney, or para-aortic lymph node involvement. No residual tumour.
Stage III	Residual tumour confined to the abdomen, or tumour biopsied or ruptured before or during surgery. Involved lymph nodes beyond para-aortic chains; tumour not completely resected.
Stage IV	Distant blood-borne metastases (usually to lung, liver, bone and/or brain). Lymph node metastases beyond the abdomen.
Stage V	Bilateral tumours at presentation.

nicians should be dissuaded from treating the occasional child with a curable cancer.

MANAGEMENT

There should be close cooperation between paediatric surgeon, radiotherapist, paediatric oncologist and pathologist to ensure that all clinicians will have the opportunity to assess each child before surgery is performed. Although full investigation is important, no attempt should be made to establish a tissue diagnosis preoperatively since renal biopsy can undoubtedly disseminate disease and worsen prognosis. Firm pre-operative diagnosis is at present impossible, though the occasional Wilms' tumour has been shown to produce a complex mucopolysaccharide in the serum, later confirmed as present in the tumour cells. This may eventually prove to be a useful tumour marker. Even in the presence of obvious metastatic disease, careful assessment of operability should always be made

since control of the primary tumour without surgery is always difficult. The advent of effective irradiation and chemotherapy have allowed surgeons to reconsider operating on children whose tumours were hopelessly inoperable at first presentation.

Guidelines for the management of Wilms' tumour are set out in Table 24.7. Surgical re-

Table 24.7. Wilms' tumour: Guidelines for management.

Stage I	Surgery and vincristine.
Stage II	Surgery; adjuvant combination chemotherapy using vincristine and actinomycin D.
Stage III	As for Stage II but whole abdominal irradiation for diffuse spread and chemotherapy includes doxorubicin.
Stage IV	Surgery and more intensive combination chemotherapy.
Stage V	Individual treatment often including bilateral renal surgery with low dose postoperative radiotherapy and adjuvant combination chemotherapy.

moval should be performed in order both to remove the tumour in its entirety, without biopsy or other disturbance of the capsule, and to assess the extent of intra-abdominal disease with careful delineation of any area of residual tumour. Enlarged lymph nodes should generally be resected or at least biopsied.

Postoperative chemotherapy with combinations of vincristine, actinomycin D and/or doxorubicin should be used (Table 24.8). However the possible roles of pre-operative chemotherapy and routine postoperative irradiation of the tumour bed remain controversial. There is a growing belief that pre-operative chemotherapy is valuable in the management of doubtfully resectable tumours, this, however has never been formally tested.

Although for 30 years or more, postoperative radiotherapy has been employed routinely as an

Table 24.8. Chemotherapy in Wilms' Tumour.

	Response rate (complete and partial) %
Single Agents	
Vincristine	70
Doxorubicin	60
Actinomycin D	40
Cyclophosphamide	35
Etoposide	30
Cisplatin	30
*Combination therapy**	
Actinomycin D and vincristine	95
Vincristine and doxorubicin	90
Vincristine, doxorubicin cyclophosphamide	90

* Response rates are approximate as these combinations have not been thoroughly tested in metastatic disease, and different combinations are used in different stages of the disease.

adjuvant to surgery, the development of effective chemotherapeutic regimens has led to a reappraisal of the role of radiotherapy.

In stage I disease, postoperative radiotherapy confers no benefit in children under the age of 2 years treated by 'adjuvant' actinomycin D and this is possibly true for older children as well.

Children with stages II and III should be treated postoperatively with combination chemotherapy and most of these children also receive postoperative radiotherapy including treatment to the whole abdomen in those with diffuse spread. There is some evidence that combination chemotherapy using vincristine, actinomycin D and doxorubicin gives a better survival rate than the use of two drugs alone.

Stage IV disease should be treated with intensive combination chemotherapy. The successful treatment of disseminated Wilms' tumour demands an aggressive approach, often requiring surgical resection of both pulmonary and hepatic metastases with multiple courses of both radiotherapy and chemotherapy. The more widespread use of chemotherapy has also led to discontinuation of total lung irradiation which in the past was a common method of treatment for mediastinal or pulmonary metastases.

In patients with bilateral (stage V) disease, treatment is usually with surgical removal of the tumour where possible, often by total nephrectomy on the more affected side and partial nephrectomy on the other. Low dose postoperative radiotherapy and chemotherapy are usually given.

Unlike neuroblastoma the routine use of chemotherapy has radically altered the outlook in this disease, which was the first of the solid tumours in which adjuvant chemotherapy was established as an important part of the initial management. Most patients tolerate this treatment without too much difficulty. Avoidance of radiotherapy wherever possible has undoubtedly reduced the long-term complications such as growth retardation within the irradiated area, scoliosis, and radiation-induced second tumours—often an unresectable and rapidly fatal sarcoma. Trials are in progress to further clarify the details of postoperative treatment. At present, important chemotherapy induced complications include nausea and vomiting, peripheral neuropathy, alopecia, and skin reactions (including recall phenomena in previously irradiated areas, following actinomycin D treatment).

Treatment of recurrent disease is always difficult because of the previous administration of chemotherapy and radiotherapy. The same agents may again be effective, particularly in cases where recurrence is late, well after discontinuation of the initial adjuvant chemotherapy. Other drugs such as cisplatin, vinblastine, bleomycin and etoposide may be of value in children resistant to first line treatment. Palliative irradiation (sometimes in combination with surgery) may also be useful for brain, lung, extradural, bony and hepatic metastases.

PROGNOSIS

The prognosis in Wilms' tumour has improved greatly as a result of routine adjuvant chemotherapy, though a better understanding of the role of surgery, radiotherapy and supportive care have also contributed. At present, the prognosis in this disease is better than for any other childhood malignancy and the overall survival rate is now 80–90% (Fig. 24.6). Several prognostic factors are known to be important, including age at diagnosis (the younger the better), histological findings such as degree of differentiation (with a better prognosis in well-differentiated tumours) and tumour stage. Prognosis for stage I disease is excellent with 5-year survival rates of at least 90%; with stage IV disease this falls to 54% (10).

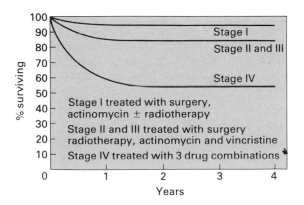

Fig. 24.6. *Survival related to stage and treatment in Wilms' tumour.*

Soft tissue sarcoma

INCIDENCE, AETIOLOGY AND CLASSIFICATION

Soft tissue sarcomas account for 7% of childhood tumours with an incidence of 0.8 per 100 000 children. Little is known of their cause although sarcomas can be produced in animals by carcinogens and RNA viruses such as the Rous sarcoma virus.

The histological types of soft tissue sarcoma in children are similar to those found in adults (see Chapter 23), but the relative frequency is different with rhabdomyosarcoma and fibrosarcoma predominating (Table 24.9).

Table 24.9. Childhood soft tissue sarcoma.

	Relative frequency (%)
Rhabdomyosarcoma	52
Fibrosarcoma (including histiocytoma)	10
Mesenchymoma	6
Synovial sarcoma	6
Liposarcoma	4
Leiomyosarcoma	2
Vascular sarcomas	5
Others	15

Rhabdomyosarcoma

This tumour is much the commonest soft tissue sarcoma of childhood. *Embryonal rhabdomyosarcoma* is the most frequent histological type with a peak incidence at 2–5 years. *Alveolar rhabdomyosarcoma* is commoner in adolescence. The tumours can arise at a variety of sites: in the head and neck (chiefly the orbit, nasopharynx, oropharynx or palate), the pelvis (particularly bladder, uterus and vagina) or less commonly, the extremities or trunk.

PATHOLOGY

There are four main histological subtypes of rhabdomyosarcoma: embryonal, alveolar, pleomorphic and mixed types. The first two account for more than 90% of all cases. Macroscopically, the tumours are usually nodular, often with a surrounding inflammatory and oedematous reaction. Although they may appear to be circumscribed, true encapsulation is very uncommon. Sarcoma botryoides has a characteristic macroscopic appearance, described as resembling bunches of grapes, which consist of mucinous polyps of tumour.

Microscopically, these tumours are highly malignant. Pathological diagnosis can be difficult, particularly if cross striation is regarded as an essential part of the histological diagnosis. Electron microscopy should always be performed if possible, since the appearances are characteristic (Fig. 24.7).

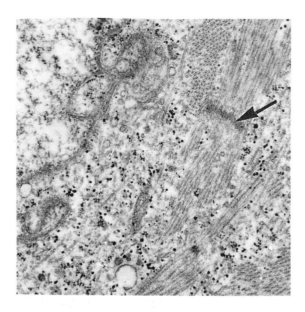

Fig. 24.7. *Electron micrograph of a portion of a rhabdomyoblast.* Thick and thin filaments are shown, and there is formation of Z bands (arrowed). (× 26 600)

Embryonal rhabdomyosarcoma is often poorly differentiated, with long slender spindle-shaped cells with a single central nucleolus and eosinophilic cytoplasm, often without obvious cross-striations. The cells usually have an irregular pattern without the cellular arrangements which are characteristic of alveolar rhabdomyosarcoma. Sarcoma botryoides is a polypoid form of embryonal rhabdomyosarcoma. The embryonal group is the commonest form of paediatric rhabdomyosarcoma and accounts for the majority of head and neck and genitourinary cases.

Alveolar rhabdomyosarcoma arises more commonly on the limbs and trunk. Microscopically these tumours have a more organized pattern and the cells tend to be separated by connective tissue bands. The typical cell is round with scanty eosinophilic cytoplasm which is sometimes vacuolated and may contain glycogen. Cross-striations are often seen, and giant multinucleate cells are common. Pleomorphic rhabdomyosarcomas are rare in childhood, and almost always arise in skeletal muscle.

All varieties are highly malignant and exhibit rapid growth with early dissemination, though embryonal rhabdomyosarcoma often presents greater problems of local recurrence. Early lymph node involvement is common, producing obvious lymphadenopathy which may be the initial presenting feature, particularly in head and neck tumours. Blood borne metastases are also frequent, particularly to lung and marrow, though other sites such as brain, liver and other soft tissue sites may also be involved.

CLINICAL FEATURES

Clinically, the commonest presentation is with a painless mass either clearly visible in the case of extremity and trunk lesions, or causing displacement as with the characteristic proptosis of orbital rhabdomyosarcoma which accounts for 30% of all head and neck cases.

In the pelvis, the commonest primary sites are the genitourinary tract and perianal area. Deep-seated tumours may cause indirect symptoms such as facial palsy and discharge from the ear with tumours in the middle ear; airway obstruction and nasal discharge from nasopharyngeal primaries and dysphagia from tumours in the oropharynx. Lymph node metastasis is common with testicular and genitourinary sites and may be the presenting sign but is very unusual with head and neck (particularly orbital) primaries.

INVESTIGATION AND STAGING

Important investigations include a chest X-ray (with whole lung tomography or CT scanning if possible); isotope, liver and bone scanning; ultrasonography and/or CT scanning of the abdomen (in patients with abdominopelvic primary tumours). In head, neck and orbital cases, detailed plain radiographs, tomography and CT scanning is essential to determine the local extent of the primary site. The most widely used staging notation is shown in Table 24.10, together with the relationship between initial stage and prognosis.

Table 24.10. Stage and prognosis in rhabdomyosarcoma in childhood.

		Prognosis (3-year survival)
Group 1	Localized disease completely resected	82%
Group 2	Localized and/or regional disease with residual microscopic tumour following local therapy	60-70%
Group 3	Regional disease with gross residual tumour after local treatment	55%
Group 4	Distant metastatic disease	30%

MANAGEMENT

As with most paediatric tumours, current management is complex, and, for the majority of patients, includes surgery, radiotherapy and chemotherapy since none of these modalities alone gives satisfactory results. This integrated multimodal approach to treatment has led to a substantial improvement in prognosis during the past 20 years (11). Until recently, radical surgical removal of the primary was always felt to be mandatory, a view which has undergone revision in recent years. Combination chemotherapy should now be used as the initial treatment, followed by local treatment with surgery and radiotherapy. Although surgery should be as complete as possible, careful judgement is required in order to avoid the risk of long-term mutilation. This has led, for example, to an increasing preference for wide excision (including compartmentectomy) rather than amputation for children with tumours of the extremities. When coupled with radical postoperative irradiation and early (adjuvant) chemotherapy this approach gives acceptably low local recurrence rates and allows for later amputation in the small number of cases where local recurrence occurs in the absence of more generalized disease.

With more deeply situated primary tumours such as nasopharynx, primary surgery plays no part other than to establish the histological diagnosis. In some of the deeply situated but more accessible abdomino-pelvic primaries, the role of surgery is more uncertain, though it is increasingly accepted that major procedures such as total cystectomy or exenteration should not be performed in the first instance since effective irradiation and chemotherapy may result in cure with far less long-term damage. Combinations of chemotherapy and irradiation are increasingly used to achieve local control in orbital rhabdomyosarcoma and it is sometimes possible to save the eye. Embryonal and alveolar rhabdomyosarcoma are relatively sensitive to irradiation (particularly embryonal rhabdomyosarcoma), though high doses are required for effective control (50-60 Gy, 5000-6000 rad, over 5-6 weeks).

Chemotherapy has now been established as an important part of treatment, both in metastatic and recurrent cases, and also as an adjuvant to local treatment. Several agents are known to produce objective responses in significant numbers of patients, including vinca alkaloids, alkylating agents, actinomycin D, doxorubicin, methotrexate and others (Table 24.11). Chemotherapy of metastatic disease usually produces only temporary remission. Treatment with combination chemotherapy is preferable using, for example, vincristine, acti-

Table 24.11. Chemotherapy in rhabdomyosarcoma in childhood.

	Response rate (complete and partial) %
Single Agents	
Vincristine	55
Actinomycin D	25
Doxorubicin	30
Cyclophosphamide	55
Mitomycin C	35
Combination chemotherapy regimens	
Vincristine, actinomycin D, cyclophosphamide	
Vincristine, actinomycin D, cyclophosphamide, doxorubicin	

nomycin D and cyclophosphamide, though actinomycin D should not be given synchronously
with radiation because of dangerous recall
phenomena, and cyclophosphamide is usually
deferred until after radiotherapy because of the
danger of myelosuppression. Adjuvant chemotherapy is usually continued for at least 12
months. Tumours in special sites may require
particular treatment strategies; for example in
parameningeal tumours prophylactic treatment
with intrathecal chemotherapy and cranial irradiation may be needed.

At present, multicentre studies in both
Europe and the United States are attempting to
provide answers to several unresolved issues
such as the need for radiotherapy, the most acceptable and effective form of adjuvant chemotherapy and the need for continued adjuvant
treatment beyond 1 year.

PROGNOSIS

With adjuvant chemotherapy, the overall survival rate has improved, and in patients with
locoregional disease (groups 1–3), 2-year survival rates of up to 80% have been reported, compared with a 2-year survival of perhaps 25%
before the era of effective chemotherapy (Table
24.10). Recurrence tends to occur early, usually
(90%) within the first 2 years. The stage of disease is the most important prognostic factor;
both the extensiveness of the primary lesion
(which will govern the likelihood of resectability) and the presence of metastases affect survival. As with other paediatric tumours, age at
presentation also affects prognosis; in one study
the median survival for children under 7 years
was 78 months, compared with 18 months for
older children (12), though the younger children
had less extensive disease at the time of diagnosis, and in general a more favourable tumour
type (predominantly embryonal rhabdomyosarcoma) than older children. Site may also be
important, and orbital tumours in general have
a better prognosis although other head and
neck tumours, particularly nasopharynx, have
a poor prognosis presumably due to their in-

accessibility, late presentation and unsuitability
for surgical resection.

Retinoblastoma

INCIDENCE AND INHERITANCE

Retinoblastoma is a rare but important
tumour, with a familial incidence. The rate
appears to have doubled over the past 40 years
and it now has a frequency of one case per
15 000 live births and accounts for about 3% of
all childhood malignancies. Its increasing incidence is due to the fact that it is an inherited
disease in which survival is increasing, which in
turn leads to an increase in the number of children born to previously affected parents.

Although most cases of retinoblastoma are
sporadic (non-familial) retinoblastoma is an important example of a congenital malignancy. It
is inherited by an autosomal dominant gene,
though some individuals can apparently carry
this defective gene without developing the
tumour. Sporadic non-familial cases are mostly
unilateral, with only a small risk that the offspring of these patients will subsequently de-

Table 24.12. Genetic counselling in retinoblastoma.

Bilateral disease is almost always familial.

Offspring of survivors of hereditary retinoblastoma,
or of bilateral sporadic cases, will have a 50%
chance of developing the tumour.

Unaffected parents with a child with unilateral disease have a 1–4% chance of having another
affected child.

Survivors of unilateral sporadic disease have a 7–
10% chance of having an affected child, and are
therefore presumed to be silent carriers.

If two or more siblings are affected there is a 50%
chance that subsequent siblings will have the
tumour.

Unaffected children from retinoblastoma families
may occasionally (5%) carry the gene but if they
have an affected child the risk in subsequent children is 50% since the parent is then identified as a
silent carrier.

---

velop the disease. However, in the occasional sporadic bilateral case, there is a 50% chance of the offspring developing the disease. In retinoblastoma families, most affected children will themselves develop bilateral disease so that in apparently unilateral familial cases, close watch must be kept on the contralateral eye. In genetic counselling (Table 24.12) it is also important to recognize that about 4% of normal parents of an affected child produce more than one child with the disease. Retinoblastoma can rarely be associated with mental retardation and cases of the tumour with severe mental retardation have been reported where there is a deletion of the long arm of chromosome. A group of patients have been reported where bilateral retinoblastoma was associated with pinealoblastoma. Other neoplasms also occur with increased frequency.

PATHOLOGY

Retinoblastoma is typically multifocal. This is presumably due to spread of tumour within the retinal layers, as well as to synchronous tumour development within different parts of the retina in cases of bilateral disease, since spread via the optic nerves and chiasm does not generally occur. The commonest route of spread, particularly of the endophytic type of tumour, is forward into the vitreous humour, and this growth within the globe tends to occur before other involvement of periglobal structures or backwards spread to the intracranial space. Retinal detachment may occur during this process, but extension of growth into the choroid does not usually occur other than with very large tumours. Invasion of the sclera may also occur, carrying a poor prognosis; the optic nerve itself may be directly invaded by the tumour via the lamina cribrosa and thence to the subarachnoid space with dissemination of tumour cells into the CSF and consequent seeding along the base of the brain.

Microscopically, retinoblastoma typically consists of an admixture of undifferentiated and small cells with deeply staining nuclei and scant cytoplasm, though larger cells are often found, sometimes with a tendency to rosette formation around the central cavity. Traditionally this was considered to be a gliomatous tumour, from glial elements derived from spongioblasts though electron microscopy has more recently suggested an origin in the photoreceptor cells.

Blood borne metastases occur, and common sites are the bone marrow, liver, lymph nodes and lungs.

CLINICAL FEATURES

Most children present under the age of 2 years, usually with a white pupil ('cats eye reflex'), or less commonly with strabismus, glaucoma, defects in visual fixation, or inflammatory changes within the eye. Any family history of retinoblastoma should immediately raise suspicion, and the most important investigation is a careful ophthalmological examination by an experienced ophthalmic surgeon. This gives an assessment of tumour site, extent, involvement of the contralateral eye and evidence of multicentricity. Only the ophthalmologist can reliably exclude important non-malignant diseases such as toxocara or retinal dysplasia, though biopsy is accepted as unwise since this may provide a pathway for tumour dissemination.

INVESTIGATION

Tumour calcification may also be present, although this may only be visible radiologically. Chest X-ray, full blood count and isotope bone scanning should be performed in all cases, with CSF examination whenever there is a suspicion of CNS involvement. Orbital CT scanning may be useful as a means of assessing extensiveness of disease.

STAGING

Size, site and multicentricity of tumour has led to the widely accepted clinical staging system which has now been in clinical use for over 25 years (Table 24.13).

Table 24.13. Staging and prognosis (% 3-year survival) in retinoblastoma.

Group I	Single or multiple tumours of size less than 4 disc diameters at or behind the equator (90–100%)
Group II	Single or multiple tumours of size 4–10 disc diameters at or behind the equator (90–100%)
Group III	Tumours anterior to the equator or a single tumour larger than 10 disc diameters at or behind the equator (70–85%)
Group IV	Multiple lesions, some greater than 10 disc diameters. This group includes any lesion extending anteriorly to the ora serrata (70–75%)
Group V	Massive tumours involving over half the retina, or tumours with vitreous seeding (35–70%)
Group VI	Residual orbital disease. Extension into the optic nerve and through the sclera (30%)

This simple system depends on ophthalmoscopic examination with accurate diagrammatic representation of the retinal lesion in relation to standard reference landmarks such as the optic nerve head, ora serrata (junction of the retina and ciliary body), etc.

TREATMENT

Treatment depends on the presenting stage. In recent years treatment philosophy has altered away from immediate or early enucleation of the more severely affected eye, to a more conservative policy with a much greater reliance on radiotherapy as the preferred local technique. The excellent results of this approach (see below) are highly dependent on careful ophthalmological assessment in every case. Eradication of tumour with preservation of vision has now become a realistic aim.

With very small tumours, cryosurgery or photo coagulation are both effective, though with tumours near the optic disc or macula, external beam irradiation is preferable because light coagulation close to these critical parts of the eye carries a risk of permanent visual damage. For these tumours, external irradiation using a single lateral field is both simple and effective.

For larger tumours (3–10 mm) brachytherapy (see Chapter 5) with radioactive cobalt plaques is frequently used; but smaller tumours near the optic disc or macula are better treated with external beam irradiation. With single tumours above 10 mm, external beam irradiation of the whole eye is the treatment of choice, and usually requires multifield treatment to ensure homogenous irradiation of the whole globe, particularly where there is a risk of vitreous seeding. Use of an anterior field allows for more adequate sparing of the contralateral eye even though the lens and cornea are unavoidably treated. This technique is also suitable where there are multiple tumours confined to one eye. A dose of 35 Gy (3500 rad) in 3–4 weeks is sufficient to control most intraocular retinoblastomas.

With obvious infiltration of the optic nerve, enucleation is preferable, though many large but non-invasive tumours have been successfully treated by external irradiation alone.

With bilateral tumours, preservation of sight is more difficult, and it is best to treat each eye individually on its own merits rather than assuming that enucleation of the worse eye will invariably be required. Where there is residual tumour in the orbit, postoperative irradiation should certainly be given to include the whole orbit and optic foramen, and in some cases where there is a risk of CNS dissemination, whole brain or even craniospinal irradiation should also be considered. A dose of 50 Gy (5000 rad) in 5 weeks is both effective and well tolerated in children requiring postoperative irradiation of the orbit, in whom the radiation tolerance of the eye is no longer a consideration. Particular care is required to ensure immobilization either by means of a head cast, or with sand bags.

In all cases of retinoblastoma treatment planning must be precise, aiming to cover all areas of disease without unnecessarily jeopardizing the lens of both the affected and the contralateral eye. Fortunately, with the radiation dose required to control most retinoblastomas (35–40 Gy (3500–4000 rad) in $3\frac{1}{2}$–4 weeks), significant complications are now uncommon, though in the early years of radiotherapy, radiation complications were frequent, often producing irreversible loss of vision. The commonest complication, cataract formation, is unavoidable when anterior beams are used, though of course not all cataracts are clinically significant and if necessary, lens extraction is fairly simple and effective. Vascular injury from irradiation, though easily visible to the ophthalmologist, rarely impairs vision though occasionally, retinal haemorrhage may result in secondary glaucoma which can be troublesome. This is particularly well recognized where a second course of irradiation has been given for recurrent disease. Irreversible damage to the orbital bones may prevent normal growth, a particular problem in infants. Finally, radiation-induced second tumours have been reported in several series, though some retinoblastoma families have a known tendency to develop second malignancies, particularly osteogenic sarcomas at any site within or distant from the irradiated volume. In one large series of nearly 400 patients, the incidence of radiation-induced tumours was over 11% (13), though many of these patients had received repeated courses of treatment, resulting in enormous doses of irradiation.

PROGNOSIS

The results of treatment are very good (Table 24.13), particularly in early cases and where specialized facilities and experienced clinicians are available. Ninety-percent cure rates are widely achieved and for one large series, children with stages I and II disease had a cure rate of 100%, and even those with stages IV and V disease had a cure rate of 75%. When conservative measures have failed, enucleation of the eye can be curative, though there is still a 10–15% overall mortality rate, due to intracranial spread or distant metastases. A few children, successfully treated, will later die from a second radiation-induced tumour (usually osteogenic sarcoma). Limitation of total radiation dose will probably reduce the incidence of this tragic complication of treatment.

For patients with high risk tumours (including those with extraocular metastases at presentation), cytotoxic chemotherapy has been used, either with single agents or with combinations of drugs. Vincristine, actinomycin D, doxorubicin, methotrexate and cyclophosphamide are the drugs most usually employed in combination chemotherapy. The results of treatment for advanced and extraocular retinoblastoma are poor and a well-designed study of adjuvant chemotherapy for these high risk tumours is desirable. Surgical or radiation cure is rare in patients with massive orbital disease or extensive optic nerve involvement at presentation. In these very advanced cases, death is equally likely to result from intracranial involvement from distant metastases, and although combination chemotherapy, whole brain irradiation and/or intrathecal chemotherapy have undoubtedly produced worthwhile responses, no cures have yet been reported.

Histiocytosis X

This is a group of disorders comprising 3–4% of paediatric tumours, whose origin is considered to be from the macrophage/monocyte series of cells. These cells arise in the bone marrow, circulate briefly as blood monocytes and then migrate to tissues where they form fixed macrophages in the liver (Kupffer cells), spleen, lung, bone marrow and tissues (histiocytes). In some ways they behave like cancers since they are often multifocal, sensitive to cytotoxic agents and irradiation, and can be fatal. A brief discussion is therefore included.

The term 'histiocytosis X' includes the spectrum of syndromes of Letterer-Siwe disease, eosinophilic granuloma and Hand-Schuller-Christian disease.

LETTERER-SIWE DISEASE

This acute disease has its onset in infancy and is characterized by hepatosplenomegaly, lymph node enlargement, thrombocytopaenia and skin rash. A greasy, scaly, scalp or nappy rash is usually the presenting feature. Widespread infiltration of the skin, liver, lungs, spleen and bone marrow gives rise to hepatic dysfunction, dyspnoea and marrow failure. Lytic lesions in bone are common. Cytotoxic drugs (vincristine, prednisolone, 6-mercaptopurine) may produce temporary improvement but the prognosis is very poor.

EOSINOPHILIC GRANULOMA

This disease forms a spectrum ranging from a single, isolated bone lesion, typically in older children, to multiple punched out bone lesions. The prognosis is worse below the age of 3 years.

Presentation is usually with bone pain or lymphadenopathy. The disease may regress spontaneously. Low dose radiotherapy is of value for localized bone lesions and cytotoxic chemotherapy will occasionally produce remissions in advanced cases. Its use is usually restricted to cases with visceral involvement.

HAND-SCHULLER-CHRISTIAN DISEASE

This disease is characterized by multiple eosinophilic granulomas. Occasionally, diabetes insipidus may occur, due to pituitary involvement as well as exophthalmos from orbital deposits. Enlargement of liver and spleen occurs as does skin infiltration, but the disease is less aggressive than Letterer-Siwe disease. As with eosinophilic granuloma, the disease may become quiescent and does not usually relapse if the activity ceases for 3–4 years. Diabetes insipidus is permanent and chronic neurological disability may occur as may cirrhosis with portal hypertension. The disease responds to chemo-

therapy; vinblastine and prednisolone are the most widely used drugs, with responses in 90% of patients.

Rare paediatric tumours

The tumours described above, the intracranial tumours of childhood, and the leukaemias and lymphomas, constitute 92% of all childhood malignancies, and the remaining 8% is made up of a variety of uncommon diseases seen only sporadically even in large paediatric centres. Some, such as hepatoblastoma and orchioblastoma are rare but 'genuine' paediatric tumours whereas other, such as adenocarcinoma of the kidney or transitional cell carcinoma of the bladder as essentially adult tumours seen very rarely in the paediatric age group. The principles of management of these rare paediatric malignancies are not yet clearly established. The importance of a joint approach with full pretreatment assessment by paediatric surgeon, radiotherapist and paediatric oncologist (working closely with a histopathologist with special experience in these tumours), cannot be emphasized too strongly.

Hepatoblastoma

This rare tumour occurs in childhood. It can be associated with anomalies such as hemihypertrophy, as well as with storage diseases and the Fanconi syndrome. The pathological features are of immature hepatic epithelial cells or a mixture of these cells with mesenchymal elements. It usually arises in the right lobe and presents with a visible asymptomatic mass which later causes pain and weight loss. Like hepatocellular carcinoma (which can also occur in children over the age of 5 years), the tumour produces AFP which may be elevated above the normal infantile range. The tumour can be demonstrated by isotopic, ultrasound and CT scanning but arteriography gives the best localization and is essential if resection is to be attempted.

The tissue diagnosis is usually made at operation when an attempt at resection is made. It does not appear possible to cure these children without complete surgical excision. Up to 75% of the liver can be removed but haemorrhage can be severe and great skill is necessary.

Postoperative chemotherapy is usually given. Doxorubicin is the most effective agent but responses are also reported to alkylating agents, cisplatin and nitrosoureas. Occasionally, unresectable cases can be made to respond to chemotherapy so that surgery can be performed, and there is growing interest in preoperative chemotherapy in this disease. Serum AFP can be used to assess response to treatment in older children.

Germ cell tumours

All of the adult tumours, germ cell tumours (see Chapters 17 & 19) are occasionally seen in childhood. In addition, specific childhood forms occur though none is common.

SACROCOCCYGEAL GERM CELL TUMOURS

These are the most common germ cell tumours of childhood and the commonest tumour of the newborn. The female:male ratio is 4:1. Clinically, there is a large swelling between the coccyx and rectum, and the tumour arises on the inner margin of the distal part of the coccyx. Approximately 10% of tumours in the newborn are malignant, but above 3 months of age, 50% are malignant. The tumour should be surgically excised but if there are malignant elements (embryonal carcinoma, choriocarcinoma) chemotherapy should be given despite its toxicity in infants.

HEAD AND NECK GERM CELL TUMOURS

Ten-percent of childhood teratomas arise in the head and neck. The sites are very variable (orbit, soft tissue, nasopharynx), and they may cause respiratory obstruction. Treatment is with surgery and chemotherapy (if malignant). Pineal teratomas are discussed in Chapter 11.

TESTICULAR GERM CELL TUMOURS

The main histological variants are the yolk sac tumour (endodermal sinus tumour, Teilum tumour, orchioblastoma), embryonal carcinoma and differentiated tumour. Below the age of 2 years, yolk sac tumours are probably less likely to metastasise than in older children. The differentiated tumours are benign. Before effective chemotherapy was available, 9% of children under 2 years old were alive 2 years after treatment, while only 25% of older children survived. This difference may be less marked since the advent of platinum-based chemotherapy. The management follows the guidelines outlined for adult testicular tumours (see Chapter 19).

SEX CORD AND STROMAL TUMOURS OF THE TESTIS

Leydig cell tumours and Sertoli cell tumours occur rarely, the Leydig cell tumour at age 4–5 years and the Sertoli cell tumour below the age of 2 years. Leydig cell tumours which may be accompanied by testicular virilization, are slow growing, and cured by orchidectomy. Sertoli cell tumours may cause feminization, and orchidectomy is adequate treatment.

Gonadoblastomas are very rare tumours, chiefly found in patients with testicular feminization (XY or XY/XO karyotype with dysgenetic gonads and feminine phenotypes). The testes may be maldescended, in which case they are present in the inguinal canals or abdomen.

OVARIAN GERM CELL TUMOURS

The classification of these tumours is discussed in Chapter 17. Dysgerminomas, embryonal carcinoma and teratoma are managed as outlined in Chapter 17; as in adults, surgery and combination chemotherapy are the major modalities though radiotherapy is important in dysgerminoma.

Gonadoblastoma develops in an abnormal gonad which is frequently indeterminate or no more than a rudimentary streak. The patients have abnormal sexual development and are either phenotypic females with virilization, or cryptorchid phenotypic males.

REFERENCES

1 Herbst, A.L., Robboy S.J., Scully R.E. & Poskanzer D.C. (1974) Clear cell adenocarcinoma of the vagina and cervix in girls: Analysis of 170 registry cases. *American Journal of Obstetrics and Gynecology* **119**, 713.

2 Li F.P., Tucker M.A. & Fraumeni J.F. (1976) Childhood cancer in sibs. *Journal of Pediatrics* **88**, 419.

3 Mäkinen J. (1972). Microscopic patterns as a guide to prognosis of neuroblastoma in children. *Cancer* **29**, 1637.

4 Breslow N. & McCann B. (1971) Statistical estimation of prognosis for children with neuroblastoma. *Cancer Research* **31**, 2098.

5 Evans A.E., D'Angio G.J. & Randolph J. (1971) A proposed staging for children of widespread neuroblastoma. *Cancer* **27**, 374.

6 D'Angio G.J., Evans A.E. & Koop C.E. (1971) Special pattern of widespread neuroblastoma with a favourable prognosis. *Lancet* **i**, 1046.

7 Koop C.E. & Johnson D.G. (1971) Neuroblastoma: An assessment of therapy in reference to staging. *Journal of Pediatric Surgery* **6**, 595.

8 Bolane R.P. (1974) Congenital and infantile neoplasia of the kidney. *Lancet* **ii**, 1497.

9 Wolff J.A. (1975) Advances in the treatment of Wilms' tumor. *Cancer* **35**, 901.

10 D'Angio G.J., Evans A.E., Breslow N., Beckwith B., Bishop H., Farewell V., Goodwin W., Leape L., Palmer N., Sinks L., Sutow. W.W., Tefft M. & Wolff J. (1981) The treatment of Wilms' tumour. Results of the second national Wilms' tumour study. *Cancer* **47**, 2302.

11 Wilbur, J.R., Sutow, W.W., Sullivan M.P. & Gottlieb J.A. (1975) Chemotherapy of sarcomas. *Cancer* **36**, 765.

12 Sutow W.W., Sullivan M.P., Reid H.L., Taylor H.G. & Griffith K.M. (1970) Prognosis in childhood rhadbomyosarcoma. *Cancer* **25**, 1384.

Chapter 25

Hodgkin's Disease

In the last 20 years the prognosis of Hodgkin's disease has greatly improved, both for patients with localized disease, who are often curable by radiotherapy, and for those with disseminated disease treated with cytotoxic drugs. Success has not only been achieved because of the introduction of entirely new methods of treatment, but also because it has become increasingly apparent how radiotherapy and chemotherapy can be employed to best advantage. There have also been improvements in staging techniques and a better understanding of the patterns of spread which have lead to more rational treatment. In this respect Hodgkin's disease has been a model which has led to improvements in management of other malignant tumours.

INCIDENCE AND EPIDEMIOLOGY

The incidence of Hodgkin's disease rises steeply from the age of 10–20 years. There is a slight fall in middle age, following by a rise after 50 years to reach a maximum at age 70 years and over (Fig. 25.1). The male to female ratio in western countries is about 1.5:1. Although the incidence varies in different parts of the world the male predominance usually holds (Table 25.1).

While the reliability of cancer statistics differs from country to country, the reported variation in incidence appears to reflect genuine differences in the frequency of the disease rather than in the accuracy of diagnosis (1). In some countries such as Colombia and Nigeria the incidence in childhood (age 5–14) is five times that

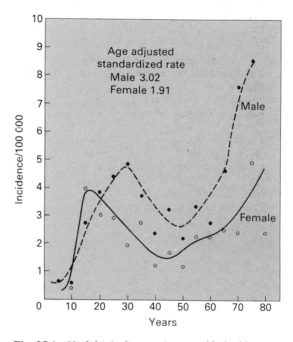

Fig. 25.1. *Hodgkin's disease.* Age specific incidence.

Table 25.1. Hodgkin's disease. Annual incidence rates (per 100 000) in various countries.

	Male	Female
England	2.2	1.3
USA		
White	2.3	1.4
Coloured	1.3	0.7
Japan	0.6	0.3
Ceylon	0.1	0.1

429

in Britain, but in adult life it is four times less common. In these countries the history also tends to be less favourable compared with Western Europe and North America. In Japan and possibly other Far East countries, the incidence appears to be substantially lower than in the West.

AETIOLOGY

Genetic, family and social factors

There have been several studies on the association of Hodgkin's disease with histo-compatibility antigens, but the results have been conflicting. In part this is due to technical problems with typing reagents and in selection of cases for analysis. In prospective studies of unselected cases, HLA-A1 has been shown to occur with a marginally increased frequency compared with controls, and HLA-A12 in younger patients with good histology.

There have been many reports of families where two or more members have developed Hodgkin's disease and sometimes the presentation has been very close in time. In the family of a patient the risk of siblings having the disease is greater than normal. The risk in siblings is possibly about six times that of the normal population and siblings of the same sex are most likely to be affected (2). The meaning of rare but dramatic clusters of cases is unknown but suggests an environmental rather than a genetic cause. There is no definite relationship with social class although there have been suggestions that it may be commoner in classes I–II.

Some studies have suggested an increased incidence of Hodgkin's disease among woodworkers in the United States, but this is not the case in Britain. Schoolmates and health care personnel have been stated to be at higher risk of exposure to a hypothetical, transmissible, causative agent. Carefully designed and controlled studies have not confirmed this.

Infections

The infectious agent which has the strongest claim to an association with Hodgkin's disease is the Epstein–Barr virus (EBV). Infectious mononucleosis (which is caused by EBV) has often been reported as occurring immediately before the presentation of Hodgkin's disease. Cells similar to Reed–Sternberg cells have been found in lymph node biopsies from patients with infectious mononucleosis. However, case-control studies (see Chapter 2) have failed to show an association, but cohort studies have usually done so although the increased risk appears marginal and these cohort studies do not constitute proof of a causal connection. The EBV genome has not been demonstrated in cultured Reed–Sternberg cells. It is possible that abnormal immune responses may make an individual more susceptible to both EBV infection and Hodgkin's disease.

There have been many attempts to find evidence that retroviruses (e.g. RNA tumour viruses, see Chapter 3) are involved in the aetiology of Hodgkin's disease. Sequences of DNA homologous with murine leukaemia virus RNA have been reported in extracts of spleen from patients with Hodgkin's disease but not in normal spleen. The interpretation of this finding is open to question, however, since neoplastic cells constitute only a small proportion of the cells in spleens involved with Hodgkin's disease.

PATHOLOGY

The Reed–Sternberg Cell

Lymph nodes from patients with Hodgkin's disease contain two categories of cells. The first is the cell which is the hallmark of the disease and which is thought to be the malignant component—the Reed–Sternberg cell or its mononuclear counterpart (Fig. 25.2). The second category consists of a pleomorphic cellular infiltrate, the composition of which varies considerably in different patients.

The malignant cells are large, often with

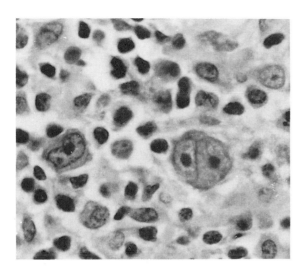

Fig. 25.2. *Section of a lymph node in Hodgkin's disease.* Showing typical binucleate Reed–Sternberg cell and mononuclear Hodgkin's cell (×400 original magnification).

slightly basophilic cytoplasm. The nuclei are usually lobulated and there may be two or more in a single cell. The classical Reed–Sternberg cell has two or more nuclei usually with large nucleoli which are acidophilic. The mononuclear variety of cell is sometimes seen in reactive inflammatory nodes and cells with a similar appearance to Reed–Sternberg cells may occasionally be found in infective lesions (infectious mononucleosis) and a variety of other lymphoproliferative disorders such as phenytoin-induced lymph node enlargement and non-Hodgkin's lymphoma. The Reed–Sternberg cells have some of the cytological characteristics of the dendritic cells which are found in the paracortical region of normal lymph nodes. In spite of intensive investigation the origin of the malignant cell in Hodgkin's disease has not yet been elucidated. The reason for, and significance of, the infiltrate of normal cells which make up the bulk of the nodal enlargement in the disorder is similarly obscure.

Classification

The histological classification which is now widely used in based on the Lukes–Butler scheme

(4) which divides the microscopic appearances into four categories:

1 *Lymphocyte predominant.* The appearances are of small lymphocytes with scarce Reed–Sternberg cells and their mononuclear variants.
2 *Nodular sclerosis.* There are broad bands of collagen (not simply fibrosis) separating cellular nodules of Hodgkin's disease.
3 *Mixed cellularity.* The infiltrate is pleomorphic with lymphocytes, macrophages, eosinophils and polymorphs.
4 *Lymphocyte depleted.* There is either diffuse fibrosis with fewer Reed–Sternberg cells, or a reticular type with numerous Reed–Sternberg cells or their mononuclear variant.

The nodular sclerosing and mixed cellularity categories make up 80–90% of all cases. Prognostically, lymphocyte predominant histology is most favourable and lymphocyte depleted least so. Mixed cellularity is generally considered to be an histological appearance with a less favourable prognosis than nodular sclerosis, but this is not the case in patients with advanced disease treated with chemotherapy. In nodular sclerosing histology it is probable that the cellular composition of the nodules also has prognostic significance (e.g. the degree of lymphocyte infiltration).

Sometimes the pathologist has great difficulty in deciding if the patient has Hodgkin's disease or not and mistakes can occur. The clinician should be very careful in cases which have atypical histology obtained from non-nodal sites, and with clinically odd presentations such as isolated disease presenting in the gut or skin. The differential histological diagnosis includes:
(a) reactive nodes with immunoblasts which may be seen in infectious mononucleosis, other herpes virus infections, or toxoplasmosis;
(b) hypersensitivity to drugs such as phenytoin;
(c) angio-immunoblastic lymphadenopathy (see Chapter 26);
(d) T cell lymphoma (see Chapter 26);
(e) metastatic melanoma;
(f) non-Hodgkins lymphoma, particularly the distinction between lymphocyte predominant

Hodgkin's disease and well-differentiated lymphocytic lymphoma.

In patients with proven Hodgkin's disease, other histological abnormalities may be found. For example at staging laparotomy, the spleen or liver may show granulomatous infiltration of unknown cause. A further example may occur after intensive chemotherapy when the lymph nodes may show an unusual appearance, with vascular invasion and atypical, lymphocyte-depleted histology with few inflammatory elements—appearances similar to a non-Hodgkin's lymphoma.

ABNORMAL IMMUNITY IN HODGKIN'S DISEASE

It has long been recognized that host defence against infection is abnormal in advanced Hodgkin's disease even before treatment. Radiotherapy and chemotherapy can impair these defence mechanisms still further. An increased susceptibility to tuberculosis was noted in 1932 and subsequently it was shown that the tuberculin skin test was frequently negative in Hodgkin's disease. These observations have been extended and it is now clear that depressed delayed-hypersensitivity reactions to a variety of antigens including Candida, mumps and histoplasmin are frequently found. These impaired responses are more common in patients with advanced disease and with constitutional symptoms. When attempts are made to induce delayed hypersensitivity to artificial antigens such as dinitrochlorobenzene (DNCB), it is frequently found that there is anergy to the antigen, particularly in patients with more advanced disease (5).

In vitro tests have not yet elucidated the nature of the defective cell-mediated immunity. There is a modest depression of blood T cell numbers in some patients with untreated advanced disease, and phytohaemagglutinin (PHA) responses are depressed, especially in more advanced cases. Depression of these responses might be due to the presence of suppressor cells in the blood, and there is evidence for a prostaglandin-mediated suppression induced by blood monocytes. Other suppressive mechanisms are possible, and the relationship between the *in vitro* tests and cutaneous anergy is far from clear. Humoral immunity is normal as judged by serum antibody levels to specific antigens. Blood B-cell numbers are occasionally slightly reduced but the numbers in the spleen may be increased.

The cause of these abnormalities remains obscure but there is little doubt that patients with Hodgkin's disease are especially susceptible to opportunistic infections. These include infections with bacteria such as pseudomonas and tuberculosis, fungi such as Candida and Aspergillus, and viruses such as *Herpes zoster* and *herpes simplex*. In all of these diseases, susceptibility is probably due to depressed cell mediated immunity.

The more advanced the disease, the greater the likelihood of anergy, but there is little clinical value in tests of immune competence as part of the routine investigation of a newly diagnosed case. The degree of spread of the disease is better assessed by more straightforward investigations.

Further depression of cell mediated immunity occurs as a consequence of treatment and is further discussed on page 449. The treatment of patients with advanced disease with cytotoxic drugs is hazardous for many reasons, one of the most important of which is the profound additional depression of immunity which may lead to fatal infection.

THE CLINICAL FEATURES

In the vast majority of cases the clinical presentation is straightforward (6). The patient has accidentally noticed an enlarged, painless lymph node in the neck or elsewhere, and a biopsy gives the diagnosis. The initial site of presentation (Fig. 25.3) includes cervical nodes (70% of all cases), axilla (25%) and inguinal area (10%). The lymph nodes usually grow slowly

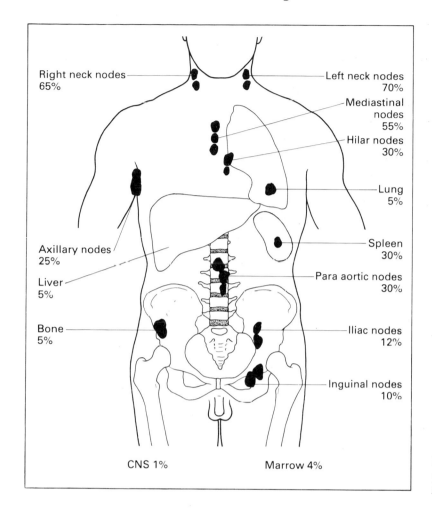

Right neck nodes
65%

Left neck nodes
70%

Mediastinal
nodes
55%

Hilar nodes
30%

Lung
5%

Axillary nodes
25%

Liver
5%

Spleen
30%

Para aortic nodes
30%

Bone
5%

Iliac nodes
12%

Inguinal nodes
10%

CNS 1%   Marrow 4%

Fig. 25.3. *Frequency of sites of involvement at presentation in patients with Hodgkin's disease.*

and are sometimes visible on photographs months or years before being noticed by a patient. Occasionally the nodes are described as growing very rapidly and sometimes they are tender if there has been a recent upper respiratory infection. The nodes may fluctuate in size with such infections and may mislead the physician into believing that the node enlargement is only inflammatory.

Twenty-five per cent of all patients have constitutional symptoms at presentation. Fever is the commonest of these and is generally of low-grade but may occasionally be hectic, up to 40°C, which usually occurs in the evening and falls to normal in the morning. In advanced disease, bouts of fever lasting 1 or 2 weeks

may occur (Pel–Ebstein fever) but this is unusual and not specific for Hodgkin's disease. Drenching sweats may occur at night, waking the patient from sleep. Lesser degrees of sweating occur in many normal individuals and are hard to evaluate. Weight loss occurs, as in any other malignancy, but is especially associated with advanced or bulky disease. The triad of constitutional symptoms (fever, sweats and >10% loss of body weight), is of very great importance since cases with one or more of these have a much poorer prognosis.

Generalized pruritus occurs in 5–10% of patients at the time of presentation, but many patients will develop this symptom during the course of the disease when it relapses. If severe, it can be a most disabling symptom, the skin becoming excoriated from scratching, especially at night. The cause is unclear although release of histamine by the tumour has been postulated. The symptom abates with successful treatment. Alcohol-induced pain is felt in involved lymph nodes in a very small number of patients (2–5%). It is aching or stabbing in nature, comes on within minutes of drinking and lasts from a few minutes to an hour (7). It is chiefly associated with mediastinal disease of nodular sclerosing histology and we have seen such a case in which the alcohol induced pain from nodes adjacent to the pericardium had the quality and distribution of myocardial ischaemia.

Other rare systemic features of Hodgkin's disease include auto-immune haemolytic anaemia (although a positive Coomb's test in the absence of haemolysis is more common) and immune thrombocytopenia. A variety of erythematous skin rashes may occur, including erythroderma, erythema multiforme, psoriasiform lesions and bullous eruptions.

Enlarged nodes may produce symptoms due to compression. Examples include limb oedema and pain due to nerve entrapment; cough, stridor or superior vena caval obstruction from mediastinal disease; obstruction of the inferior vena cava or the ureters by para-aortic nodes; obstructive jaundice due to nodes in the porta hepatis. Internal mammary node enlargement may give rise to a chest wall mass in the parasternal region. In contrast to non-Hodgkin's lymphoma the tonsil and Waldeyer's ring are rarely involved, and when this does occur it is usually associated with upper cervical node involvement.

Hodgkin's disease occasionally presents as a pulmonary lesion and then must be distinguished from infection or other bronchial neoplasms by sputum cytology, culture and biopsy. Endobronchial Hodgkin's disease is very rare—the clinical features being wheezing and haemoptysis. Much more commonly, pulmonary infiltration occurs from direct spread from enlarged hilar or mediastinal nodes. Pulmonary nodules of Hodgkin's disease are easily missed on conventional chest X-rays, and whole-lung tomograms or CT scans are very useful when the diagnosis is in doubt. Pleural infiltration usually presents as an effusion, and is nearly always associated with mediastinal and pulmonary disease. If the mediastinal disease is massive, the pleural effusion may be due to lymphatic obstruction rather than direct invasion by tumour. The same is true for chylous effusions. A diagnosis of pleural infiltration can only be made reliably by biopsy or by a CT scan showing nodules of tumour in the pleura or subpleural lung. Cytological examination is usually unrewarding since Reed–Sternberg cells are rarely found.

Bone marrow involvement occurs at presentation in approximately 5% of patients and is nearly always associated with widespread disease elsewhere, and with constitutional symptoms. The diagnosis is by marrow trephine biopsy. The number of positive routine marrow biopsies in patients with early stage disease is very small, but a normal blood count does not preclude involvement in those with advanced disease. Marrow involvement is, however, more likely if there is anaemia, thrombocytopenia or leucopenia. The disease is focal within the marrow so false negative biopsies are frequent.

Occasionally the bones are involved in a more localized way by Hodgkin's disease, either by direct spread from adjacent nodes, or by metastatic spread (in which case there is usually widespread disease elsewhere). The commonest histology is nodular sclerosis. The presentation is with pain, the serum alkaline phosphatase is elevated, X-rays may show either osteoblastic or osteolytic lesions, and an isotope bone scan is positive. A solitary bone deposit does not necessarily indicate Stage IV disease (i.e. diffuse involvement of an extranodal tissue, see Table 15.2) and may respond to local treatment, with a good prognosis.

Skin and subcutaneous infiltration are uncommon as presenting features but may occur in the context of aggressive disease over lymph node masses or in their drainage areas. The nodules of tumour are often painless but may ulcerate. Subcutaneous lesions may occur in the breasts. Primary cutaneous Hodgkin's disease is a great rarity.

When Hodgkin's disease involves the central nervous system it is usually spinal rather than cerebral. This is a rare presentation and usually occurs by extension through the intervertebral foramina from adjacent lymph nodes to cause epidural compression. The clinical features are of root pain, parasthesiae or spinal cord compression. Both are medical emergencies because there is a serious risk of paraplegia (see Chapter 8). Laminectomy and radiotherapy are the normal methods of diagnosis and treatment. If the diagnosis is known, prompt treatment with radiotherapy alone is usually adequate. Compression of the spinal cord may be localized and does not necessarily constitute an indication for chemotherapy. Rarely, Hodgkin's disease may present with leptomeningeal spread, with a clinical syndrome of basal malignant meningitis causing cranial nerve palsies, or symptoms and signs of raised intracranial pressure.

The gut is rarely the primary site of Hodgkin's disease and the diagnosis should be viewed with suspicion, since gastro-intestinal non-Hodgkin's lymphomas are so much more common. Nevertheless, there are isolated cases of the disease arising in the oesophagus, stomach, small and large bowel. The presentation is usually indistinguishable from other tumours at these sites. When the disease occurs in the small bowel it usually affects the terminal ileum and may cause malabsorption syndrome.

The urinary tract is seldom clinically involved, and the commonest manifestation is ureteric compression with hydronephrosis. It is very unusual for direct renal infiltration to be clinically apparent. Rarely, cases of nephrotic syndrome occur, which are due to immune complex glomerulonephritis or to compression of the renal veins by tumour masses.

Hodgkin's disease may be accompanied by paraneoplastic syndromes. In the central nervous system, patients may rarely develop progressive multifocal leucoencephalopathy. This is a relentless, fatal, demyelinating disorder, now known to be caused by a papovavirus and characterized by dementia, disorientation and focal signs leading to coma and death (see Chapter 2). Subacute cerebellar degeneration has also been recorded, with progressive ataxia, especially truncal ataxia, due to degeneration of Purkinje cells in the vermis. The Guillain-Barré syndrome occurs in the disease, more commonly than would be expected by chance. There are a few cases of segmental, granulomatous, angiitis in the brain, which may respond to treatment of Hodgkin's disease and which are possibly related to varicella-zoster infection. These paraneoplastic syndromes are discussed further in Chapter 9.

PATTERNS OF SPREAD

In early Hodgkin's disease some lymph node groups are much more commonly involved than others (Fig. 25.3). By far the commonest site of presentation is the neck, while involvement of mesenteric nodes is rare. Following localized treatment, adjacent lymph nodes are the most frequent sites of relapse, a finding which led to the introduction of extended field radiotherapy. In more detailed analyses, certain patterns of spread have been found (bilateral cervical node enlargement is unusual unless there is also mediastinal disease; mediastinal disease is itself frequently associated with involved neck nodes). Nodular sclerosing Hodgkin's disease in the mediastinum is more frequently found in women and is not usually associated with subdiaphragmatic disease. Splenic involvement is uncommon when the presentation is with isolated inguinal node enlargement. In the abdomen the coeliac plexus is the commonest site of node involvement (8).

When the disease involves the liver or bone marrow, splenic disease is nearly always present; involvement of the liver with sparing of the spleen is so unusual that the pathological findings should be questioned. It is not clear if splenic involvement is a source of dissemination although vascular invasion in splenic Hodgkin's disease may signify a worse prognosis.

STAGING CLASSIFICATION

As with many cancers, the adoption of a generally agreed staging notation has been of immense value for a number of reasons. First, because it has encouraged clinicians to compare like with like in trials of treatment; second, because stage correlates closely with prognosis; and finally because it focuses attention, in individual cases of the disease, on the importance of knowing the degree of spread of the disorder before considering the treatment options. Nevertheless, it is surprising how commonly the process of 'staging the patient' is regarded as an end in itself without regard to the value of the information gained by what are often expensive, uncomfortable and sometimes dangerous investigations. Understanding the full extent of the disease is only important if it will influence treatment. In Hodgkin's disease this is often, but not always, the case. The Ann Arbor classification (9) is widely used as a description of clinical or pathological stage and is outlined in Table 25.2. This staging notation (with explanatory notes) is used throughout this Chapter.

There is a distinction to be made between the anatomical description of the extent of the disease on the basis of clinical examination, routine chest X-ray, lymphangiography and isotope scans (clinical stage) and the description based on information obtained by biopsy and laparotomy (pathological stage). The former is obviously likely to under-estimate the extent of the disease especially in patients with more aggressive disease and those with constitutional symptoms.

When comparison is made between the results of clinical and pathological staging (based on laparotomy) it is generally found that

Table 25.2. Ann Arbor staging classification for Hodgkin's disease.

Staging Classification

Stage I	Involvement of a single lymph node region or of a single extra-lymphatic site or organ.
Stage II	Involvement of two or more node regions on the same side of the diaphragm, or of a localized extranodal involvement and one or more lymph node regions on the same side of the diaphragm (IIE).
Stage III	Involvement of lymph nodes on both sides of the diaphragm which may include the spleen (IIIS) or a localized extranodal site (IIIE) or both (IIISE).
Stage IV	Diffuse involvement of one or more extralymphatic organs.

Notes

1 Suffix A = no constitutional symptoms. Suffix B = constitutional symptoms present. These are fevers, night sweats and/or loss of 10% or more of body weight over 6 months. Pruritus is not included.

2 Localized extranodal involvement can at times be difficult to distinguish from Stage IV disease. A good working rule is that localized spread means that the lesion in question could still be treated with radiotherapy.

3 Stage III disease can be usefully subdivided according to the extent of intra-abdominal node involvement. Stage III_1 means involvement of spleen, splenic, coelic or portal nodes or any combinations of these. Stage III_2 means involvement of para-aortic, iliac or mesenteric nodes with or without upper abdominal disease.

4 In the case of the marrow or liver, diffuse involvement means the demonstration of any amount of unequivocal Hodgkin's disease since localized spread at these sites is not recognized and radiotherapy not regarded as a treatment option.

for each clinical stage there is a 25–30% chance of error as judged by pathological stage (Table 25.3). While most of these errors are the result of underestimation of the extent of disease using clinical criteria, some patients in whom

Table 25.3. Clinical *vs* laparotomy (pathological) staging. Data from Kaplan (13) and other sources.

	Positive at laparotomy	Negative at laparotomy
Spleen		
Clinically*+ve	50	50
Clinically −ve	24	76
Overall	28	72
Liver		
Clinically +ve	6	94
Clinically −ve	2	98
Overall	3	97
Abdominal Nodes		
Clinically +ve	73	27
Clinically −ve	14	86
Overall	29	71

*Clinically positive means definitely abnormal lymphogram, hepatomegaly or splenomegaly.

disease is judged to be widespread, are shown to have less extensive disease on pathological stage. An example of this 'downstaging' of disease is seen in patients who have a palpable spleen but no evidence of histological involvement at laparotomy.

INVESTIGATION

Haematology and biochemistry

Full blood counts are normal in most patients with localized nodal disease without constitutional symptoms (stages IA and IIA). Mild anaemia, polymorphonuclear leucocytosis and a high ESR are more common with advanced disease. The anaemia is usually normochromic or slightly hypochromic and is typical of the anaemia of chronic disease. Rarely, auto-immune haemolytic anaemia may occur at presentation. Lymphopenia usually signifies advanced disease but eosinophilia, which occurs in a few patients, has no prognostic significance. The ESR is a somewhat unreliable guide to extent and activity of disease but a high ESR (above 40) is usually associated with more widespread disease.

Liver enzymes and plasma bilirubin are often abnormal with hepatic involvement but isolated, modest elevation in aspartate transaminase or glutamyl transpeptidase sometimes occur in the absence of proven involvement. The plasma alkaline phosphatase is often elevated and is more likely to be so in advanced disease. Usually it is the liver isoenzyme which is responsible but bone phosphatase may sometimes be contributory. An elevated alkaline phosphatase is not conclusive evidence of extensive disease if it is an isolated finding.

Routine X-rays

CHEST X-RAY

The chest X-ray is an essential examination. Enlargement of mediastinal and bronchopulmonary lymph nodes is very common and the anatomical distribution of the lymph node groups is shown in Fig. 25.4. Mediastinal ad-

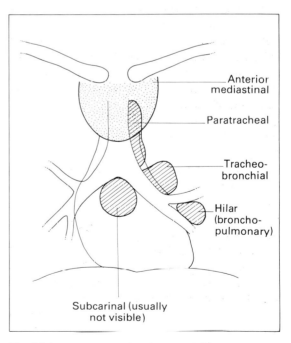

Fig. 25.4. *Anatomical distribution of the major lymph node groups which may be involved in Hodgkin's disease.*

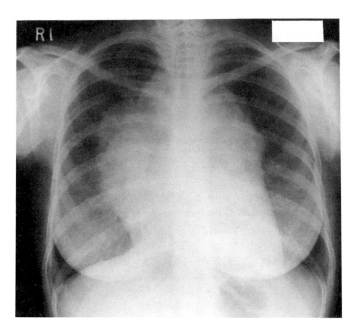

Fig. 25.5. *Chest X-ray showing a very large, well-defined mediastinal mass.* The patient was a woman of 22, with nodular sclerosing Hodgkin's disease.

enopathy is particularly common in women with nodular sclerosing disease. Massive mediastinal node enlargement may occur, leading to superior vena caval obstruction (Fig. 25.5). The thymus may be involved and often the mass projects laterally to the right and is seen anteriorly on lateral films. The bronchopulmonary lymph nodes may be enlarged with more subtle radiological changes. Usually there is associated mediastinal node enlargement.

The pulmonary changes may be due to compression of a bronchus, direct intrapulmonary extension from a lymph node mass or, less commonly, to localized intrapulmonary Hodgkin's disease. Bronchial compression may cause atelectasis of a whole lobe with associated consolidation within the collapsed area. Direct extension from lymph nodes (Fig. 25.6) is not infrequent. In patients who have been treated with radiation to mediastinal nodes, extension of the disease into the lung may be very difficult to distinguish radiologically from radiation pneumonitis and fibrosis. Tuberculosis and other infections may produce similar radiolog-

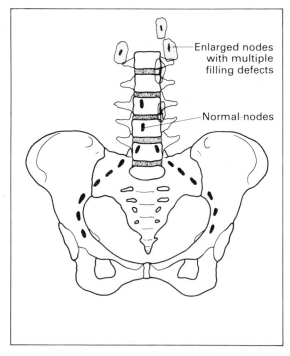

Fig. 25.6. *Diagrammatic representation of enlarged nodes shown on a lymphogram.* The X-ray would show enlargement, displacement from the midline and a lace-like texture.

ical appearances. A chest X-ray may also show enlargement of the cardiac shadow due to a pericardial effusion, or erosion of a rib or the sternum due to local extension from lymph nodes.

LYMPHOGRAPHY

In this technique lymphatic channels on the dorsum of each foot are outlined by a subcutaneous injected of a green or blue dye. The lymph channels are cannulated, and low viscosity contrast material is injection slowly. X-rays of the pelvis and abdomen are taken at the time of injection and the next day. The hazards of the technique are that it is uncomfortable for the patient; sites of cannulation may become infected; local extravasation of contrast material may occur, and lymphocysts may develop, particularly at a site of previous inguinal node biopsy. In addition hypersensitivity reactions to the dye or contrast material can occur, and the contrast material embolizes in the lungs causing a transient reduction in diffusing capacity. This may be dangerous in patients with underlying lung disease which is therefore a relative contra-indication to the investigation.

The filling films show the lymphatic channels and nodes. There are usually anastamosis from each side at the level of the para-aortic nodes. The nodes are seldom shown clearly above L1

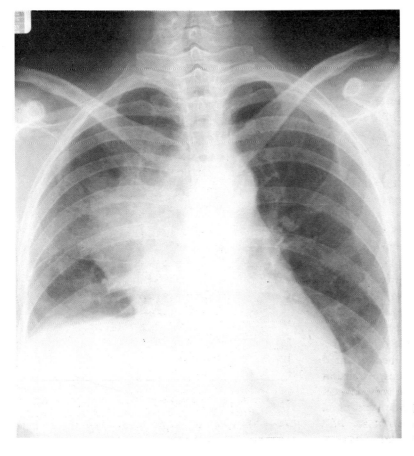

Fig. 25.7. *Involvement of hilar nodes with extension into the lung on the right.*

but occasionally the thoracic duct can be seen and the left supraclavicular nodes are often outlined. Most information about the lymph nodes is obtained from the films at 48 hours. Normally the lymph nodes are 1–2.5 cm in size and homogeneous in texture. In the inguinal nodes there may be filling defects perhaps due to previous infections. These can be confusing when the technique is being used to look for metastatic cancer (e.g. melanoma). In lymphomas isolated filling defects are not the typical finding. Usually the affected node enlarges diffusely so that the contrast material takes on a 'foamy' or 'lacey' appearance (Fig. 25.7). When the node is completely replaced by disease it may not opacify or may show a thin rim of contrast material. This can stay in the node for weeks or months and therefore be useful as a means of assessing response or progression. There are several limitations of lymphography. First, some lymph groups are not normally outlined, such as the obturator, high para-aortic, splenic, renal hilar, mesenteric and porta hepatis nodes. Second, it gives no information about the spleen. Third, the technique and its interpretation depends on the skill and experience of the radiologist. Finally, some lymphographic appearances cannot be evaluated without follow-up films.

Other imaging techniques

CT SCANNING OF THORAX AND ABDOMEN

Thoracic CT scan will determine whether there is intrapulmonary spread of disease with greater accuracy than whole-lung tomograms, and in particular it will demonstrate small pulmonary and subpleural nodules of tumour.

Involvement of mediastinal nodes is delineated by the technique. Although in practice, treatment decisions are not often altered by the routine application of thoracic CT scans; the additional information may lead to a change in treatment policy and the scans are of value in the planning of involved field radiotherapy.

In the abdomen, CT scanning is probably less sensitive than lymphography in demonstrating abnormal pelvic, iliac and lower para-aortic nodes, but it can be useful in the upper abdomen, where lymphography is of limited value. Small foci of hepatic or splenic disease cannot be demonstrated. CT scanning of the abdomen is especially valuable if it shows widespread disease in asymptomatic patients, because the management will be altered.

ULTRASOUND EXAMINATION OF THE ABDOMEN

Ultrasound examination may demonstrate enlarged nodes and may be of value in the upper abdomen (see Chapter 4). The technique depends critically on the experience of the radiologist, so that assessment of its accuracy and value in routine use is difficult. In experienced hands the technique can be invaluable, particularly since it is entirely non-invasive and can be easily repeated.

Both ultrasound and CT scanning may alter treatment policy, but are not as accurate as laparotomy and give no information about microscopic spleen involvement.

ISOTOPE SCANNING

In asymptomatic patients with localized disease, liver scans seldom give useful information. Even in patients with constitutional symptoms and mildly abnormal liver function tests, the correlation between liver scans and laparotomy findings is poor. Occasionally a grossly abnormal scan will indicate the need for chemotherapy in a doubtful case, but such instances are rare.

Bone scanning may be useful in demonstrating isolated areas of involvement and is cheaper and more reliable that plain X-rays as a screening procedure. The information obtained from routine use is limited, but if there is bone pain, it is an essential investigation, since a positive scan may change treatment policy if the cause of the abnormality is Hodgkin's disease. The areas shown up on scan must be examined radiologically since increased uptake on a bone scan has many causes including degenerative joint disease or previous trauma. Both gallium scanning with ^{67}Ga and scanning with bleomycin labelled with ^{111}In have been advocated as techniques for indicating sites of involvement in lymph nodes, but the accuracy and resolving power of the techniques is low.

CONTRAST RADIOLOGY

Barium studies of the stomach and bowel are unnecessary unless there are clear symptoms requiring investigation. In the stomach the usual radiological appearance of Hodgkin's disease is of a mass indenting the barium, occasionally with appearances suggesting ulceration. In the small and large bowel the typical appearance is of a long segment of infiltration with a coarse and distorted mucosal pattern and thickening of the bowel wall. The involvement may be patchy and discontinuous.

Intravenous urography (i.v.u.) was performed in the past as a means of demonstrating para-aortic node involvement by displacement of the ureters or kidneys. Most radiologists still obtain an i.v.u. on the second day of a lymphogram, since very large nodes may not take up lymphographic contrast material. Its use as a separate investigation has been superceded by modern imaging techniques.

PERCUTANEOUS BIOPSY

Some of the indications for percutaneous biopsy have already been discussed. Marrow trephine biopsy is an essential investigation in patients with stage III disease and in all those with constitutional symptoms, since a positive result will mean that further investigation is not necessary in order to decide treatment. It may be difficult to decide whether the marrow is involved since typical Reed–Sternberg cells may not be present. The mononuclear Hodgkin's cell may be found and may be sufficient for

diagnosis. The involvement is usually focal so there are considerable sampling errors.

Percutaneous liver biopsy is not a reliable investigation since Hodgkin's disease may be focal within the liver. It can be useful in selected cases with abnormal liver function tests, constitutional symptoms or hepatomegaly, and if positive, may remove the need for further staging procedures. There may be a considerable problem in interpreting liver biopsy material even if obtained at laparotomy. Focal mononuclear infiltrates are frequently found, and pathologists are usually reluctant to diagnose the disease on the basis of occasional malignant-looking mononuclear cells. In both liver and marrow, noncaseating granulomata may be found, the cause of which is unknown, and these should not be confused with Hodgkin's disease.

STAGING LAPAROTOMY AND SPLENECTOMY

The introduction of laparotomy and splenectomy by Kaplan, Rosenberg and co-workers at Stanford in the 1960's showed that, even in patients with clinical, localized (stage I or II) supradiaphragmatic disease, there was a significant chance of finding disease below the diaphragm. Since then there has been considerable debate about the necessity for this procedure in newly diagnosed Hodgkin's disease and recently the tendency has been towards a more conservative approach in some patients.

The technical aspects of the laparotomy are very important. It is not a procedure for the non-specialist general surgeon because the information obtained may then be sub-optimal. The para-aortic lymph node chain is exposed and biopsies taken from as high and as low as possible. The spleen is removed, splenic hilar nodes are biopsied, as are iliac nodes if possible. The porta hepatis is carefully inspected. Wedge biopsies are taken from the lobes of the liver, and trephine biopsy from the iliac crest. One or both ovaries may be moved and repositioned, usually in a more central position (oophoropexy), in anticipation of possible pelvic node irradiation, since a central position allows shielding from irradiation without compromising the dose to iliac lymph nodes.

The diagnostic yield of laparotomy and splenectomy is shown in Table 25.3. Demonstration of occult disease is mainly in the spleen and para-aortic nodes. In most studies, about 40% of patients have been shown to have been 'understaged' clinically, as judged by subsequent laparotomy and splenectomy. After an adequate staging procedure, the chances of subsequent relapse in the abdomen are 10%. The questions which therefore arise are:

Can we select the patients who should undergo the procedure?

Can we devise treatment strategies which make this operation unnecessary?

What are the immediate and long-term hazards of laparotomy and splenectomy?

There is no purpose to be served by a staging laparotomy and splenectomy if no change in the proposed treatment will follow. There is no known therapeutic benefit from removing a diseased spleen. For this reason patients who are known beyond doubt to have stage IIIB, IVA and IVB disease on the basis of clinical evidence and preliminary investigations, should not be subjected to laparotomy since drug treatment will be used (see below). The aim of the laparotomy is to help in the planning of the areas to be irradiated and, in some cases, to decide whether chemotherapy should be used in place of, or in addition to, radiotherapy. In those centres where it is routine practice to use chemotherapy for massive mediastinal disease and stage IIIA disease (Table 25.2), a laparotomy is also unnecessary.

In clinically localized disease above the diaphragm, a laparotomy will disclose subdiaphragmatic disease in 40% of patients. It is probable that in patients presenting in this way but not subjected to laparotomy, extended field radiation above and below the diaphragm, with irradiation of the spleen, produces as good relapse-free survival as radiation fields planned on the basis of laparotomy findings. Some centres have therefore employed these extensive radiation fields in preference to laparotomy. The disadvantage of this approach is that many patients will be overtreated with radiotherapy since only a minority will have intra-abdominal disease. High dose radiation over an extended field has a considerable morbidity (see below) and this approach is not generally used. In other centres, it is still the practice, in disease localized to one side of the neck or to the mediastinum, to treat without laparotomy on the basis that in these patients the chances of finding disease are small and that if relapse occurs in the abdomen, effective salvage treatment is available. Many oncologists do not take this view, arguing that there is a risk of occult splenic involvement and that this may give rise to disseminated disease, putting the patient at risk. However, it is not clear that a policy of limited assessment followed by radiotherapy, with chemotherapy if relapse occurs, will lead to reduced survival. The risks of laparotomy are small. The operative mortality in experienced hands is less than 1%. On the other hand, the procedure adds to the patient's discomfort and means that the treatment has been prolonged by a stay in hospital and convalescence. There is also a risk of morbidity associated with the procedure, such as subphrenic abscess, chest infection and venous thrombosis.

The long-term sequelae of splenectomy have been the subject of much investigation. In children below the age of 12 years, splenectomy seems unwise since the risk of bacterial infection, particularly with *Haemophilus influenzae* and *Streptococcus pneumoniae*, is increased. The problem is that patients with Hodgkin's disease are susceptible to infection by virtue of the immune suppression caused by the disease and its treatment. There seems little doubt that splenectomy adds to this susceptibility in children, and may also do so in adults although this is less well documented. It is not known whether prophylactic oral penicillin is of value in preventing late bacterial infection, although it is frequently recommended.

TREATMENT

It is important that physicians treating patients with Hodgkin's disease realize that there is now a good chance of cure for all patients, even when they present with extensive disease. The mainstay of treatment of localized disease is radiotherapy, with chemotherapy for advanced disease, and combined modality treatment in particular clinical situations. Chance of cure depends on when the patient first presents. Careful assessment of the best treatment strategy is critical at this stage. While many patients can still be cured after relapse, recurrence of disease usually worsens the outlook.

In the last 15 years the methods of using radiotherapy and drugs have changed considerably. An understanding of the principles of these treatments in the disease is important in planning the correct approach in each patient.

Principles of radiotherapy

The development of megavoltage equipment has allowed greater doses to be given over a wider area without intolerable damage to normal intervening tissues (see Chapter 5). Like all lymphomas, Hodgkin's disease is highly sensitive to radiotherapy, so that modest doses are generally adequate. The probability of long-term control (Fig. 25.8) at the irradiated site is

dependent on dose (10). The dose–response relationship is, however, less clear with doses above 30–35 Gy. It is uncertain whether the dose which is needed to eradicate clinically inapparent disease in adjacent nodes is the same or less than that required for enlarged nodes and big tumour masses. The usual practice at the present time is to treat both the involved and adjacent fields to the same dose level—usually in the region of 40 Gy in 25 daily fractions—though in some centres the uninvolved adjacent areas are treated to a lower dose, usually 35 Gy over 4 weeks.

There has been considerable debate over many years as to whether it is preferable to treat only the sites of clinical involvement (involved field, IF) or whether to extend the field to adjacent nodes (extended field, EF). The debate shifts its ground as new procedures such as staging laparotomy and combination chemotherapy are introduced and as 'salvage' treatment becomes more effective for relapse. For example, in patients with clinically localized cervical node disease, the possible advantage of

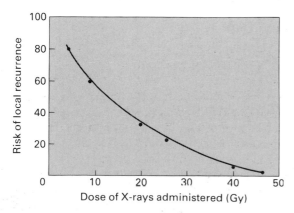

Fig. 25.8. *The relationship between local recurrence rate and dose of radiation administered.*

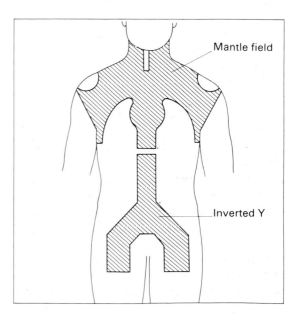

Fig. 25.9. *Mantle and inverted Y fields.* These are commonly employed fields. In this case the patient has been splenectomized.

EF radiotherapy such as the mantle field (Fig. 25.9) is less apparent if these patients do not have a staging laparotomy, since some of them will have undiagnosed (and therefore untreated) intra-abdominal disease and an even wider field would be necessary to treat these cases. Furthermore, now that chemotherapy for relapse after radiation failure is so much more successful than it was at the time when EF radiation was first introduced, the long-term survival advantage for EF rather than IF is much less apparent. The radiation fields most commonly employed are the mantle field for treating disease in the neck, mediastinum and axillae, and the inverted Y field for nodes in the para-aortic and iliac regions (Fig. 25.9). The lungs, larynx and humeral heads are shielded. When large mediastinal masses are irradiated the field is often progressively contracted as resolution occurs, to avoid irradiating large volumes of lung (see Chapter 5).

Principles of chemotherapy

A wide variety of cytotoxic agents show activity against Hodgkin's disease. The approximate response rates obtained with the different drugs, when used as single agents in advanced disease, are shown in Table 25.4.

When cytotoxic drugs are used as single agents the likelihood of a complete response is small and, if obtained, the response is not usually sustained for more than a few months even if the same drug or another is continued. Single agent chemotherapy is therefore palliative and not curative. The use of a single cytotoxan drug impairs the subsequent response to other drugs either alone or in combination. Complete lack of 'cross-resistance' is unusual. For this reason the prior administration of single agent chemotherapy is a grave mistake if there is a chance of cure with combination therapy.

The major step forward, therefore, was the evolution of modern combination chemotherapy in the 1960s. The drug regimen which has been most widely employed is the MOPP schedule introduced by DeVita and colleagues (11). The details of this and other commonly employed regimens are given in Table 25.5 with the approximate response rates. A total of six cycles of chemotherapy produces responses in a far higher proportion of cases than is seen with single agent treatment, even when the latter is given in high dosage with curative intent. Equally important, most of the responses are complete and in most cases are sustained when chemotherapy is stopped. Figure 25.10 shows the proportion of relapse-free patients after

Table 25.4. Approximate % response rates to cytotoxic drugs.

	Complete response	Partial response	Total
Alkylating agents			
Nitrogen mustard	10	50	60
Cyclophosphamide	10	45	55
Chlorambucil	15	45	60
Vinca alkaloids			
Vincristine	30	30	60
Vinblastine	30	30	60
Other agents			
Prednisolone	0	60	60
Procarbazine	30	35	65
Doxorubicin	10	30	40
Bleomycin	5	30	35
CCNU	5	40	45

Table 25.5. Combination chemotherapy regimes and approximate response rates (%).

		Complete response	Partial response	Total
MOPP (28 day cycle)		70	10	80
Mustine	6 mg/m² days 1,8 i.v.			
Vincristine (Oncovin)	2 mg (max) or 1.4 mg/m² days 1,8 i.v.			
Procarbazine	100 mg/m² days 1–19 p.o.			
Prednisolone	40 mg/m² days 1–14 p.o.			
MVPP (42 day cycle)		70	10	80
Mustine	6 mg/m² days 1,8 i.v.			
Vinblastine	6 mg/m² days 1,8 i.v.			
Procarbazine	100 mg/m² days 1–14 p.o.			
Prednisolone	40 mg days 1–14 p.o.			
ChlVPP (28 day cycle)		70	15	85
Chlorambucil	6 mg/m² days 1–14 p.o.			
Vinblastine	6 mg/m² days 1,8 i.v.			
Procarbazine	100 mg/m² days 1–14 p.o.			
Prednisolone	40 mg days 1–14 p.o.			
ABVD (28 day cycle)		70	10	80
Doxorubcin (Adriamycin)	25 mg/m² days 1,15 i.v.			
Bleomycin	10 mg/m² days 1,15 i.v.			
Vinblastine	10 mg/m² days 1,15 i.v.			
DTIC	375 mg/m² days 1,15 i.v.			

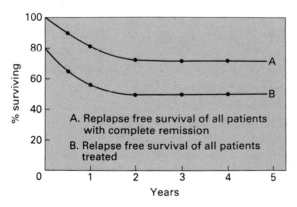

Fig. 25.10. *Relapse-free survival using MOPP chemotherapy.* Note: later relapses do occur and approximately 50% of all patients are relapse-free at 10-years.

A. Replapse free survival of all patients with complete remission

B. Relapse free survival of all patients treated

treatment with MOPP. Previously untreated patients have a 40–50% chance of long-term relapse-free survival with MOPP and other regimens and may be cured. The likelihood of achieving sustained complete response seems to be somewhat less in men, in patients over the age of 40 years and in those with marked constitutional symptoms. In these patients, alternating regimens of different drugs (i.e. MOPP and ABVD) may improve response and survival (12). Response rate, duration, and survival are much worse if the patient has previously been treated with single or multiple drug therapy. Previous radiotherapy does not seem to jeopardize response although the toxicity may be greater (see below). The general principles of administration of the drugs are discussed in Chapter 6.

The response to chemotherapy is usually rapid with disappearance of fever and reduction in tumour masses. Following six cycles of treatment there appears to be little advantage in maintenance chemotherapy with MOPP, although the use of a different regimen such as ABVD may prove to increase remission duration. If relapse occurs after MOPP, temporary improvement may be obtained by further treatment with MOPP. With the use of a different regimen (such as ABVD) prolonged survival is occasionally achieved, especially in those patients who relapse after having been treated with MOPP previously and are now in remission.

Single agent chemotherapy still has a place in the management of Hodgkin's disease only when it has been decided that intensive treatment is inappropriate or offers no chance of cure. Examples include elderly patients with associated general medical problems, and patients who have relapsed after previous intensive chemotherapy. In these patients, steroids will often suppress fever and restore appetite, whilst alkylating agents given intravenously or orally may control the disease for many months with little toxicity. Vinca alkaloids are also useful in this situation, vincristine being especially valuable if there is marrow depression.

MANAGEMENT AS DETERMINED BY STAGE

In the following discussion, guidelines are given as to the management of Hodgkin's disease at presentation according to clinical and pathological stage. Clinical practise varies considerably, so a consensus view is presented and difficult areas of management are considered separately.

CLINICAL STAGE IA, IIA; PATHOLOGICAL STAGE IA, IIA

In this category patients have one or more groups of nodes involved on one side of the diaphragm, and investigation including laparotomy and splenectomy has failed to show disease elsewhere. For this group of patients radiotherapy produces excellent results (Fig. 25.11). The usual practice for patients with cervical and mediastinal disease is to irradiate the mantle field (Fig. 25.9) to a dose of 40–44 Gy in 20–25 fractions. For those presenting with inguinal

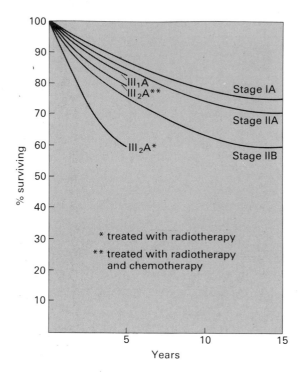

Fig. 25.11. *Survival related to stage in Hodgkin's disease.* Figures are approximate and incorporate results using different treatment strategies.

node disease the inverted Y field is generally used. The use of chemotherapy in localized disease and the treatment of massive mediastinal disease are discussed separately.

CLINICAL STAGE IA, IIA; PATHOLOGICAL STAGE UNKNOWN

Although the practice of staging laparotomy and splenectomy as part of the management of individual patients has grown and has much to commend it, it is not universal and in some patients the risk of the procedure may be considered unacceptable. The best method of management when laparotomy has not been performed is a matter of considerable controversy. Three treatment strategies have been advocated.

1 To treat with either mantle field or IF irradiation only, and to rely on salvage irradiation or chemotherapy on relapse. The advantage of

this approach is that it avoids overtreatment of a large number of patients especially those with good histology in whom the risk of occult intra-abdominal disease is small. However, the question of whether treatment on relapse is as effective as early treatment is as yet unanswered. Diminished survival with delayed treatment has been reported, but mostly from trials conducted in the days before combination chemotherapy.

2 To treat with total nodal irradiation (TNI) including the spleen. This is associated with good results but many patients will be overtreated by this approach, and if systemic relapse occurs soon after TNI, the toxicity of chemotherapy may be very considerable.

3 To treat with mantle radiotherapy followed by six cycles of MOPP, or with chemotherapy followed by irradiation. Again many patients will be over-treated and the long-term sequelae of radiotherapy and chemotherapy are worrying (see below). Long-term disease-free survival is usually obtained and this approach may be safest especially if the histology is poor. There is an increasing tendency to use chemotherapy first.

The policy for this group of patients will, therefore, vary in different institutions. Some centres do not perform laparotomies on clinical stage IA and IIA patients preferring to treat all of them by **2** or **3** above. In Britain many centres will adopt strategy **1**.

CLINICAL STAGE IA, IIA, IIIA; PATHALOGICAL STAGE IIIA

In this category patients have presented with localized disease but laparotomy has demonstrated spread to spleen and/or lymph nodes in the abdomen. The distinction between $IIIA_1$ and $IIIA_2$ is useful in deciding on treatment within the IIIA category as a whole. In this group stage $IIIA_1$ patients (see Table 25.2) can be treated with TNI, reserving chemotherapy for relapse, but stage $IIIA_2$ patients fare less well with this approach and their prognosis appears to be improved by adding chemotherapy to the TNI.

The morbidity of TNI and MOPP is, however, considerable but the differences in survival (Fig. 25.11) indicate that chemotherapy is necessary. A recent trial has indicated that chemotherapy alone may be as effective as TNI and chemotherapy in stage IIIA.

CLINICAL STAGE IIB, IIIB; PATHOLOGICAL STAGE IIIB, IVB, OR UNKNOWN

The patient presents with constitutional symptoms and widespread disease, or with more localized disease (IIB), and is either found to have extensive disease at laparotomy or the pathological stage is unknown. The mainstay of treatment is chemotherapy with MOPP or a similar regimen. In poor prognosis patients (see principles of chemotherapy above) there may prove to be an advantage in treatment with alternating 'non cross-resistant' drugs such as ABVD but this remains to be seen. Although pathological stage IIB disease (an unusual category) can be treated with EF radiotherapy alone, the risk of relapse is high and if IF radiotherapy is used the results are very poor, early relapse being very likely.

Clinical problems

There are a number of problems in management which occur frequently and which do not fall readily into any of the above categories.

MASSIVE MEDIASTINAL DISEASE

It is not uncommon to find a huge mediastinal mass in a relatively asymptomatic patient, in which the mass, on chest X-ray, occupies more than one-third of the transverse diameter of the chest or is greater than 10 cm across (Fig. 25.5). Several studies have suggested that it is difficult to control the disease by radiation alone and that early chemotherapy improves both relapse-free survival and overall survival. At present the data are somewhat conflicting, but many physicians would treat such patients with both radiotherapy and combination chemotherapy using MOPP or one of its variants. If chemotherapy is used it avoids the need for laparotomy. The usual practice is to give chemotherapy first, allowing a smaller volume to be irradiated.

COMBINED MODALITY TREATMENT IN PATHOLOGICAL STAGE IA AND IIA

In early disease the use of chemotherapy in addition to radiotherapy has been the subject of considerable investigation and is by no means standard practice. To date it can be said that while relapse-free survival is better than with radiotherapy alone, overall survival is not improved because 'salvage' treatment is increasingly effective on relapse. IF radiotherapy and chemotherapy without laparotomy may prove to be as effective in early disease as EF radiotherapy after full staging procedures. At present there is no definite indication for using chemotherapy early in IA and IIA disease although some centres do so if there are many (>5) groups of nodes involved.

TREATMENT ON RELAPSE

If patients who have been treated with radiotherapy relapse with widespread disease or with marked constitutional symptoms, then chemotherapy is the mainstay of treatment. If relapse appears to be localized, and potentially curable by radiotherapy, it is important to reassess the extent of the disease. This will usually mean liver and marrow biopsy, chest X-ray, CT scan of the abdomen and/or refill lymphogram, and in selected cases, a laparotomy. The circumstances depend on the extent of previous staging investigations and treatment. For many patients, relapse does not mean that they cannot be cured, but it is often the case that the first relapse is the last chance of definitive treatment.

HODGKIN'S DISEASE IN CHILDHOOD

There is no evidence that Hodgkin's disease carries a worse prognosis in childhood and current results are as good or better than in adults. The disease appears particularly sensitive to chemotherapy in children. There are, however, several problems in management of the disease in young children. First, high dose radiation profoundly affects bone growth and for example in the case of vertebrae, the child's prospect of reaching a normal height is reduced (see Chapter 8). Second, in children, splenectomy is associated with an increased risk of bacterial infection, particularly with pneumococci. Third, the long-term consequences of treatment in childhood are not yet fully understood.

In children with clinical stage I, with minimal disease, the yield of staging laparotomy is small. Such patients can be treated by IF irradiation without laparotomy, with good results. For children with clinical stage II and III disease and with bulky stage I disease, extended field irradiation produces a relapse-free survival of about 50% at 5-years. However there is a strong argument for treatment with low dose (20–25 Gy) extended field irradiation, with six cycles of MOPP or equivalent often given as three cycles before and after radiotherapy. Relapse-free 5-year survival of about 80% is achieved by this means and staging laparotomy is avoided. It is not clear if chemotherapy alone is as effective as the combined modality treatment. As in adults, chemotherapy is the mainstay of treatment of stage IIIB and IV disease.

HODGKIN'S DISEASE DURING PREGNANCY

Occasionally Hodgkin's disease is diagnosed for the first time during pregnancy. If this happens during the first 20 weeks, it is probably best to advise termination and then to proceed to the usual evaluation and treatment. During the last trimester, if the patient is not ill, it is possible to wait until delivery before investigation and treatment. More difficult problems arise if the pregnancy is advanced (20 weeks or more) and the disease is progressing and/or the patient is constitutionally unwell, or if the pregnancy is early but termination is refused.

In a woman in advanced pregnancy in whom treatment cannot be delayed until delivery because the disease is advanced or growing rapidly, it is probably best to treat with combination chemotherapy. There are several reports of normal full-term children being born to women who have received combination chemotherapy during pregnancy but clearly it is prudent to postpone such treatment for as long as possible. Single agent chemotherapy was used in the past but this is not good practice since there is little to suggest that the adverse effects on the foetus are less, and there is a grave problem of worsening the long-term prognosis by single agent therapy. If a woman refuses termination early in pregnancy and has progressive disease, chemotherapy should be delayed as long as possible to allow the early, crucial stages of foetal development to proceed. If the patient has apparently localized supradiaphragmatic disease but it is felt inadvisable to wait until after delivery, localized radiotherapy is given and full investigation is deferred. In this situation, where a decision has to be made between chemotherapy and irradiation, abbreviated staging using ultrasound and a lymphogram with one X-ray exposure can be helpful.

If a woman with previously diagnosed, investigated and treated for Hodgkin's disease relapses during pregnancy, then similar considerations apply. In women who have been successfully treated for Hodgkin's disease there is no evidence that pregnancy will provoke recurrence or adversely affect prognosis.

Toxicity of treatment

The toxicity of radiotherapy and chemotherapy has been dealt with in general terms in Chapters 5 and 6. The following brief account specifically concerns Hodgkin's disease.

ACUTE TOXICITY OF CHEMOTHERAPY

Bone Marrow Depression is a common accompaniment of all standard chemotherapeutic regimens in Hodgkin's disease. Most centres make dosage reductions in response to depressed blood counts, rather than delay the cycle, although delay may be necessary on occasions. The toxicity tends to be cumulative and particular care should be taken as treatment progresses, especially in the elderly, in those who have received EF radiotherapy in the past and in ill patients with extensive disease. After TNI the problem is particularly severe since over 50% of the adult haemopoietic marrow is within the irradiation field. Recovery of the marrow after TNI takes years, and is often incomplete, so chemotherapy should be introduced with caution in these patients.

Immunosuppression Treatment adds to the depression of cell-mediated immunity (CMI) which is commonly present in advanced disease. Lymphopenia is an invariable consequence of EF irradiation and persists for several months after treatment. Depression of CMI is induced by most cytotoxic agents, especially alkylating agents and steroids. For this reason *Herpes zoster* and *Herpes simplex* are very common in heavily treated patients and may be life-threatening. Less common nowadays is reactivation of tuberculosis, but other opportunistic infections such as pneumocystis, cytomegalovirus and aspergillosis are occasionally seen.

LONG-TERM COMPLICATIONS OF RADIATION

Radiation pneumonitis, leading to fibrosis, is a relatively common complication if the radiation dose is above 40 Gy. For this reason very large mediastinal masses require special consideration. Chemotherapy is often used to produce tumour shrinkage before irradiation, though it is not clear whether it is sufficient to irradiate the residual volume only. For smaller nodal areas complication is exceptionally rare.

Occasionally mediastinal irradiation may cause pericarditis with a pericardial effusion which usually resolves. This may cause pain but is usually asymptomatic. Constrictive pericarditis is an extremely uncommon complication of mediastinal irradiation using modern techniques. Radiation damage to coronary arteries seems to be very rare.

Clinical hypothyroidism is an infrequent (5%) complication of mantle field irradiation, although transiently elevated TSH levels are more frequent (30%). Radiation damage to the bowel following infradiaphragmatic irradiation may rarely occur giving rise to diarrhoea (sometimes bloody), steatorrhoea and intestinal obstruction. It is related to both the volume and the total dose administered. It is more likely to occur if the bowel has been tethered in one site by previous inflammation or surgery.

In the CNS the commonest symptom of radiation damage is Lhermitte's syndrome of tingling and parasthesiae in the legs, often provoked by neck flexion. This usually passes off with no sequelae. Transverse myelitis should not occur with modern planning techniques. Very high repeated doses over peripheral nerves can rarely lead to peripheral neuropathy usually within 1–5 years.

Impaired spermatogenesis occurs with doses of irradiation as low as 50 cGy and is more rapid, complete and long lasting with higher doses, being invariable and often permanent above 5 Gy (see Chapter 5). During pelvic irradiation, with effective shielding, the dose should be below 100 cGy. The dose which causes permanent cessation of ovarian function is higher than for the testis. Oophoropexy is sometimes carried out at staging laparotomy to bring the ovaries out of a possible pelvic irradiation field (see above).

LONG-TERM COMPLICATIONS OF MOPP
(SEE CHAPTER 6)

Female fertility may be depressed after MOPP but the effect is inconsistent. Persistent amenorrhoea and the onset of the menopause are more likely to occur in older women. Amenorrhoea frequently occurs during treatment but normal menstruation usually returns and many patients have had children after treatment. There are worrying anecdotes of foetal abnormalities as a result of such pregnancies but the risk is not clear. The hazard of teratogenicity during chemotherapy on the other hand is usually regarded as an indication for termination.

Azoospermia is almost inevitable after MOPP or its variants. Procarbazine and the alkylating agents appear to be responsible. Recovery from sterility is rare. Sperm storage prior to chemotherapy is advisable for men who are concerned about the effects of fertility.

During the first 5 years after MOPP chemotherapy the cumulative risk of herpes zoster is approximately 15% and is 50% after MOPP with TNI. Disseminated zoster (9%) is more common in those receiving combined modality treatment than with chemotherapy or radiation alone (2%). Bacterial infections, especially pneumococcal, occur more often, particularly in children, patients over 50, and possibly in those who have had splenectomy.

SECOND MALIGNANCIES

In recent years it has become apparent that following chemotherapy for Hodgkin's disease, there is an increased risk of developing a second cancer. The association is best documented for acute non-lymphocytic leukaemia (ANL). At present, the risk of developing ANL in the 7 years after chemotherapy alone, or combined modality treatment, is approximately 6%. However, in patients over the age of 40 years, the risk of ANL appears to be higher. Other miscellaneous tumours occur less often, possibly no more frequently than by chance. Both alkylating agents and procarbazine are potential carcinogens, but the cause of the increased incidence of ANL is not known. ANL may be less common after ABVD; however, this regimen has been introduced into clinical practice more recently than MOPP, and since the leukaemia risk is highest more than 5 years after chemotherapy, it is too soon to assume that ABVD is not leukaemogenic. The risk of leukaemia relates to survivors rather than those treated. It is important to appreciate that the risk of dying of Hodgkins's disease is far greater than the hazard of a second malignancy.

REFERENCES

1 Correa P. & O'Connor GT (1971) Epidemiologic patterns of Hodgkin's disease. *International Journal of Cancer* **8**, 192.
2 Grufferman S.G., Cole P., Smith P.G. & Lukes R.J. (1977) Hodgkin's disease in siblings. *New England Journal of Medicine* **296**, 248.
3 Smith P.G., Pike M.C., Kinlen L.J., Jones A. & Harris R. (1977) Contacts between young patients with Hodgkin's disease. A case-control study. *Lancet* **2**, 59.
4 Lukes R.J. & Butler J.J. (1966) The pathology and nomenclature of Hodgkin's disease. *Cancer Research* **26**, 1063.
5 Eltringham J.R. & Kaplan H.S. (1973) Impaired delayed hypersensitivity responses in 154 patients with untreated Hodgkin's disease. *National Cancer Institute Monography* **36**, 107.
6 Ultman J.E. & Moran E.M. (1973) Clinical course and complications in Hodgkin's disease. *Archives of Internal Medicine* **131**, 332.
7 Atkinson M.K., Austin D.E., McElwain T.J. & Peckham M.J. (1976) Alcohol pain in Hodgkin's disease. *Cancer* **37**, 895.
8 Irving M. (1973) The role of surgery in the management of Hodgkin's disease. *British Journal of Surgery* **62**, 853.
9 Carbone P.P., Kaplan H.S., Musshoff K., Smithers D.W. & Tubiana M. (1971) Report of the committee on Hodgkin's disease staging. *Cancer Research* **31**, 1860.
10 Kaplan H.S. (1966) Evidence for a tumorical dose level in the radiotherapy of Hodgkin's disease. *Cancer Research* **26**, 1221.
11 DeVita V.T., Serpick A. & Carbone P.P. (1970) Combination chemotherapy in the treatment of advanced Hodgkin's disease. *Annals of Internal Medicine* **73**, 881.
12 Long D.L., Young R.C. & DeVita V.T. (1982) Chemotherapy for Hodgkin's disease: the remaining challenges. *Cancer Treatment Reports* **66**, 925.

FURTHER READING

Kaplan H.S. (1980) *Hodgkin's disease.* (2nd edn) Harvard University Press. A masterpiece of experience, lucidity and scholarship, and an unsurpassed source of reference.

Chapter 26

Non-Hodgkin's Lymphomas

INCIDENCE AND AETIOLOGY

Non-Hodgkin's lymphomas are a heterogeneous group of neoplasms which occur mainly in the elderly population. The age-specific incidence is shown in Fig. 26.1. There are marked geographical variations in the incidence of these tumours. Burkitt's lymphoma, for example, is common in Africa and rare in the United States and Britain, while in the Middle East intestinal lymphoma is much more common than in Britain.

A variety of medical conditions is associated with an increased tendency to develop lymphoma (Table 26.1). It is of interest that many of these diseases are associated with depressed immunity, either congenital, as in Wiskott-Aldrich syndrome and ataxia telangiectasia, or acquired, as in the lymphoma which occurs in renal transplant recipients and AIDS. In Sjögren's syndrome and in rheumatoid arthritis, the lymphoma appears to arise independently of immunosuppressive therapy.

Careful follow-up of patients on long-term immunosuppressive drugs for autoimmune dis-

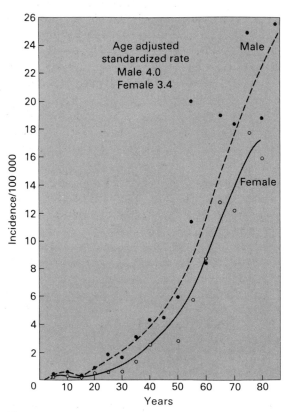

Fig. 26.1. *Age-specific incidence of non-Hodgkin's lymphoma.*

Table 26.1. Disorders predisposing to development of lymphoma.

Congenital
    Chediak-Higashi syndrome
    Ataxia-Telangiectasia
    Wiscott-Aldrich syndrome
    Swiss-type agammaglobulinaemia
    Klinefelter's syndrome
    Coeliac disease
    Bloom's syndrome
    X-linked lymphoproliferative disease

Acquired
    Chronic immune suppression
      (e.g. Renal allograft recipients)
    Sjögrens syndrome
    Rheumatoid Arthritis
    Common variable hypogammaglobulinaemia
    Acquired Immune Deficiency Syndrome (AIDS)

ease or to prevent renal allograft rejection, have shown that there is an increased incidence of lymphoma (1). Curiously in Wiskott-Aldrich syndrome and in renal allograft recipients there is a particular tendency to develop an intracerebral immunoblastic lymphoma. This tumour is rarely seen except in these patients. It is not clear whether immunosuppressive therapy is itself carcinogenic, or whether it permits activity of another oncogenic agent, such as Ebstein-Barr virus, in a chronically immunosuppressed patient. An increased risk of lymphoma has been reported in the survivors of the atom bomb explosion in Hiroshima, and in those patients who have been irradiated in early adult life for ankylosing spondylitis.

Recently, in cases of Burkitt's lymphoma, a series of characteristic translocations of immunoglobulin genes has been described. There is reciprocal translocation of the variable region of the immunoglobulin heavy chain locus on chromosome 14 and a portion of chromosome 8, and the lambda chain locus on chromosome 22 and kappa locus on chromosome 2 may also be reciprocally translocated to chromosome 8. Of great interest is the recent finding that in Burkitt's cells the cellular homologue of the retrovirus oncogene, c-myc, has been located in the long arm of chromosome 8 which is involved in these translocations (see Chapter 3). Furthermore, there is increased expression of c-myc in Burkitt's cells in culture. This provides some evidence for the controlling influence of these genes during oncogenesis. In other types of lymphoma chromosome defects have not been demonstrated consistently.

There is a strong association between serological evidence of Epstein-Barr virus (EBV) and Burkitt's lymphoma. In White children with Burkitt's lymphoma there is no serological association with EBV though cultured lymphoma cells from many American and all African children express Epstein-Barr virus nuclear antigen EBNA, (2). In areas of Africa where Burkitt's lymphoma is endemic, most children have evidence of past infection with EBV as shown by serum antibody to EBV. The majority of these children do not develop Burkitt's lymphoma, so it is assumed that some other factor is operating to produce the tumour and that the EBV has a permissive role in its development.

Similar difficulties in interpretation surround the role of the newly described non-Hodgkin's T cell leukaemia/lymphoma virus (HTLV1). In 1977 a T cell leukaemia/lymphoma was described in Japan, and in 1981 a retro-virus was isolated from T cell cultures from these tumours. Subsequently it was shown that antibodies to HTLV1 are usually present in patients with this disorder, but not detected in patients with non T cell lymphomas. Antibodies were, however, sometimes present in relatives of patients with the disease. At the same time, workers in the United States isolated a retrovirus from cultures of lymphoma T cells taken from a patient with a cutaneous T cell lymphoma. Subsequently, similar viruses have been isolated from a wide variety of T cell tumours. T cell lymphoma has been described in Caribbeans in which the patients have antibody to HTLV1 in the serum, and HTLV1 coded antigens can be demonstrated on the surface of the tumour T cells. Curiously, many of these patients have hypercalcaemia. It is not clear what the role of HTLV1 is in the production of the tumours.

In summary, in spite of intriguing circumstantial evidence, at the present time it is not possible to be certain what role viral infections play in the aetiology of non-Hodgkin's lymphomas.

Finally, phenytoin can cause a lymphoma-like syndrome (see p. 467). This may subside spontaneously after removal of the drug. However, a small proportion of cases go on to develop a progressive lymphoma and it is possible that the drug is instrumental in its development.

PATHOLOGY

There is a bewildering profusion of terminology to describe the pathological appearance of non-Hodgkin's lymphoma. This has come about because the enormous growth of knowledge in cellular immunology in the last decade has led to attempts to classify the tumour according to what is known about normal lymphocyte development. At the same time conventional pathological descriptions of the diseases have been developed and refined to accommodate the widely differing clinical features and prognosis. Attempts have also been made to combine both pathological and immunological descriptions, and immunocytochemical staining of fresh-frozen biopsy material is increasingly employed for accurate diagnosis. This has led to increasing difficulty for the clinician and general pathologist. What follows, therefore, is a brief guide to the basis of the immunological contribution to our understanding of these diseases, followed by a synopsis of how the diseases are described in pathological terms.

During foetal life precursors of T lymphocytes are formed and migrate to the thymus, and thence to the developing lymph nodes and spleen. Maturation into mature T cells takes place at various stages especially in the thymus. The sequence of maturation can be defined by their surface antigen structure. Monoclonal antibodies to T cell surface antigens have been

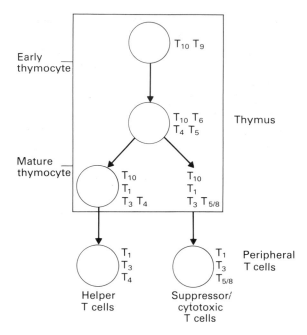

Fig. 26.2. *T cell surface phenotype during maturation in the thymus.* The T cell antigens are identified by monoclonal antibodies and are helpful in categorizing the various forms of T cell lymphoma and leukaemia.

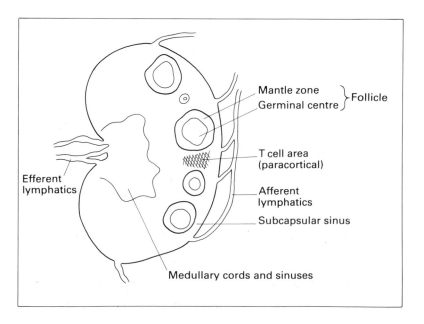

Fig. 26.3. *Lymph node structure.*

especially helpful in this respect. The sequence of maturation is shown in Fig. 26.2. By the time the T cell leaves the thymus its function as a helper cell or cytotoxic/suppressor cell is established.

In the lymph nodes the T cells lodge in the paracortical region (Fig. 26.3) and around the central arterioles in the spleen. Some T cells recirculate from the lymphatic system to the blood and thence from the blood back to the lymph nodes where they enter the paracortical region through post-capillary venules.

Early B lymphocytes are formed in the foetal liver and subsequently in the bone marrow. From there they migrate to the lymph nodes. They are found in the follicles which consist of an outer mantle zone of small lymphocytes, and a germinal centre composed of cells where the nucleus is either irregular in shape or large and round. The cells with a nucleus of irregular outline are called cleaved cells or *centrocytes* and those with a large round nucleus, non-cleaved or *centroblasts*. Some B lymphocytes recirculate between nodes and blood. After contact with antigen B cells transform into antibody-secreting plasma cells.

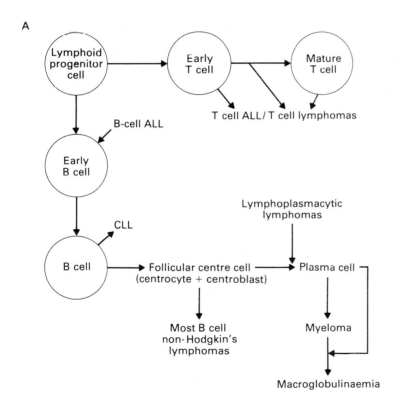

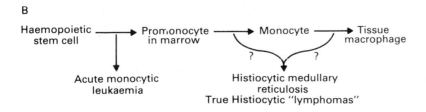

Fig. 26.4. *Simplified scheme of cell origin of non-Hodgkin's lymphomas.* (A) Origin of B cell and T cell lymphomas. (B) Origin of macrophage tumours.

Macrophages, or mononuclear phagocytes, are formed from pluripotent haemopoietic stem cells in the marrow. They are liberated into the blood stream as monocytes and lodge in tissues at sites of inflammation (histiocytes). They also play a part in repopulating the 'fixed' tissue phagocytic cells—Kupffer cells, splenic, alveolar and peritoneal macrophages. The antigen-presenting cells (dendritic cells) in lymph nodes and spleen may also be part of the mononuclear phagocyte system. A simplified guide to the stage in differentiation of lymphocytes and macrophages to which various non-Hodgkin's lymphomas and leukaemias correspond is shown in Fig. 26.4 and a synopsis of the immunological classification of lympho-reticular neoplasms is shown in Table 26.2.

In the early 1970s it was realized that the majority of lymphomas were derived from cells of the follicular centre and consisted of either centrocytes (cleaved cells) or centroblasts (non-cleaved cells), or a mixture of the two. As immunological techniques developed, more individual cell types were identified within the lymphomas and classification developed accordingly. The following cell types have been identified: small lymphocytes (B and T), lymphoplasmacytic cells, plasma cells, centrocytes (small and large), centroblasts (small and large), immunoblasts (B and T), and lymphoblasts (B and T).

B cell neoplasms make up the majority of non-Hodgkin's lymphomas (Table 26.2). The most common are all the follicular lymphomas which are derived from the B cell of the follicle centre. However these cells do not always form follicles and may also give rise to a diffuse lymphoma.

T cell lymphomas probably constitute about 10% of non-Hodgkin's lymphomas (Table 26.2). The T cell lymphomas can be divided into three broad categories:
1 cutaneous lymphomas
2 Thymic lymphomas
3 Peripheral T cell lymphoma
Morphologically they are diffuse with a wide variety of cellular morphology.

It is not yet clear how many of these tumours are neoplasms of malignant macrophages. Those which are, should not strictly speaking, be called lymphomas (4). The term histiocytic lymphoma which was introduced by Rappaport is now regarded as erroneous since many of the tumours which he described are B cell neoplasms. There is still uncertainty about how frequently true macrophage (histiocytic) tumours occur. Recent histochemical evidence has suggested that they may account for 5% of diffuse large-cell lymphomas (Table 26.2).

Table 26.2. Cell of origin of lymphomas.

B Cell Tumours	T Cell tumours
Follicular lymphomas of centrocytes and centroblasts	Cutaneous T cell lymphoma
Diffuse lymphomas centroblastic, centrocytic, immunoblastic	T cell lymphoma of mediastinum with convoluted nuclei
Lymphoplasmacytoid (Waldenström's)	Peripheral T cell lymphoma
Chronic lymphatic leukaemia	Other lymphoblastic and immunoblastic lymphomas usually of diffuse type
Burkitt's lymphoma	
Heavy chain disease	*Macrophage tumours* Some diffuse large cell 'lymphomas'
	Histiocytic medullary reticulosis
	Histiocytosis X

Although the immunological classification of lymphoma is logical and in many respects superior, the pathological diagnosis in most departments rests on conventional light microscopical appearances (Fig 26.5). The Rappaport system divided the lymphomas according to whether there was nodule formation or the node was diffusely replaced by tumour. The term 'nodular' is sometimes used synonymously with 'follicular'. In most instances the pattern is due to the formation of follicles by the neoplastic cells and the term follicular rather than nodular should be used to describe these tumours. These categories (follicular and diffuse) were then divided according to cell type: well-differentiated lymphocytic; poorly differentiated lymphocytic; mixed lymphocytic and histiocytic; histiocytic and undifferentiated. The term 'histiocytic' was a misnomer (see above) but the classification emphasized the prognostic significance of the microscopic appearances. The follicular lymphomas had a good prognosis and lymphocytic lymphomas a better outlook than histiocytic or undifferentiated. This scheme is still widely used.

Recently, a panel of distinguished pathologists have devised a working formulation which

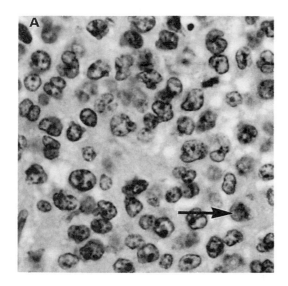

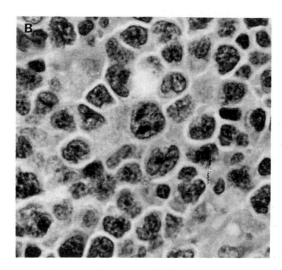

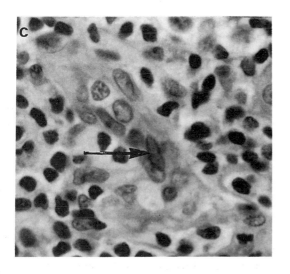

Fig. 26.5. *Histological appearances in non-Hodgkin's lymphoma.* (Original magnification ×400.) (A) Follicle centre cell lymphoma predominantly containing centrocytes but with scattered centroblasts (arrowed). (B) Follicle centre cell lymphoma composed principally of centroblasts. (C) Peripheral T cell lymphoma showing proliferating high endothelial venules (arrowed) and a mixture of small and large lymphocytes, some with clear cytoplasm, others showing an irregular nuclear outline.

allows some cross-reference between the classifications (5). It has been criticized for not being immunologically based but it is given here because it is likely to be used increasingly. This formulation was not intended to supplant existing classifications but to allow increasingly bewildered clinicians to steer their way through the maze of classifications and terms used in publications, text books and by their local pathologists. The formulation is given in Table 26.3.

One major difficulty with any classification is that within a single lymph node, or group of nodes, areas of follicular or diffuse change may both occur, and both small and large cells are often found. Furthermore, follicular lympho-

Table 26.3. Working formulation for clinical usage (with alternative terminology in italics)

Low Grade Malignancy
A   Diffuse small cell differentiated lymphocytes, consistent with chronic lymphatic leukaemia. Plasmacytoid features may be present.

B   Follicular. Small cleaved cells—*centrocytes*. Some diffuse areas.

C   Follicular mixed small and large cleaved cells. Some diffuse areas.

Intermediate Grade Malignancy
D   Follicular. Large centrocytes and centroblasts—*cleaved and non-cleaved*. Diffuse areas.

E   Diffuse. Small cleared cell—*centrocytic*.

F   Diffuse. Small and large cell—*small and large centrocytic and centroblastic*.

G   Diffuse. Large cleaved and non-cleaved cells—*large centrocytes and centroblasts*.

High Grade
H   Diffuse large cell, immunoblastic type.
I   Diffuse lymphoblastic cells sometimes convoluted.
J   Diffuse small non-cleaved cells—*centroblasts*.

Other
   Mycosis fungoides

   Unclassifiable

   Plasmacytomas—*extramedullary*

mas frequently evolve into diffuse large cell forms in the course of their natural history.

A rule of thumb with respect to prognosis is that the greater the degree of follicle formation the better, and that small well-differentiated lymphocytes are associated with a better prognosis than lymphoblastic, immunoblastic or other large cell types.

CLINICAL FEATURES

Non-Hodgkin's lymphomas usually arise in peripheral lymph nodes, but may also develop at a wide variety of extra-nodal sites. The clinical features of extra-nodal lymphomas are described later (see p. 468).

PRESENTATION OF NODAL DISEASE

Painless enlargement of a lymph node is the most frequent presentation of non-Hodgkin's lymphoma, and the commonest site is the neck. Sometimes the nodes fluctuate in size which can lead to delay in diagnosis. Non-Hodgkin's lymphomas tend to be more widespread at presentation than Hodgkin's disease and to be present at more unusual lymph node sites, for example, Waldeyer's ring. Although the presentation is usually straightforward the enlarging lymph node mass may cause initial symptoms due to compression, for example, swelling of the arm or leg, simulating deep venous thrombosis, or superior vena caval obstruction.

Retroperitoneal lymph node enlargement can cause backache and obstructive renal failure, and nodes in the porta hepatis may cause obstructive jaundice. Widespread infiltration of the liver is usually accompanied by weight loss, anorexia and fever.

Even without liver involvement, constitutional symptoms are not infrequent with weight loss, night sweats and fever. Intra-abdominal lymphoma may present with fever of unknown origin, especially if there is hepatic or narrow involvement.

Clinical examination must be meticulous. The neck should be carefully examined and it is often easier to determine the extent of disease in the neck if the examination is carried out from behind the patient. Node enlargement should be sought in the pre- and post-auricular regions, in the occiput, the supra- and infraclavicular areas, and deep behind the sternomastoid. The axilla should be carefully examined both in the apex and the walls. Epitrochlear nodes are often missed. In the abdomen the size of the liver and spleen should be noted and an attempt made to examine abdominal and retroperitoneal nodes by deep palpation. The inguinal nodes are often slightly enlarged in normal individuals but pathological inguino-femoral nodes may extend downwards into the medial aspect of the thigh. Examination of the oro- and nasopharynx should be a routine, as should rectal examination which may lead to detection of large masses of pelvic nodes.

Diagnosis and investigation of nodal lymphomas

The diagnosis is by node or tissue biopsy. Although there is usually little difficulty about the diagnosis, other conditions may simulate lymphoma (see p. 465) especially at extranodal sites, and precise immunological classification is becoming increasingly important in management. For these reasons a lymph node biopsy should be regarded as an important clinical investigation and not as a trivial affair. The biopsy should not be left to a junior surgeon. Too often inexperienced surgeons biopsy a superficial node, which shows reactive hyperplasia, or a node in the neck or groin which may not be obviously abnormal. If there is a deeper clearly pathological node this should be removed. Nowadays, immunohistochemistry is helping a great deal in diagnosis, particularly in distinguishing large cell lymphomas from anaplastic carcinoma, and in the diagnosis of T cell tumours. Some of these investigations can only

be done on fresh or frozen tissue so the biopsy should not be placed in formaldehyde and the pathologist will advise as required. If the node shows reactive hyperplasia or an equivocal result one should not hesitate to biopsy another node if the clinical suspicion is high. If the nodes are in an inaccessible site it may be necessary to proceed to laparotomy or mediastinotomy. It is often better to do this than to repeatedly biopsy equivocally enlarged peripheral nodes.

Staging notation

The staging notation is the same as that employed for Hodgkin's disease (see Table 25.2). Unlike Hodgkin's disease the great majority of patients will have Stages III and IV disease at presentation.

In the investigation of non-Hodgkin's lymphoma there are certain routine tests which are inexpensive, harmless, and sometimes rewarding and these should be performed. A chest X-ray may show hilar, mediastinal or paratracheal node enlargement. Parenchymal lung lesions are less common as are pleural effusions, but the latter occur not infrequently when there is massive mediastinal disease. Occasionally the effusion is chylous due to rupture of lymphatics in the mediastinum. Lung infiltrates and effusions which contain lymphoma cells usually occur when there is associated mediastinal or hilar disease.

The blood count may show anaemia, which is usually normochromic and typical of the anaemia of chronic disease (with a low serum iron and iron-binding capacity). Occasionally it is due to auto-immune haemolysis and a Coombs' test and reticulocyte count should be performed if this is suspected. The blood film may show circulating lymphoma cells. However immunological methods may detect a malignant population which is not apparent on the blood smear and the proportion of patients with blood involvement will certainly prove to be higher than the present 10% of cases identified by the blood film. Recent methods of demonstrating monoclonality in B cells have been applied to bone marrow and have suggested a high level (30–50%) of involvement in both follicular and diffuse lymphomas. An abnormal blood film implies marrow disease, but this may not always be detected on aspiration and biopsy. Conversely marrow involvement on biopsy is not always associated with an abnormal peripheral blood picture. The blood urea and electrolytes should be measured to exclude renal failure. The liver enzymes should also be measured since a rise in alkaline phosphatase and transaminases may indicate liver infiltration and the alkaline phosphatase and bilirubin may be elevated if there are nodes in the porta hepatis causing compression.

Other investigations include ultrasound or CT scanning of the abdomen or pelvis to demonstrate intra-abdominal or pelvic disease, an intravenous urogram if there is evidence of renal impairment and X-rays and bone scan if there is bone pain or tenderness at a particular site. Lymphography has been widely used to demonstrate pelvic and para-aortic nodes. Most patients (80%) with nodular lymphoma have abnormal lymphograms, and approximately 60% of those with diffuse lymphoma. Unlike Hodgkin's disease, a positive lymphogram is also associated with increased likelihood of disease in mesenteric nodes in the porta hepatis, and with involvement of liver and spleen. CT scanning is a less troublesome alternative to lymphography and has about the same sensitivity. It has the advantage of being able to demonstrate nodal masses in the mesentery and in the upper abdomen—sites poorly demonstrated by lymphography.

How far should these tests be done as a routine and combined with more invasive tests such as liver or marrow biopsy? This depends on what the treatment strategy is to be. If there is a prospect that the disease is localized and the patient might be cured by radiotherapy, extensive investigation is needed to define the true extent of the disease. But if the treatment is to be with palliative local radiotherapy, for example in an elderly patient with clinically local-

ized disease, then invasive investigations are meddlesome. If the histology and clinical features indicate widespread poor prognosis disease then intensive chemotherapy will be used and it becomes irrelevant to persist with unpleasant investigations like lymphography. In other words, one should ask oneself the question 'will I learn something from this investigation which will affect my decision about management or prognosis?'

Most cases of non-Hodgkin's lymphoma presenting as nodal disease should be regarded as widespread, irrespective of histology (6). Typical results of investigation of nodal disease are shown in Table 26.4 and 26.5. This shows that for both nodular and diffuse lymphomas it is likely that there will be evidence of disease on lymphography, and a not inconsiderable

Table 26.4. Investigation of nodal non-Hodgkin's lymphoma (% positive). (From Chabner *et al* (6), with permission.)

Lymphomas	Lymphogram	Marrow biopsy*	Liver biopsy*
Follicular	90%	30%	20%
Diffuse	60–80%	30%	20%

*The proportion of marrow and liver biopsies showing disease will be higher if more sensitive tests for demonstrating tumour B lymphocytes are used.

Table 26.5. Change in stage after investigation of nodal non-Hodgkin's lymphoma. (From Chabner *et al.* (6), with permission.)

	Stage			
	I	II	III	IV
Clinical	10	20	45	25
After lymphography*	7	13	55	25
After bone marrow**	6	10	34	50
After liver biopsy**	6	10	24	60

*Lymphography shows that many clinical stage I and II patients are stage III.
**Marrow and liver biopsy shows that many stage III patients are stage IV.

chance of detecting disease in the marrow or liver. While 30% of patients had *clinically* localized (stages I and II) at presentation, after sequential investigation the proportion had fallen to only 16%. Laparotomy makes little contribution to assessment of spread compared with less invasive investigations—a situation which is different from Hodgkin's disease. Laparotomy is not therefore performed for staging purposes in non-Hodgkin's lymphoma, and is only carried out for diagnosis or if there is a intra-abdominal lymphoma presenting as a surgical emergency. The chances of the disease being localized are small, yet of the 30% with clinically localized disease, nearly half (16%) will still have localized disease after investigation so that there may yet be a place for radiotherapy in this group (this point is discussed further below).

The management of non-Hodgkin's lymphoma presenting as nodal disease

RADIATION THERAPY

Non-Hodgkin's lymphomas are extremely sensitive to radiation. There is, however, a distinction to be made between local control of the disease by radiation therapy, and alteration of the natural history and cure. While local control may be permanently achieved by radiation, there are very few patients who are cured by this treatment alone. This is because nodal non-Hodgkin's lymphoma is nearly always a generalized disease at presentation. There are however a minority of patients (10–15%) who have genuinely localized disease stages I and II (see Table 26.5). These patients can be treated and sometimes cured by radiotherapy. In diffuse large cell lymphoma, a small proportion of patients will have true stage I disease and in this group there is a 90% chance of long term disease-free survival using radiotherapy alone. With Stage II disease the proportion free of relapse at 5 years falls to 40%. Doses of 35–40 Gy are usually given, and there is no evidence that extended field irradiation produces

better results than involved field (i.e. treatment of the abnormal node group alone). It should, however, be pointed out that stages I and II non-Hodgkin's lymphoma of diffuse high-grade type can also be successfully treated with combination chemotherapy. For this reason, in a young or middle aged adult, most physicians would prefer to use combination chemotherapy in stage II disease rather than rely on the accuracy of anatomical staging.

With localized (stages I and II) indolent (follicular) lymphomas approximately 70% will be disease free at 10 years using radiotherapy. These patients are not cured by the treatment and relapse at another site will almost certainly occur in time. As our ability to detect microscopic disease in the marrow improves it may be possible to define with greater accuracy the minority of patients with genuinely localized disease in whom radiotherapy is a potentially curative treatment.

Although the curative role of radiotherapy in diffuse and follicular non-Hodgkin's lymphomas is limited, there are many indications for its use as palliation. Many patients with follicular lymphoma present with very large lymph node masses causing compression of a limb or of structures such as the superior vena cava. These symptoms may be rapidly relieved by radiotherapy. Since these tumours are extremely sensitive to chemotherapy, compressive symptoms might also be relieved by that means. In the elderly in particular, localized palliative radiotherapy is a particularly useful form of treatment which will bring relief quickly. In using radiotherapy it is wise to keep the radiation field as small as possible since widespread irradiation will increase the toxicity of any chemotherapy which may need to be given subsequently.

Radiotherapy has also been used as a systemic treatment in widespread nodal non-Hodgkin's lymphoma of intermediate grade. Total body irradiation (TBI) has been given with a low dose rate, typically 5–15 rad three times a week, to a total dose of 100–150 rad. This treatment is profoundly myelosuppressive and it is often necessary to interrupt it. Randomized prospective comparisons have shown that the treatment is approximately equal to the combination of cyclophosphamide, vincristine and prednisolone (COP) but its use in advanced nodal non-Hodgkin's lymphoma has gradually declined as combination chemotherapy regimens have become more effective. Intensive treatments using higher doses of TBI in one or several fractions, in conjunction with autologous or allogeneic bone marrow transplantation, are presently being investigated.

SINGLE AGENT CHEMOTHERAPY IN NODAL NON-HODGKIN'S LYMPHOMA

A variety of drugs is effective in non-Hodgkin's lymphoma and the activity of single agents is shown in Table 26.6. The most useful drugs are

Table 26.6. Single agent chemotherapy in non-Hodgkin's lymphoma.

Drug	Approximate Response rate (%)
Cyclophosphamide	55
Chlorambucil	40
Doxorubicin	55
Vincristine	60
Prednisolone	60
Bleomycin	40
Methotrexate*	30–60
Etoposide	45

* Methotrexate response rate is dose dependent.

alkylating agents, with a response rate of approximately 50%. Cyclophosphamide is the most widely used; the schedule of administration varying with the type of lymphoma. Of the other agents vinca alkaloids, prednisolone and anthracyclines (particularly doxorubicin) are the mainstay of treatment. Responses to very high dose methotrexate are reportedly as high as 70%, but this is probably an overestimate.

Etoposide and bleomycin are also useful agents with response rates of the order of 40%.

In the advanced, diffuse (intermediate and high grade) non-Hodgkin's lymphoma there is now no place for single agent chemotherapy, except in the elderly where palliation is required or in those with some other intercurrent disease which makes combination chemotherapy impossible. No patients are cured with single agent chemotherapy and in this group of diseases the prognosis with single drug treatment is bad, most patients dying within 18 months (Fig. 26.6). The position is rather different in advanced, follicular low-grade non-Hodgkin's lymphomas. These diseases are often indolent, and when treated palliatively with localized radiotherapy or single agent chemotherapy, 50% of patients are alive at 5 years (Fig. 26.6). There are, however, difficulties in treating patients with follicular lymphomas with single agent chemotherapy. Although comparisons with combination chemotherapy have shown that there is little survival advantage for the combination compared with the single agent (7), low dose single agent treatment has the disadvantage that with its repeated use, drug resistance will have emerged and further chemotherapy will then be difficult when the disease progresses, as it often does, into a more aggressive form. Low dose chlorambucil is particularly likely to produce long-term bone marrow depression. For this reason some authors have advocated that patients with stages III and IV follicular lymphoma who have no particular clinical problem, should be left untreated until such time as the nodes progressively enlarge and cause symptoms (8). Though such a policy is logical, many patients dislike having very large nodal masses and there is as yet no evidence that patients with diffuse transformation of follicular lymphoma can indeed be cured by combination chemotherapy.

At the present time for elderly patients with follicular lymphoma, there is every reason to recommend an expectant policy using single agent chemotherapy or radiotherapy for properly staged stage I and II disease and single

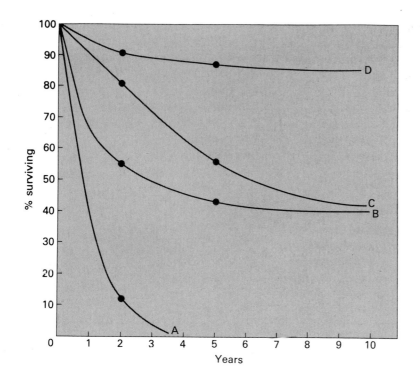

Fig. 26.6. *Prognosis in nodal non-Hodgkin's lymphoma.* (A) Diffuse intermediate and high-grade disease treated with single agent chemotherapy. (B) Diffuse intermediate and high-grade disease treated with combination chemotherapy. (C) Follicular low-grade disease, treated with single agent, or combination chemotherapy. (D) Carefully staged 'true' stage 1 disease (intermediate and some high-grade) treated with radiotherapy and chemotherapy.

agent chlorambucil or cyclophosphamide for stage III and IV disease if the symptoms warrant it. In these patients there is no advantage in using combination chemotherapy from the outset. Occasionally however, one sees young patients with follicular lymphoma in whom a median survival of 5 years can only be regarded as disastrous. It is not clear if intensive combination chemotherapy will manage to cure any of these patients, and in most centres it is still the usual policy to treat them like elderly patients with this desease, with single agent chemotherapy and radiation according to the clinical problem.

COMBINATION CHEMOTHERAPY IN NODAL NON-HODGKIN'S LYMPHOMA

In advanced, nodal, diffuse non-Hodgkin's lymphomas, there is now clear evidence that combination chemotherapy is superior to single agent treatment in both response rate and long-term disease-free survival. A variety of combination regimens has been introduced. MOPP (see Chapter 25) has been widely used in these diseases, as in Hodgkin's disease, although the evidence that procarbazine is an active agent in non-Hodgkin's lymphoma is limited. Other regimens (Table 26.7) are BACOP, M-BACOD and CHOP, all of which can produce complete responses in 60–85% of patients. Of the complete responders approximately 80% will be alive at 5-years, but the prognosis for those who do not achieve a complete response is very bad, most patients being dead in 2 years. The proportion of complete responders, and of long-term survivors, depends on the stage and on some clinical features. The prognosis is worse in men, in those with a large intra-abdominal mass, and patients with marrow or liver disease (9). In stage III and IVB patients, the proportion of responses falls to 60% and 35% respectively. In stages I and II disease, the use of combination chemotherapy is associated with long-term disease-free survival in over 90% of patients.

Table 26.7. Combination chemotherapy regimens in advanced nodal non-Hodgkin's lymphoma.

Acronym	Drugs	Clinical response	Survival at 5 years (all patients)
CHOP	Cyclophosphamide, doxorubicin, vincristine, prednisolone	64%	40%
Pro MACE, MOPP	VP16-213, methotrexate, doxorubicin, cyclophosphamide, prednisolone with mustine, vincristine, procarbazine, prednisolone	75%	70%
M-BACOD	Methotrexate, bleomycin, doxorubicin, cyclophosphamide, vincristine, dexamethasone	71%	70%
COMLA	Cyclophosphamide, vincristine, methotrexate, cytosine arabinoside	60%	55%
CHOP-Bleo	As for CHOP with bleomycin	75%	40%

Recent studies from the National Cancer Institute using an aggressive alternating regimen (ProMACE-MOPP, Table 26.7) have produced long-term survival in 70% of patients. Similar results are reported for the M-BACOD regimen.

The use of these regimens requires considerable skill. Myelosuppression is common with all of them and deaths from this cause occurred in 10% of patients in the first ProMACE-MOPP programme. High dose methotrexate (in the M-BACOD programme) requires folinic acid rescue to be carefully supervized or prolonged pancytopenia will occur.

The follicular lymphomas respond to combination chemotherapy but there is no evidence that prognosis is improved by these regimens. Trials comparing a single agent with regimens such as CVP have shown no advantage for the combination programme at 5 years. On the other hand, 5 years may not be long enough to allow such a distinction to be made, and CVP would no longer be regarded as the most effective regimen for the treatment of a non-Hodgkin's lymphoma.

Recently, there has been growing interest in the use of very high dose chemotherapy in patients with stages III and IV high grade non-Hodgkin's lymphoma, who are not going into remission or who have relapsed after combination chemotherapy. This technique involves the use of autologous bone marrow to lessen the period of aplasia. It is not yet clear whether worthwhile results can be obtained using this approach.

Treatment of thymic and peripheral (nodal) T cell lymphoma

The majority of T cell lymphomas occur in adolescence and early adult life. Typically, they present with a large mediastinal mass due to the thymic origin of the disease (Sternberg sarcoma). Some patients present as a nodal non-Hodgkin's lymphoma behaving in a clinically aggressive fashion. With increasing recognition of these tumours and the use of immunological markers, it has become clear that 5–10% of adult lymphomas are of T cell type.

In childhood the T cell lymphomas are often

associated with marrow infiltration and the distinction from T cell acute lymphoblastic leukaemia (T-ALL) is not clear cut. Indeed some children with T-ALL will be found to have a mediastinal mass on chest X-ray or on tomography.

Histologically the mediastinal T cell lymphomas are characterized by diffuse histological appearance with sheets of malignant cells which typically have convoluted nuclei. The use of immunological techniques will usually show that the cells form rosettes with sheep red blood cells (a T cell marker) and they will usually stain with anti-T cell reagents although the less differentiated tumours may fail to exhibit typical T cell markers.

Clinically these T cell lymphomas are usually highly aggressive, with a short history and with constitutional symptoms. The mediastinal mass not infrequently causes superior vena caval obstruction. The marrow is often involved although low levels of marrow infiltration are hard to detect since there are no tests for the clonal origin of T cells (as there are with B cells which show restriction of the tumour cells to a single light chain type). A small number of T cells are normally found in the bone marrow, and it may be very difficult to determine whether these are tumour cells or not. The thymic T cell lymphomas also frequently spread to the central nervous system, particularly the leptomeninges and along the nerve sheaths as they leave the spinal cord. Root lesions, lymphomatous meningitis, nerve palsies, and raised intracranial pressure are the result of central nervous system involvement in these diseases as in acute leukaemia.

Because of the widespread dissemination, staging procedures are not really required for T cell lymphomas apart from examination of the bone marrow and cerebrospinal fluid.

The prognosis of T cell lymphomas appears to be bad. Certainly in childhood and adolescence the outlook is poor. It is not yet clear whether there will be variants of peripheral T cell tumours in adult life, some of which may be associated with a better prognosis. At the present time they are linked together in a single category of very poor prognosis lymphomas.

Following the development of the LSA$_2$L$_2$ protocol by Wollner and colleagues (10) which proved very successful in childhood lymphoblastic lymphoma (see p. 477), attempts have been made to treat thymic and peripheral T cell lymphomas along similar lines. Recent studies have shown that long-term survival can be obtained in adolescence and young adults with T cell lymphomas using modifications of the LSA$_2$L$_2$ protocol. It consists of an intensive induction regimen followed by a consolidation programme including central nervous system prophylaxis, and then by a long-term cyclical maintenance therapy. It is by no means clear which parts of this treatment are necessary for successful treatment of T cell lymphomas, and certainly a great deal of skill and care is required in the use of therapy of this type.

In recent years there has been some interest in a bone marrow allotransplantation for young patients with thymic T cell lymphoma. Some patients who have been treated in this way in second remission have been long survivors, but if such treatment is to be successful it is likely that it will need to be used during the first remission phase. Similarly, autotransplantation with massive chemotherapy has recently been introduced, but it is too early to assess the usefulness of such treatment regimens.

Lymph node enlargement simulating lymphoma

A variety of conditions may present with lymph node enlargement clinically indistinguishable from either Hodgkin's disease or non-Hodgkin's lymphoma. The histological appearance may be similar to lymphoma but the patient may in fact be suffering from a non-malignant condition. These conditions are a trap for the unwary clinician or pathologist. The main sources of diagnostic difficulty are given in Table 26.8. It is convenient to classify these diseases according to whether the histological pattern is follicular or diffuse.

Table 26.8. Lymph node enlargement simulating lymphoma.

Follicular histology
Reactive hyperplasia
Rheumatoid arthritis and related arthritides
Angiofollicular hyperplasia
Toxoplasmosis

Diffuse histology
Phenytoin sensitivity
Dermatopathic lymphadenopathy
Angioimmunoblastic lymphadenopathy with
    dysproteinaemia
Metastatic carcinoma

Other histologies
Sinus histiocytosis with massive lymph node
    enlargement
Infectious mononucleosis
Cat scratch fever
Metastatic carcinoma (especially melanoma)

FOLLICULAR HISTOLOGICAL APPEARANCES

Reactive hyperplasia Reactive lymphoid follicles within the lymph node may vary considerably in size and in shape, however the germinal follicles are usually clearly defined and the mantle zone of small lymphocytes well preserved. In a follicular lymphoma the follicles often coalesce and have a less well demarcated margin, and the cells within the nodule are usually much more uniform in type. In a reactive lymph node macrophages are usually visible within a germinal centre. Reactive hyperplasia caused by infection (including syphilis), or inflammatory conditions such as rheumatoid arthritis, may produce considerable diagnostic difficulties. Immunohistochemistry is of great help in making the distinction. In non-Hodgkin's lymphoma of B cell type there will be surface immunoglobulin of a single light chain type (light chain restriction). In reactive hyperplasia the B cells in the germinal centres are polyclonal and there is no restriction of light chain type. Reactive hyperplasia is also found in the syndrome of persistent lymphadenopathy which may develop into Acquired Immune Deficiency Syndrome (AIDS).

Angiofollicular hyperplasia This condition was first clearly delineated by Castleman who described a small number of patients with benign hyperplastic mediastinal lymph nodes which resembled thymomas. Subsequently, lymph nodes with similar histology were found at other sites and more recently, a syndrome with fever, anaemia and hyperglobulinaemia has been recognized in association with this lesion. Two types have been recognized. The first is called the hyaline-vascular type; this is the most common variety. There is usually a single rounded mass of nodes with small follicular centres in which vessels are present, surrounded by sheaths of hyalinized collagen. The second type is the so-called plasma cell type in which there are large numbers of mature plasma cells between the follicles. The lymphoid sinuses are usually effaced but follicular centres present, either of normal or large size.

The disease can occur at any stage and in either sex. Within the chest, most of the enlarged nodes are along the tracheo-bronchial tree or in the mediastinum, but intrapulmonary masses also occur. Usually the disease is asymptomatic but occasionally cough, dyspnoea and chest pain can be produced by compression, and pleural effusion may also develop. In the hyaline-vascular type there are seldom any haematological abnormalities. Lesions may remain static for many years and are usually cured by surgical excision. The disease does not respond well to radiation. In the plasma cell type, anaemia, an elevated sedimentation rate, hyperglobulinaemia and hypoalbuminaemia may all occur. Clinical features of fever, sweating, fatigue and leucocytosis have also been described. The symptoms may not settle after surgical removal of the lesion. The disease may be multicentric and associated with severe immune deficiency.

Toxoplasmosis The lymph node shows reactive hyperplasia with small aggregates of epithelioid cells in the interfollicular areas intruding on the follicular centre.

DIFFUSE HISTOLOGICAL APPEARANCES

In these conditions, the lymph node architecture is replaced by a diffuse proliferation of immunoblasts. The erroneous diagnosis which is usually made is of a diffuse poorly differentiated non-Hodgkin's lymphoma. The major areas of diagnostic difficulty are discussed below.

Phenytoin hypersensitivity. Generalized enlargement of lymph nodes may occur in patients taking hydantoin drugs. The lymph node shows either a diffuse or follicular hyperplasia with large numbers of immunoblasts and infiltration with eosinophils, neutrophils and plasma cells. Typical Reed-Sternberg cells are not seen but a mistaken diagnosis of Hodgkin's disease may be made. Associated with this syndrome may be other features of hydantoin hypersensitivity including skin rash, eosinophilia and neutropenia. It is not clear whether this condition can develop into a lymphoma, but there appear to be well documented cases where the lesions have not regressed after stopping phenytoin and a recurrent lymphoma has developed.

Dermatopathic lymphadenopathy. A variety of chronic inflammatory conditions of the skin may cause enlargement of draining lymph nodes of sufficient size to simulate lymphoma. When biopsied, the lymph nodes show a fairly typical histological appearance. The paracortex (T zone) of the node is widened and contains numerous interdigitating reticulum cells (which are resident antigen presenting cells). Eosinophils, plasma cells and immunoblasts may be present. This condition is often seen in association with cutaneous T cell lymphoma and it may be difficult to decide whether the node involvement is due to infiltration with lymphoma or to dermatopathic lymphadenopathy.

Immunoblastic (angioimmunoblastic) lymphadenopathy. In this syndrome the presentation is with malaise, fever and lymph node enlargement which is accompanied by polyclonal gammopathy and sometimes Coombs positive haemolytic anaemia. The lymph node architecture is destroyed with proliferation of high endothelial venules, numerous immunoblasts, plasma cells and eosinophils. Large numbers of epithelioid histiocytes may be present. Clinically, the disease may be localized to one or more lymph nodes for a prolonged period but usually there is more generalized involvement of the spleen, liver, abdominal nodes and bone marrow. The disease may develop into an aggressive non-Hodgkin's lymphoma of T cell type with a fatal outcome. It is unwise to treat these patients in the early phase of the disease, particularly as many of them are elderly and the tempo of the disease can be slow. Intensive chemotherapy does not produce durable regression of the disease or any alteration in its outcome. A complete response to corticosteroids is associated with a better prognosis.

Metastatic carcinoma. Deposits of undifferentiated carcinoma (particularly undifferentiated adenocarcinoma and metastatic carcinoma) may simulate malignant lymphomas of large cell type. Metastatic small cell carcinoma of the lung may be confused with lymphocytic lymphoma. The use of immunohistochemical techniques (especially with monoclonal antibodies against common leucocyte antigens) has greatly helped in the distinction between metastatic carcinoma and lymphoma.

OTHER HISTOLOGIES

There is a variety of other causes of lymph node enlargement in which the histological appearances are very variable, which may cause diagnostic difficulty.

Sinus histiocytosis with massive lymph node enlargement. This curious disease is characterized by grossly enlarged lymph nodes and soft tissue infiltrates particularly of skin, orbit and nasopharynx. It typically affects young children, especially black children, but adults are sometimes affected. In addition to massive lymph node enlargement, the patient may be generally unwell with fever and malaise. The blood shows neutrophil leucocytosis, an elevated ESR and polyclonal hypergammaglobulinaemia. The lymph node and skin histology is characteristic. The lymph sinuses are markedly distended and are filled with histiocytes with round nuclei and prominent nucleoli. The cytoplasm is large and often vacuolated, appearing foamy and filled with lipid. Within the cytoplasm there may be ingested lymphocytes, plasma cells or erythrocytes.

Infectious mononucleosis. This disease, which is caused by the Epstein-Barr virus, results in a proliferation of lymphoid tissue which can sometimes be so intense as to simulate a lymphoma. The lymph node contains numerous atypical lymphoid cells which are immunoblasts, and may resemble Reed-Sternberg cells very strongly.

Cat scratch fever. This disease is accompanied by fever and regional lymph node enlargement. The clinical diagnosis may not be apparent and occasionally a lymph node biopsy is taken; this shows microabscesses with necrosis and neutrophil infiltration.

EXTRA-NODAL PRESENTATION OF NON-HODGKIN'S LYMPHOMA

Non-Hodgkin's lymphomas may present at a variety of extra-nodal sites, and when they do there are particular problems in diagnosis and management. In addition to presentation at an extra-nodal site, there may be involvement of these sites at a time when the nodal lymphoma relapses and disseminates. In this latter circumstance, this is usually part of a generalized spread of the disease. Treatment will be palliative if there has been intensive previous chemotherapy.

The account which follows concerns the management of non-Hodgkin's lymphoma presenting at an extranodal site, in the absence of clinically overt disease elsewhere.

Gastro-intestinal lymphoma

Lymphomas may occur at any site in the gastro-intestinal tract but the small intestine and stomach are most frequently involved. The aetiology and pathogenesis are not well understood. The gut-associated lymphoid tissue in a normal individual shows a well defined pattern of lymphocyte traffic. Immunoglobulin bearing cells in the follicle centre of small intestinal lymphoid nodules (Peyer's patches) migrate into the blood stream and return to the lamina propria of the small bowel where they differentiate to plasma cells. A similar 'homing' mechanism may take place with gastric and large bowel lymphocytes and with lymphocytes bearing immunoglobulin of other classes.

SMALL BOWEL LYMPHOMA

Lymphoma of the small intestine represents the most common gut tumour of children below the age of 10 years and there is a rise in incidence in adults above the age of 50 years. There is a slight male preponderance (M:F,1.5:1) and there are two predisposing conditions. In long standing untreated coeliac disease there is an increased incidence of intestinal lymphoma, and in this situation the lymphoma has now been shown to be of T cell type and the bowel is usually widely involved. In the Middle East, there is a high incidence of intestinal lymphoma which is usually preceded by a diffuse plasma cell and lymphocytic proliferation in the small bowel, known as immunoproliferative disease of the small intestine. During this early phase there is an excess production by the plasma cells of the heavy chain of IgA—the alpha chain (alpha chain disease). At this early stage, the disease may respond to treatment with antibiotics, but it subsequently progresses and a B cell lymphoma develops which may be rapidly evolving. The secretion of alpha heavy chains in the blood may disappear at this stage.

In the typical case of intestinal lymphoma in Europeans, no predisposing cause has been detected. The neoplasm arises in the lymphoid tissues of the mucosa of the bowel, invades and ulcerates the mucosa, and penetrates through the bowel wall to the serosal surface. Often the lymphoma is localized to a single area of bowel, but occasionally multiple discrete lesions are present. Involvement of the small bowel is not uniform and coincides with a gradual increase in frequency of lymphoid tissues in the lower small bowel. The tumour is therefore rare in the duodenum, increases in frequency further down the jejunum and is most common in the ileum. It spreads to involve adjacent lymph nodes near the intestine and at the root of the mesentery. As the neoplasm increases in size, it causes intestinal obstruction. Occasionally perforation of the small bowel occurs and curiously this is very often in an area of small bowel above the site of the neoplasm. Histologically, most small bowel lymphomas are of the diffuse large cell type, but in adults some of the lymphomas may be follicular. In keeping with the general rarity of follicular lymphomas in children, this type is exceptional in childhood. The lymphoma which arises in coeliac disease is more likely to do so in untreated patients after many years. The intestine is diffusely involved and the malignant cell is derived from T cells. This rare form of lymphoma responds poorly to treatment with chemotherapy.

In small bowel lymphoma the presentation is usually with subacute or acute intestinal obstruction with colicky abdominal pain, vomiting and constipation. There may be diarrhoea or even malabsorption but this is unusual. Gastro-intestinal haemorrhage occurs, usually of a chronic type leading to iron deficiency anaemia. When perforation occurs the clinical picture is typical of perforation of the bowel at any site. Occasionally patients may present with ascites, usually chylous in nature, but sometimes it is due to widespread dissemination of intraperitoneal lymphoma. When the disease

has become more extensive within the abdomen, there may be fever and anaemia, and intestinal lymphoma is a cause of pyrexia of unknown origin.

The diagnosis is usually made at laparotomy or by a barium follow-through examination which may show infiltration of the bowel wall with ulceration and segments of narrowing above which are areas of bowel dilatation.

The management of non-Hodgkin's lymphoma of the small intestine is often difficult. This is in part due to the fact that the disease often presents as an acute surgical emergency and may be operated on by an inexperienced surgeon and adequate resection not carried out. Nevertheless, the prognosis is dependent on an adequate surgical excision of the tumour. A simple system of staging related to prognosis has been advocated by Crowther and Blackledge (11) and is shown in Table 26.9.

Table 26.9. Staging of intestinal lymphoma.

1A	Single tumour confined to gut
1B	Two or more tumours confined to gut
2A	Local node involvement
2B	Local extension to adjacent structures
2C	Local tumour with perforation and peritonitis
3	Widespread lymph node enlargement
4	Disseminated tumour (to liver, spleen and elsewhere)

All cases should be further staged with chest X-ray and bone marrow aspiration. A liver biopsy should be performed during the laparotomy. Complete local excision of the tumour with the cut ends free of disease, and without involvement of mesenteric nodes, will frequently result in a cure, and the role of radiation therapy and adjuvant chemotherapy is still to be determined in this type of case. If the lymphoma has a follicular histology and complete excision has been carried out, then it is probable that no further treatment is needed. If, as is more likely, there is local node involvement and the histology is of a diffuse large cell type, most oncologists would treat the patient further and in recent years the tendency has been to use combination chemotherapy rather than to attempt to control the disease by local radiation. Without combination chemotherapy the 5-year survival of diffuse lymphomas of the gut is about 20%, and of follicular lymphomas about 50%, but this clearly depends on the stage.

The combination of drugs usually employed will include cyclophosphamide, vincristine, doxorubicin and prednisolone in various regimens as for diffuse non-Hodgkin's lymphomas at other sites (Table 26.7). In children, the likelihood of CNS involvement is small and it does not appear that prophylactic treatment of the central nervous system is an essential part of management (see p. 472).

NON-HODGKIN'S LYMPHOMA OF THE STOMACH

Lymphoma of the stomach is an uncommon tumour, comprising less than 0.5% of all gastric neoplasms. The patient is usually middle-aged or elderly but the disease can affect young adults. The tumour is composed of follicular centre cells and may be follicular or diffuse. Some tumours appear to spread early to adjacent lymph nodes, but others are localized and remain a largely mucosal neoplasm. As with small intestinal lymphoma, it is possible that the lymphoid cells in this type of tumour are specifically 'gastric' B lymphocytes, with the property of homing to gastric mucosa with little tendency to spread or lodge in other sites until late in the disease.

The presentation of gastric lymphoma is similar to that of adenocarcinoma of the stomach with nausea, anorexia and upper abdominal discomfort being the chief symptoms and occasionally haematemesis, or chronic iron deficiency anaemia being associated. A barium meal shows a large gastric ulcer, or appearances similar to adenocarcinoma of the stomach. On endoscopy, a malignant ulcer is usually seen, but occasionally the appearances can simulate a benign gastric ulcer. Biopsy evidence can be misleading since the specimen may show small lymphocytes which are hard to distinguish from an inflammatory infiltrate.

Treatment of gastric lymphoma is by surgical resection where possible. The histopathologist can help in deciding on the site of resection by examining multiple endoscopic biopsies and determining the upper level of the malignant infiltration. Postoperative radiotherapy is usually given but this policy may need reappraisal since if the tumour has been completely resected further treatment may not be necessary. Treatment with combination chemotherapy is usually preferred if there is a risk of dissemination. This is more likely in the large cell diffuse type of tumour and if there is involvement of adjacent lymph nodes. Chemotherapy will then be along similar lines to an advanced non-Hodgkin's lymphoma occurring in a nodal site, with drug combinations usually including cyclophosphamide, vincristine, doxorubicin and prednisolone.

Non-Hodgkin's lymphoma of bone

Non-Hodgkin's lymphoma frequently invades the marrow and may sometimes cause localized bone lesions with pain, vertebral collapse and pathological fractures. Occasionally non-Hodgkin's lymphoma presents as a bone lesion and most of these cases are of large cell lymphoma formerly called 'reticulum cell sarcoma of bone'. Sometimes the lesion is localized with no evidence of non-Hodgkin's lymphoma at other sites, even after extensive investigations. In children, isolated lymphoma of bone may be mistaken for Ewing's sarcoma. Immunohistochemical studies will usually resolve any diagnostic difficulty. In most cases of non-Hodgkin's lymphoma of bone the lesion is confined to one bone and a long bone is usually affected. The antecedent history is often very long and the lesions are often very large with extensive soft tissue infiltration. Radiotherapy (40–45 Gy) produces local control in 90% of cases and in general should encompass the whole bone and soft tissue. Fifty-percent of non-Hodgkin's lymphomas presenting in bone are cured by local radiotherapy but dissemination to other bones and through the bone marrow is not infrequent. For this reason, careful pre-treatment staging should be undertaken including bone marrow examination and abdominal CT scan. In the elderly it is reasonable to use radiotherapy in the first instance if there is no evidence of dissemination on investigation, but in children and young adults combination chemotherapy is usually given in addition.

CNS involvement with lymphoma

Primary lymphomas of the brain and spinal cord occur but are rare. Usually the CNS is involved as part of the pattern of spread of generalized disease and there is a particular tendency for the CNS to be involved in diffuse lymphomas especially of childhood, of T cell type and when there is marrow involvement.

PRIMARY LYMPHOMA OF THE BRAIN

This uncommon tumour occurs more frequently in renal allograft recipients and in those on long-term immunosuppressive therapy. The tumour has been given a variety of names such as reticulum cell sarcoma and microglioma. The histological appearances are usually of a follicular centre cell lymphoma with both centrocytic and centroblastic forms. Lymphoplasmacytic types also occur. They arise in the cerebrum in 70% of cases, cerebellum and brain stem (25% of cases), and are rare in the spinal cord. They tend to be multicentric, and perivascular infiltration is common. Although rare in the spinal cord, seeding into the CSF occasionally occurs late in the disease. The patients do not usually show lymphoma elsewhere at presentation or later in the disease so that, apart from bone marrow and CSF examination, detailed staging investigations are not usually necessary (12).

Treatment is with radiotherapy but the disease can be difficult to control, local relapse being common even after doses as high as 45–50 Gy. Spinal irradiation is usually recommended. There are too few data to know whether intrathecal methotrexate or systemic chemotherapy will improve results.

SECONDARY LYMPHOMA OF THE CNS

Involvement of the CNS occurs in about 9% of all cases of non-Hodgkin's lymphoma (12). The clinical presentation is either with lymphomatous meningitis (55%) or with extradural compression (45%), see Fig. 26.7. The great majority of patients have diffuse large cell (centroblastic) lymphoma or diffuse centrocytic lymphoma as the primary disease. Light microscopical evidence of involvement of the bone marrow at diagnosis is present in 70% of cases and this is probably an underestimate if more sensitive tests of involvement are undertaken. The patients usually have advanced nodal spread at diagnosis, and involvement of retroperitoneal nodes is common. Lymphomatous involvement of the CNS is particularly frequent in childhood lymphomas and in lymphomas of T cell type.

The clinical presentation of lymphomatous meningitis is with cranial nerve palsies, mental confusion and raised intracranial pressure. Root lesions frequently occur due to compression and perivascular infiltration. The most important diagnostic test is lumbar puncture. The CSF is examined cytologically and if possible, surface markers (light chain restriction, T cell markers) should be identified in an attempt to distinguish the cells from reactive lymphocytes which might be found in tuberculous or fungal meningitis which may be part of the differential diagnosis.

Epidural compression usually occurs in the thoracic spine, but nerve roots may be compressed including the cauda equina. These patients usually have retroperitoneal lymphoma and sometimes intra-vertebral deposits. The clinical syndrome is with a paraparesis and is a medical emergency whose management is discussed in Chapter 8.

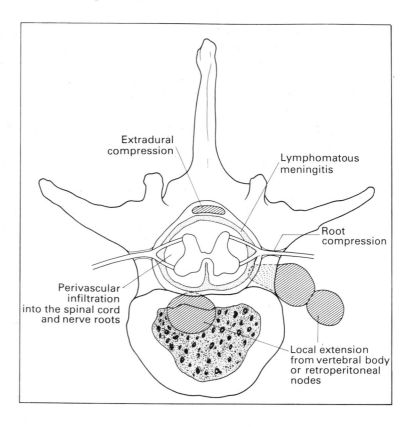

Extradural
compression

Lymphomatous
meningitis

Root
compression

Perivascular
infiltration
into the spinal cord
and nerve roots

Local extension
from vertebral body
or retroperitoneal
nodes

Fig. 26.7. *Involvement of the spinal cord with lymphoma.* Extradural compression may result from lymphomatus involvement of the vertebral body or by extension from para-aortic nodes. Leptomeningeal infiltration is probably haematogenous and is particularly common when bone marrow is involved.

Lymphomatous meningitis is a serious complication and very few patients in whom it has developed will be cured. The management is with intrathecal chemotherapy using methotrexate in combination with cytosine arabinoside and craniospinal irradiation. Patients at high risk (many childhood lymphomas and T cell lymphomas in childhood and adolescence) should receive prophylactic treatment of the CNS with intrathecal methotrexate and craniospinal irradiation in an attempt to avoid this complication. Although it has been argued (13) that adult patients with large cell and undifferentiated lymphomas should receive CNS prophylaxis it does not in fact appear that the incidence of CNS disease in adults is rising as survival improves with chemotherapy (as it did in childhood leukaemia). Newer regimens for systemic treatment often include methotrexate and other drugs which penetrate the CSF and these may confer adequate protection. Alternatively, the risk of CNS disease in adults may be lower than had been predicted.

Non-Hodgkin's lymphoma of Waldeyer's ring

Non-Hodgkin's lymphoma may present in the lymphoid tissue of the oropharynx and nasopharynx, in the absence of clinical evidence of disease elsewhere. The histology may be follicular or diffuse, centroblastic or centrocytic. The presentation is with difficulty in swallowing and nasal congestion. There may be enlargement of cervical lymph nodes, or evidence of disease elsewhere.

Approximately 20% of patients have localized disease (stage I) and 40% have involvement of cervical nodes (stage II). Lymphangiography will demonstrate that half of the patients with stage II disease have involved abdominal nodes (stage III). Approximately 50% of patients have stage III disease at presentation, and 10% of patients, stage IV disease (in bone marrow or liver). Patients who present with stage I disease do not usually prove to have more extensive disease on investigation (14).

The gastro-intestinal tract may be involved, and a barium meal and follow-through should be performed as part of the initial investigations.

For patients with disease localized to Waldeyer's ring and cervical nodes, treatment is usually with radiotherapy. Many patients (possibly 60%) will be free of disease at 5–10 years. For patients with stage III and IV disease, treatment is with chemotherapy, but it is not clear if the prognosis has been greatly improved by modern regimens. In the past, most of these patients had died before 5 years (14).

Ocular non-Hodgkin's lymphoma

Uncommonly the conjunctiva and the orbit can be the site of development of NHL. Orbital lymphomas present with unilateral proptosis, external ocular palsy and visual disturbance. Conjunctival lymphoma presents with swelling of the lid and visible tumour.

These tumours are uncommon, and their prognosis is not known with certainty (15). They must be distinguished from the more frequent benign lymphoid proliferations which affect the eye. They are usually treated with local radiotherapy, but systemic spread probably occurs in about half the cases.

Cutaneous non-Hodgkin's lymphoma

The skin is a frequent site of secondary spread of NHL of all types. It is usually involved in the context of disseminated and often drug resistant disease. Clinically there are subcutaneous lumps or papular infiltrates in the dermis. The treatment is of the underlying disease where possible. Superficial X-rays are very helpful in controlling troublesome lesions and elec-

tron therapy is useful for widespread cutaneous infiltrates.

The skin may also be the site of a primary lymphoma and in recent years it has become apparent that these are often T cell in origin. The two major syndromes are *mycosis fungoides* and *Sezary's syndrome*.

MYCOSIS FUNGOIDES

This rare disease is uncommon in Blacks and has an equal sex incidence. The onset is usually at 40–60 years of age, though many cases may have a long history with an origin much earlier in life. There are three well recognized stages in the clinical evolution, although in individual cases, they are often not easily separable.

In the *erythematous* or *pre-tumour* stage there is a rash which may resemble psoriasis with fine red scaly patches. There are often poikilodermatous changes which suggest the diagnosis. This phase may last for many years and the diagnosis can only be substantiated by biopsy. There is acanthosis, parakeratosis and clusters of histiocytes (Darier-Pautrier abscesses).

In the *infiltrative* or *plaque* stage there are indurated plaques. Microscopically there is infiltration of the upper dermis and epidermis with lymphoma cells which are helper T cells. In the cases seen in Britain there is usually no significant lymph node enlargement. If the nodes do enlarge, they may show 'dermatopathic lymphadenopathy (p.467) and, later, clear evidence of tumour infiltration.

In the *tumour* stage the lesions enlarge and ulcerate. Involvement of internal organs may occur.

Treatment in the first stage is symptomatic with antipruritic agents. Steroid creams and topical nitrogen mustard have also been used. More advanced lesions, if not too infiltrated, can be treated with psoralens with UV light (PUVA). Wide-field irradiation is the treatment usually used in the mycotic stage. Whole-body electron therapy is increasingly preferred in order to avoid treatment of deeper structures. Visceral involvement is very difficult to treat effectively. Responses to combination chemotherapy occur but are seldom sustained. Median survival from the time of biopsy is about 5 years.

SEZARY'S SYNDROME

The original description was of patients with generalized erythrodermia and large atypical lymphocytes in the blood. The latter are now known to be T cells (of helper type). The skin shows infiltration with T cells. Lymph node enlargement and hepatomegaly may be present. The disorder can be regarded as a disseminated form of mycosis fungoides. The patient complains of intense itching, the skin becomes red and thickened and may be swollen. Hair is lost and palmar hyperkeratosis occurs with dystrophy and loss of nails. The circulating cells were called *'cellules monstreuses'* by Sezary. They do not infiltrate the marrow until late in the disease. Hepatosplenomegaly may occur and there may be lymph node enlargement.

Chemotherapy may produce remissions when the disease is widely disseminated, but the patient is not cured. Combination chemotherapy is usually employed. Responses to PUVA occur as in mycosis fungoides.

Non-Hodgkin's lymphoma of the thyroid

These tumours usually present as a rapidly enlarging thyroid mass in a middle-aged or elderly woman (16). They are associated with Hashimoto's thyroiditis, and areas of thyroiditis may be found in the gland on biopsy. Histologically they are usually diffuse large cell tumours which are generally of B cell type. Follicular and plasmacytoid forms are unusual, and T cell tumours are rare. The evolution of the disease in a gland affected by autoimmune disease is reminiscent of the development of lymphomas in Sjögren's syndrome. The mass does not take up radioactive iodine and cannot be distinguished clinically from other thyroid cancers. Diagnosis is made by biopsy or thyroidectomy. Radical

surgery has little role in management however, since the tumours are sensitive to radiotherapy.

Staging investigations are necessary since the prognosis is excellent with local treatment if the disease is confined to the gland. These investigations should include chest X-ray, abdominal CT scan and/or lymphogram, and marrow aspiration and biopsy. Relapse in the gut is relatively frequent and a small bowel barium examination may be useful.

If there is no local extension of the tumour from the gland, and no evidence of involvement of adjacent nodes radical radiotherapy (30–40 Gy in 3–4 weeks) including the gland and adjacent nodes will cure 90% of patients. Only 50% of patients with local and nodal extension will be cured, and the prognosis is also worse over the age of 65 years. Adjuvant chemotherapy should therefore be considered in these cases, and is clearly necessary for patients with more widespread disease. It seems likely that T cell tumours will also require chemotherapy. There are, as yet, little data to show whether chemotherapy will improve the prognosis.

Non-Hodgkin's lymphoma of the testis and ovary

NHL of the testis is usually a diffuse large cell (centroblastic) lymphoma. The patients are generally over the age of 50 years—an age when seminoma and teratoma are uncommon (17). The tumours are mostly unilateral but there is a considerable risk of contralateral involvement. Presentation is with a painless enlargement of the testis. After investigation most patients are found to have stages I or II disease (Ann Arbor system, Table 25.2). The disease has a tendency to spread to abdominal nodes and to Waldeyer's ring. Occasionally CNS relapse occurs.

Staging investigations should include lymphangiogram and/or CT scan of the abdomen, and bone marrow examination. Localized disease (IE and IIE) can be adequately treated with radiotherapy to the pelvic and para-aortic lymph nodes. Bilateral or advanced (stages III and IV) disease carries a bad prognosis and systemic chemotherapy is required.

NON-HODGKIN'S LYMPHOMA IN CHILDHOOD

Incidence and Aetiology

Non-Hodgkin's lymphomas (NHL) are rather more common in children than Hodgkin's disease (1.5:1) and are the third most frequent childhood cancer. Approximately 0.6 per 100 000 children below 15 years develop the disease each year with a peak onset age 6–10 years (Fig. 26.1). A variety of inherited diseases predispose to childhood NHL (Table 26.1). The other aetiological factors as discussed in the section on adult NHL.

Pathology

The distinction between childhood NHL and leukaemia is to some extent a semantic one. Many childhood lymphomas spread to the bone marrow and the frequency of diagnosis of marrow involvement is increasing as techniques for the demonstration of monoclonality of B cells (e.g. light-chain restriction) are improving. A convention is to regard >25% infiltration as compatible with lymphoma. The lymph nodes almost always show diffuse involvement and follicular patterns are very rare. The main types are shown in Table 26.10. Diffuse lymphoblastic lymphoma is the commonest type. Some of these tumours show a convoluted nuclear morphology, form rosettes with sheep red blood cells, and react with anti-T cell reagents, i.e. are

Table 26.10. Pathology of childhood non-Hodgkin's lymphoma.

Diffuse lymphoblastic lymphoma B cell, T cell
Diffuse large cell immunoblastic lymphoma
True 'histiocytic' lymphoma
Burkitt's lymphoma
Undifferentiated

T cell tumours. Others show surface Ig, i.e. are B cell tumours. Other tumours have neither T nor B markers.

Childhood NHL has a greater tendency to involve extra-nodal sites such as the gut, bone marrow and CNS. The lymph nodes of Waldeyer's ring and the mediastinum are frequently involved. The distribution of the main mass of disease at presentation is shown in Table 26.11 and a staging system in Table 26.12.

Table 26.11. Distribution of main primary site of disease in children with non-Hodgkin's lymphoma (%).

Intra-abdominal	30
Peripheral nodes	25
Mediastinal	22
Skeleton	7
Nasopharynx	10
Subcutaneous	3.5
Epidural	1
Thyroid	0.5
Testis	0.5
Breast	0.5

Table 26.12. A simple staging system for childhood non-Hodgkin's lymphoma and Burkitt's lymphoma.

Stage	Description
Non-Hodgkin's lymphoma	
I	One nodal site excluding mediastinum
II	Two or more nodal sites on one side of the diaphragm, excluding the mediastinum
III	Mediastinal mass or nodes on both side of the diaphragm
IV	Any of the above with liver, CNS or marrow involvement
Burkitt's lymphoma	
A	Single extra-abdominal site
B	Multiple extra-abdominal sites
C	Intra-abdominal tumour
D	Intra-abdominal tumour with extra-abdominal sites

Childhood B cell lymphomas

The majority of NHL in childhood are B cell tumours. These diffuse lymphomas are either of large cell type or consist of small non-cleaved cells. The large cell lymphomas are usually found in boys and are often extra-nodal occurring in the nasopharynx, lung, mediastinum, bone, soft tissues and tonsils.

The small non-cleaved cell lymphomas are either Burkitt's lymphoma, or a form in which the cells are more pleomorphic. Burkitt's lymphoma occurs predominantly in Africa but is occasionally seen in Western countries. In Africa the presentation is usually with jaw or orbital tumours which grow rapidly. Other sites of involvement include the ovaries, retroperitoneal tissues, kidneys and glandular tissues such as breast and thyroid. Lymph node and marrow invasion is infrequent. Spread to the CNS is common and occurs early, often with paraplegia and cranial nerve palsy. A staging system, which relates to prognosis is shown in Table 26.12. In Western countries Burkitt's lymphoma is more likely to present with an abdominal mass, or with enlarged cervical nodes. Marrow involvement is more frequent than in African cases.

Many childhood B cell lymphomas are generalized diseases with a risk of marrow and CNS involvement. However, some cases have a lower risk of meningeal spread. These cases include localized tumours of the gut, and patients with localized nodal disease. With localized gut lymphoma it is not clear if any treatment should be given after a complete resection, but it is the usual practice to treat with chemotherapy. CNS prophylaxis does not appear to be necessary in these cases.

Childhood T cell lymphomas

These tumours almost always present with anterior mediastinal or cervical node enlargement. They disseminate rapidly to the bone marrow, the central nervous system, and to the testes. The cells may have convoluted nuclei and focal acid phosphatase activity in the cytoplasm. They usually exhibit T cell markers, forming rosettes with sheep erythrocytes and reacting with T cell monoclonal antibodies.

The patients are usually males and there may be superior vena cava obstruction at presentation which may need urgent treatment (usually with steroids and vincristine) before the diagnostic biopsy can be taken. This therapy can make subsequent diagnosis difficult, but the situation may be life-threatening and aggravated by biopsy under anaesthetic. Marrow failure from infiltration, or CNS symptoms, may be the presenting feature.

Diagnosis and investigation of childhood non-Hodgkin's lymphoma

Diagnosis is by lymph node or tissue biopsy. Initial staging investigations should be performed quickly since progress of the disease may be rapid. A marrow aspiration and biopsy should be performed and the CSF examined for cells. Biochemical tests of liver and kidney function are necessary with measurement of plasma calcium and urate since the tumour lysis syndrome (see Chapter 8) may occur when treatment starts.

Precise immuno-histochemical definition of the tumour is now often possible. Although at present the relationship to prognosis is not clear, in the next few years the application of these techniques may allow a more precise definition of risk and therefore lead to greater precision in selecting treatment.

Treatment of non-Hodgkin's lymphoma in childhood

T CELL AND B CELL LYMPHOMAS
(EXCLUDING BURKITT'S LYMPHOMA)

During the 1960s the prognosis of acute lymphoblastic leukaemia in childhood was improving rapidly with the use of more intensive drug regimens and prophylactic treatment of the CNS. Childhood lymphomas were however still rapidly fatal, 85% of children dying within 1 year and only 10–15% surviving 5 years.

In 1971, Wollner and her colleagues at the Memorial Sloan-Kettering Cancer Center in

New York proposed a protocol of treatment for childhood lymphomas based on ideas derived from treatment of leukaemia. This protocol known as LSA_2L_2 has greatly improved management and 5-year survival of 70–80% is now obtained with few children relapsing beyond this time (10). The LSA_2L_2 protocol has the following components.

1 An intensive induction regimen using cyclophosphamide, vincristine, doxorubicin, prednisolone and intrathecal methotrexate.

2 A consolidation phase using antimetabolites—cytosine arabinoside, thioguanine, asparaginase.

3 A maintenance phase lasting 1 year, using sequential alternating pairs of drugs.

The results of protocols of this type are shown in Fig. 26.8. Survival is better in stages I and II disease.

It is not clear if early stage disease can safely be treated less intensively. In a randomized study in paediatric non-Hodgkin's lymphoma of all stages comparing the LSA_2L_2 protocol with a slightly less aggressive regimen (COMP), the Children's Cancer Study Group in the United States found little difference between the two treatments, and better disease-free survival at 2-years for localized disease (81%) than for generalized disease (46%). Although the results with COMP are excellent with localized disease, it seems unwise to reduce the amount of chemotherapy given to these children if they have advanced disease. In non-localized disease the LSA_2L_2 protocol proved better than COMP regimen for patients with lymphoblastic disease. Lymphoblastic lymphoma in childhood tends to present with mediastinal disease and includes many cases of T cell lymphoma. Non-lymphoblastic disease tends to be more localized and have an intra-abdominal presentation.

Other regimens have been used, some of which include cranial irradiation as prophylactic CNS treatment. With the LSA_2L_2 protocol, using intrathecal methotrexate only, the incidence of CNS relapse is about 16%. The incidence is probably lower when cranial irradiation is used in addition. The risk of CNS disease

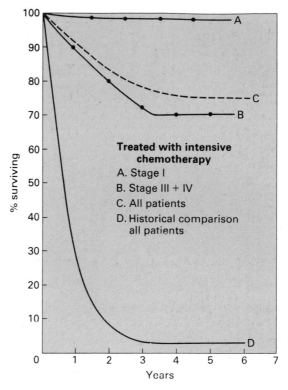

Fig. 26.8. *Results of intensive chemotherapy of lymphoma in childhood.*

appears to be low for those with Stage I nodal disease, and those whose intra-abdominal lymphoma has been resected.

BURKITT'S LYMPHOMA

The agents usually employed in treating this disease are cyclophosphamide, vincristine, methotrexate and prednisolone (COMP). Almost all children will have a complete remission but 50% will relapse. Cure is still possible if CNS relapse occurs, but many regimens now include some form of CNS prophylaxis.

Children who survive 2 years will probably be cured. The 2 year disease-free survival figures for each stage (Table 26.12) are A and B 80%; C 65%; D 40%. In Stage C it is advisable to remove as much bulk as possible before treatment. With 90% removed the results approach those for stage A. More aggressive regimens are being developed for Stage D cases including very high dose chemotherapy with autologous bone marrow transplantation.

TUMOUR LYSIS SYNDROME

This syndrome of hyperuricaemia and renal failure is particularly likely to occur in patients with Burkitt's lymphoma, those with large intra-abdominal tumours, and with T cell tumours with a large mediastinal mass. The cause, prevention and treatment of tumour lysis syndrome are discussed in Chapter 8.

REFERENCES

1 Penn I. (1975) The incidence of malignancies in transplantation recipients. *Transplant Proceedings* **8**, 323.

2 Anderson M. & Klein G. (1976) Association of Epstein-Barr viral genomes with American Burkitt lymphoma. *Nature* **260**, 357.

3 Lukes R.J. & Collins R.D. (1974) Immunological characterization of human malignant lymphomas. *Cancer* **34**, 1488.

4 Golde D. & Cline M.J. (1973) A review and re-evaluation of the histiocytic disorders. *American Journal of Medicine* **55**, 49.

5 Classification of non-Hodgkin's lymphomas. Summary and description of a working formulation for clinical usage. *Cancer* **49**, 2112.

6 Chabner, B.A., Johnson, R.E., Young, R.C., Canellos G.P., Hubbard S.P., Johnson S.K. & DeVita V.T. (1976) Sequential non-surgical and surgical staging of non-Hodgkin's lymphoma. *Annals of Internal Medicine* **85**, 149.

7 Lister, T.A., Cullen, M.H., Beard, M.E., Brearley R.L., Whitehouse J.M.A., Wrigley P.F.M., Stansfeld A.G., Sutcliffe S.B.J., Malpas J.S. & Crowther D.F. (1978). Comparison of combined and single agent chemotherapy in non-Hodgkin's lymphoma of favourable histological type. *British Medical Journal* **1**, 533.

8 Portlock C.S. & Rosenberg S.A. (1979) An initial therapy for stage III and IV non-Hodgkin's lymphoma of favourable histologic types. *Annals of Internal Medicine* **90**, 10.

9 Fisher R.I., DeVita, V.T., Johnson B.L., Simon R. & Young R.C. (1977) Prognostic factors for advanced diffuse histiocytic lymphoma following treatment with combination chemotherapy. *American Journal of Medicine* **63**, 177.

10 Wollner N., Exelby P.R. & Liberman P.H. (1979) Non-Hodgkins lymphoma in children: a progress report on the original patients treated with LSA_2-L_2 protocol. *Cancer* **44**, 1190.

11 Blackledge G., Bush H., Dodge O.G. & Crowther D.F. (1979) A study of gastro-intestinal lymphoma. *Clinical Oncology* **5**, 209.

12 Levit L.J., Dawson D.M., Rosenthal D.S. & Moloney W.C. (1980) CNS involvement in the non-Hodgkin's lymphomas. *Cancer* **45**, 545.

13 Bunn P.A., Schein P.S., Banks P.M. & DeVita V.T. (1976) Central nervous system complication in patients with diffuse histiocytic and undifferentiated lymphoma: leukaemia revisited. *Blood* **47**, 3.

14 Banfi A., Bonadonna G., Ricci S.B., Milani F., Molinari R., Marfardini S. & Zucali R. (1972) Malignant lymphomas of Waldeyer's ring: natural history and survival after radiotherapy. *British Medical Journal* **3**, 140.

15 Knowles D.M. & Jakobiec F.A. (1982) Ocular adnexa lymphoid neoplasms. *Human Pathology* **13**, 148.

16 Burke J.S., Butler J.J. & Fuller L.M. (1977) Malignant lymphomas of the thyroid. *Cancer* **39**, 1587.

17 Duncan P.R., Checa F., Gowing F.C., McElwain T.J. & Peckham M.J. (1980) Extranodal non-Hodgkin's lymphoma presenting in the testicle. *Cancer* **45**, 1578.

Chapter 27

Myeloma and Other Paraproteinaemias

MYELOMA

Incidence and aetiology

Myeloma (multiple myeloma, myelomatosis plasma cell myeloma) is a disease of the elderly. The incidence rises with age and is commonest in patients aged 65 and over (Fig. 27.1). It is almost twice as common in males. There is an annual incidence of approximately 3 per 100 000 and the disease is twice as common in American Blacks as in Whites. Family clusters have been reported, and there is an increased incidence in first degree relatives. Use of serum electrophoresis as a screening test reveals a far higher incidence of paraproteinaemia (a monoclonal immunoglobulin band), and up to 3% of an asymptomatic elderly population (70 years and older) have a monoclonal gammopathy detected by this means. Most of these patients will have benign paraproteinaemia (see p. 489) but a minority have, or subsequently develop, asymptomatic myeloma. An increased incidence has been reported in a group of American radiologists, presumably due to life-long radiation exposure, and also in survivors of Nagasaki and Hiroshima with a delay of 20 years.

Pathogenesis

IMMUNOGLOBULIN ABNORMALITIES

Multiple myeloma is one of a group of B lymphocyte neoplasms which are characterized by continued synthesis and release of immunoglobulins (Table 27.1). In myeloma there is neoplastic proliferation of a clone of B lymphocytes resulting in the formation of large numbers of immature plasma cells which infiltrate the bone marrow and which can occasionally be found in the blood. The oncogenic event

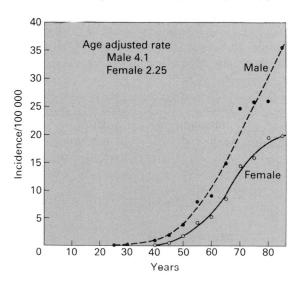

Fig. 27.1. *Age-specific incidence of myeloma in Britain.*

Table 27.1. Immunoglobulin producing neoplasms.

Benign
Benign monoclonal gammopathy
Cold agglutinin disease

Malignant
Myeloma
Waldenström's macroglobulinaemia
Primary amyloidosis
Non-Hodgkin's lymphomas
Heavy chain diseases (γ, α or μ)

479

may however occur earlier in the B cell differentiation pathway but clonal expansion, giving rise to the clinical syndrome, occurs at the plasma cell stage (Fig. 27.2). Production of large amounts of a monoclonal immunoglobulin is, therefore, a finding characteristic of multiple myeloma. Calculations of growth rate in myeloma has indicated that the disease has usually been present for several years before the tumour has expanded sufficiently to cause symptoms (1).

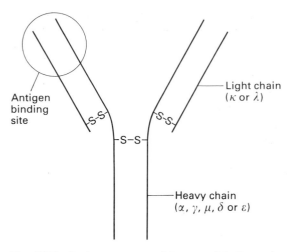

Fig. 27.3. *Basic structure of immunoglobulin molecules.* Two light chains are joined by disulphide bonds to two heavy chains. These are also joined by a variable number of disulphide bonds. The heavy chain varies in each immunoglobulin class, but light chains do not.

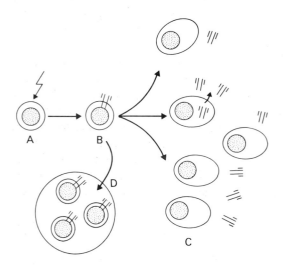

Fig. 27.2. *Pathogenesis of myeloma.* (A) Oncogenic event in a B cell. (B) Expansion of a clone of malignant B cells. (C) Proliferation of plasma cells leading to bone lesions and production of paraprotein. (D) Suppression of normal B cells leads to hypogammaglobulinaemia.

The basic structure of normal immunoglobulins consists of two polypeptide light chains (with molecular weights of 22 000) and two heavy chains (molecular weights of 55 000–70 000). These are held together by covalent (disulphide) and non-covalent bonds (Fig. 27.3). There is variability in heavy chain structure, with five separate types of heavy chain—γ, α, μ, δ and ε (Fig. 27.3). These differences form the basis of the five classes of immunoglobulin, IgG, IgA, IgM, IgD, IgE. However, there are only two types of light chain—kappa (κ) and

lambda (λ). IgG, IgD and IgE are found in the plasma as single molecules with a molecular weight of 160 000–200 000. IgM is a macroglobulin (molecular weight 900 000) synthesized as a pentamer of IgG structure. IgA is formed by plasma cells in the gut and respiratory tract, and is therefore found in external secretions such as saliva, tears, bronchial and gastro-intestinal mucosa, as well as in the blood. It has an important role in primary defence against invading pathogens.

Normal immunoglobulins are diverse in their detailed structure since they are synthesized in response to a variety of antigenic stimuli. Each immunoglobulin molecule recognizes one antigenic structure only, and the portion of the molecule which confers this specificity is known as the idiotypic determinant. It is located at the highly variable antigen binding site (Fig. 27.3). By contrast, in myeloma the product of the neoplastic plasma cell clone is an immunoglobulin of a single homogeneous structure (i.e. a single idiotype). This tumour product is called a myeloma protein or M-protein (not to be confused with IgM), or paraprotein. There is always

Table 27.2. Paraprotein frequency in myeloma.

Immunoglobulin class	Frequency (%)
IgG	55
IgA	24
Bence-Jones only	15
IgM*	2
IgD	2
Biclonal	1
None detected	1

*Excluding Waldenström's macroglobulinaemia

light-chain restriction, that is, to either κ or λ type.

In most patients with myeloma, whole immunoglobulin molecules are usually synthesized, but there may be a disproportionate production of one component so that free light or heavy chains may be produced. In approximately 1% of patients with multiple myeloma no monoclonal protein can be detected in the plasma or urine. In these patients (often termed non-secretors) the myeloma cells can sometimes be shown to contain abnormal heavy or light chains in the cytoplasm which are not secreted.

When free light chains are secreted into the blood, they cross the glomerular membrane and are therefore detectable in the urine. They have the unusual property of producing a cloudy precipitate when the urine is heated to 50–60°C, with dissociation of the precipitate as the temperature is raised near boiling point. Excre-tion of free light chains (sometimes called Bence-Jones protein after Henry Bence-Jones who described it in 1850), occurs in 40–50% of all cases of myeloma, and may be the only detectable abnormal protein since about 25% of patients with myeloma do not synthesize complete immunoglobulin molecules. It is detected nowadays by immunoelectrophoresis of the urine.

The major classes of immunoglobulin have differing physical properties and when there is excess production these properties may be clinically relevant since many aspects of the disease are attributable to the physical characteristics or deposition of the immunoglobulin itself. For example, IgM has a high molecular weight and hyperviscosity syndrome is not uncommon (see below). IgA molecules polymerize in the plasma and will also cause hyperviscosity. Excess light chains may be deposited in the renal tubule and contribute to renal failure (see p. 455. Polymerization of light chains is one component of amyloid which also contributes to renal disease. The incidence of the different types of myeloma protein roughly parallels the concentrations of normal serum immunoglobulins (Table 27.2) and reflects the number of plasma cells normally found in each group. IgG myeloma is the commonest type, followed by IgA. IgM production is rarely due to a true myeloma but is usually part of Waldenström's macroglobulinaemia (see p. 490). IgD meloma is very uncommon, and IgE exceedingly rare. More than 5×10^9 plasma cells must be present

Table 27.3. Prognostic features in myeloma.

Good	Poor
Haemoglobin > 10 g/dl	Haemoglobin < 8.5 g/dl
Serum calcium normal	Serum calcium > 2.9 mmol/l
No bone lesions	More than 3 bone lesions
Low paraprotein level	High paraprotein level
IgG < 50 g/l	IgG > 70 g/l
IgA < 30 g/l	IgA > 50 g/l
Urine light chains < 4 g/24 hours	Light chains > 12 g/24 hours
Plasma urea < 8 mmol/l	Urea > 8 mmol/l

for the paraprotein to be detectable as a discrete immunoglobulin band.

In myeloma an assessment of tumour mass can be made using a formula which includes haemoglobulin, calcium, presence of multiple bone lesions, paraprotein concentration and blood urea (Table 27.3). Patients with a large tumour mass ($>0.5 \times 10^{12}$ cells), have a worse prognosis and respond less frequently to chemotherapy.

Depression of production of normal immunoglobulin is a characteristic feature of the disease and one which helps to differentiate it from benign monoclonal gammopathy (p. 489). It occurs most frequently and profoundly in IgG myeloma, and to a lesser extent in cases producing Bence-Jones protein only. The mechanism of suppression of normal Ig production is not clear. This depression affects all classes of normal immunoglobulin and contributes greatly to susceptibility to bacterial infection.

There are many other causes of monoclonal immunoglobulin production (Table 27.4).

Table 27.4. Causes of monoclonal gammaglobulinaemia other than myeloma.

Monoclonal gammopathy of unknown significance (MGUS)

Non-lymphoid and lymphoid malignancy
Carcinoma of breast, gastrointestinal tract, ovary, bladder, prostate and others
Soft tissue sarcomas
Melanoma
Lymphoma
Waldenström's macroglobulinaemia

Autoimmune diseases
Rheumatoid arthritis
Polyarteritis nodosa

---

are discussed on pp. 489–491. One disorder in particular, benign monoclonal gammopathy (BMG), also called monoclonal gammopathy of unknown significance (MGUS), is very common in the elderly and may cause diagnostic difficulty, particularly as it may later progress to myeloma.

PATHOLOGICAL FEATURES

In myeloma there is infiltration of the bone marrow and bone by malignant plasma cells (Fig. 27.4). These cells are round or oval, often with an eccentrically placed nucleus like their normal counterpart. The cytoplasm is densely basophilic, due to the RNA which produces the paraprotein, with a clear perinuclear zone where the Golgi apparatus is situated. Immunoglobulin is present in the rough endoplasmic reticulum. Abnormal forms are often present

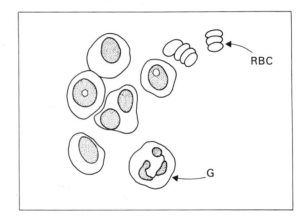

Fig. 27.4. *A clump of myeloma cells in bone marrow.* The cells are often large and sometimes contain more than one nucleus. The nucleus may be eccentrically placed or central. Red cells (RBC) are shown forming rouleaux due to the paraprotein; a granulocyte is also shown (G).

and these cells are large and may be bi- or tri-nucleate sometimes with more than one nucleolus and the nucleus eccentrically placed. These abnormal forms may be diagnostically helpful when the degree of infiltration is small. The marrow infiltration is often patchy, unlike leukaemia—hence the name multiple myeloma—a small tumour mass. The histological diagnosis is highly probable when the level of infiltration exceeds 20% of all nucleated marrow cells, but the diagnosis is not excluded by lesser degrees of involvement. The bone becomes destroyed by the tumour. Typically the lesions are lytic

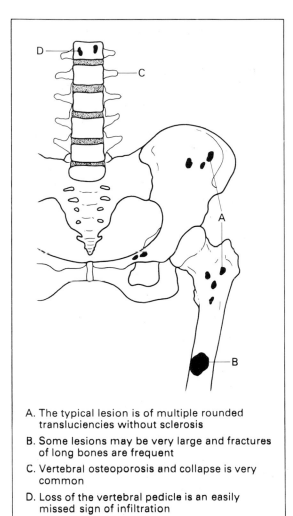

A. The typical lesion is of multiple rounded transluciencies without sclerosis

B. Some lesions may be very large and fractures of long bones are frequent

C. Vertebral osteoporosis and collapse is very common

D. Loss of the vertebral pedicle is an easily missed sign of infiltration

Fig. 27.5. *Diagrammatic representation of bone lesions in myeloma.*

and fractures are common (Fig. 27.5). The mechanism of lysis is not fully understood but osteoclastic activating factors produced by the myeloma or mature B cells have been described. Any bone can be affected and common sites include vertebrae, pelvis, skull, ribs and proximal long bones.

The kidney is affected in several ways (Fig. 27.6). First, light chains are taken up by distal renal tubular cells which are a major site of catabolism of normal light chains. The massive load of light chains results in tubular damage and large casts of light chains and albumin fill the tubule and obstruct the nephron, imposing a further load on the remaining nephrons. Specific defects in tubular reabsorption may occur, possibly due to the protein aggregation in renal tubule cells and leading to tubular reabsorptive defects with leakage of amino acids, glucose, potassium and phosphate (acquired Fanconi syndrome).

Second, amyloid deposition in the blood vessels of the glomerulus occurs in 10% of patients. It is especially common in those cases where light chains alone are produced. In myeloma (but not in all other circumstances), this protein consists in part of polymerized light chain fragments. Lambda light chains are much more likely to lead to amyloid formation. Other features of the disease which contribute to renal impairment include hypercalciuria and nephrocalcinosis, urate deposition and renal tubular leakage. Urinary tract infection is common and pyelonephritis may develop. Together, these processes constitute 'myeloma kidney'.

Occasionally there is deposition of malignant plasma cells in soft tissues producing localized swellings. This typically occurs late in the disease when there is a large tumour mass. Skin, lymph nodes, liver and spleen are the commonest sites.

Clinical features

Patients with multiple myeloma may be asymptomatic for many years, before presenting with weakness, bone pain, anorexia and other symptoms due either to abnormal proliferation of the malignant plasma cells, to direct effects of the abnormal immunoglobulin, or to hypercalcaemia.

In many patients, diffuse bone pain is the major complaint and skeletal abnormalities are present in about two-thirds of patients with multiple myeloma. The pain is typically dull or aching, and often felt in the spine, ribs or pelvis. Pathological fractures are common and acute

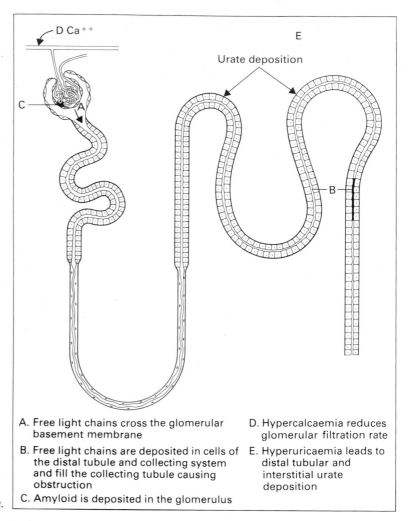

A. Free light chains cross the glomerular basement membrane

B. Free light chains are deposited in cells of the distal tubule and collecting system and fill the collecting tubule causing obstruction

C. Amyloid is deposited in the glomerulus

D. Hypercalcaemia reduces glomerular filtration rate

E. Hyperuricaemia leads to distal tubular and interstitial urate deposition

Fig. 27.6. *Renal damage in myeloma.*

back pain from a vertebral crush fracture is a frequent first presentation of myeloma. This may lead to acute cord compression (see Chapter 8).

Typical radiological appearances include generalized osteoporosis (particularly evident in the dorsal and lumbar spine and sacro-iliac area), and punched out osteolytic lesions, with little or no sclerosis (Fig. 27.5), though osteoblastic lesions are occasionally seen. Full radiological skeletal survey will often reveal unsuspected bone lesions and should always be performed at diagnosis. In addition to the ribs, vertebrae, and hips, these lesions are frequently found in the skull, where they are usually asymptomatic until they reach a large size. Biopsy of these sites reveals heavy infiltration with abnormal plasma cells.

Many patients present with fatigue and lassitude due to anaemia and recurrent bacterial infection due to immuneparesis. Nausea, anorexia and dehydration may be due to hypercalcaemia and lead to deteriorating renal function.

Hyperviscosity syndrome may develop in patients in whom the type and level of abnormal immunoglobulin contributes to an increase in plasma viscosity. This is most commonly seen in patients with Waldenström's macroglobulinaemia (see below) but also occurs in patients with myeloma especially with IgA and IgM paraproteins. Clinically, this syndrome consists of neurological symptoms, chiefly vertigo, confusion, transient ischaemic episodes; retinopathy with distended retinal veins, haemorrhages and papilloedema; and hypervolaemia with increased vascular resistance. A bleeding tendency is frequently due to both thrombocytopenia and a clotting disturbance whose pathogenesis is not clearly understood, but often due to interference of the coagulation system by the paraproteins. Although at presentation the platelet count is not usually below $50 \times 10^9/1$, coating of platelets by abnormal immunoglobulin may lead to reduced platelet aggregation. This may lead, in turn, to an abnormally prolonged bleeding time with purpura, epistaxis, mucosal bleeding and retinal haemorrhage. A positive Hess test, reduced thromboplastin generation time and defective clot retraction may occur.

In addition to cord compression from direct involvement of the vertebrae by myeloma, patients often suffer other neurological complications. Direct extradural involvement may occur through involvement of nerve roots via the intervertebral foramina. Soft tissue deposits may occur in the orbit or base of skull, leading to proptosis or cranial nerve palsies. Carpal tunnel syndrome may occur, and is thought to be due to amyloid infiltration. Patients may occasionally develop a mixed polyneuropathy and rarely-multifocal leucoencephalopathy (see Chapter 9).

Lymphadenopathy, hepatomegaly and splenomegaly are not usually present but may develop later in the course of the disease. Megaloblastic anaemia can occur, possibly due to defective folate metabolism, though many patients have some degree of macrocytosis with no megaloblastic change and the cause is uncertain. Recurrent infection is a common feature of the disease and is frequently one of the presenting complaints. Leucopenia predisposes to infection, as does the generalized depression of normal immunoglobulins. This immunoglobulin abnormality frequently fails to become normal even with 'successful' treatment which may depress the monoclonal immunoglobulin band. Some patients also have impairment of phagocytosis and cellular immune responses.

The plasma volume may be high as a result of the increase in total plasma protein. This will contribute to the anaemia even when the total red cell mass is near normal. Congestive cardiac failure is occasionally encountered. The M-band is also responsible, by direct coating of erythrocytes, for the raised ESR and erythrocyte rouleaux formation which are so characteristic of multiple myeloma. Typically the ESR is $> 80\,\text{mm/hr}$. Bone marrow involvement is almost always demonstrable, though the distribution may be patchy, and for diagnostic purposes, direct biopsy of a tender area is more likely to be positive. Some haematologists advise against sternal marrow puncture in patients with myeloma, in view of the extreme fragility of bone and the danger of inadvertently entering the mediastinum. It is usually best to sample tender, or radiologically abnormal areas, wherever possible. Abnormal plasma cells can account for up to 95% of the nucleated cell population.

Hypercalcaemia is a common feature, chiefly attributable to the bone destruction from abnormal plasma cell proliferation although other factors which activate osteoclasts have been described in myeloma (3). Approximately one-third of patients have an abnormally elevated plasma calcium at diagnosis, and the majority of patients develop hypercalcaemia during the course of the illness. Hypercalciuria is even more frequent. Hypercalcaemia may be of sufficient severity to require emergency treatment (see Chapter 9). The symptoms include polyuria, polydipsia, constipation, nausea, vomiting, dehydration and mental confusion.

Impaired renal function is common. Its pathogenesis has been described above. It is important to realize that once hypercalcaemia and renal impairment have developed, a vicious circle becomes established in which there is

worsening renal function, increasing hypercalcaemia, further dehydration with falling
glomerular filtration rate, and increasing tubular obstruction and dysfunction from light
chain deposition. This is a medical emergency
and its management is described below.

Diagnosis

In a typical case when there are bone lesions,
anaemia, paraproteinaemia, hypercalcaemia
and marrow involvement, there is no diagnostic
difficulty. In less florid cases, the differential
diagnosis can be difficult and may include:

1   other causes of anaemia, bone pain and hypercalcaemia such as metastatic cancer;
2   other causes of paraproteinaemia such as
monoclonal gammopathy of unknown significance (MGUS), occult primary tumours (Table
27.4), Wäldenstrom's macroglobulinaemia or
lymphomas;
3   other causes of lytic lesions in bone such as
breast or bronchial carcinoma;
4   other causes of spinal cord compression
such as metastatic cancer;
5   other causes of anaemia and raised ESR
such as connective tissue diseases;
6   solitary plasmacytomas (see below).

The diagnosis may sometimes be difficult
especially if there is minimal marrow involvement, no detectable paraprotein, or a solitary
bone lesion on skeletal X-rays. In doubtful
cases the marrow examination may have to be
repeated. However, if there is no pressing indication for treatment, a period of observation
may allow the diagnosis to be established more
easily (Table 27.5).

Treatment

When patients with myeloma present with
dangerous manifestations such as dehydration,
hypercalaemia and/or spinal cord compression,
the first treatment should be to correct the
metabolic disturbance or serious local problem
(see Chapter 9). Intravenous fluid replacement,
correction of hypercalcaemia, local irradiation

Table 27.5. Important investigations in myeloma.

Haematological
 Full blood count ESR
 Marrow aspiration and biopsy
 Serum viscosity

Biochemical
 Urea and electrolytes, creatinine clearance
 Serum calcium
 Serum albumin
 Quantitative immunoglobulins
 Immunoelectrophoresis
 Twenty-four hour urine for light chains and total
   protein and calcium excretion
 β_2 microglobulins—plasma/urine

Radiological
 Skeletal survey

and sometimes decompressive laminectomy
should, in these circumstances, take precedence.
In the majority of patients, however, the
presenting clinical syndrome is more slowly
evolving and, in contrast to these clinical emergencies there will be time to confirm the diagnosis before instituting treatment.

CHEMOTHERAPY

Chemotherapy, using continuous or intermittent alkylating agents, is the mainstay of treatment for multiple myeloma and has improved
the median survival time from 6-12 months
(untreated) to 2-3 years (4). Intermittent therapy with oral melphalan ($7 mg/m^2 \times 4$-7 days
given every 6 weeks) is the most widely used
agent. The addition of oral prednisolone (1 mg/
kg body weight daily $\times$ 4-7 days with each
course of melphalan) has slightly improved the
remission rate (4). However, prednisolone is
avoided in myeloma patients who have severe
osteoporosis. This combined oral therapy is
generally well tolerated although some patients
complain of nausea or steroid side-effects. In
long survivors, there is undoubtedly a small risk
of development of acute myeloblastic leukaemia related to chronic melphalan therapy (5);
this fatal complication has chiefly been noted in

patients on long term daily melphalan therapy rather than pulsed intermitent courses of treatment. Cyclophosphamide (75-150 mg daily by mouth) is sometimes used for patients who show no improvement with melphalan. Other agents such as vincristine, doxorubicin or nitrosoureas have been used to induce remission (5), but this approach has not been convincingly shown to give superior results to the standard melphalan/prednisolone combination. Table 27.6 summarizes results of recent trials of chemotherapy (6, 7).

Most patients with myeloma will respond to oral chemotherapy, with improvement in symptoms, particularly pain, tenderness and hypercalcaemia. The paraprotein level generally falls within the first three cycles of chemotherapy, though the immune paresis of the unaffected immunoglobulins usually takes longer to recover, and may never do so. Other parameters such as haemoglobin, albumin and blood urea may return to normal limits and can be useful for monitoring progress. In patients who respond to chemotherapy, it is rarely necessary to continue the initial treatment beyond 6-9

courses, since little further is to be gained. By this time the patient will either have entered a 'plateau' phase, in which no further reduction of the paraprotein occurs, or the patient's immunoglobulin levels will be normal and treatment can reasonably be discontinued. In some cases the patient's paraprotein level will have risen throughout the early courses of melphalan/prednisolone therapy, in which case it is clearly necessary to consider alternative treatment.

After discontinuation of oral first line chemotherapy, patients should be carefully monitored since further treatment will always be required, though sometimes only after many months or years. If treatment with melphalan/prednisolone or other first line chemotherapy is discontinued following a well-documented response, it is usually worth reinstituting the same therapy at the point of relapse since a second response is usually seen. Relapse is usually readily detectable by a rise in the monoclonal immunoglobulin band, although some patients become symptomatic again without such a rise. Further supportive therapy with blood transfusion,

Table 27.6. Chemotherapy trials in multiple myeloma (5, 6, 7). New regimens compared with melphalan/prednisolone.

Drug combination	% Response	Median survival (months)
All cases		
BCNU, cyclophosphamide and prednisolone	49	36
Melphalan and prednisolone	52	36
MeCCNU, vincristine, melphalan and prednisolone	70	41
Melphalan and prednisolone	58	39
Vincristine, BCNU, melphalan, cyclophosphamide and prednisolone	74	33
Melphalan and prednisolone	57	29
Early stage disease		
MeCCNU, vincristine, melphalan and prednisolone	85	48
Melphalan and prednisolone	69	43

antibiotics or palliative radiotherapy is often required if the patient becomes anaemic, develops infections or painful bony lesions.

Second-line chemotherapy in myeloma remains unsatisfactory, though successes have been claimed with combinations of doxorubicin, vincristine, nitrosoureas and other agents (8). Responses to secondary chemotherapy are usually of short duration, and at the cost of inflicting more undesirable side-effects than are seen with melphalan/prednisolone. In an elderly population, careful judgement is always required before considering such treatment and it is important to establish that no further response can be obtained with first-line chemotherapy.

RADIOTHERAPY

Radiotherapy is of great value in multiple myeloma and is often required as part of the initial treatment, particularly for patients who present with painful bone deposits in the vertebrae or long bones especially if there is a likelihood of pathological fracture or cord compression. Radiotherapy is the most important modality in myelomatous spinal cord compression either alone or in combination with neurosurgical decompression. Myelography should be performed if possible to define the full extent of the compression. Treatment should be started early at the onset of radicular pain. If delayed until signs of paraparesis have developed, the outcome is worse. For lytic deposits of long bones, radiotherapy is often combined with internal fixation particularly where a weight-bearing long bone is affected. Since myeloma deposits are relatively radiosensitive, large doses are rarely required.

For spinal deposits, a total of 30 Gy (3000 rad) in 10 fractions over 2 weeks is commonly employed. Although shorter treatments, 5 Gy (500 rad) × 5 fractions over 1 week are effective, many radiotherapists prefer to avoid the risks of short fractionation regimens where significant portions of the spinal cord are included in the volume (see Chapter 5 for a fuller

discussion of radiation myelitis). In myeloma, lengthy portions of cord are often unavoidably treated. At other sites, treatment with shorter fractionation regimens is often used. Single fractions, 8–12 Gy (800–1200 rad) are effective and safe, which is of particular value in myeloma since patients often require frequent courses of treatment at multiple sites.

Success has recently been claimed with systemic or hemibody irradiation in myeloma (8), and there seems little doubt that treatment can be effective in patients with symptomatic relapse who are no longer responsive to standard chemotherapy treatment. Our practice is to offer treatment to the upper half of the body to a dose of 7.5 Gy (750 rad), followed 6–8 weeks later by treatment to 10 Gy (1000 rad) to the lower half of the body (or vice versa). Toxicity includes acute nausea and vomiting, diarrhoea and alopecia. Pulmonary complications are unusual if the dose to the upper half of the body is kept below 8.0 Gy (800 rad). The whole of the face, from the point of the chin to the supraorbital ridge can be shielded from treatment in order to avoid painful mucositis and parotitis, and we do not usually irradiate the cranium unless troublesome lytic skull deposits are present.

Prognosis

Many patients with myeloma experience remissions and relapses requiring careful judgement for optimal choice and timing of therapy. Some patients survive for 10 years or more, requiring little in the way of chemotherapy, but radiotherapy and general support measures. Such patients usually have a low tumour burden based on simple criteria (Table 27.3). Large retrospective analyses of patients with myeloma have shown that tumour burden is a good predictor of response and survival (9). Median survival in the best prognostic categories is approximately 5 years, compared with only 6 months in the worst groups (Fig. 27.7). Since many patients with myeloma eventually develop renal failure, it is not surprising that

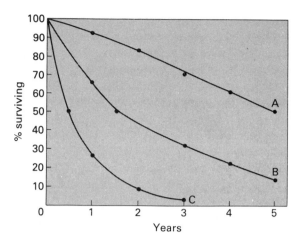

A. Low tumour mass (median survival 5 years)
B. Intermediate mass (median survival 2 years)
C. High tumour mass (median survival 6 months)

Fig. 27.7. *Prognosis in myeloma related to tumour mass.*

simple measures of renal function represent the most important single prognostic criterion at diagnosis. Apart from recurrence and increasingly severe renal dysfunction, the other important group of myeloma complications results from progressive pancytopenia both from crowding of normal elements by abnormal plasma cells, and also from therapy. Anaemia often requiring transfusion at an ever decreasing interval, infection and thrombocytopenia with bleeding are all common and contribute to ill-health and eventually to death. Occasionally, hypercalcaemia may become totally resistant to treatment.

SOLITARY PLASMACYTOMA

Solitary plasmacytoma is a single plasma cell lesion, found either in bone or soft tissue (particularly nasal or oral cavity, bowel or bronchus) with the typical histological finding of malignant plasma cell infiltration, as in multiple myeloma. In many patients, no other evidence of myeloma develops provided adequate local treatment with radiotherapy is given. However,

solitary plasmacytomas can be the initial manifestation of myeloma and these patients should be carefully investigated since a proportion with apparently solitary lesions will prove to have multiple myeloma at the outset. Patients with true solitary plasmacytomas should be followed up regularly since a proportion of them will undoubtedly develop myeloma later, though latent periods of several years are not unusual. This progression is more common in those who present with a plasmacytoma in bone than in those where the site is extramedullary. There is no proven benefit in aggressive treatment of solitary plasmacytomas with chemotherapy in the expectation that this will prevent the development of generalized myeloma.

MONOCLONAL GAMMOPATHY OF UNKNOWN SIGNIFICANCE (MGUS)

There are many diseases in which a monoclonal immunoglobulin band is found but without evidence of a plasma cell neoplasm (Table 27.4). The commonest cause, and the one which creates greatest diagnostic confusion is MGUS, which is a disease of the elderly. It is common, with a prevalence of 0.5% in adults over 40 years and 3% over 70 years. MGUS accounts for 40% of all paraproteinaemias. The concentration of monoclonal immunoglobulin is usually less than 30 g/l. A large majority (85%) have an IgG paraprotein. There is no other abnormality of plasma proteins or symptoms of the kind found in patients with multiple myeloma. Bence-Jones protein is occasionally found. The ESR is sometimes raised. MGUS requires no treatment though a small proportion (less than 20%) will eventually develop myeloma. Until recently this condition was known as benign monoclonal gammopathy.

MACROGLOBULINAEMIA

This group of conditions is characterized by the production of monoclonal IgM. The causes are given in Table 27.7.

Table 27.7. Causes of macroglubulinaemia.

Benign
    Benign macroglobulinaemia
    Cold agglutinin disease

Neoplasms
    Waldenström's macroglobulinaemia
    IgM myeloma
    Non-Hodgkin's lymphomas
    Chronic lymphatic leukaemia

Benign macroglobulinaemia follows a similar course to other forms of MEUS (see above).

Cold agglutinin disease is a disease of the elderly in which the patients suffer from vascular disturbances in the extermities due to intracapillary agglutination of red cells in parts of the body exposed to cold. A deep blue-violet discolouration may occur (acrocyanosis) which may lead to gangrene. In addition, a moderate haemolysis is usually present.

Physical examination reveals little in the way of abnormalities apart from the spleen being slightly enlarged. The disease is due to a monoclonal IgM which has the property of being a cold agglutinin. If simple measures—gloves or mittens and warm boots—are inadequate, treatment with alkylating agents can be helpful.

WALDENSTROM'S MACROGLOBULINAEMIA

This condition, which occurs in the elderly, is characterized by bone marrow infiltration, with lymphoid cells which have the appearance of an 'intermediate' form between lymphocytes and plasma cells (lymphoplasmacytoid). There is enlargement of lymph nodes, liver and spleen. Unlike IgM myeloma, bone lesions are uncommon though diffuse osteoporosis may occur. There is production of a monoclonal IgM, often in very large amounts, sometimes producing hyperviscosity.

The patient presents with ill-health and weakness. The symptoms of hyperviscosity may predominate with headache, mental confusion,

retinal haemorrhages and renal impairment. Renal disease is less common than in myeloma. The macroglobulin may produce haemolytic anaemia or act as a cold agglutinin. It may produce haemorrhage by interaction with platelets and clotting factors. Purpura and bleeding are not infrequent. Investigations reveal anaemia, variable thrombocytopenia, a raised serum IgM and occasionally immune paresis.

Treatment and prognosis

The disease is only slowly progressive and, in the absence of symptoms treatment can be withheld. Chlorambucil or cyclophosphamide, given in a small daily dose, usually produce regression of lymphadenopathy and a fall in IgM levels. Steroids are of little value.

Since IgM is intravascular, plasmapheresis will produce reduction of viscosity and is essential if clinical hyperviscosity is present. It should be repeated until chemotherapy reduces IgM production. The prognosis is variable, but average survival is 3–4 years from diagnosis.

HEAVY CHAIN DISEASES

These diseases are lymphocyte neoplasms in which there is production of incomplete heavy chains of immunoglobulin, without light chains. The first patient was described by Franklin in 1964 (10). So far, only γ, α and μ heavy chain diseases have been described. Interestingly, each has distinct clinical features.

γ-Heavy chain disease

γ-heavy chain disease usually effects elderly patients, producing lymphadenopathy, tonsillar enlargement, palatal oedema, and hepatosplenomegaly. Bone lesions are unusual. Occasionally there are associated auto-immune diseases such as systemic lupus erythematosus or Sjögren's syndrome. Anaemia is common but the bone marrow may not show any diagnostic features. The lymph nodes may be replaced with lymphoplasmacytoid cells, but may not be diagnostic. The γ-heavy chain fragment is found in serum or urine and there may also be immune paresis.

Chemotherapy is usually minimally effective. Although this disease may occasionally regress without treatment, survival time is usually not greater than 3 years.

α-Heavy chain disease

This important disease is the commonest of the heavy chain diseases and is chiefly found in young Mediterranean adults and in the populations of the Middle East and South America. It is a disease of the small bowel although occasionally the stomach, large bowel and postnasal space are affected. Typically, the disease occurs in adults aged 20–30 years. There is frequently a history of gastro-intestinal disturbance extending over many years, and some patients have been previously diagnosed as having immune proliferative disease of the small intestine. Because of massive lymphoid infiltration of the bowel, severe malabsorption and diarrhoea develop and, although the histological appearances may initially not appear to be malignant, a true lymphoma usually develops.

α-heavy chains are present in the blood but their detection is difficult. The marrow is not involved and liver, spleen and lymph nodes is not enlarged. The diagnosis is made by small bowel biopsy. Treatment with cytotoxic chemotherapy at the stage of frank lymphoma is only temporarily effective. Whole abdominal irradiation has sometimes been used. Before this stage, treatment with oral tetracycline may produce long remissions.

μ-Heavy chain disease

In this very rare disease, μ-heavy chains are found in the plasma. The clinical disease is longstanding chronic lymphatic leukaemia, or a non-Hodgkin's lymphoma, usually with marked visceral organomegaly, and treatment is similar to that used for these diseases.

REFERENCES

1 Durie B.G.M., Salmon S.E. & Moon T.E. (1980) Pretreatment tumour mass cell kinetics and prognosis in multiple myeloma. *Blood* **55**, 364–72.

2 Alexanian R., Balcerzak S., Bonnet J.D., Gehan E.A., Haut A., Hewlett J.S. & Monto R.W. (1975) Prognostic factors in multiple myeloma. *Cancer* **36**, 1192.

3 Mundy G.R., Raisz L.G., Cooper R.A., Schechter G.P. & Salmon S.E. (1974) Evidence for the secretion of an osteoclast stimulating factor in myeloma. *New England Journal of Medicine* **291**, 1041–6.

4 Medical Research Council (1980) Report on the second myelomatosis trial after 5 years of follow up. *British Journal of Cancer* **42**, 823.

5 Alexanian R., Salmon S., Bonnet J., Gehan E., Haut A. & Weick J. (1977) Combination chemotherapy for multiple myeloma. *Cancer* **40**, 2765–71.

6 Pavlovsky S., Saslavsky J. & Tezanos Pinto M. (1980) A randomised trial of melphalan and prednisolone versus melphalan, prednisolone, cyclophosphamide, MeCCNU and vincristine in untreated multiple myeloma. *Journal of Clinical Oncology* **2**, 836–40.

7 Barlogie B., Smith L. & Alexanian R. (1984) Effective treatment of advanced multiple myeloma refractory to alkylating agents. *New England Journal of Medicine* **310**, 1353–6.

8 Tobias J.S., Richards J.D.M., Blackman G.M., Joannides T., Trask C.W.L. & Nathan J.I. (1985) Hemibody irradiation in multiple myeloma. *Radiotherapy and Oncology* **3**, 11–16.

9 Woodruff R.K., Wadsworth J., Malpas J.S. & Tobias J.S. (1979) Clinical staging in multiple myeloma. *British Journal of Haematology* **42**, 199–205.

10 Franklin E.C., Lowenstein J., Bigelow B. & Meltzer M. (1964) Heavy chain disease. A new disorder of serum gammaglobulin. *American Journal of Medicine* **37**, 332.

Chapter 28
Leukaemia

Leukaemias are neoplastic proliferations of white blood cells. Although uncommon, they have been the subject of detailed investigation because of the insights they give into aetiology and pathogenesis of the malignant process. The intensive chemotherapy which has been responsible for the increasing cure rate in acute leukaemia has served as an example for the treatment of other malignancies. Allogeneic bone marrow transplantation was developed as a treatment for acute leukaemia and is now under investigation as a method of treatment in other neoplasms. For these reasons, the principles of management are described in this chapter, but more detailed discussion and guidance is given in articles and books mentioned on page 509.

Incidence and aetiology

In childhood (below 15 years of age), acute lymphoblastic leukaemia (ALL) accounts for 80% of all cases, acute myeloblastic leukaemia (AML) and its variants accounting for 17% of the remainder, and chronic granulocytic leukaemia (CGL) approximately 3%. The death rate from acute leukaemia in the population is approximately 7 per 100 000. The disease is slightly more common in males (3:2), and its incidence over the last decade appears to have been constant. Acute leukaemia is most common in the elderly (Fig. 28.1A & B), and over 15 years of age, 85% of cases are AML. In adults, AML and ALL have a very similar prognosis, but childhood ALL has different clinical features and a much better prognosis than adult ALL, or AML at any age.

A variety of aetiological factors have been implicated. Ionizing irradiation is leukaemogenic. Survivors of the Hiroshima and Nagasaki atom bombs have an increased risk of leukaemia and the risk is greater for those who were near the centre of the explosions. AML and CGL are the most frequent types. The increased incidence began 2 years after the explosion and then declined after 6 years (Fig. 28.1C). There is an increased risk of AML in patients treated with extended field irradiation for Hodgkin's disease, especially if this is combined with cytotoxic drugs (see Chapter 25). Cytotoxic agents are themselves leukaemogenic as shown by the increased incidence of leukaemia following alkylating agent therapy for ovarian and other cancers. Low dose chronic administration of alkylating agents frequently causes myelodysplastic changes, and some of these patients go on to develop AML often with chromosomal abnormalities. Benzene and possibly its derivatives are known to predispose to the development of both aplastic anaemia and acute leukaemia.

Viral causes of leukaemia have long been postulated but to date there is no firm evidence of a causal role for any virus. RNA viruses (retroviruses, see Chapter 3) are the most likely candidates. Recently, seroepidemiological evidence has implicated a retrovirus in the pathogenesis of T cell leukaemia in Japan and T cell lymphoma in the Caribbean (see Chapter 3).

Certain genetic abnormalities predispose to the development of leukaemia. Many familial

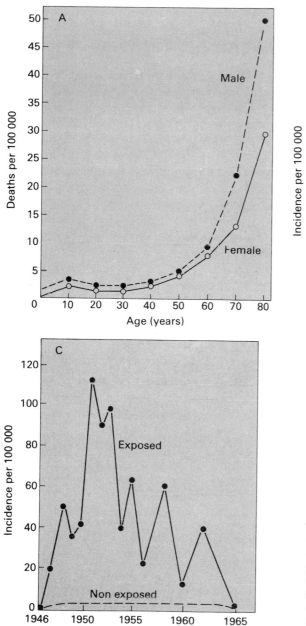

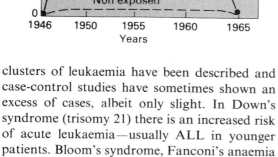

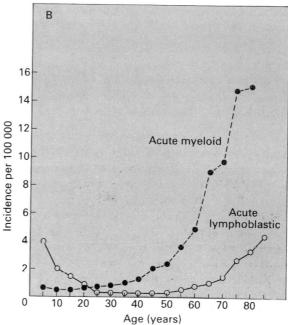

Fig. 28.1. *Incidence of leukaemia.* (A) Age-specific death rates from leukaemia of all types in England (1979). (B) Age-specific incidence rates of acute lymphoblastic and myeloblastic leukaemia (3rd National Cancer Survey USA 1969–71). (C) Leukaemia incidence in Hiroshima from 1946 onwards, in exposed and non-exposed individuals. (From Wintrobe M. (1980) *Blood Pure and Eloquent* p. 528. McGraw Hill. With permission).

clusters of leukaemia have been described and case-control studies have sometimes shown an excess of cases, albeit only slight. In Down's syndrome (trisomy 21) there is an increased risk of acute leukaemia—usually ALL in younger patients. Bloom's syndrome, Fanconi's anaemia and ataxia-telangiectasia are all autosomal recessive diseases characterized by chromosome breakage and an increased risk of leukaemia. A defective DNA repair mechanism may be responsible. AML is the usual leukaemia in Fanconi anaemia, and ALL in ataxia-telangiectasia.

Cytogenetic abnormalities are frequently found in leukaemic cells and these are discussed below.

THE ACUTE LEUKAEMIAS

Pathology and classification

In recent years there has been a considerable growth of knowledge about the maturation of haemopoietic and lymphoid cells. Acute leukae-mias often retain many of the cytoplasmic and membrane characteristics of their normal counterparts, so it is possible to relate the various types of acute leukaemia to a particular stage of myeloid or lymphoid maturation. A simplified scheme is shown in Fig. 28.2.

The diagnosis is made from blood and mar-row films and careful staining and preparation are essential. In the typical case there are leu-kaemic blasts in the blood and the marrow is packed with uniform-looking blast cells. Cases

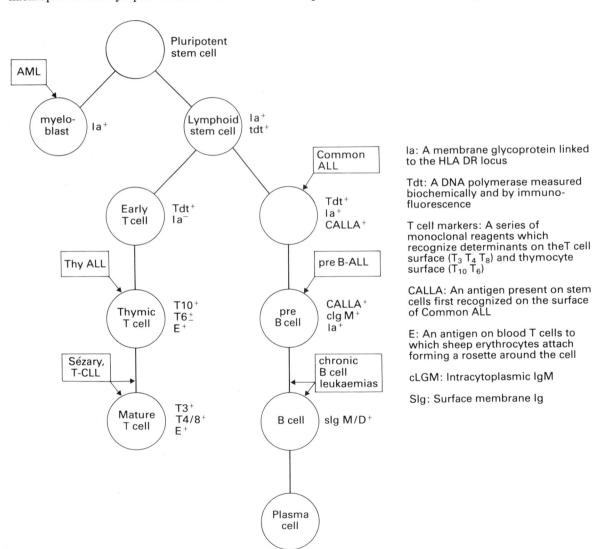

Fig. 28.2. *Maturation of haemopoietic and lymphoid cells in relation to types of leukaemia.*

of ALL almost always show these appearances but in adult AML the leukaemic process may be much more subtle with few blasts in the blood. The marrow must show over 30% of blasts for the diagnosis to be made with confidence. When there are less than 20% blasts the diagnosis of myelodysplastic state is usually made (see p. 500).

In recent years the acute leukaemias have been subdivided on morphological grounds using a scheme devised by an Anglo-French cooperative group (1). An outline is given in Table 28.1. With the exception of acute promyelocytic leukaemia, the prognostic significance of this subdivision is doubtful.

Table 28.1. A Morphological classification of acute leukaemia (1).

AML
- M1 myeloblastic (no maturation, undifferentiated)
- M2 myeloblastic (some maturation)
- M3 hypergranular promyelocytic
- M4 myelo-monocytic
- M5 monocytic
- M6 erythroleukaemia

ALL
- L1 small monomorphic cells
- L2 large heterogeneous cells
- L3 Burkitt-like

In AML, the myeloblasts may contain Auer rods which are pink staining rod-like inclusions which are probably aberrant forms of the cytoplasmic granules found in normal granulocyte precursors. These granules are often prominent in the cytoplasm in AML and are particularly frequent and often large in the M3 variety (hypergranular promyelocytic leukaemia). In monocytic leukaemia (M5) the blasts are large with abundant cytoplasm and in erythroleukaemia (M6) there are erythroblasts and myeloblasts in the marrow.

The commonest form of ALL (L1) is characterized by scanty cytoplasm and fewer nucleoli. In the less common form (L2) the blasts

are larger, with a larger nucleolus. This form, which is more common in adults, is more easily mistaken for AML and may account for some cases designated as undifferentiated leukaemia.

Cytochemical stains help to determine the type of leukaemia if there is doubt. The commonly used stains are shown in Table 28.2.

Table 28.2. Cytochemical stains in AML and ALL.

Stain	AML	ALL	
Sudan Black	+	−	
Peroxidase	+	−	
PAS	+/−	+	('block' positivity)
Acid phosphatase	+	−	in c ALL/+ in T ALL

Note: in undifferentiated leukaemia many or all of these stains may be negative. PAS positivity is sometimes present in AML and is not always positive in ALL. Non specific esterase (NSE) is used to identify monocytic components.

These stains may help to confirm the diagnosis in doubtful cases. In occasional instances of undifferentiated acute leukaemia, the cytochemical stains are unhelpful. Some further help in diagnosis may be obtained by using the membrane markers shown in Fig. 28.2. In ALL in particular, these markers may help to distinguish common ALL from T cell ALL and Burkitt's lymphoma (Table 28.3).

Chromosomal abnormalities are frequent in acute leukaemia. In AML, abnormalities are found in half of all cases using conventional karyotypic analysis, but in almost all cases sensitive when banding techniques are employed. The abnormalities include structural defects such as translocations and deletions, and abnormal numbers of chromosomes. In AML chromosomes 5, 7, 8, 15, 17 and 21 are most frequently affected. In promyelocytic leukaemia a specific translocation (15q+; 17q−) is found in 50% of cases.

In ALL the most important finding is that the Ph' chromosome (see p. 505) is present in 20% of cases, with the same translocation (9q+; 22q−) as in classical chronic granulocytic leu-

Table 28.3. Markers of ALL in childhood.

Markers*	Common ALL	T cell ALL	B cell ALL
Anti T cell antibodies (against early T cells)	−	+	−
Erythrocyte rosettes	−	+	−
Anti-CALLA antibody	+	−	+
Acid phosphatase	−	+	−
TdT	+	+	+
Anti-1a antibody	+	−	+
Cytoplasmic IgM	−	−	+

* See Fig. 28.2 for explanation of markers

kaemia (CGL). After treatment some cases may become like CGL. Other abnormal karyotypes are less frequent than in adult AML.

Clinical features and management of acute leukaemias

ACUTE LYMPHOBLASTIC LEUKAEMIA (ALL) IN CHILDHOOD

The disease usually presents at the age of 4–5 years, and the symptoms are due to marrow infiltration causing anaemia, thrombocytopenia, infection and bone pain, especially in long bones. As with other forms of acute leukaemia the history is of a few weeks of malaise, sometimes with fever even in the absence of obvious infection. Oral and pharyngeal ulceration may occur and bone pains are frequent. Although petechiae are often found on examination, presentation with other haemorrhagic phenomena is less common.

On examination the child is usually pale. There may be lymph node enlargement, splenomegaly and slight hepatic enlargement. The bones may be tender on pressure particularly over the sternum. Skin petechiae are common (and may also be seen on the palate) and as haemorrhages in the eye, either in the retina or as larger sub-hyaloid haemorrhages. Skin infiltration with leukaemia is uncommon and

takes the form of plaques of tumour of purple colour.

Occasionally the patient has symptoms of meningeal involvement at presentation. This usually manifests itself as headache, vomiting and neck stiffness. Cranial nerve palsies may occur as in other forms of malignant meningitis (see Chapter 8).

Investigation usually reveals anaemia, thrombocytopenia and an elevated total white cell count (WBC) with numerous lymphoblasts. In 40% of cases, the total WBC is not elevated but blasts are usually present. 'Aleukaemic leukaemia' is a term used to describe those cases where blasts are not present in the blood film (approximately 5% of cases). In all cases a bone marrow examination is essential, with cytochemical and immunological studies when possible (as outlined above). A chest X-ray is usually normal, but in T cell ALL, may show a mediastinal mass due to thymic enlargement. This form of ALL is common in adolescent boys. Bone X-rays are not infrequently abnormal and the typical abnormality is of radiolucent bands in the metaphyseal region. Diffuse demineralization also occurs, and discrete osteolytic lesions.

Biochemical investigation may show a raised uric acid due to rapid proliferation and death of leukaemic cells. A lumbar puncture may show leukaemic cells even though there may be no clinical evidence of disease in the CNS (see p. 497).

Treatment: remission induction and consolidation. The mainstay of treatment is chemotherapy, which should be instituted as soon as possible. Because of the rapid breakdown of tumour which may produce the tumour lysis syndrome (see Chapter 8) the patient should be hydrated and given allopurinol in order to prevent secondary hyperuricaemia. The principles of chemotherapy of ALL are shown in Fig. 28.3.

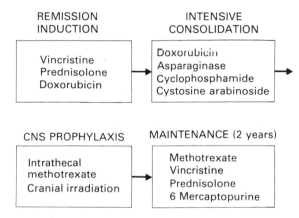

Fig. 28.3. *Outline of management of acute lymphoblastic leukaemia in childhood.*

Haematological and clinical remission is induced with vincristine, prednisolone and doxorubicin. With this regimen 75% of patients remit within 3 weeks and the remission is achieved with little toxicity and recovery of normal haematopoiesis.

Following the induction of complete or partial remission, the treatment is intensified by using drugs such as asparaginase, an anthracycline (daunorubicin or doxorubicin), cytosine arabinoside and cyclophosphamide. These drugs are myelosuppressive but at this stage the bone marrow has recovered following the elimination of most of the leukaemic population.

Prophylaxis of CNS disease. The importance of CNS prophylaxis was demonstrated in the early 1970s (2). Before that time, infiltration of the meninges by leukaemic cells was responsible for relapse in half of all cases. The lymphoblasts infiltrate the meninges diffusely and extend to the spinal meninges and sheaths of cranial nerves. Clinical presentation is with symptoms of raised intracranial pressure: headache, nausea and vomiting, with a stiff neck and papilloedema. Convulsions may occur and cranial nerve palsies (particularly VII, VI and III) often develop, and may be the first sign. The diagnosis is made on lumbar puncture when leukaemic blasts are found. The risk of coning from the lumbar puncture is small.

Prophylactic treatment greatly diminishes the frequency of CNS relapse. Nowadays the usual regimen is cranial irradiation (18 Gy, 1800 rad, in 8–10 fractions over 2 weeks) together with intrathecal methotrexate ($10 \, mg/m^2 \times 4$ over the same period). Established CNS disease (which now occurs in 5–10% of cases) is treated by intrathecal methotrexate twice weekly with cranial irradiation to a higher dose (often 24 Gy, 2400 rad, over 2–3 weeks), together with or followed by spinal irradiation. Lasting control of CNS disease is however unusual. Intrathecal cytosine arabinoside is also used in patients who are thought to be resistant to methotrexate.

CNS prophylaxis is sometimes followed after 1–2 months, by a transient syndrome of somnolence and lethargy. Several reports have suggested that there may later be a degree of intellectual impairment and personality change, possibly associated with cerebral atrophy.

Treatment and prophylaxis of testicular disease. Relapse in the testis is common and is one reason for the worse prognosis of ALL in boys. It occurs in about 25% of prepubertal boys but is less common in older children. Relapse may not be clinically apparent at first—swelling and hardness being late signs. It is usually bilateral and testicular biopsy shows peritubular leukaemic infiltration. Treatment is by testicular irradiation, generally to a dose of the order of 24 Gy (2400 rad) in 2–3 weeks. The role of prophylactic testicular irradiation is still undecided.

Maintenance therapy. The consensus of opinion is that maintenance therapy should be continued for at least 2 years. 6MP and methotrexate are the most widely used drugs, often in conjunction with vincristine and prednisolone. In cases with poor prognostic features (Table 28.4) more aggressive regimens have been used as intermittent pulsed therapy. At the end of treatment a testicular biopsy is sometimes performed, if prophylactic irradiation has not been given, to detect occult disease. Relapse at any site is unusual beyond 1 year after treatment has been stopped.

Treatment on relapse. Bone marrow relapse is treated by an attempt to induce a second remission. Although this is often possible, few patients are cured and in this group, bone marrow transplantation should be considered.

If relapse occurs in the CNS despite prophylaxis, a further remission may be obtained with more intrathecal methotrexate or craniospinal irradiation. Methotrexate can also be given through an Ommaya or Rickham reservoir which allows direct delivery of the drug into the cerebral ventricular system. Systemic relapse is inevitable, and further systemic treatment is usually given.

Prognosis. The important prognostic features are given in Table 28.4. Survival is better in girls than in boys and is shown in Fig. 28.4.

ACUTE LYMPHOBLASTIC LEUKAEMIA IN ADULTS

The clinical features are similar to those in children except for the greater percentage of patients with a mediastinal mass. Above the age of 12 years, ALL has a significantly worse prognosis. More cases (20%) are Ph′ positive and at least some cases represent chronic granulocyte leukaemia presenting in the acute phase. Only 30% are common ALL, 12% are B cell ALL, 8% T cell ALL, and 30% of cases are unclassifiable (null cell ALL). Although the prognosis appears to be as poor as in adult acute myelo-

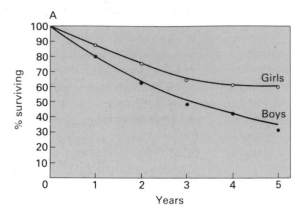

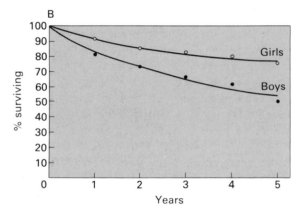

Fig. 28.4. *Relapse-free survival (A) and overall survival (B) in acute lymphoblastic leukaemia in children.*

blastic leukaemia (AML), adult ALL is usually regarded separately because CNS relapse is as common as in childhood ALL.

The treatment of adult ALL is similar to the childhood disease with the following modifications.

1 Induction treatment is more intense with regimens which include anthracyclines and asparaginase.

2 More intensive 'consolidation' therapy with cytosine arabinoside and anthracyclines.

3 CNS prophylaxis and maintenance are similar to childhood ALL but testicular relapse is less frequent and prophylactic treatment is not given.

Table 28.4. Prognostic factors in childhood ALL.

Factors	Prognosis	
	Good	Poor
Age	3–7	other ages
Sex	girls	boys
Total white count	$<20 \times 10^9/l$	$>20 \times 10^9/l$
Cell type	common ALL	T cell or B cell
Remission	In first 3 weeks	Later remission
CNS disease at presentation	absent	present

ACUTE MYELOBLASTIC LEUKAEMIA (AML)

In most cases the history and physical findings are similar to those in ALL (see above). Bone pain and radiological evidence of bone infiltration are less common in AML, and CNS disease is very unusual at presentation. Lymph node enlargement is also less frequently found than in ALL.

In myelomonocytic (M4, Table 28.1) and monocytic (M5) leukaemia gum infiltration is common leading to gum 'hypertrophy'. Skin infiltrates are common in these forms and associated features are a high total WBC and high serum and urinary lysozyme which is liberated from the tumour.

Pallor, hepatosplenomegaly, purpura and bone tenderness are the most common physical signs. The white count is often elevated with myeloblasts usually demonstrable (see p. 494). Confirmation of the diagnosis is made by bone marrow examination and the use of special stains when appropriate (Table 28.2).

Treatment: remission induction. The aim is to induce a complete marrow and clinical remission. To do this, intensive therapy is normally needed with blood, platelet and antibiotic support during the period of hypoplasia which is the inevitable accompaniment of the chemotherapy (see Chapter 8). Combinations of cytosine arabinoside, daunorubicin and 6-thioguanine are used (Fig. 28.5). The blast count usually falls rapidly in the blood and

bone marrow with suppression of normal haematopoiesis. The mortality of this stage is now about 10% when skilled support is available. During the hypoplastic period further cytotoxic therapy is often needed if the marrow still

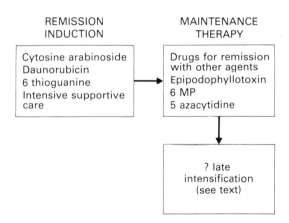

Fig. 28.5. *Outline of management of acute myeloblastic leukaemia.*

shows disease, and this intensifies the hypoplasia and increases the risk. Regular bone marrow examination is therefore essential.

The induction of remission is therefore a highly skilled procedure, best carried out in a unit where the nursing and medical staff are experienced in the problems of bone marrow failure. Careful attention to fluid and electrolyte problems is essential as is prompt diagnosis and treatment of infection (see Chapter 8). Prophylactic treatment of the CNS is not usually given.

Maintenance therapy. Although continued cytotoxic therapy probably prolongs the duration of remission, it is uncertain if it contributes to survival. Nevertheless most regimens include a period of maintenance therapy. The agents used are cyclophosphamide, cytosine arabinoside, methotrexate, 6MP, daunrorubicin and etoposide. In recent years there has been considerable interest in allogeneic bone marrow transplantation and in 'late intensification' of remission with autologous bone marrow transplantation (see below).

Treatment of relapse. Although induction of a second remission is possible in patients who have relapsed after treatment has been discontinued, these remissions are usually short-lived. Patients who relapse while on treatment may have a worse prognosis, but an attempt at remission induction is usually made.

CNS relapse is treated in a similar fashion to ALL (see above).

Supportive care. Blood product support is essential during the intensive phase of remission induction. As discussed in Chapter 8, platelet transfusion has been a major advance in prevention of death from haemorrhage. The indications for platelet transfusion are discussed on p. 123. A falling platelet count below $20 \times 10^9/1$ is an indication for transfusion, as are haemorrhagic manifestations with counts below $40 \times 10^9/1$.

Blood transfusions are essential for anaemia but should be avoided if possible if the white blood count is very high (over $100 \times 10^9/1$) because leucostasis in cerebral vessels may occur. Chemotherapy and, if necessary, leucapheresis, should be used to reduce the white count before transfusion. Granulocyte transfusions are usually only considered if there is life-threatening infection unresponsive to antibiotics (see Chapter 8). During intensive treat-

ment an indwelling intravenous line ('Hickman' line) running subcutaneously may be of great help particularly in children, and in adults with difficult veins.

During the period of remission induction several steps are taken to try to prevent infection. Patients should be instructed to wash carefully with particular attention to the perineal region. Dental and oral sepsis should be treated promptly. Food should be cooked and clean—fresh salads are best avoided. Regular examination of the mouth, skin and perineum are essential and swabs taken from these sites regularly to detect pathogens such as *klebsiella* or *pseudomonas*. Co-trimoxazole is given prophylactically in some units, and has the advantage that it gives considerable protection against the opportunistic pathogen *Pneumocystis carinii*.

Most patients will develop fever at some stage during the period of neutropenia. The management of infection in the neutropenic patient is discussed in Chapter 8. Often no bacteriological diagnosis is made. Most fatal infections are from gram-negative organisms. Fungal infections may occur. They are very dangerous and can be extremely difficult to diagnose. Opportunistic infections cause considerable diagnostic difficulty in a patient with fever and pulmonary infiltration (see Chapter 8). Fungal infection, *Pneumocystis carinii*, and less commonly, cytomegalovirus and other viral infections must be considered.

After blood cultures have been taken at the onset of fever, wide spectrum intravenous antibiotic therapy is begun. Such regimens usually include an aminoglycoside and a cephalosporin, and metronidazole is often added particularly if there is clinical deterioration after 24 hours. If there are pulmonary infiltrates, treatment with high dose co-trimoxazole for pneumocystis, amphotericin B for fungal infection and acyclovir for *Herpes simplex*, should be considered.

Myelodysplastic syndromes (MDS)

These include a range of disorders, usually of unknown aetiology, characterized by one or more peripheral cytopenias, with a cellular marrow showing morphological evidence of disordered haematopoiesis. This may include ring sideroblasts, hypogranular polymorphs with abnormally segmented nuclei, and increased numbers of early myeloid cells. MDS have an inherent tendency to progress to acute leukaemia and for this reason the syndromes were often referred to as preleukaemia.

MDS are classified according to the major abnormality present, but it should be appreciated that there is often more than one abnormality and that precise categorization may be difficult and arbitrary. When ring sideroblasts are the prominent abnormality a diagnosis of sideroblastic anaemia is usually made, and when blast cells are present in modest numbers the disease is labelled as refractory anaemia with an excess of blasts. This has a particular propensity to develop into acute leukaemia and it is synonymous with the term smouldering leukaemia.

Most MDS are treated with supportive measures only and chemotherapy is deferred until the development of overt acute leukaemia.

Bone marrow transplantation in acute leukaemia

The early 1970s saw the beginning of attempts to treat refractory acute leukaemia by marrow ablation using total body irradiation (TBI) and cyclophosphamide, followed by marrow transplanted from an HLA matched donor (usually a relative). This technique is known as allogeneic bone marrow transplantation (BMT). In 1977 the group in Seattle under the leadership of E. D. Thomas reported their experience of allogeneic BMT in 110 patients with relapsed acute leukaemia (3). Most patients died in the first year from relapse, of a syndrome of skin rash, diarrhoea and metabolic disturbance known as graft versus host disease (GVHD). However, about 10% of patients survived more than 2 years suggesting that there was a possibility of cure.

Since that time there has been intensive interest in this treatment, and several issues are being investigated at present.

At what point in treatment should BMT be used? There is general agreement that the results in relapsed AML are poor and that BMT will only have a useful role in AML in first remission (4). In the case of ALL in childhood there is a prospect for cure after first relapse and a second remission can usually be induced. BMT is therefore usually considered in second remission. In adult ALL and poor prognosis childhood ALL, BMT is usually considered in first remission.

Does BMT offer an advantage over the best AML therapy now available? Conventional therapy has been improving and the relative advantages of BMT and conventional treatment may change in the next few years.

Can GVHD be avoided? GVHD appears to be mediated by immunologically competent cells (probably T lymphocytes) in the donor marrow. Attempts have been made to prevent GVHD by careful matching of donors, by the use of cyclosporin A, which damages proliferating T cells and by trying to remove T lymphocytes from the donor marrow using monoclonal antibodies or physical separation techniques.

Is it possible to perform BMT with a partially mismatched graft? Only a minority of patients have a sibling who is a completely matched donor. A panel of tissue-typed donors is one way to try and get round this restriction, but another way is to use mismatched marrow. GVHD is then very severe but attempts are being made to avoid this by the methods described above.

Is TBI and cyclosphosphamide the best anti-leukaemia treatment or would other drugs be more effective? Many other regimens are currently being tested.

The results of BMT are therefore changing and the following is an assessment of the present position.

1 In ALL grafted in 1st and 2nd remission 30–45% of patients are alive at 2–4 years. Death

is from leukaemic relapse, GVHD, infection and pneumonitis. Pneumonitis may be due to total body irradiation or opportunistic infection, and is a major problem in management.

2 In AML grafted in 1st remission, approximately 40% of patients are alive at 3 years. Death from leukaemic relapse may be less common than in ALL.

3 In some series the overall survival curves, in both AML and ALL, do not show a plateau. Late leukaemic relapse remains a problem.

4 GVHD occurs in 30–60% of patients but newer methods of treatment and prevention may be reducing its frequency and severity.

5 The frequency of relapse of leukaemia in AML appears to be higher when patients have had a transplant from an identical twin compared with a matched donor. If true, this suggests that the graft itself may have an effect on suppressing leukaemic proliferation (graft *vs* leukaemia effect).

THE CHRONIC LEUKAEMIAS

There are two main forms of chronic leukaemia: chronic lymphocytic (lymphatic) leukaemia (CLL) and chronic granulocytic (myeloid) leukaemia (CGL). CLL is exceptionally rare below 40 years of age, whilst CGL can occur at any age, although it is commoner in middle and old age.

Chronic lymphocytic leukaemia

This disease is nearly always a chronic neoplastic proliferation of small B lymphocytes. This B cell is probably early in the B cell differentiation pathway (Fig. 28.2). The immunoglobulin classes IgM and IgD are present in small amounts on the cell membrane but no cytoplasmic Ig can be detected. Nevertheless at some stage in the disease, free light chains can be found in the urine in many patients. Since the tumour is a clonal proliferation each cell bears the same immunoglobulin molecule with the same type of light chain. Although clonal, B-CLL may not be a homogeneous disease.

About 5% of cases are of T cell type, usually a suppressor T cell phenotype (T8). The condition is indolent and differs from B-CLL in being associated with less peripheral node enlargement and less suppression of normal immunoglobulin synthesis.

CLINICAL FEATURES

Over 25% of patients have no symptoms at the time of diagnosis. The disease is discovered because of lymphocytosis noted on a blood count taken for another reason, or because enlargement of lymph nodes or spleen is detected on routine physical examination. In other patients the symptoms are due to noticeably enlarged lymph nodes in the neck or elsewhere, fatigue and malaise due to mild anaemia, infection due to immunosuppression, pain from an enlarged spleen or bruising and bleeding due to thrombocytopenia.

Physical examination reveals painless enlarged lymph nodes which are rubbery and mobile. Many node groups are affected (unlike most lymphomas) and the spleen is often palpable. Massive splenomegaly is unusual at presentation and splenic infarction is less frequent than in CGL.

The diagnosis is made on the blood count. This shows a raised total white count which may even be as high as $500–1000 \times 10^9/l$ but is more usually below $100 \times 10^9/l$. The diagnosis must be considered when the lymphocyte count is above $10 \times 10^9/l$. The differential count shows a great excess of small lymphocytes which usually have a normal morphology but which are sometimes larger with less mature-looking nuclei. Cleaved nuclei suggest the diagnosis of follicular-centre cell lymphoma rather than CLL (see Chapter 26). Prolymphocytic leukaemia cells (see p. 504) are larger with more cytoplasm and a distinct prominent nucleolus. Hairy cells (see p. 505) are usually easily distinguished. If the diagnosis is in doubt it may be necessary to undertake a lymph node biopsy which in CLL shows diffuse infiltration with small well-differentiated lymphocytes, or a marrow aspiration and biopsy which may show focal collections of lymphoma cells in follicular lymphoma but which shows a marked diffuse increase in small well-differentiated lymphocytes in CLL. A blood film is all that is necessary for diagnosis in the great majority of cases.

Occasionally the lymphocytosis is slight and it is then not clear if the patient has a reactive lymphocytosis or CLL. This problem can now often be solved by examining the cell surface for light chain restriction. In CLL all the cells are identical and are restricted to one light chain type (kappa or lambda), while both light chain types are represented in a reactive lymphocytosis.

Anaemia is variable and when present indicates extensive marrow infiltration. Autoimmune haemolytic anaemia sometimes occurs. The platelet count may be low as a result of marrow infiltration, hypersplenism, chemotherapy and occasionally anto-immune thrombocytopenia. There is suppression of immunoglobulin synthesis in many patients, with marked hypogammaglobulinaemia which leads to increased susceptibility to infection.

STAGING

It may seem contradictory to stage a leukaemia (see Chapter 4). However, it has been shown that a simple staging classification, based on clinical findings and blood count, has prognostic value (5). This staging notation is shown in Table 28.5. The worse prognostic categories (III and IV) have greater degrees of marrow failure at presentation.

TREATMENT

There is no cure for CLL and it is not even clear if treatment greatly influences survival. The careful use of treatment undoubtedly produces symptomatic benefit. This comes from reduction of the leukaemia mass and consequent improvement in marrow function. Asymptomatic patients should not be treated. Clear indications for treatment include troublesome symptoms of fatigue, greatly enlarged nodes especially if causing pressure, splenic discomfort and marrow failure causing anaemia and thrombocytopenia. Most patients requiring treatment will have stage II–IV disease.

Drug treatment. Alkylating agents (especially chlorambucil and cyclophosphamide) and steroids are the mainstay of treatment. Steroids (usually prednisolone) are useful in patients developing marrow failure (anaemia, thrombocytopenia) since they do not suppress haemopoiesis. In a patient with anaemia, prednisolone 30–40 mg can be given daily by mouth for 2–3 weeks followed by an alkylating agent. Chlorambucil is given either as a low dose (2–4 mg/day) continuously, or intermittently at a dose

Table 28.5. Staging of chronic lymphocytic leukaemia.

Stage	Definition	Median survival (months)
0	No enlarged nodes or spleen, Hb >11 g/dl, platelets $<100 \times 10^9/l$ lymphocytes $<15 \times 10^9/l$	150
I	As stage 0 with enlarged nodes	100
II	As stage 0 with enlargement of spleen or liver	70
III	As 0, I or II; Hb <11 g/dl	20
IV	As 0, II, or III; platelets $<100 \times 10^9/l$	20

of about 10 mg daily 2 weeks on, 2 weeks off. The treatment is continued until the symptoms and signs of the disease have regressed to a considerable extent, and then discontinued. A prolonged period of stable disease may then follow before progression which will then require further treatment. Repeated chemotherapy will ultimately contribute to bone marrow failure.

Radiotherapy. Splenic irradiation is sometimes used often to a dose of 10 Gy (1000 rad) in 6–8 fractions over 2 weeks. The lymphocyte count falls and the spleen shrinks. Peripheral nodes may diminish in size. The treatment may produce temporary control of the disease, but myelosuppression can be troublesome particularly if the spleen (and therefore the treatment field) is very large. If there are painful enlarged lymph nodes these can also be treated effectively by irradiation. Whole-body irradiation, given as small doses to a total of 1.0–1.5 Gy (100–150 rad) in 10–20 fractions has also been used for CLL, but is very myelosuppressive and responses are often not maintained. Extracorporeal irradiation of the blood lowers the lymphocyte count but is not a useful treatment and is now seldom used.

Splenectomy. Occasionally anaemia and thrombocytopenia seem to be due more to the sequestration of cells in the very large spleen than to marrow failure. If splenic irradiation has been effective but relapse occurs, splenectomy might then be considered. The surgical risks are not negligible but in carefully selected patients the operation can give benefit.

Leucapheresis. A cell separator can be used to reduce a grossly elevated white count. This is necessary before blood transfusion which may otherwise cause stasis of white cells in cerebral vessels. The procedure can also be used to tide patients over a period before other treatments such as chemotherapy begin to work.

Treatment of infection. The hypogammaglobulinaemia renders patients highly susceptible to bacterial infection. Febrile illnesses such as upper respiratory infections should be treated promptly with antibiotics and patients warned of their susceptibility. Immune globulin is sometimes given prophylactically to patients who have recurrent infections. Penicillin is usually given prophylactically to patients who have been splenectomized or who have had an episode of pneumococcal infection.

PROGNOSIS

In this elderly population death frequently occurs from other causes. Infection contributes to mortality and as the disease progresses, marrow failure develops, increasing the likelihood of infection and bleeding. A median survival of 5 years has been noted in several series, and there is little evidence that it is improving. Survival is closely related to initial stage of disease (Table 28.5).

Second cancers are possibly more common in CLL than in the general population. A small proportion of patients die from an aggressive malignant transformation with fever, weight loss, and rapidly increasing tumour containing large undifferentiated cells. This syndrome (Richter's syndrome) is unusual and most patients do not develop a transformation of the disease as a terminal event, unlike CGL (see below).

Prolymphocytic leukaemia

This uncommon disease occurs in the elderly. The presentation is like CLL but without much lymph node enlargement and with marked splenomegaly. The white count is high ($> 100 \times 10^9/1$). The white cells are larger than CLL cells, with more cytoplasm and a single prominent nucleolus. The cells are B cells with bright staining for surface immunoglobulin, although occasional T cell variants have been described.

Treatment is with chemotherapy and splenic irradiation. Combination chemotherapy is usually used with regimens similar to those used in high-grade non-Hodgkin's lymphoma (see Chapter 26).

Hairy cell leukaemia (leukaemic reticuloendotheliosis)

This disease occurs more commonly in men (M:F 4:1) aged 50–70 years and is characterized by anaemia, thrombocytopenia and neutropenia, splenomegaly and the presence of cells in the blood which have unusual cytoplasmic villi—so called hairy cells. There is little enlargement of lymph nodes and constitutional symptoms (fever, night sweats) are very unusual unless there is an intercurrent infection due to the neutropenia.

There has been considerable debate as to the nature of the hairy cell. B cell markers (surface Ig) are often present and the current view is that the cell is an activated clonal B lymphocyte. The cells contain tartrate-resistant acid phosphatase.

Splenectomy benefits many patients, with improvement of the platelet count, but patients without splenomegaly and with heavy marrow infiltration do not benefit from the operation. The response to chemotherapy is less certain and intensive chemotherapy carries the risk of infection and is seldom helpful. The prognosis is very variable, some patients surviving several years. Death is from infection and bleeding. Alpha interferon is undoubtedly effective in many cases with reduction of peripheral cytopenia and splenomegaly, but its long-term value is uncertain.

Chronic granulocytic leukaemia

Chronic granulocytic leukaemia (CGL) is a disease of great interest to oncologists because in the majority of patients it is associated with a specific, acquired chromosomal defect and also after a period of slow progression the disease transforms into a more malignant variety of leukaemia.

The chromosomal defect is the Philadelphia chromosome (Ph'), which is a translocation of part of the long arm of chromosome 22 to chromosome 9. This defect was described in 1960 (6). The amount of the chromosome which is lost varies between patients and occasionally the translocation is to another chromosome than 9. The Ph' chromosome is found in megakaryocytes and erythroblasts as well as granulocyte precursors but not in mature lymphocytes. In the untreated disease almost every cell in the marrow is Ph' positive but the normal marrow precursors are not eliminated since after intensive therapy Ph' negative cells may reappear. The tumour is clonal in origin since in heterozygotes for the enzyme G6PD all the Ph'+ve cells contain the same isoenzyme.

The Ph'+ve clone proliferates at the expense of the normal marrow progenitors. This proliferation proceeds slowly but the clone appears genetically unstable and transformation to a more malignant form is inevitable; this is accompanied by further karyotype abnormalities.

Not all patients with CGL have the Ph' chromosome in the leukaemic cells. The 20% of cases that do not appear to, have a somewhat different clinical picture (see below).

CLINICAL FEATURES

These are shown in Table 28.6. The patient may be asymptomatic and the diagnosis made on a routine blood count, but fatigue, anaemia, weight loss and splenic pain eventually occur. Bruising and bleeding may develop. Abdominal pain may be due to stretching of the splenic capsule or may be acute and pleuritic if there has been splenic infarction. Peptic ulceration is ten times more common than in the general population.

On examination there is usually splenomegaly and often sternal tenderness. The spleen is often considerably enlarged with a splenic 'notch' palpable. Hepatomegaly and purpura may be present and retinal haemorrhages are not infrequent.

INVESTIGATION

The white blood count is grossly elevated with an increase in all stages of the granulocyte series,

Table 28.6. Clinical and laboratory findings in CGL.

	Frequency
Symptoms and Signs	
Malaise and fatigue	80%
Weight loss	60%
Bruising and bleeding	40%
Abdominal discomfort	40%
Splenomegaly	95%
Bone tenderness	70%
Hepatomegaly	50%
Purpura	25%
Typical laboratory findings	
Anaemia	9–12 g/dl
WBC	$25–1000 \times 10^9/l$
granulocytes	40%
metamyelocytes	10%
myelocytes	30%
promyelocytes	5%
myeloblasts	3%
Platelets	
$<150 \times 10^9/l$	10% of cases
$150–400 \times 10^9/l$	40% of cases
$>400 \times 10^9/l$	50% of cases

particularly myelocytes. Promyelocytes and myeloblasts are present in smaller numbers than myelocytes unless the presentation of the disease is with acute transformation ('blast crisis'). There is a variable degree of anaemia and the platelet count may be high (because of excess production of abnormal platelets) or low (because of hypersplenism and marrow failure). The diagnosis can usually be made from the blood film and the bone marrow examination

(although usually performed) does not contribute to diagnosis. It shows an expanded hypercellular marrow with an increase in the myeloid series, with an excess of early forms.

Leucocyte alkaline phosphatase is low or absent, and the Ph' chromosome can be demonstrated in metaphases in cultured marrow cells. The greatly increased turnover of myeloid cells leads to hyperuricaemia.

Patients who are Ph'−ve usually show more anaemia, a less high white blood count, more numerous monocytes in the blood and more abnormal myeloid forms.

THE EVOLUTION OF CGL (Fig 28.6)

As the leukaemic mass increases, the spleen enlarges and the patient becomes progressively more anaemic. The white blood cell count doubles every 3–12 months. With treatment (see below) the white blood count falls and a stable 'plateau' may then be reached with the patient off treatment. Eventually the white count will rise again and with treatment will improve. Gradually the 'remissions' become shorter and the recurrences more rapid. Finally an aggressive disease develops with drug resistant splenomegaly or rising white count showing blastic transformation (Fig. 28.6C). The clinical picture is now dominated by an acute leukaemia which responds poorly to treatment and with a fatal outcome in a few months.

The transformation is usually accompanied by malaise, splenic enlargement, skin deposits, bone pain which may be localized, and a rising

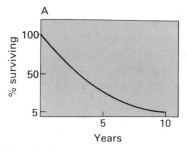 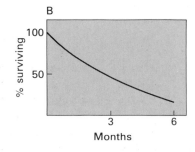 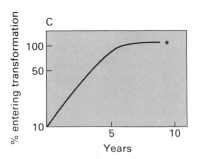

Fig. 28.6. *Survival in chronic granulocytic leukaemia.* (A) Overall survival; (B) Survival after transformation (months); (C) % entering transformation.

blast count. It may be more insidious, the disease showing only a progressive loss of control from chemotherapy and sometimes with features of myelosclerosis. This progressive change is known as 'terminal metamorphosis'. In practical terms it is defined as the time when, for whatever reason, the primary form of treatment has to be abandoned.

The transformation is usually into AML but recently it has become clear that 20% of cases show transformation into ALL in which the blast cells are Ph′ +ve. The ALL is of the common ALL phenotype (see p. 497). This most interesting finding implies that the malignancy affects a very early progenitor cell. It is now known that about 20% of cases of adult ALL are Ph′ +ve.

TREATMENT OF CGL IN CHRONIC PHASE (Fig. 28.7)

Several drugs are effective in the chronic phase. Busulphan is the drug most widely used, and is given by mouth. It is given at a dose of 0.07 mg/kg (4–5 mg) daily until the white count falls to about $20 \times 10^9/1$. It is important to stop treatment at this point because the myelosuppressive effect of busulphan is delayed so the WBC may fall further, until it begins to rise again later. The rise in count may be very slow and treatment may not need to be re-started for months or even years. Some physicians prefer to give larger doses of busulphan (60–100 mg) as a single dose at 6 week intervals. Although the white blood count usually falls slowly with busulphan, in some patients there is a more rapid reduction and they may even become pancytopenic.

With repeated treatments the recovery of the white blood count becomes more rapid and the duration of the plateau, or 'remission', shorter. There is no evidence that other drugs such as 6-thioguanine or hydroxyurea alter this sequence of events. Side-effects of busulphan (see Chapter 6) include skin pigmentation and pulmonary fibrosis.

Drug treatment produces symptomatic and

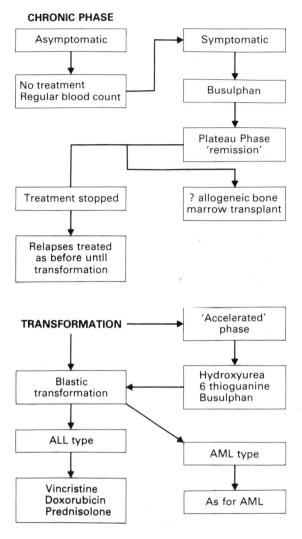

Fig. 28.7. *Outline of management of chronic granulocytic leukaemia.*

haematological improvement in almost all patients. The leukaemic mass is reduced with a fall in white blood count, reduction in spleen size, improvement in marrow function with a rise in haemoglobin, and a consequent amelioration of symptoms of fatigue and malaise. In spite of this, the cells in the marrow remain Ph′ +ve and the transformation of the disease is not prevented. Indeed the extent to which survival is improved by chemotherapy is not clear. Because treatment is palliative it can be safely delayed in patients who have no symptoms and in whom the diagnosis has been made as a result of a blood count taken for some other reason.

TREATMENT OF ACCELERATED AND TRANSFORMED CGL

As the speed of relapse increases the spleen usually starts to enlarge and marrow failure, due both to the disease and its treatment, becomes apparent. Changing from busulphan to hydroxyurea (1–2 g/day) may produce temporary benefit. If there is massive splenomegaly which is thought to contribute to anaemia and thrombocytopenia splenectomy may be helpful provided that blastic transformation has not yet occurred.

Blastic transformation is usually to AML and is often treated as such unless the patient is infirm or elderly. In those cases where ALL supervenes, treatment is as for adult ALL. In both cases the prognosis is very bad. Remissions may be obtained but median survival is only 3 months (Fig. 28.7B).

BONE MARROW TRANSPLANTATION IN CGL

Allogeneic bone marrow transplantation (BMT) has been used in both blastic transformation and in chronic phase. The results of BMT in blastic transformation are very disappointing although occasional patients have had a return of normal Ph′−ve haemopoiesis for several months. Allogeneic BMT has been more successful when carried out in chronic phase, and sustained remissions have been achieved with Ph′−ve haemopoiesis. Although early results are encouraging it remains to be seen if this will prove to be a useful contribution to management.

Allogeneic BMT can only be carried out if there is a histocompatible donor and if the patient is below the age of 45. When there is no donor, attempts have been made to harvest the patient's (Ph′+ve) bone marrow in the chronic phase, preserve it in liquid nitrogen, and, when blastic transformation occurs, to treat the patient with ablative therapy (usually total-body irradiation and chemotherapy) and reinfusion of the preserved marrow. In some patients the chronic phase has been restored but it is not yet clear how long this will last or how often the procedure can be repeated.

PROGNOSIS OF CGL

Less than 5% of patients survive 5 years (Fig. 28.6). The long-term survival of patients undergoing allogeneic BMT in chronic phase remains to be determined.

PH′−VE CGL

These patients differ from Ph′+ve CGL in having a greater degree of splenomegaly at presentation, more profound anaemia and a lower total white count. The blood film reveals more abnormal neutrophils and monocytes, and fewer myelocytes. The disease appears to run a more rapid course than Ph′+ve CGL with a median survival of only 18 months in some series (7). Treatment is along the same lines as Ph′+ve CGL.

Eosinophilic leukaemia

This disease is characterized by eosinophilia sometimes accompanied by anaemia, neutropenia and thrombocytopenia. There may be cough associated with transient pulmonary infiltration and non-bacterial endocarditis occurs leading to heart failure.

The disease may be difficult to distinguish from other forms of chronic eosinophilia and the diagnosis of leukaemia may be hard to establish. Acute blastic transformation of the disease occurs in some patients and the response to treatment is poor.

REFERENCES

1 Bennett J.M., Catovsky D., Daniel M-T., Flandrin G., Galton D.A.G., Gralnick H.R. & Sultan C. (1976) Proposals for the classification of the acute leukaemias. *British Journal of Haematology* **33**, 451.

2 Hustu H.O., Aur R.F.A., Verzosa M.S., Simone J.V. & Pinkel D. (1973) Prevention of central nervous system leukaemia by irradiation. *Cancer* **32**, 585.

3 Thomas E.D., Flournoy N., Buckner C.D., Clift R.A., Fefer A., Heiman P.E. & Storb R. (1977) Cure of leukaemia by marrow transplantation. *Leukaemia Research* **1**, 67–70.

4 Powles R.L., Morganstern G., Clink H.M., *et al.* (1980) The place of bone marrow transplantation in acute myelogenous leukaemia. *Lancet* **i**, 1047.

5 Rai K.R., Sawitsky A., Cronkite E.P., Chanana A.D., Levy R.N. & Pasternack B.S. *et al.* (1975) Clinical staging of chronic lymphocytic leukaemia. *Blood* **46**, 219.

6 Nowell P.C. & Hungerford D.A. (1960) A minute chromosome in human chronic granulocytic leukaemia. *Science* **132**, 1497.

7 Whang-Peng J., Canellos G.P., Carbone P.P., & Tjio J.H. (1968) Clinical implications of cytogenetic variants in chronic myelocytic leukaemia (CML) *Blood* **32**, 755.

FURTHER READING

Richards J.D.M., Linch D.C. & Godstone A.H. (1983) *A Synopsis of Haematology*. Wright, Bristol.

Wintrobe M.M., Lee G.R., Boggs D.R. Bithell T.C., Foerster J., Athens J.W. & Lukens J.N. (1981) *Clinical Hematology* (8th edn.) Lea and Febiger, Philadelphia.

Index